4. Traumatic Disorders

坎贝尔骨科手术学
运动医学

Campbell's Operative Orthopaedics

第 14 版
（影印版）

Frederick M. Azar, MD

James H. Beaty, MD

人民卫生出版社
·北 京·

图书在版编目（CIP）数据

坎贝尔骨科手术学.运动医学：英文/（美）弗雷德里克·M.阿扎尔（Frederick M. Azar），（美）詹姆斯·H.比蒂（James H. Beaty）主编.—影印本.—北京：人民卫生出版社，2021.12

ISBN 978-7-117-32515-8

Ⅰ.①坎… Ⅱ.①弗… ②詹… Ⅲ.①骨科学–外科手术–英文②运动医学–外科手术–英文 Ⅳ.①R68 ②R87

中国版本图书馆 CIP 数据核字（2021）第 242981 号

人卫智网	www.ipmph.com	医学教育、学术、考试、健康，购书智慧智能综合服务平台
人卫官网	www.pmph.com	人卫官方资讯发布平台

图字：01–2021–6747 号

坎贝尔骨科手术学
运 动 医 学
Kanbeier Guke Shoushuxue
Yundong Yixue

主　　编：Frederick M. Azar　James H. Beaty
出版发行：人民卫生出版社（中继线 010-59780011）
地　　址：北京市朝阳区潘家园南里 19 号
邮　　编：100021
E - mail：pmph @ pmph.com
购书热线：010-59787592　010-59787584　010-65264830
印　　刷：三河市宏达印刷有限公司（胜利）
经　　销：新华书店
开　　本：889×1194　1/16　印张：22
字　　数：1048 千字
版　　次：2021 年 12 月第 1 版
印　　次：2022 年 1 月第 1 次印刷
标准书号：ISBN 978-7-117-32515-8
定　　价：329.00 元

坎贝尔骨科手术学
运动医学

Campbell's Operative Orthopaedics

第 14 版

（影印版）

Frederick M. Azar, MD

Professor
Department of Orthopaedic Surgery and Biomedical Engineering University of
Tennessee–Campbell Clinic
Chief of Staff, Campbell Clinic
Memphis, Tennessee

James H. Beaty, MD

Harold B. Boyd Professor and Chair
Department of Orthopaedic Surgery and Biomedical Engineering University of
Tennessee–Campbell Clinic
Memphis, Tennessee

Editorial Assistance

Kay Daugherty *and* **Linda Jones**

人民卫生出版社
·北 京·

Elsevier (Singapore) Pte Ltd.
3 Killiney Road,
#08–01 Winsland House I,
Singapore 239519
Tel:（65）6349–0200; Fax:（65）6733–1817

ELSEVIER

This English Reprint of Part XIII from Campbell's Operative Orthopaedics, 14E by Frederick M. Azar and James H. Beaty was undertaken by People's Medical Publishing House and is published by arrangement with Elsevier (Singapore) Pte Ltd.

Part XIII from Campbell's Operative Orthopaedics, 14E by Frederick M. Azar and James H. Beaty由人民卫生出版社进行影印，并根据人民卫生出版社与爱思唯尔（新加坡）私人有限公司的协议约定出版。

ISBN: 978–7–117–32515–8

Notice

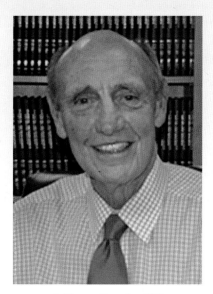

S. Terry Canale, MD

It is with humble appreciation and admiration that we dedicate this edition of *Campbell's Operative Orthopaedics* to Dr. S. Terry Canale, who served as editor or co-editor of five editions. He took great pride in this position and worked tirelessly to continue to improve "The Book." As noted by one of his co-editors, "Terry is probably the only person in the world who has read every word of multiple editions of *Campbell's Operative Orthopaedics.*" He considered *Campbell's Operative Orthopaedics* an opportunity for worldwide orthopaedic education and made it a priority to ensure that each edition provided valuable and up-to-date information. His commitment to and enthusiasm for this work will continue to influence and inspire every future edition.

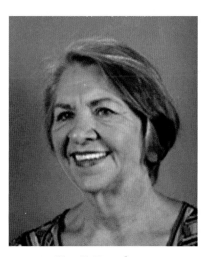

Kay C. Daugherty

It is with equal appreciation and regard that we dedicate this edition to Kay C. Daugherty, the managing editor of the last nine editions *Campbell's Operative Orthopaedics*. Over the last 40 years, she has faithfully and tirelessly edited, reshaped, and overseen all aspects of publication from manuscript preparation to proofing. She has a profound talent to put ideas and disjointed words into comprehensible text, ensuring that each revision maintains the gold standard in readability. Each edition is a testament to her dedication to excellence in writing and education. A favorite quote of Mrs. Daugherty to one of our late authors was, "I'll make a deal. I won't operate if you won't punctuate." We are grateful for her many years of continual service to the Campbell Foundation and for the publications yet to come.

FREDERICK M. AZAR, MD
Professor
Director, Sports Medicine Fellowship
University of Tennessee–Campbell Clinic
Department of Orthopaedic Surgery and
  Biomedical Engineering
Chief-of-Staff, Campbell Clinic
Memphis, Tennessee

JAMES H. BEATY, MD
Harold B. Boyd Professor and Chair
University of Tennessee–Campbell Clinic
Department of Orthopaedic Surgery and
  Biomedical Engineering
Memphis, Tennessee

MICHAEL J. BEEBE, MD
Instructor
University of Tennessee–Campbell Clinic
Department of Orthopaedic Surgery and
  Biomedical Engineering
Memphis, Tennessee

CLAYTON C. BETTIN, MD
Assistant Professor
Director, Foot and Ankle Fellowship
Associate Residency Program Director
University of Tennessee–Campbell Clinic
Department of Orthopaedic Surgery and
  Biomedical Engineering
Memphis, Tennessee

TYLER J. BROLIN, MD
Assistant Professor
University of Tennessee–Campbell Clinic
Department of Orthopaedic Surgery and
  Biomedical Engineering
Memphis, Tennessee

JAMES H. CALANDRUCCIO, MD
Associate Professor
Director, Hand Fellowship
University of Tennessee–Campbell Clinic
Department of Orthopaedic Surgery and
  Biomedical Engineering
Memphis, Tennessee

DAVID L. CANNON, MD
Associate Professor
University of Tennessee–Campbell Clinic
Department of Orthopaedic Surgery and
  Biomedical Engineering
Memphis, Tennessee

KEVIN B. CLEVELAND, MD
Instructor
University of Tennessee–Campbell Clinic
Department of Orthopaedic Surgery and
  Biomedical Engineering
Memphis, Tennessee

ANDREW H. CRENSHAW JR., MD
Professor Emeritus
University of Tennessee–Campbell Clinic
Department of Orthopaedic Surgery and
  Biomedical Engineering
Memphis, Tennessee

JOHN R. CROCKARELL, MD
Professor
University of Tennessee–Campbell Clinic
Department of Orthopaedic Surgery and
  Biomedical Engineering
Memphis, Tennessee

GREGORY D. DABOV, MD
Assistant Professor
University of Tennessee–Campbell Clinic
Department of Orthopaedic Surgery and
  Biomedical Engineering
Memphis, Tennessee

MARCUS C. FORD, MD
Instructor
University of Tennessee–Campbell Clinic
Department of Orthopaedic Surgery and
  Biomedical Engineering
Memphis, Tennessee

RAYMOND J. GARDOCKI, MD
Assistant Professor
University of Tennessee–Campbell Clinic
Department of Orthopaedic Surgery and
  Biomedical Engineering
Memphis, Tennessee

BENJAMIN J. GREAR, MD
Instructor
University of Tennessee–Campbell Clinic
Department of Orthopaedic Surgery and
  Biomedical Engineering
Memphis, Tennessee

JAMES L. GUYTON, MD
Associate Professor
University of Tennessee–Campbell Clinic
Department of Orthopaedic Surgery and
  Biomedical Engineering
Memphis, Tennessee

JAMES W. HARKESS, MD
Associate Professor
University of Tennessee–Campbell Clinic
Department of Orthopaedic Surgery and
  Biomedical Engineering
Memphis, Tennessee

ROBERT K. HECK JR., MD
Associate Professor
University of Tennessee–Campbell Clinic
Department of Orthopaedic Surgery and
  Biomedical Engineering
Memphis, Tennessee

MARK T. JOBE, MD
Associate Professor
University of Tennessee–Campbell Clinic
Department of Orthopaedic Surgery and
  Biomedical Engineering
Memphis, Tennessee

DEREK M. KELLY, MD
Professor
Director, Pediatric Orthopaedic Fellowship
Director, Resident Education
University of Tennessee–Campbell Clinic
Department of Orthopaedic Surgery and
  Biomedical Engineering
Memphis, Tennessee

SANTOS F. MARTINEZ, MD
Assistant Professor
University of Tennessee–Campbell Clinic
Department of Orthopaedic Surgery and
  Biomedical Engineering
Memphis, Tennessee

ANTHONY A. MASCIOLI, MD
Assistant Professor
University of Tennessee–Campbell Clinic
Department of Orthopaedic Surgery and
  Biomedical Engineering
Memphis, Tennessee

BENJAMIN M. MAUCK, MD
Assistant Professor
Director, Hand Fellowship
University of Tennessee–Campbell Clinic
Department of Orthopaedic Surgery and
  Biomedical Engineering
Memphis, Tennessee

MARC J. MIHALKO, MD
Assistant Professor
University of Tennessee–Campbell Clinic
Department of Orthopaedic Surgery and
  Biomedical Engineering
Memphis, Tennessee

WILLIAM M. MIHALKO, MD PhD
Professor, H.R. Hyde Chair of Excellence in
  Rehabilitation Engineering
Director, Biomedical Engineering
University of Tennessee–Campbell Clinic
Department of Orthopaedic Surgery and
  Biomedical Engineering
Memphis, Tennessee

ROBERT H. MILLER III, MD
Associate Professor
University of Tennessee–Campbell Clinic
Department of Orthopaedic Surgery and
    Biomedical Engineering
Memphis, Tennessee

G. ANDREW MURPHY, MD
Associate Professor
University of Tennessee–Campbell Clinic
Department of Orthopaedic Surgery and
    Biomedical Engineering
Memphis, Tennessee

ASHLEY L. PARK, MD
Clinical Assistant Professor
University of Tennessee–Campbell Clinic
Department of Orthopaedic Surgery and
    Biomedical Engineering
Memphis, Tennessee

EDWARD A. PEREZ, MD
Associate Professor
University of Tennessee–Campbell Clinic
Department of Orthopaedic Surgery and
    Biomedical Engineering
Memphis, Tennessee

BARRY B. PHILLIPS, MD
Professor
University of Tennessee–Campbell Clinic
Department of Orthopaedic Surgery and
    Biomedical Engineering
Memphis, Tennessee

DAVID R. RICHARDSON, MD
Associate Professor
University of Tennessee–Campbell Clinic
Department of Orthopaedic Surgery and
    Biomedical Engineering
Memphis, Tennessee

MATTHEW I. RUDLOFF, MD
Assistant Professor
Co-Director, Trauma Fellowship
University of Tennessee–Campbell Clinic
Department of Orthopaedic Surgery and
    Biomedical Engineering
Memphis, Tennessee

JEFFREY R. SAWYER, MD
Professor
Co-Director, Pediatric Orthopaedic
    Fellowship
University of Tennessee–Campbell Clinic
Department of Orthopaedic Surgery and
    Biomedical Engineering
Memphis, Tennessee

BENJAMIN W. SHEFFER, MD
Assistant Professor
University of Tennessee–Campbell Clinic
Department of Orthopaedic Surgery and
    Biomedical Engineering
Memphis, Tennessee

DAVID D. SPENCE, MD
Assistant Professor
University of Tennessee–Campbell Clinic
Department of Orthopaedic Surgery and
    Biomedical Engineering
Memphis, Tennessee

NORFLEET B. THOMPSON, MD
Instructor
University of Tennessee–Campbell Clinic
Department of Orthopaedic Surgery and
    Biomedical Engineering
Memphis, Tennessee

THOMAS W. THROCKMORTON, MD
Professor
Co-Director, Sports Medicine Fellowship
University of Tennessee–Campbell Clinic
Department of Orthopaedic Surgery and
    Biomedical Engineering
Memphis, Tennessee

PATRICK C. TOY, MD
Associate Professor
University of Tennessee–Campbell Clinic
Department of Orthopaedic Surgery and
    Biomedical Engineering
Memphis, Tennessee

WILLIAM C. WARNER JR., MD
Professor
University of Tennessee–Campbell Clinic
Department of Orthopaedic Surgery and
    Biomedical Engineering
Memphis, Tennessee

JOHN C. WEINLEIN, MD
Assistant Professor
Director, Trauma Fellowship
University of Tennessee–Campbell Clinic
Department of Orthopaedic Surgery and
    Biomedical Engineering
Memphis, Tennessee

WILLIAM J. WELLER, MD
Instructor
University of Tennessee–Campbell Clinic
Department of Orthopaedic Surgery and
    Biomedical Engineering
Memphis, Tennessee

A. PAIGE WHITTLE, MD
Associate Professor
University of Tennessee–Campbell Clinic
Department of Orthopaedic Surgery and
    Biomedical Engineering
Memphis, Tennessee

KEITH D. WILLIAMS, MD
Associate Professor
University of Tennessee–Campbell Clinic
Department of Orthopaedic Surgery and
    Biomedical Engineering
Memphis, Tennessee

DEXTER H. WITTE III, MD
Clinical Assistant Professor in
    Radiology
University of Tennessee–Campbell Clinic
Department of Orthopaedic Surgery and
    Biomedical Engineering
Memphis, Tennessee

PREFACE

When Dr. Willis Campbell published the first edition of *Campbell's Operative Orthopaedics* in 1939, he could not have envisioned that over 80 years later it would have evolved into a four-volume text and earned the accolade of the "bible of orthopaedics" as a mainstay in orthopaedic practices and educational institutions all over the world. This expansion from some 400 pages in the first edition to over 4,500 pages in this 14th edition has not changed Dr. Campbell's original intent: "to present to the student, the general practitioner, and the surgeon the subject of orthopaedic surgery in a simple and comprehensive manner." In each edition since the first, authors and editors have worked diligently to fulfill these objectives. This would have not been possible without the hard work of our contributors who always strive to present the most up-to-date information while retaining "tried and true" techniques and tips. The scope of this text continues to expand in the hope that the information will be relevant to physicians no matter their location or resources.

As always, this edition also is the result of the collaboration of a group of "behind the scenes" individuals who are involved in the actual production process. The Campbell Foundation staff—Kay Daugherty, Linda Jones, and Tonya Priggel—contributed their considerable talents to editing often confusing and complex author contributions, searching the literature for obscure references, and, in general, "herding the cats." Special thanks to Kay and Linda who have worked on multiple editions of *Campbell's Operative Orthopaedics* (nine editions for Kay and six for Linda). They probably know more about orthopaedics than most of us, and they certainly know how to make it more understandable. Thanks, too, to the Elsevier personnel who provided guidance and assistance throughout the publication process: John Casey, Senior Project Manager; Jennifer Ehlers, Senior Content Development Specialist; and Belinda Kuhn, Senior Content Strategist.

We are especially appreciative of our spouses, Julie Azar and Terry Beaty, and our families for their patience and support as we worked through this project.

The preparation and publication of this 14th edition was fraught with difficulties because of the worldwide pandemic and social unrest, but our contributors and other personnel worked tirelessly, often in creative and innovative ways, to bring it to fruition. It is our hope that these efforts have provided a text that is informative and valuable to all orthopaedists as they continue to refine and improve methods that will ensure the best outcomes for their patients.

Frederick M. Azar, MD
James H. Beaty, MD

CONTENTS

CHAPTER 1

KNEE INJURIES

Robert H. Miller III, Frederick M. Azar

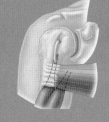

ANATOMY

The knee is one of the most frequently injured joints because of its anatomic structure, its exposure to external forces, and the functional demands placed on it. Basic to an understanding of knee injuries is an understanding of the normal knee anatomy. Although much emphasis has been placed on the ligaments of the knee, without the supporting action of the associated muscles and tendons, the ligaments are not enough to maintain knee stability. The structures around the knee have been classified into three broad categories: osseous structures, extraarticular structures, and intraarticular structures.

OSSEOUS STRUCTURES

The osseous structures of the knee consist of three components: the patella, the distal femoral condyles, and the proximal tibial plateaus, or condyles. The knee is called a hinge joint, but actually it is more complicated than that, because in addition to flexion and extension its motion has a rotary component. The femoral condyles are two rounded prominences that are eccentrically curved. Anteriorly, the condyles are somewhat flattened, which creates a larger surface for contact and weight transmission. The condyles project very little in front of the femoral shaft but markedly so behind. The groove found anteriorly between the condyles is the patellofemoral groove, or trochlea. Posteriorly, the condyles are separated by the intercondylar notch. The articular surface of the medial condyle is longer than that of the lateral condyle, but the lateral condyle is wider. The long axis of the lateral condyle is oriented essentially along the sagittal plane, whereas the medial condyle usually is at about a 22-degree angle to the sagittal plane.

The expanded proximal end of the tibia forms two rather flat surfaces, condyles or plateaus, that articulate with the femoral condyles. They are separated in the midline by the intercondylar eminence with its medial and lateral intercondylar tubercles. Anterior and posterior to the intercondylar eminence are the areas that serve as attachment sites for the cruciate ligaments and menisci. The posterior lip of the lateral tibial condyle is rounded off where the lateral meniscus slides posteriorly during flexion of the knee.

The articular surfaces of the knee are not congruent. On the medial side, the femur meets the tibia like a wheel on a flat surface, whereas on the lateral side, it is like a wheel on a dome. Only the ligaments acting in concert with the other soft-tissue structures provide the knee with the necessary stability.

The patella is a somewhat triangular sesamoid bone that is wider at the proximal pole than at the distal pole. The articular surface of the patella is divided by a vertical ridge, resulting in a smaller medial and a larger lateral articular facet, or surface. With the knee in extension, the patella rides above the superior articular margin of the femoral groove. In extension, the distal portion of the lateral patellar facet articulates with the lateral femoral condyle, but the medial patellar facet barely articulates with the medial femoral condyle until complete flexion is approached. At 45 degrees of flexion, contact moves proximally to the midportion of the articular surfaces. In complete flexion, the proximal portions of both facets are in contact with the femur; and during flexion and extension, the patella moves 7 to 8 cm in relation to the femoral condyles. With complete flexion, more pressure is applied to the medial facet.

Trauma that affects these osseous structures and their relationship with each other frequently causes derangement of the joint. Restoration of these structures is essential to restoration of the function of the knee.

EXTRAARTICULAR TENDINOUS STRUCTURES

The important extraarticular structures supporting and influencing the function of this joint are the synovium, capsule, collateral ligaments, and musculotendinous units that span the joint. The musculotendinous units are principally the quadriceps mechanism, the gastrocnemius, the medial and lateral hamstring groups, the popliteus, and the iliotibial band.

The four components of the quadriceps mechanism form a three-layered quadriceps tendon that inserts into the patella. The tendon of the rectus femoris flattens immediately above the patella and becomes the anterior layer, which inserts at the anterior edge of the proximal pole. The tendon of the vastus intermedius continues downward as the deepest layer of the quadriceps tendon and inserts into the posterior edge of the proximal pole. The middle lamina is formed by the confluent edges of the vastus lateralis and vastus medialis. The fibers of the medial retinaculum formed from the aponeurosis of the vastus medialis insert directly into the side of the patella to help prevent lateral displacement of the patella during flexion. The patellar tendon takes its origin from the apex or distal pole of the patella and inserts distally into the tibial tuberosity.

The gastrocnemius, the most powerful calf muscle, spans the posterior aspect of the knee in intimate relationship with the posterior capsule to insert on the posterior aspect of the medial and lateral femoral condyles.

Pes anserinus is the term for the conjoined insertion of the sartorius, gracilis, and semitendinosus muscles along the proximal medial aspect to the tibia. These primary flexors of the knee have a secondary internal rotational influence on the tibia and help protect the knee against rotary and valgus stress. Their counterpart on the lateral side of the knee is the strong biceps femoris insertion into the fibular head, lateral tibia, and posterolateral capsular structures. This muscle is a strong flexor of the knee that also produces simultaneous strong external rotation of the tibia. It provides rotary stability by preventing forward dislocation of the tibia on the femur during flexion. Its contributions to the arcuate ligament complex at the posterolateral corner of the knee also provide varus and rotary stability. The iliotibial tract, the posterior third of the iliotibial band, inserts proximally into the lateral epicondyle of the femur and distally into the lateral tibial tubercle (Gerdy's tubercle). It thus forms an additional ligament that is contiguous anteriorly with the vastus lateralis and posteriorly with the biceps. The iliotibial band moves forward in extension and backward in flexion but is tense in both positions. During flexion, the iliotibial band, the popliteal tendon, and the lateral collateral ligament (LCL) cross each other, whereas the iliotibial band and biceps tendon remain parallel to each other as in extension, all serving to enhance lateral stability (Fig. 1.1).

The popliteus muscle has three origins, the strongest of which is from the lateral femoral condyle. Other important origins are from the fibula (popliteofibular ligament) and from the posterior horn of the lateral meniscus. The femoral

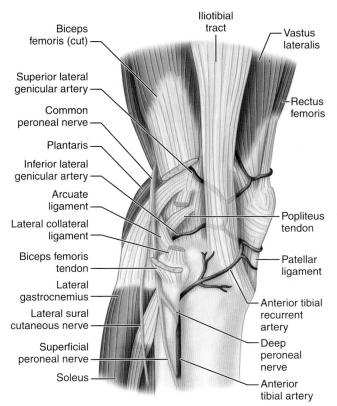

FIGURE 1.1 Tendinous and neurovascular structures of lateral side of knee.

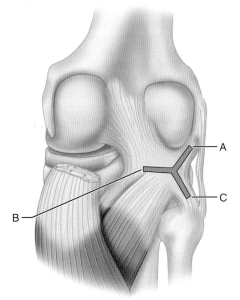

FIGURE 1.2 Popliteus muscle with its tripartite origin. Main tendon attached to lateral condyle of femur *(A)*. Attachment to posterior horn of lateral meniscus *(B)*. Attachment to fibular head *(C)*.

and fibular origins form the arms of an oblique Y-shaped ligament, the arcuate. The arms are joined together by the capsule and meniscal origin. The arcuate ligament is not a separate ligament but is a condensation of the fibers of the origin of the popliteus (Fig. 1.2). With electromyographic studies, Basmajian and Lovejoy found that the popliteus muscle is a prime medial rotator of the tibia during the initial stages of

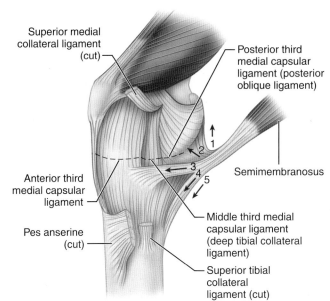

FIGURE 1.3 Medial supporting structures of knee. *1,* Oblique popliteal ligament; *2,* posterior capsule and posterior horn of medial meniscus; *3,* anterior or medial tendon of semimembranosus; *4,* direct head of semimembranosus; *5,* distal portion of semimembranosus tendon (see text).

flexion and also acts to withdraw the meniscus during flexion. In addition, it supplies rotary stability to the femur on the tibia and aids the posterior cruciate ligament (PCL) in preventing forward dislocation of the femur on the tibia.

The semimembranosus muscle is especially important as a stabilizing structure around the posterior and posteromedial aspects of the knee. It has five distal expansions (Fig. 1.3). The first is the oblique popliteal ligament (OPL), which passes from the insertion of the semimembranosus on the posteromedial aspect of the tibia obliquely and laterally upward toward the insertion of the lateral gastrocnemius head (Fig. 1.4A). It acts as an important stabilizing structure on the posterior aspect of the knee. The semimembranosus helps tighten this ligament with contraction (Fig. 1.4B). When the OPL is pulled medially and forward, it tightens the posterior capsule of the knee. This maneuver can be used to tighten the posterior capsule in the posteromedial corner of the knee in surgical repair. A second tendinous attachment is to the posterior capsule and posterior horn of the medial meniscus. This tendinous slip helps tighten the posterior capsule and pulls the medial meniscus posteriorly during knee flexion. The anterior or deep head continues medially along the flare of the tibial condyle and inserts beneath the superficial medial collateral ligament (MCL) just distal to the joint line. The direct head of the semimembranosus attaches to the tubercle on the posterior aspect of the medial condyle of the tibia just below the joint line. This tendinous attachment provides a firm point in which sutures can be anchored for posteromedial capsular repair. The distal portion of the semimembranosus tendon continues distally to form a fibrous expansion over the popliteus and fuses with the periosteum of the medial tibia. The semimembranosus, through its muscle contraction, tenses the posterior capsule and posteromedial capsular structures, providing significant stability. Functionally, it acts as a flexor of the knee and internal rotator of the tibia.

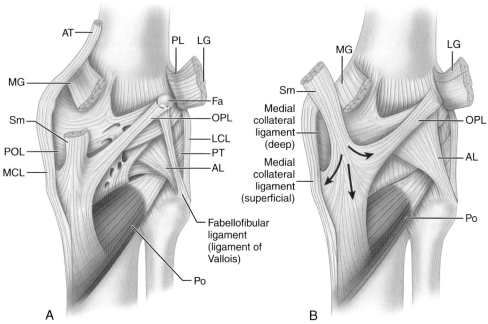

FIGURE 1.4 **A,** Triangular arrangement of passive elements in posterior capsule of knee crucial for rotary stability. **B,** Posterior view of knee showing ligamentous reinforcement of posterior capsule. Oblique popliteal ligament is dynamically stabilized by semimembranosus muscle and arcuate ligament by popliteus muscle. *AL,* Arcuate ligament; *AT,* anterior tibial; *Fa,* fabella; *LCL,* lateral collateral ligament; *LG,* lateral gastrocnemius muscle; *MCL,* medial collateral ligament; *MG,* medial gastrocnemius muscle; *OPL,* oblique popliteal ligament; *PL,* plantaris longus muscle; *Po,* popliteus muscle; *POL,* posterior oblique collateral ligament; *PT,* popliteal tendon; *Sm,* semimembranosus.

The medial extensor expansion, or medial retinaculum, is a distal expansion of the vastus medialis aponeurosis. It attaches along the medial border of the patella and patellar tendon and distally inserts into the tibia. It functions as the medial tracking support of the patella in the patellofemoral groove. It covers and may blend into the anteromedial capsular ligament. Contraction of the vastus medialis helps tighten the anterior portion of the medial capsular ligament.

The lateral extensor expansion, or lateral retinaculum, is an extension of the vastus lateralis attaching to the iliotibial band, which helps tense this band as the knee extends and the iliotibial band moves forward. Imbalance between the lateral and medial retinacular structures often is present in patellar subluxations and dislocations.

In addition to these musculotendinous units that directly span the knee, abnormalities in the orientation and alignment of the foot, as well as deficiencies in the hip flexors and abductors, can influence the alignment and function of the knee and must be considered in evaluation and rehabilitation of this joint.

EXTRAARTICULAR LIGAMENTOUS STRUCTURES

The joint capsule and the collateral ligaments are the principal extraarticular static stabilizing structures. The capsule is a sleeve of fibrous tissue extending from the patella and patellar tendon anteriorly to the medial, lateral, and posterior expanses of the joint. The menisci are attached firmly at the periphery to this capsule, especially so medially and less so laterally. Laterally, the passage of the popliteal tendon through the popliteal hiatus to its origin on the femoral condyle produces a less secure meniscal attachment than is present medially. The medial capsule is more distinct and well defined than its lateral counterpart. The capsular structures, along with the medial and lateral extensor expansions of the powerful quadriceps musculature, are the principal stabilizing structures anterior to the transverse axis of the joint. The capsule is especially reinforced by the collateral ligaments and the medial and lateral hamstring muscles, as well as by the popliteus muscle and the iliotibial band posterior to the transverse axis.

The anteromedial and anterolateral portions of the capsule are relatively thin structures but are reinforced by the medial and lateral patellar retinacular expansions and also laterally by the iliotibial band and medially by reinforcing bands extending from the patella as the medial patellofemoral ligament and the medial patellotibial ligament. The medial patellofemoral ligament is more important for patellar stability and runs from the patella near the junction of the middle and superior thirds to the medial femoral epicondyle. Laterally, there are corresponding lateral patellofemoral and lateral patellotibial ligaments supporting the tracking of the patella.

The anteromedial and anterolateral portions of the capsule are significant in protecting the anteromedial and anterolateral aspects of the knee against subluxation and rotational excesses.

In their classic study of knee anatomy, Warren and Marshall divided the knee into three layers. *Layer I* includes the deep fascia or crural fascia; *layer II* is composed of the

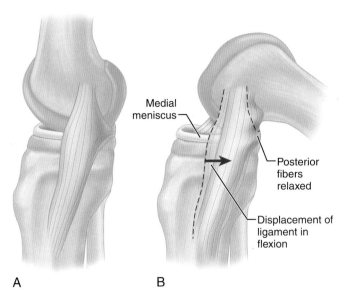

FIGURE 1.5 Joint stripped to reveal medial collateral ligament. **A,** Anterior, posterosuperior, and posteroinferior portions of ligament are tense with joint in extension. **B,** On flexion and extension, ligament glides backward and forward on tibia; in flexion, posterior oblique portions are relaxed. Note that ligament attaches 4 to 5 cm distal to joint.

superficial MCL, various structures anterior to this ligament, and the ligaments of the posteromedial corner; and *layer III* is made up of the capsule of the knee joint and the deep MCL.

■ MEDIAL SIDE ANATOMY

Robinson et al. performed a cadaver study of the medial side of the knee, dividing the anatomy into thirds extending circumferentially from the medial edge of the patellar tendon to the medial edge of the medial head of the gastrocnemius posteriorly. They identified three distinct ligamentous components that cross the joint line: the superficial MCL, the deep MCL, and the posteromedial capsule. The anterior third reaches from the medial edge of the patella tendon to the anterior edge of the superficial MCL. The superficial MCL composes the middle third. The posterior third extends from the posterior edge of the superficial MCL to the medial head of the gastrocnemius and makes up the posterior medial corner.

▎MEDIAL COLLATERAL LIGAMENT

The MCL is a long, rather narrow, well-delineated structure lying superficial to the medial capsule and capsular ligaments, originating on the medial epicondyle and inserting 7 to 10 cm below the joint line on the posterior half of the medial surface of the tibial metaphysis deep to the pes anserinus tendons. It has been referred to as the superficial tibial collateral ligament or the superficial portion of the MCL. Biomechanical studies have shown that it provides the principal stability to valgus stresses. It glides forward over the side of the femoral condyle in extension and posteriorly in flexion (Fig. 1.5). The long fibers of the MCL are the primary stabilizers of the medial side of the knee against valgus and external rotary stress. The anterior fibers of the ligament tighten as the knee flexes, with fibers more posteriorly becoming slack (Fig. 1.6).

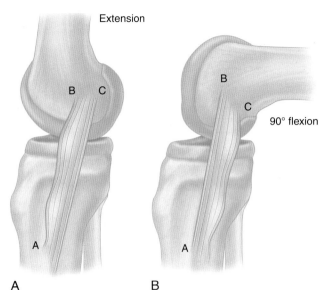

FIGURE 1.6 **A** and **B,** Fibers of medial collateral ligament. Points *A* and *B* are at anterior border of long fibers. *C* is 5 mm posterior to *B* (see text).

▎MIDMEDIAL CAPSULE

The midmedial capsule is reinforced and thickened by vertically oriented fibers and has often been referred to as the deep layer of the MCL. It originates from the femoral condyle and epicondyle and inserts just below the tibial articular margin. It is divided into a meniscofemoral portion, extending from the meniscal attachment to the femoral origin, and the meniscotibial portion, extending as the coronary ligament of the meniscus to its tibial insertion. The meniscofemoral portion is the much longer and stronger of these two divisions. The midmedial capsule resists valgus and rotary stresses.

▎POSTEROMEDIAL CORNER

The posteromedial corner of the knee has five major components: the posterior oblique ligament (POL), the semimembranosus tendon and its expansions, the OPL, the posteromedial joint capsule, and the posterior horn of the medial meniscus.

Hughston described this POL as a thickening of the medial capsular ligament attached proximally to the adductor tubercle of the femur and distally to the tibia and posterior aspect of the capsule. The distal attachment is composed of three arms: (1) the prominent central, or tibial, arm, which attaches to the edge of the posterior surface of the tibia close to the margin of the articular surface and central to the upper edge of the semimembranosus tendon; (2) the superior, or capsular, arm, which is continuous with the posterior capsule and the proximal part of the OPL; and (3) the poorly defined inferior, or distal, arm, which attaches distally both to the sheath covering the semimembranosus tendon and to the tibia just distal to the direct insertion of the semimembranosus tendon (Figs. 1.7 to 1.10).

The central portion is the thickest and probably the most important arm of the ligament, originating in the region of the adductor tubercle (the origin has also been described as being posterior and distal to the adductor tubercle) and coursing posteriorly and obliquely to insert at the posteromedial corner of the tibia near the insertion of the direct head of

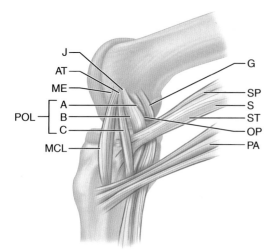

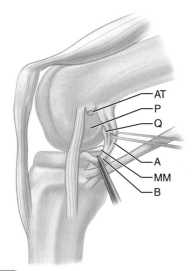

FIGURE 1.7 Posteromedial corner of the knee. *A,* Superior or capsular arm of posterior oblique ligament *(POL); AT,* Adductor tubercle; *B,* central or tibial arm of posterior oblique ligament; *C,* superficial arm of posterior oblique ligament; *G,* gastrocnemius muscle; *J,* common ligament of origin of posterior oblique ligament; *MCL,* medial collateral ligament; *ME,* medial epicondyle; *OP,* oblique popliteal ligament; *PA,* pes anserinus; *S,* common tendon of semimembranosus; *SP,* portion of semimembranosus tendon that becomes oblique popliteal ligament; *ST,* portion of semimembranosus tendon that goes to posteromedial corner of tibia.

FIGURE 1.8 Common origin of posterior oblique ligament has been dissected from adductor tubercle *(AT).* Capsular arm *(A)* is retracted posteriorly and tibial arm *(B)* distalward. *P,* Intraarticular portion of femoral condyle; *Q,* attachment of tibial arm of posterior oblique ligament to posteromedial corner of medial meniscus *(MM).*

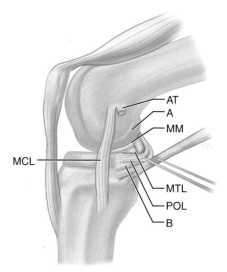

FIGURE 1.9 Posteromedial aspect of knee. Femoral attachment of posterior oblique ligament is divided and ligament is retracted posteriorly. Capsular arm *(A)* forms portion of posterior capsule (see text and previous illustrations).

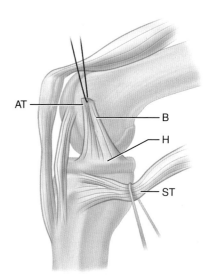

FIGURE 1.10 By pulling central or tibial arm *(B)* of posterior oblique ligament proximally toward its insertion on adductor tubercle *(AT)* while tibial arm of semimembranosus tendon *(ST)* is retracted posteriorly and inferiorly, firm broad attachment *(H)* of central arm of posterior oblique ligament to tibia is visible beneath and deep to semimembranosus tendon (see text and previous illustrations).

the semimembranosus tendon. The superior, or more proximal, arm of the POL passes posteriorly, blending with the posterior capsule and the OPL as it separates from the semimembranosus tendon. The inferior and distal groups of fibers pass superficially over the insertion of the semimembranosus tendon, attach to the tibia and fascia inferiorly, and probably have little functional importance.

As previously described, the semimembranosus tendon has five expansions: (1) the direct arm, (2) the anterior or deep arm, (3) the arm to the POL or capsular arm, (4) the arm to the OPL, and (5) the expansion to the popliteus aponeurosis or the inferior arm.

The OPL is a broad fascial band originating from the capsular arm of the POL and the lateral expansion of the semimembranosus to cross the posterior aspect of the knee. It passes laterally and proximally toward the lateral femoral condyle. Laterally it attaches to the meniscofemoral portion of the posterior capsule and to the fabella.

The posteromedial capsule begins posterior to the superficial and deep MCL. Posteriorly, the deep MCL blends with and becomes inseparable from the central arm of the POL. The central arm forms a thick fascial reinforcement of both the meniscofemoral and meniscotibial portions of the posteromedial capsule with an additional attachment to the medial meniscus.

The posterior horn of the medial meniscus is the last component of the posteromedial corner. It is linked to the posteromedial capsule, the deep MCL, the POL, and the semimembranosus expansion. The contributions to knee stability are well known, serving as a chock block on the tibial plateau. Absence of the posterior horn increases instability in both anterior cruciate ligament (ACL) and PCL deficient knees.

The posteromedial portion of the medial capsular ligamentous complex is especially important for valgus and rotational stability to the knee. The posteromedial capsule and POL become progressively relaxed as the knee flexes; however, with active contraction of the semimembranosus muscle, each of the three arms of the POL is tense. Therefore, both kinetic and static stabilizing effects are obtained from this portion of the medial capsular ligament, even with the knee flexed. In knee ligament reconstruction, this important part of the posteromedial complex is as essential as any other structures requiring attention if stability is to be restored. A precise understanding of anatomy and function is required for repair or reconstruction of this posteromedial complex. The central arm of the POL must be tightened in surgical repair or reconstruction, or passive stability cannot be attained regardless of any other surgical procedures.

▌LATERAL COLLATERAL LIGAMENT

The LCL attaches to the lateral femoral epicondyle proximally and to the fibular head distally. The LCL has an average femoral attachment slightly proximal (1.4 mm) and posterior (3.1 mm) to the lateral epicondyle. In a cadaver study, Kamath et al. identified the origin of the LCL as 58% across the width of the condyle and 2.3 mm distal to the Blumensaat line, with less than 5 mm variance from the mean in all specimens. Distally, it is attached 8.2 mm posterior to the anterior aspect of the fibular head. It is more of a tendinous structure than a wide ligamentous band. It is of prime importance in stabilizing the knee against varus stress with the knee in extension. As the knee goes into flexion, the LCL becomes less influential as a varus-stabilizing structure.

▌ILIOTIBIAL BAND

In addition to the lateral ligaments and lateral capsular structures, stability depends on the iliotibial band, the biceps tendon, and the popliteal tendon. The iliotibial band inserts into the lateral epicondyle of the femur and then passes in its broad expansion between the lateral aspect of the patella and the more posterior location of the biceps femoris to insert into the lateral tibial (Gerdy's) tubercle. Thus it acts as a supplemental ligament across the lateral aspect of the joint. This band moves anteriorly as the knee extends and slides posteriorly as the knee flexes but remains tense in all knee positions. With flexion, the iliotibial band, the popliteal tendon, and the LCL cross each other, thereby greatly enhancing lateral stability. The biceps tendon functions as a lateral stabilizer by contributing to the arcuate complex and by being a powerful flexor and external rotator of the tibia on the femur. The popliteal tendon courses from the posterior aspect of the tibia through the popliteal hiatus and attaches deep to, and somewhat anterior to, the femoral insertion of the LCL.

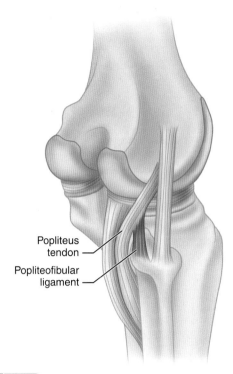

Popliteus tendon

Popliteofibular ligament

FIGURE 1.11 Popliteofibular ligament arises from posterior part of fibula to join popliteal tendon just above musculotendinous junction.

▌POPLITEAL TENDON

Warren et al. identified a strong direct attachment of the popliteal tendon to the fibula, which has been called the popliteal fibular fascicle and the fibular origin of the popliteus muscle. These researchers called this structure the popliteofibular ligament because it connects the fibula to the femur through the popliteal tendon (Fig. 1.11). This ligament is located deep to the lateral limb of the arcuate ligament; it originates from the posterior part of the fibula and posterior to the biceps insertion and joins the popliteal tendon just proximal to its musculotendinous junction. Thus the popliteus muscle-tendon unit is a Y-shaped structure with a muscle origin from the posterior part of the tibia, a ligamentous origin from the fibula, and a united insertion on the femur. The popliteal tendon has a constant, broad-based femoral attachment at the most proximal and anterior fifth of the popliteal sulcus. The popliteal tendon attachment on the femur is always anterior to the LCL. The average distance between the femoral attachments of the popliteal tendon and the LCL is 18.5 mm. The popliteofibular ligament has two divisions, anterior and posterior. The average attachment of the posterior division is 1.6 mm distal to the posteromedial aspect of the tip of the fibular styloid process, and the anterior division attaches 2.8 mm distal to the anteromedial aspect of the tip of the fibular styloid process. Selective cutting studies confirmed that the popliteal tendon attachments to the tibia and the popliteofibular ligament are important in resisting posterior translation, varus rotation, and external rotation.

■ LATERAL SIDE ANATOMY

Seebacher, Inglis, Marshall, and Warren defined three distinct layers of the lateral structures of the knee. The most superficial layer, or layer I, has two parts: (1) the iliotibial tract and its expansion anteriorly and (2) the superficial portion of the

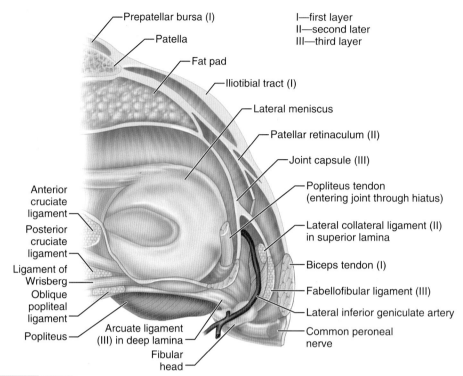

— Prepatellar bursa (I)
— Patella
— Fat pad
— Iliotibial tract (I)

I—first layer
II—second later
III—third layer

— Lateral meniscus
— Patellar retinaculum (II)
— Joint capsule (III)
— Popliteus tendon
(entering joint through hiatus)
— Lateral collateral ligament (II)
in superior lamina
— Biceps tendon (I)
— Fabellofibular ligament (III)
— Lateral inferior geniculate artery
— Common peroneal
nerve

Anterior
cruciate
ligament
Posterior
cruciate
ligament
Ligament of
Wrisberg
Oblique
popliteal
ligament
Arcuate ligament
(III) in deep lamina
Popliteus
Fibular
head

FIGURE 1.12 View of right knee joint from above after removal of right femur. Note three layers of lateral side and division of posterolateral part of capsule (layer III) into deep and superficial laminae, which are separated by lateral inferior genicular vessels.

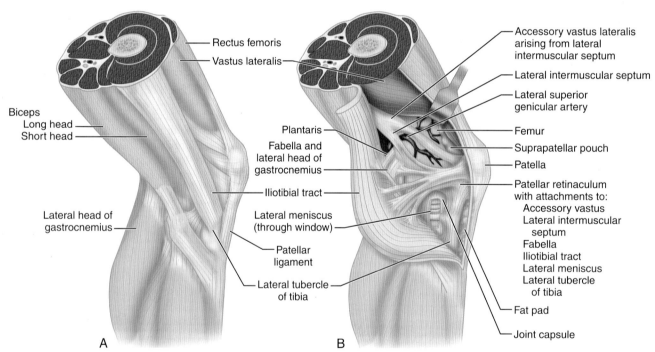

— Rectus femoris
— Vastus lateralis

Biceps
Long head
Short head

Lateral head of
gastrocnemius

Plantaris
Fabella and
lateral head of
gastrocnemius
Iliotibial tract
Lateral meniscus
(through window)
Patellar
ligament
Lateral tubercle
of tibia

— Accessory vastus lateralis
arising from lateral
intermuscular septum
— Lateral intermuscular septum
— Lateral superior
genicular artery
— Femur
— Suprapatellar pouch
— Patella
— Patellar retinaculum
with attachments to:
Accessory vastus
Lateral intermuscular
septum
Fabella
Iliotibial tract
Lateral meniscus
Lateral tubercle
of tibia
— Fat pad
— Joint capsule

A   B

FIGURE 1.13 Layers I and II of structures of lateral side of knee. **A,** Major constituents of layer I: iliotibial tract and superficial portion of expansion of biceps. **B,** Layer I has been incised and peeled back from lateral margin of patella, showing layer II. Layer II includes vastus lateralis and its expansions, as well as patellofemoral and patellomeniscal ligaments.

biceps femoris and its expansion posteriorly (Figs. 1.12 and 1.13). The peroneal nerve lies on the deep side of layer I, just posterior to the biceps tendon. Layer II is formed by the retinaculum of the quadriceps, most of which descends anterolaterally and adjacent to the patella.

ANTEROLATERAL LIGAMENT

Although Segond identified the anterolateral ligament (ALL) in 1879, it was believed to be a variant of the LCL and of little importance. More recently, however, a number of cadaver, radiographic, and biomechanical studies have established it as a distinct ligament important to knee stability. One study identified a network of peripheral nerves, suggesting a proprioception function of the ALL. Claes et al., in 2013, identified the ALL in 40 of 41 cadaver knees, finding that the ligament had consistent origin and insertion sites in 97% of specimens. Despite the number of studies devoted to investigation of the ALL, its exact structure and function are not clearly defined. Although most studies agree on the location of the ALL tibial insertion halfway between Gerdy's tubercle (average 18 to 25 mm posterior to it) and the fibular head (average 17 to 24 mm anterior to it), the femoral insertion site is not firmly established. Two anatomic variations have been described: posterior and proximal to the insertion of the LCL and anterior and distal to it. The position of the ALL relative to the popliteus tendon also is controversial. Claes et al. and Cavaignac et al. described the ALL origin as proximal and posterior to the popliteus tendon; Vincent et al. described it as being anterior to the tendon. In a systematic review of the literature, Van der Watt et al. concluded that the ALL is an extraarticular structure with a clear course from the lateral femoral epicondylar region, running anteroinferiorly to the proximal tibia at a site midway between Gerdy's tubercle and the head of the fibula (Table 1.1 and Fig. 1.14). The mean width of the ALL at the lateral joint was found to be 6.7 mm, with a thickness of about 2 mm.

The location and appearance of the ALL have been delineated on radiographs (Fig. 1.15), MRI (Fig. 1.16), and ultrasound, as well as intraoperative observation. Reported sensitivity of MRI ranges from 51% to 98%. In their cadaver ultrasound study, Cavaignac et al. found that the entire ALL was visible from its proximal insertion to its distal insertion, with excellent agreement between ultrasound and anatomic findings.

Several studies have suggested that the primary function of the ALL is to provide anterolateral stability, preventing the proximal-lateral tibia from subluxation anteriorly relative to the distal femur, with the stabilizing force most significant at 30 and 90 degrees of knee flexion. It also has been implicated in lateral meniscal tears and Segond fractures.

In numerous articles detailing the anatomy of the lateral side of the knee, LaPrade and co-investigators described the structures from superficial to deep. The first structure encountered is the iliotibial band, a thick fascial sheath inserting on the anterolateral aspect of the lateral tibial plateau at Gerdy's tubercle. The iliotibial band has three layers. The superficial layer appears first and, after splitting this layer, deeper fibers adhere to the lateral supracondylar tubercle of the femur and blend into the lateral intramuscular septum. These layers are called the deep and capsule-osseous layers or "Kaplan fibers." An anterior band, the iliopatellar band, curves anteriorly and inserts onto the lateral aspect of the patella.

The deep layer begins 6 cm proximal to the lateral femoral epicondyle, at the termination of the lateral intermuscular septum, and connects the medial border of the superficial iliotibial layer to the distal termination of the lateral intermuscular septum of the distal femur. Medial and distal to the deep layer, the capsule-osseous layer originates from the region of the lateral intermuscular septum and the fascia over the lateral gastrocnemius and plantaris muscles, creating a sling over the lateral femoral condyle. This structure blends with the short head of the biceps femoris in a region known as the confluence of the short head of the biceps femoris and

the capsule-osseous layer. Distally, it inserts onto the lateral tibial tuberosity, just posterior and proximal to Gerdy's tubercle. This lateral sling is the structure most surgeons attempt to reconstruct in extraarticular ACL reconstructions.

The biceps femoris has two insertions: the long and short heads. The long head has five major insertions at the knee, two tendinous and three fascial. The tendinous components are the direct arm, which inserts onto the lateral aspect of the fibula styloid, and the anterior arm, which courses lateral to the lateral collateral ligament (LCL) and inserts onto the lateral tibial plateau. A small biceps femoris bursa separates this arm from the LCL. The three fascial components are the reflected arm and the anterior and lateral aponeurotic expansions. The latter connects the long and short heads of the biceps femoris to the posterolateral aspect of the LCL.

The short head divides into six components consisting of direct, capsular, and anterior tendinous arms and three nontendinous attachments. The three tendinous arms are the most important. The direct arm attaches to the posterolateral aspect of the fibular styloid. The capsular arm attaches to the posterolateral aspect of the capsule and just lateral to the tip of the fibular styloid, providing a stout attachment between the posterolateral capsule, the lateral gastrocnemius tendon, and the capsule-osseous layer of the iliotibial band. The most distal edge of the capsular arm is the fabellofibular ligament, which spans from the lateral edge of the fabella, distally and laterally, to attach to the fibular head just posterior to the posterior division of the popliteofibular ligament. The anterior arm passes medial to the LCL and inserts with the meniscotibial portion of the midthird lateral capsular ligament onto the proximal-lateral tibia. This insertion site is the location of the Segond fracture seen in association with ACL injuries.

The surgeon should be mindful that the peroneal nerve lies deep and posterior to the biceps femoris tendon, passing 1.5 to 2 cm distal to the fibular styloid as it travels along the lateral aspect of the fibular head.

The LCL is the primary static stabilizer to varus stress of the knee between 0 and 30 degrees of flexion. It also provides resistance to external rotation of the tibia, primarily near extension. The femoral attachment is extracapsular and lies 1.4 mm proximal and 3.1 mm posterior to the lateral epicondyle. The LCL is approximately 70 mm long and inserts on the lateral aspect of the fibular head 8.2 mm posterior to the anterior border of the fibula and 28.4 mm antero-inferior to the proximal tip of the fibular styloid. At surgery, the LCL can be identified by making an incision parallel to the fibers of the long head of the biceps tendon superficial to the proximal aspect of the fibular head exposing the biceps bursa which encompasses the LCL.

POPLITEUS MUSCLE AND LIGAMENT

The popliteus muscle is obliquely oriented, originating from the posteromedial aspect of the proximal tibia. The tendon passes proximally through the popliteal hiatus in the coronary ligament where it becomes intraarticular and inserts into the popliteal sulcus of the lateral femoral condyle. It is usually found in the most anterior one fifth and proximal half of the sulcus. It has also been located 18.5 mm distal and anterior to the femoral insertion of the LCL and 15.8 mm distal and anterior to the lateral femoral epicondyle. The popliteus has multiple other insertion sites. The ligamentous insertion on the fibula is composed of the anterior and posterior

TABLE 1.1

Structure of Anterolateral Ligament

STUDY	ORIGIN	COURSE	INSERTION	CHARACTERISTICS
Claes et al.	Lateral femoral epicondyle	Depth of lateral tibial synovial recess measured 6.5 ± 1.5 mm	Anterolateral proximal tibia Gerdy's tubercle to ALL: 22 mm Fibular head to ALL: 21.3 mm	Gerdy's tubercle to Segond fracture: 22.4 mm Insertion width: 11.3 mm
Helito et al.	1.9 ± 1.4 mm anterior and 4.1 ± 1.1 mm distal to LCL Lateral radiograph: 47% from anterior condyle and 3.7 mm inferior to Blumensaat line AP radiograph: 15.8 mm from posterior bicondylar line	Not stated	4.4 ± 0.8 mm distal to anterolateral proximal tibia, at a point 42% of the way from the fibular head to Gerdy's tubercle Lateral radiograph: 53% from anterior tibial plateau AP radiograph: 7.0 mm from tibial joint line	Not stated
Helito et al.	Lateral femoral condyle, immediately anterior to LCL	Anteroinferior, superficial to popliteal tendon Bifurcation 3.0 mm proximal to lateral meniscus	7.0 mm distal to lateral tibial plateau	Thin linear structure with thickness between 1 and 3 mm
Rezansoff et al.	Near lateral femoral epicondyle, at a point on a line drawn from the posterior femoral cortical line and just inferior to the Blumensaat line	Not stated	24.7 mm from Gerdy's tubercle and 11.5 mm distal to lateral tibial plateau, at a point between a line along the posterior tibial cortex and a parallel line from the apex of the tibial spine, intersecting a perpendicular line from the apex of the posterior tibial condyles	Not stated
Caterine et al.	Two variations: (1) proximal and posterior to lateral epicondyle and (2) anterior and distal to lateral epicondyle	Obliquely within capsule to insert on tibia. Deep attachment to lateral meniscus	Midway between head of fibula and Gerdy's tubercle	Intracapsular ligamentous thickening of anterolateral capsule
Dodds et al.	8 mm proximal and 4.3 mm posterior to lateral femoral epicondyle	Superficial to LCL and capsule with branching attachments to meniscus	Midway between head of fibula and Gerdy's tubercle	Extracapsular ligamentous structure
Cianca et al.	Not stated	Over lateral meniscus, traveling obliquely and parallel to ITT	Inferior to proximal lateral edge of tibia, posterior and proximal to Gerdy's tubercle	Easiest to identify with 90 degrees of flexion and internal rotation of knee, resulting in ligament being taut
Helito et al.	2.2 ± 1.5 mm anterior and 3.5 ± 2.1 mm distal to LCL	Bifurcation present at 52.5% of its length (proximal to distal), attaching to lateral meniscus	4.4 ± 1.1 mm distal to lateral tibial plateau, at a point 38% of way from fibular head to Gerdy's tubercle	Length: 37.3 ± 4.0 mm Width: 7.4 ± 1.7 mm Thickness: 2.7 ± 0.6 mm Histology: dense connective tissue with arranged fibers and little cellular material
Claes et al.	Lateral femoral epicondyle, anterior to LCL, proximal and posterior to insertion of popliteus	Oblique anteroinferior to proximal tibia Attachment to meniscus	In middle of a line connecting Gerdy's tubercle and tip of fibular head	Length: 41.5 mm (flexion), 38.5 mm (extension) Width: 8.3 mm (origin), 6.7 mm (joint line), 11.2 mm (insertion) Thickness: 1.3 mm (joint line)

Continued

TABLE 1.1

Structure of Anterolateral Ligament—cont'd

STUDY	ORIGIN	COURSE	INSERTION	CHARACTERISTICS
Vincent et al.	Lateral femoral epicondyle	Obliquely anteroinferiorly toward lateral meniscus and tibial plateau	Proximal anterolateral tibia, 5 mm from articular cartilage, posterior to Gerdy's tubercle	Collagenous fibers with dense core and parallel orientation Width: 8.2 mm Thickness: 2 to 3 mm Length: 34.1 mm
Vieira et al.	Lateral supraepicondylar region bordering lateral edge of lateral epicondyle	Oblique course toward proximal tibia	Laterally to Gerdy's tubercle	Well-defined ligamentous structure
Patella et al.	1.5 cm anterior and superior to lateral epicondyle	Oblique anteroinferior course	1.5 cm posteriorly to Gerdy's tubercle	Ligamentous structure composed of a superficial and deep bundle
Campos et al.	Lateral femoral epicondyle	Oblique anteroinferior course	Lateral midportion of proximal tibia	Thick band of tissue between ITT and LCL at level of lateral tibial plateau
Irvine et al.	Not stated	Not stated	Midway between Gerdy's tubercle and head of fibula	Ligamentous structure, strong enough to cause avulsion fracture off proximal tibia
Terry et al.	Near lateral epicondyle	Oblique course toward proximal tibia	Just posterior to Gerdy's tubercle on lateral tibial tuberosity	Distinct ligamentous structure
Dietz et al.	Not stated	Not stated	A point between Gerdy's tubercle and fibular head	Can cause avulsion off tibial condyle (optimal radiograph is straight AP radiograph)
Fulkerson and Gossling	Lateral epicondyle, just anterior to origin of gastrocnemius	Anteroinferior course	Proximal tibia immediately anterior to fibular head	Not stated
Johnson	Lateral femoral epicondyle	Not stated	Proximal tibia	Strong ligamentous structure
Hughston et al.	Lateral femoral epicondyle	Not stated	Tibial joint margin	Technically strong ligament

ALL, Anterolateral ligament; *AP*, anteroposterior; *LCL*, lateral collateral ligament; *ITT*, iliotibial tract.
From Van der Watt L, Khan M, Rothrauff BB, et al: The structure and function of the anterolateral ligament of the knee: a systematic review, *Arthroscopy* 31:569, 2015.

popliteofibular ligaments, which arise from the popliteus tendon at its musculotendinous junction, forming a "Y" configuration also known as the arcuate ligament. These ligaments provide a strong connection between the popliteus tendon and the fibula. The more important posterior division (and the one typically reconstructed in posterolateral corner injuries) inserts 1.6 mm distal to the tip of the fibular styloid process on its posterior medial downslope. The anterior division inserts anterior to the posterior arm and medial to the FCL typically 2.8 mm distal to the anteromedial aspect of the fibular styloid process. The popliteus also has attachments to the lateral meniscus known as the three popliteomeniscal fascicles, which contribute to the dynamic stability of the lateral meniscus.

The popliteus is a dynamic internal rotator of the tibia and provides dynamic and static stability to the knee primarily in response to external tibial rotation. The popliteofibular ligament is a static stabilizer of the lateral and posterolateral knee resisting varus, external rotation, and posterior tibial

translation. The popliteus and popliteofibular ligament are vital components of any posterolateral reconstruction.

The deepest layer is the joint capsule, which is divided into superficial and deep laminae. The superficial layer is the original capsule embryologically; it encompasses the LCL and ends posteriorly at the fabellofibular ligament. The deep capsular layer is phylogenetically younger and results from the fibula receding from the lateral femur during early embryonic development. It extends posterolaterally and forms the coronary ligament and the hiatus for the popliteus tendon. It travels along the lateral meniscus and spans from the junction of the popliteus muscle and tendon to its termination at the popliteofibular ligament. The capsule can be divided into three sections: anterior, lateral, and posterior. The anterior section extends from the patellar tendon to the anterior border of the popliteus tendon insertion on the femur. The lateral capsule extends from the anterior border of the popliteus tendon to the lateral gastrocnemius attachment. The posterior capsule attaches to the femur

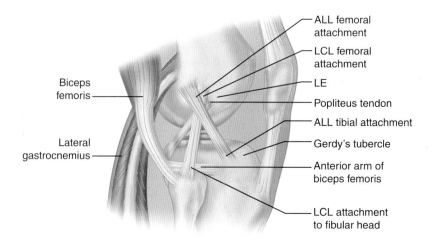

FIGURE 1.14 Lateral view, right knee: osseous landmarks and attachment sites of main structures of lateral knee (iliotibial band and non-anterolateral-ligament related capsule removed). Femoral attachment of anterolateral ligament is located posterior and proximal to lateral collateral ligament; it courses anterodistally to its anterolateral tibial attachment approximately midway between center of Gerdy's tubercle and the anterior margin of fibular head. *ALL*, Anterolateral ligament; *LCL*, lateral collateral ligament; *LE*, lateral epicondyle. (Redrawn from Kennedy MI, Claes S, Fuso FA, et al: The anterolateral ligament: an anatomic, radiographic, and biomechanical analysis, *Am J Sports Med* 43:1606, 2015.)

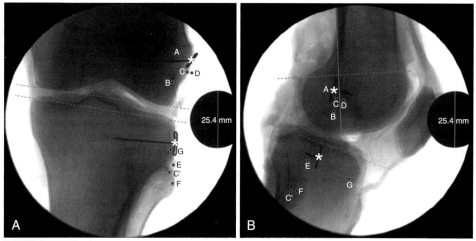

FIGURE 1.15 Anteroposterior **(A)** and lateral **(B)** radiographs illustrating relationship of femoral and tibial anterolateral ligament attachments *(*)* to lateral gastrocnemius tendon *(A)*, popliteus tendon *(B)*, femoral attachment of the lateral collateral ligament *(C)* and lateral epicondyle *(D)*, anterior arm of short head of biceps femoris *(E)*, anterior margin of fibular head *(F)*, and Gerdy's tubercle *(G)*. (From Kennedy MI, Claes S, Fuso FA, et al: The anterolateral ligament: an anatomic, radiographic, and biomechanical analysis, *Am J Sports Med* 43:1606, 2015.)

proximal to the articular margin of the lateral femoral condyle. It is covered by the muscular origins of the plantaris and lateral gastrocnemius muscle and tendon. Distally, it blends with the musculotendinous junction of the popliteus and the posterior division of the popliteofibular ligament. The midthird capsular ligament is a thickening of the lateral capsule of the knee and is divided into the meniscofemoral and meniscotibial components similar to the deep MCL on the medial side of the knee. It is thought to be an important secondary stabilizer to varus instability, and the meniscotibial portion helps stabilize the lateral meniscus anterior to the popliteal hiatus.

INTRAARTICULAR STRUCTURES

The principal intraarticular structures of importance are the medial and lateral menisci and the anterior and PCLs. Numerous functions have been assigned to the menisci, some known and some hypothetical. Among these functions are distribution of joint fluid, nutrition, shock absorption, deepening of the joint, stabilization of the joint, and a load-bearing or weight-bearing function. The cruciate ligaments function as stabilizers of the joint and axes around which rotary motion, both normal and abnormal, occurs. They restrict the backward and forward motion of the tibia on the femur and assist in the control of both medial and lateral rotation of the tibia on the femur. External rotation of the tibia produces an unwinding of the ligaments, and internal rotation produces a winding up of the cruciate ligaments (Fig. 1.17). Further discussion of their specific functions is presented in the section on cruciate ligament injuries.

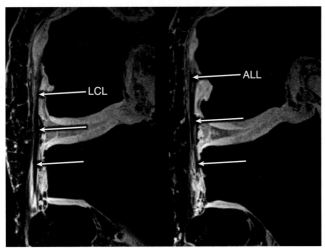

FIGURE 1.16 Coronal magnetic resonance images of right knee demonstrating the anatomic location of lateral collateral ligament *(LCL)* on left and anterolateral ligament *(ALL)* on right, located more anteriorly to lateral collateral ligament. (From Van der Watt L, Khan M, Routhrauff BB, et al: The structure and function of the anterolateral ligament of the knee: a systematic review, *Arthroscopy* 31:569, 2015.)

MECHANICS

Both menisci are displaced slightly forward in full extension and move backward as flexion proceeds. The anchorage of the medial meniscus permits less mobility than of the lateral meniscus, possibly explaining why injuries are more common to the medial meniscus than to the lateral meniscus. The action of the popliteus muscle laterally and the semimembranosus muscle medially retracting the menisci posteriorly also helps prevent the menisci from becoming entrapped during movements of the knee. The menisci are described as moving with the femoral condyles with flexion and extension but moving with the tibia with rotary movements.

The mechanical axis of the femur does not coincide with its anatomic axis because a line traversing the center of the hip joint and the center of the knee forms an angle of 6 to 9 degrees with the axis of the shaft of the femur. The mechanical axis generally passes near the center of the normal knee joint. Significant deviations from this mechanical axis may be present with genu varum or genu valgum deformity. The medial and lateral femoral condyles have different configurations. The lateral condyle is broader in the anteroposterior and the transverse planes than the medial condyle, and the medial condyle projects distally to a level slightly lower than the lateral condyle. This distal projection helps compensate for the inclination of the mechanical axis in the erect position so that the transverse axis lies near the horizontal.

Since the medial femoral condyle articular surface is smaller than the lateral, during rotary movements it describes a smaller arc than the lateral condyle, thereby producing

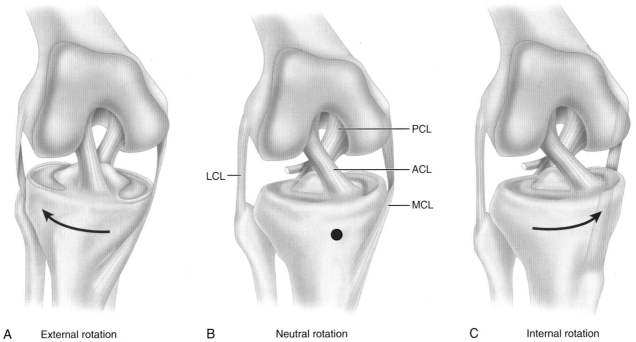

A   External rotation   B   Neutral rotation   C   Internal rotation

FIGURE 1.17 In addition to their synergistic functions, cruciate and collateral ligaments exercise basic antagonistic function during rotation. **A,** In external rotation, it is collateral ligaments that tighten and inhibit excessive rotation by becoming crossed in space. **B,** In neutral rotation, none of four ligaments is under unusual tension. **C,** In internal rotation, collateral ligaments become more vertical and are more lax, whereas cruciate ligaments become coiled around each other and come under strong tension. *ACL,* Anterior cruciate ligament; *LCL,* lateral collateral ligament; *MCL,* medial collateral ligament; *PCL,* posterior cruciate ligament.

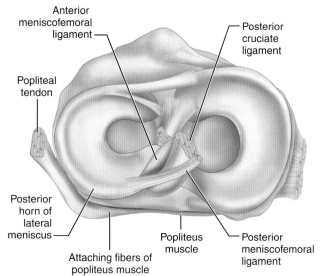

FIGURE 1.18 Superior view of tibial condyles after removal of femur. Lateral meniscus is smaller in diameter, thicker around its periphery, wider in body, and more mobile; posteriorly, it is attached to medial femoral condyle by either anterior or posterior meniscofemoral ligament, depending on which is present, and to popliteus muscle.

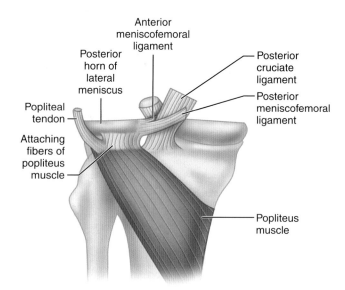

FIGURE 1.19 Posterior view of knee after removal of femur. Posteriorly, lateral meniscus is attached to either anterior or posterior meniscofemoral ligament, depending on which is present, and to popliteus muscle.

two types of motion during flexion and extension. The knee thus possesses features characteristic of both a ginglymus (hinge joint) and a trochoid (pivot joint) articulation. The joint permits flexion and extension in the sagittal plane and some degree of internal and external rotation when the joint is flexed. No rotation is possible when the knee is in full extension.

The complex flexion-extension motion is a combination of rocking and gliding. The rocking motion is demonstrable in the first 20 degrees of flexion, after which the motion becomes predominantly of the gliding type. This transition from one form of motion to the other is gradual but progressive. The rocking motion in the first 20 degrees of flexion better meets the requirements for stability of the knee in the relatively extended position, whereas the gliding motion as the joint unwinds permits more freedom for rotation.

The articular surface of the medial condyle is prolonged anteriorly, and as the knee comes into the fully extended position, the femur internally rotates until the remaining articular surface on the medial condyle is in contact. The posterior portion of the lateral condyle rotates forward laterally, thus producing a "screwing home" movement, locking the knee in the fully extended position. When flexion is initiated, unscrewing of the joint occurs by external rotation of the femur on the tibia. As previously mentioned, the rotary movement responsible for screwing and unscrewing of the knee joint occurs around an axis that passes near the medial condyle of the femur and is greatly influenced by the PCL.

Normal flexion and extension are from 0 to 140 degrees, but 5 to 10 degrees of hyperextension is often possible. With the knee flexed to 90 degrees, passive rotation of the tibia on the femur can be demonstrated up to 25 or 30 degrees; this passive rotation varies with each individual. The extent of internal rotation always exceeds that of external rotation, and no rotation is possible with the knee fully extended. Sagittal displacement of the tibia on the fixed femur is detectable in both the anterior and posterior directions when the knee is flexed. Under normal conditions, the extent of the excursion should not exceed 3 to 5 mm. When the knee is extended, lateral (abduction–adduction) motion at the knee joint occurs to a limited extent; this motion varies with individual characteristics but should not exceed 6 to 8 degrees. In the hyperextended position, no lateral motion is present. In the flexed position, more lateral motion is possible but should never exceed 15 degrees.

MENISCI
FUNCTION AND ANATOMY

Meniscal function is essential to the normal function of the knee joint. As stated in the previous section on anatomy, various functions have been attributed to the menisci, some of which are known or proved and others that are theorized. The menisci act as a joint filler, compensating for gross incongruity between femoral and tibial articulating surfaces (Figs. 1.18 and 1.19). So located, the menisci prevent capsular and synovial impingement during flexion-extension movements. The menisci are believed to have a joint lubrication function, helping to distribute synovial fluid throughout the joint and aiding the nutrition of the articular cartilage. They contribute to stability in all planes but are especially important rotary stabilizers and are probably essential for the smooth transition from a pure hinge to a gliding or rotary motion as the knee moves from flexion to extension.

Radiographic changes, as described by Fairbank, appear after meniscectomy and include narrowing of the joint space, flattening of the femoral condyle, and formation of osteophytes. Narrowing of the joint space initially is caused by removal of the spacer effect of the meniscus (approximately 1 mm); it is further narrowed by a reduction in the contact area in the absence of the meniscus. When the medial meniscus is removed, the contact area is reduced by approximately 40%; in other words, the contact area is 2.5 times greater when the meniscus is present. The larger contact area provided by the

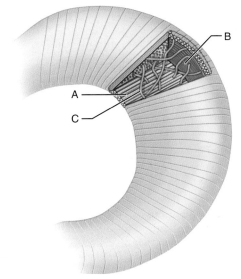

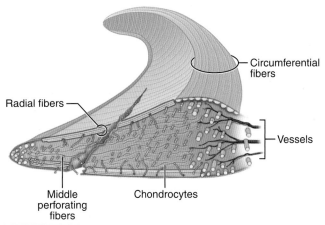

FIGURE 1.22 Cross section of meniscus showing direction of longitudinal tear. Note that direction of tear usually is oblique rather than vertical.

FIGURE 1.20 Pattern of collagen fibers within meniscus. Radial fibers (A). Circumferential fibers (B). Perforating fibers (C).

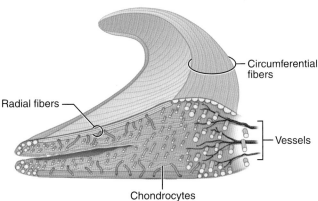

FIGURE 1.21 Cross section of meniscus showing horizontal cleavage split.

meniscus reduces the average contact stress acting between the bones. The menisci are thus important in reducing the stress on the articular cartilage; they prevent mechanical damage to both the chondrocytes and the extracellular matrix. Increased contact stress resulting from decreased contact area may produce bone remodeling, producing a flattened femoral condyle. Softening of the joint cartilage also results in increased joint space narrowing and osteophyte formation.

The menisci have long been assumed to have shock- or energy-absorbing functions. Significant weight-bearing or load-transmitting forces are carried by the menisci, from 40% to 60% of the superimposed weight in the standing position. Thus, if normal and intact menisci spare the articular cartilage from compressive loads, then perhaps this partly explains the high incidence of osteoarthritis after removal of the meniscus.

The effects of meniscectomy on joint laxity have been studied for anteroposterior and varus-valgus motions and rotation. These studies indicated that the effect on joint laxity depends on whether the ligaments of the knee are intact and whether the joint is bearing weight. In the presence of intact ligamentous structures, excision of the menisci produces small increases in joint laxity. When combined with

ligamentous insufficiency, these increased instabilities caused by meniscectomy are greatly exaggerated. In an ACL-deficient knee, medial meniscectomy has been shown to increase tibial translation by 58% at 90 degrees, whereas primary anterior and posterior translations were not affected by lateral meniscectomy. Anatomically, the capsular components that attach the lateral meniscus to the tibia do not affix the lateral meniscus as firmly as they do the medial meniscus. These results indicate that in contrast to the medial meniscus, the lateral meniscus does not act as an efficient posterior wedge to resist anterior translation of the tibia on the femur. Therefore, in knees that lack an ACL, the lateral meniscus is subjected to forces different from those that occur on the medial side; forces in the medial meniscus increase significantly in response to an anterior tibial load after transection of the ACL. This may account for the different patterns of injury of the lateral and medial menisci in knees with ACL deficiency.

Biomechanical studies have shown that under loads of up to 150 kg, the lateral meniscus appears to carry 70% of the load on that side of the joint; whereas on the medial side, the load is shared approximately equally by the meniscus and the exposed articular cartilage. Medial meniscectomy decreases contact area by 50% to 70% and increases contact stress by 100%. Lateral meniscectomy decreases contact area by 40% to 50% but dramatically increases contact stress by 200% to 300% because of the relative convex surface of the lateral tibial plateau.

The menisci are crescents, roughly triangular in cross section, that cover one half to two thirds of the articular surface of the corresponding tibial plateau. They are composed of dense, tightly woven collagen fibers arranged in a pattern providing great elasticity and ability to withstand compression. The major orientation of collagen fibers in the meniscus is circumferential; radial fibers and perforating fibers also are present. The arrangement of these collagen fibers determines to some extent the characteristic patterns of meniscal tears (Figs. 1.20 to 1.22). When meniscal samples are tested by application of a force perpendicular to the fiber direction, the strength is decreased to less than 10% because collagen fibers function primarily to resist tensile forces along the direction of the fibers. The circumferential fibers act in much the same way as metal hoops placed around a pressurized

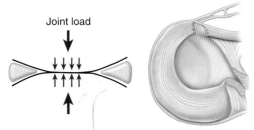

FIGURE 1.23   Role of hoop tension in menisci. Hoop tension developed in menisci acts to keep them between bones.

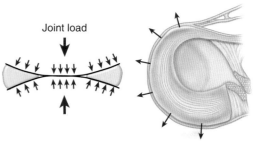

FIGURE 1.24   Role of hoop tension in menisci. Single cut to radial edge eliminates hoop tension and allows menisci to move out from between bones.

wooden barrel. The tension in the hoops keeps the wooden staves in place (Figs. 1.23 and 1.24). The compression of the menisci by the tibia and the femur generates outward forces that push the menisci out from between the bones. The circumferential tension in the menisci counteracts this outward or radial force. These hoop forces are transmitted to the tibia through the strong anterior and posterior attachments of the menisci. Hoop tension is lost when a single radial cut or tear extends to the capsular margin; in terms of load bearing, a single radial cut through the meniscus may be equivalent to meniscectomy.

The peripheral edges of the menisci are convex, fixed, and attached to the inner surface of the knee joint capsule, except where the popliteus is interposed laterally; these peripheral edges also are attached loosely to the borders of the tibial plateaus by the coronary ligaments. The inner edges are concave, thin, and unattached. The menisci are largely avascular except near their peripheral attachment to the coronary ligaments. The inferior surface of each meniscus is flat, whereas the superior surface is concave, corresponding to the contour of the underlying tibial plateau and superimposed femoral condyle.

The medial meniscus is a C-shaped structure larger in radius than the lateral meniscus, with the posterior horn being wider than the anterior. The anterior horn is attached firmly to the tibia anterior to the intercondylar eminence and to the ACL. Most of the weight is borne on the posterior portion of the meniscus. The posterior horn is anchored immediately in front of the attachments of the PCL posterior to the intercondylar eminence. Its entire peripheral border is firmly attached to the medial capsule and through the coronary ligament to the upper border of the tibia.

The lateral meniscus is more circular in form, covering up to two thirds of the articular surface of the underlying tibial plateau. The anterior horn is attached to the tibia medially in front of the intercondylar eminence, whereas the posterior horn inserts into the posterior aspect of the intercondylar eminence and in front of the posterior attachment of the medial meniscus. The posterior horn often receives anchorage also to the femur by the ligament of Wrisberg and the ligament of Humphry and from fascia covering the popliteus muscle and the arcuate complex at the posterolateral corner of the knee. The inner border, like that of the medial meniscus, is thin, concave, and free. The tendon of the popliteus muscle separates the posterolateral periphery of the lateral meniscus from the joint capsule and the FCL. The tendon of the popliteus is enveloped in a synovial membrane and forms an oblique groove on the lateral border of the meniscus.

The lateral meniscus is smaller in diameter, thicker in periphery, wider in body, and more mobile than the medial meniscus. It is attached to both cruciate ligaments and posteriorly to the medial femoral condyle by either the ligament of Humphry or the ligament of Wrisberg, depending on which is present; it is also attached posteriorly to the popliteus muscle (see Figs. 1.18 and 1.19). It is separated from the LCL by the popliteal tendon. In contrast, the medial meniscus is much larger in diameter, is thinner in its periphery and narrower in body, and does not attach to either cruciate ligament. It is loosely attached to the medial capsular ligaments.

The menisci follow the tibial condyles during flexion and extension, but during rotation they follow the femur and move on the tibia; consequently, the medial meniscus becomes distorted. Its anterior and posterior attachments follow the tibia, but its intervening part follows the femur; thus it is likely to be injured during rotation. However, the lateral meniscus, because it is firmly attached to the popliteus muscle and to the ligament of Wrisberg or of Humphry, follows the lateral femoral condyle during rotation and therefore is less likely to be injured. In addition, when the tibia is rotated internally and the knee flexed, the popliteus muscle, by way of the arcuate ligament, draws the posterior segment of the lateral meniscus backward, thereby preventing the meniscus from being caught between the condyle of the femur and the plateau of the tibia.

The vascular supply to the medial and lateral menisci originates predominantly from the lateral and medial geniculate vessels (both inferior and superior). Branches from these vessels give rise to a perimeniscal capillary plexus within the synovial and capsular tissue. The plexus is an arboroid network of vessels that supplies the peripheral border of the meniscus throughout its attachment to the joint capsule (Fig. 1.25). These vessels are oriented in a predominantly circumferential pattern with radial branches directed toward the center of the joint (Fig. 1.26). Microinjection techniques have shown that the depth of peripheral vascular penetration is 10% to 30% of the width of the medial meniscus and 10% to 25% of the width of the lateral meniscus. The medial and lateral geniculate arteries, along with their branches, supply vessels to the menisci through the vascular synovial covering of the anterior and posterior horn attachments. A small reflection of vascular synovial tissue also is present throughout the periphery of the menisci at both the femoral and tibial attachments and extends for a short distance (1 to 3 mm).

The meniscus is a relatively acellular structure with predominately fibroblast-like cells in the peripheral vascular zone and chondrocyte-like cells in the avascular zone. Knees

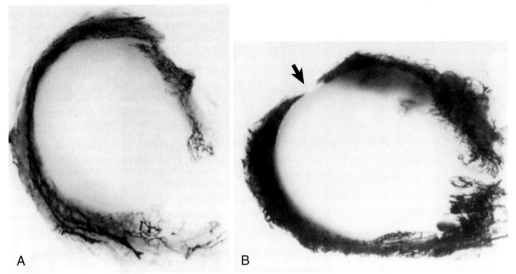

FIGURE 1.25 Superior aspect of medial **(A)** and lateral **(B)** menisci after vascular perfusion with India ink and tissue clearing by modified Spalteholz technique. Note vascularity at periphery of meniscus, as well as at anterior and posterior horn attachments. Absence of peripheral vasculature at posterolateral corner of lateral meniscus *(arrow)* represents area of passage of popliteal tendon.

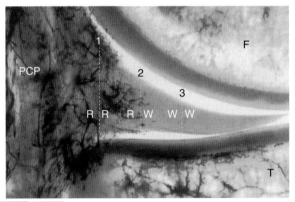

FIGURE 1.26 Frontal section of medial compartment of knee. Branching radial vessels from perimeniscal capillary plexus *(PCP)* can be seen penetrating peripheral border of medial meniscus. *F,* Femur; *T,* tibia. Three zones of meniscal vascularity are shown: *1 RR,* red-red is fully within vascular area; *2 RW,* red-white is at border of vascular area; and *3 WW,* white-white is within avascular area. (From Arnoczky SP, Warren RF: Microvasculature of the human meniscus, *Am J Sports Med* 10:90, 1982.)

with traumatic or degenerative meniscal tears have synovial fluid that contains degradative enzymes, including metalloproteinases and aggrecanases, which contribute to meniscal degeneration through proteoglycan and collagen degradation. Biologic augmentation strategies are designed to promote a healing environment and disrupt the degradative cascade.

MENISCAL HEALING AND REPAIR

The vascular supply to the meniscus determines its potential for repair. The peripheral meniscal blood supply is capable of producing a reparative response similar to that observed in other connective tissues because of a perimeniscal capillary plexus that supplies the peripheral 10% to 25% of the menisci. Meniscal tears have been classified on the basis of

their location in three zones of vascularity—red (fully within the vascular area), red-white (at the border of the vascular area), and white (within the avascular area)—and this classification indicates the potential for healing after repair (see Fig. 1.21 and section on surgical repair of torn menisci).

After injury within the peripheral vascular zone, a fibrin clot that is rich in inflammatory cells forms. Vessels from the perimeniscal capillary plexus proliferate throughout this fibrin scaffold and are accompanied by the proliferations of differentiated mesenchymal cells. The lesion is eventually filled with cellular fibrovascular scar tissue that glues the wound edges together and appears continuous with the adjacent normal meniscal fibrocartilage. Vessels from the perimeniscal capillary plexus as well as the proliferative vascular pannus from the synovial fringe penetrate the fibrous scar to provide a marked inflammatory response. Experimental studies in animals have shown that complete radial lesions of the meniscus are completely healed with a young fibrocartilaginous scar by 10 weeks, although several months are required for maturation to fibrocartilage that appears normal.

Several reports described excellent results after primary repair of lesions at the periphery of the meniscus; because results of repair of tears in partially vascular or avascular areas are not as predictable, techniques have been developed to improve vascularity in meniscal repair. Techniques for open suture of peripheral tears of the meniscus are presented in this chapter, and those for arthroscopic suture are described in other chapter.

Controversy exists about the ability of a meniscus or a meniscus-like tissue to regenerate after meniscectomy. It is now generally accepted that for a meniscus to regenerate to any extent, the entire structure must be resected to expose the vascular synovial tissue; or, in subtotal meniscectomy, the excision must extend to the peripheral vasculature of the meniscus. Subtotal excisions of the meniscus within the avascular central half of the meniscus do not show any regeneration potential. The frequency and degree of regeneration of the meniscus have

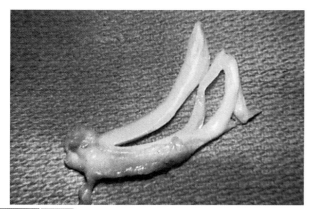

FIGURE 1.27 Two tears of medial meniscus: classic bucket-handle tear and tear of posterior peripheral part.

not been determined precisely. Many surgeons believe that only the peripheral rim regenerates after total meniscectomy and that the quality of regenerated meniscus does not compare with that of original meniscus (see discussion of regeneration of menisci after excision).

MECHANISM OF TEAR

Traumatic lesions of the menisci are produced most commonly by rotation as the flexed knee moves toward an extended position. The medial meniscus, being far less mobile on the tibia, can become entrapped between the condyles, and injury can result. The most common location for injury is the posterior horn of the meniscus, and longitudinal tears are the most common type of injury. During vigorous internal rotation of the femur on the tibia with the knee in flexion, the femur tends to force the medial meniscus posteriorly and toward the center of the joint. A strong peripheral attachment posteriorly may prevent the meniscus from being injured, but if this attachment stretches or tears, the posterior part of the meniscus is forced toward the center of the joint, is caught between the femur and the tibia, and is torn longitudinally when the joint is suddenly extended. The length, depth, and position of the tear depend on the position of the posterior horn in relation to the femoral and tibial condyles at the time of injury. If this longitudinal tear extends anteriorly beyond the MCL, the inner segment of the meniscus is caught in the intercondylar notch and cannot return to its former position; thus a classic bucket-handle tear with locking of the joint is produced (Fig. 1.27).

The same mechanism can produce a posterior peripheral or a longitudinal tear of the lateral meniscus; the lateral femoral condyle forces the anterior half of the meniscus anteriorly and toward the center of the joint, and this strain in turn may tear the posterior half of the meniscus from its peripheral attachment. When the joint is extended, a longitudinal tear results. Because of its mobility and structure, the lateral meniscus is not as susceptible to bucket-handle tears; however, because it is more sharply curved and is neither attached to, nor controlled by, the LCL, the lateral meniscus sustains incomplete transverse tears more often than does the medial meniscus.

Menisci with peripheral cystic formation or menisci that have been rendered less mobile from previous injury or disease may sustain tears from less trauma. Congenital anomalies of the menisci, especially discoid lateral meniscus, may predispose to either degeneration or traumatic laceration. Likewise, areas of degeneration that develop as a result of aging cannot withstand as much trauma as healthy fibrocartilage. Abnormal mechanical axes in a joint with incongruities or ligamentous disruptions expose the menisci to abnormal mechanics and thus can lead to a greater incidence of injury. Congenitally relaxed joints and those with inadequate musculature, especially the quadriceps, probably are at significantly greater risk of meniscal injuries, as well as other internal derangements.

CLASSIFICATION OF MENISCAL TEARS

Numerous classifications of tears of the menisci have been proposed on the basis of location or type of tear, etiology, and other factors; most of the commonly used classifications are based on the type of tear found at surgery. These are (1) longitudinal tears, (2) radial and oblique tears, (3) horizontal cleavage tears, (4) complex tears which are a combination of longitudinal and cleavage tears, (5) tears associated with cystic menisci, and (6) tears associated with discoid menisci.

More recently, investigators have focused on two versions of the previously described tear patterns: the posterior root tear, which is a type of radial tear at the posterior root attachment of the meniscus, and the ramp lesion, which is a form of longitudinal tear at the menisco-capsular junction or the menisco-tibial attachment of the meniscus. Both tear types are thought to lead to increased anterior instability in ACL-deficient knees, as well as increased contact forces and early arthritis with posterior root tears.

The most common type of tear is the longitudinal tear, usually involving the posterior segment of either the medial or the lateral meniscus. Before the extensive use of arthroscopy for diagnosis and treatment of meniscal injuries, tears of the medial meniscus in most series were approximately five to seven times more common than those of the lateral meniscus. However, as use of the arthroscope has increased, allowing more thorough inspection of both menisci, more lateral meniscal tears have been diagnosed. The two types are believed to occur with almost equal frequency. Tears within the meniscus itself can be complete or incomplete. Most involve the inferior rather than the superior surface of the meniscus. Small tears limited to the posterior horn are not capable of producing locking but will cause pain, recurrent swelling, and a feeling of instability in the joint. Extensive longitudinal tears can cause mechanical locking if the central portion of the meniscus is displaced into the intercondylar notch. A pedunculated fragment may result if either the posterior or anterior attachment of the bucket-handle fragment becomes detached.

Transverse, radial, or oblique tears can occur in either meniscus but more commonly involve the lateral meniscus. These usually are located at the junction of the anterior and middle thirds and, as previously pointed out, tend to occur when forces separate the anterior and posterior segments of the meniscus, stretching the inner concave border and resulting in a transverse tear. Because the lateral meniscus is more of a circle and has a shorter radius, the inner free edge is more easily torn radially than its medial counterpart. Radial tears also can result from degenerative changes within the meniscus itself or from injury or conditions such as cystic changes at the periphery that render the meniscus less mobile. Both radial and longitudinal complex tears may be found and may follow degeneration or repeated traumatic episodes.

Cysts of the menisci are frequently associated with tears and are nine times more common on the lateral than on the medial side. The most common cause is trauma that produces degeneration and secondary mucinous and cystic changes in the periphery of the meniscus; when inflammatory changes follow, the meniscus may become less mobile during flexion, extension, and rotary motions and thus more susceptible to additional longitudinal or radial tearing.

Discoid menisci are abnormal and, because of hypermobility and the bulk of the tissue between the articular surfaces, they are vulnerable to compression and rotary stresses. Degeneration within the discoid meniscus, as well as tears, may develop. The diagnosis often is made incidentally on MRI and occasionally at the time of arthroscopy, since the discoid meniscus may not produce significant symptoms until some derangement of the meniscus occurs.

■ DIAGNOSIS

The diagnosis of a meniscal tear can be difficult even for an experienced orthopaedic surgeon. Use of a careful history and physical examination and supplementation of standard radiographs in specific instances with special imaging techniques and arthroscopy can keep errors in diagnosis of tears of the menisci to less than 5%.

When a meniscus has been injured, capsular and ligamentous structures and the articular surfaces also often have been injured. For simplicity, tears of the menisci are discussed here as though they always are isolated injuries, but evidence of other injuries always must be sought. Disorders that can produce symptoms similar to those of a torn meniscus must be kept in mind and, to avoid error, a detailed, careful, systemic history and physical examination supplemented with appropriate imaging studies are indicated, especially if symptoms and findings are not quite typical of a torn meniscus.

A history of specific injury may not be obtained, especially when tears of abnormal or degenerative menisci have occurred. This scenario is noted most often in a middle-aged person who sustains a weight-bearing twist on the knee or who has pain after squatting. Occasionally, an overweight middle-aged patient with mild-to-moderate knee arthritis describes a painful pop in the back of the knee when loading the knee, such as stepping up. In this scenario, the pop represents failure of the posterior root of the meniscus. Tears of normal menisci usually are associated with more significant trauma or injury but are produced by a similar mechanism: the meniscus is entrapped between the femoral and tibial condyles in flexion, tearing as the knee is extended. Patients with tears in degenerative menisci may recall symptoms of mild catching, snapping, or clicking, as well as occasional pain and mild swelling in the joint. Once the tear in the meniscus becomes of significant size, more obvious symptoms of giving way and locking may develop.

The syndromes caused by tears of the menisci can be divided into two groups: those in which there is locking and the diagnosis is clear and those in which locking is absent and the diagnosis is more difficult. The first group requires little discussion because the symptoms and findings have been described many times elsewhere. However, locking may not be recognized unless the injured knee is compared with the opposite knee, which should exhibit the 5 to 10 degrees of recurvatum that normally is present. The injured knee can be locked and still extend to neutral position. This presentation may be seen with a chronic bucket-handle tear when the tear has elongated sufficiently to allow the meniscal fragment to displace far enough into the notch so that knee extension is no longer impaired. Locking usually occurs only with longitudinal tears and is much more common with bucket-handle tears, usually of the medial meniscus. A very peripheral tear of the lateral meniscus may cause locking, even though the MRI appears normal. The patient will describe an episode when the knee locks in more flexion (sometimes approaching 70 degrees) and is associated with lateral-side knee pain. Often this is preceded by the patient having placed the knee in a highly flexed position, such as sitting on the knee, sitting tailor fashion, kneeling, or squatting. When the patient is able to unlock the knee, it usually occurs with an audible clunk and a visible jerk to the knee. The pain will lessen but soreness along the lateral joint line persists. When the MRI appears normal, the history may be the only clue to the diagnosis. Locking of the knee must not be considered pathognomonic of a bucket-handle tear of a meniscus; an intraarticular tumor, an osteocartilaginous loose body, and other conditions can cause locking. Regardless of its cause, locking that is unrelieved after aspiration of the hemarthrosis and a period of conservative treatment may require surgical treatment. A serious error is failure to distinguish locking from false locking. False locking occurs most often soon after an injury in which hemorrhage around the posterior part of the capsule or a collateral ligament with associated hamstring spasm prevents complete extension of the knee. Aspiration and a short period of rest until the reaction has partially subsided usually differentiates locking from false locking of the joint.

If a patient does not have locking, the diagnosis of a torn meniscus is more difficult even for the most astute surgeon. Degenerative tears often present in this fashion. These tears result from repetitive physiologic forces leading to gradual wear of the meniscus, commonly resulting in horizontal cleavage or complex tears accompanied by osteoarthritic changes of the joint. A patient typically gives a history of several episodes of trouble referable to the knee, often resulting in effusion and a brief period of disability but no definite locking. A sensation of "giving way" or snaps, clicks, catches, or jerks in the knee may be described, or the history may be even more indefinite, with recurrent episodes of pain and mild effusion in the knee and tenderness along the joint line after excessive activity. The clinician should also be mindful that mechanical symptoms may result from osteoarthritis when rough, incongruous surfaces catch on each other instead of gliding smoothly. When they are well understood, the following clues can be important in the differential diagnosis in this second group: a sensation of giving way, effusion, atrophy of the quadriceps, tenderness over the joint line (or the meniscus), and reproduction of a click by manipulative maneuvers during the physical examination.

A sensation of giving way is in itself of little help in diagnosis because it can occur in other disturbances of the knee, especially loose bodies, chondromalacia of the patella, instability of the joint resulting from injury to the ligaments or from weakness of the supporting musculature, especially the quadriceps, or any painful stimulus. When this symptom results from a tear in the posterior part of a meniscus, the patient usually notices this on rotary movements of the knee and often associates it with a feeling of subluxation or "the joint jumping out of place." When giving way is a result of other causes, such as quadriceps weakness, it usually is noticeable during simple flexion of the knee against resistance, such as in walking down stairs.

Effusion indicates that something is irritating the synovium; therefore, it has limited specific diagnostic value.

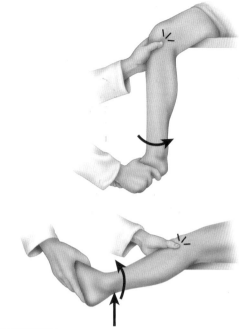

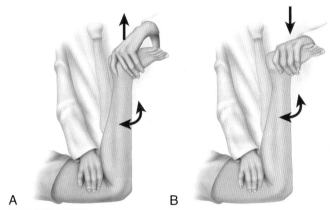

The sudden onset of effusion after an injury usually denotes a hemarthrosis, and it can occur when the vascularized periphery of a meniscus is torn. Tears occurring within the body of a meniscus or in degenerative areas may not produce a hemarthrosis. Repeated displacement of a pedunculated or torn portion of a meniscus can cause sufficient synovial irritation to produce a chronic synovitis with an effusion of a nonbloody nature. Thus, the time at onset and the characteristics of the effusion are of value in assessing the knee, but the absence of an effusion or hemarthrosis does not rule out a tear of the meniscus.

Atrophy of the musculature around the knee, especially of the vastus medialis component of the quadriceps mechanism, suggests a recurring disability of the knee but does not indicate its cause.

Probably the most important physical finding is localized tenderness along the medial or lateral joint line or over the periphery of the meniscus. This most often is located posteromedially or posterolaterally, because most meniscal tears are in the posterior horn areas. The meniscus itself is without nerve fibers except at its periphery; therefore, the tenderness or pain is related to synovitis in the adjacent capsular and synovial tissues.

■ DIAGNOSTIC TESTS

Clicks, snaps, or catches, either audible or detected by palpation during flexion, extension, and rotary motions of the joint, can be valuable diagnostically, and efforts should be made to reproduce and accurately locate them. If these noises are localized to the joint line, the meniscus most likely contains a tear. Similar noises originating from the patella, the quadriceps mechanism, the patellofemoral groove, or arthritic joint surfaces must be differentiated. Numerous manipulative tests have been described, but the McMurray test and the Apley

grinding test probably are most commonly used. All basically involve attempts to locate and to reproduce crepitation that results as the knee is manipulated.

The *McMurray test* (Fig. 1.28) is probably best known and is carried out as follows. With the patient supine and the knee acutely and forcibly flexed, the examiner can check the medial meniscus by palpating the posteromedial margin of the joint with one hand while grasping the foot with the other hand. Keeping the knee completely flexed, the leg is externally rotated as far as possible and then the knee is slowly extended. As the femur passes over a tear in the meniscus, a click may be heard or felt. The lateral meniscus is checked by palpating the posterolateral margin of the joint, internally rotating the leg as far as possible, and slowly extending the knee while listening and feeling for a click. A click produced by the McMurray test usually is caused by a posterior peripheral tear of the meniscus and occurs between complete flexion of the knee and 90 degrees. Popping, which occurs with greater degrees of extension when it is definitely localized to the joint line, suggests a tear of the middle and anterior portions of the meniscus. The position of the knee when the click occurs thus may help locate the lesion. A McMurray click localized to the joint line is additional evidence that the meniscus is torn; a negative result of the McMurray test does not rule out a tear.

The *grinding test,* as described by Apley, is carried out as follows. With the patient prone, the knee is flexed to 90 degrees and the anterior thigh is fixed against the examining table. The foot and leg are then pulled upward to distract the joint and rotated to place rotational strain on the ligaments (Fig. 1.29A); when ligaments have been torn, this part of the test usually is painful. Next, with the knee in the same position, the foot and leg are pressed downward and rotated as the joint is slowly flexed and extended (Fig. 1.29B); when a meniscus has been torn, popping and pain localized to the joint line may be noted. Although the McMurray, Apley, and other tests cannot be considered diagnostic, they are useful enough to be included in the routine examination of the knee.

Tears of one meniscus can produce pain in the opposite compartment of the knee. This is most commonly seen with posterior tears of the lateral meniscus. This phenomenon is not understood. The use of MRI has minimized initial exploration of the wrong compartment.

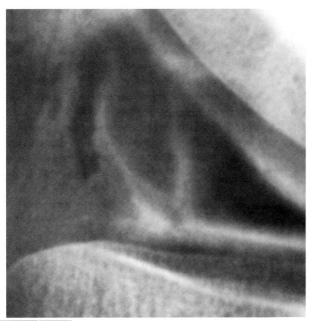

FIGURE 1.30 Arthrogram of knee showing tear of meniscus.

Another useful test, the *squat test,* consists of several repetitions of a full squat with the feet and legs alternately fully internally and externally rotated as the squat is performed. Pain usually is produced on either the medial or lateral side of the knee, corresponding to the side of the torn meniscus. Pain in the internally rotated position suggests injury to the lateral meniscus, whereas pain in the external rotation suggests injury to the medial meniscus. However, the localization of the pain to either the medial joint line or the lateral joint line is a much more dependable localizing sign than the position of rotation.

Karachalios et al. described a test for early detection of meniscal tears *(Thessaly test)* for which they reported diagnostic accuracy rates of 94% in detecting tears of the medial meniscus and 96% in the detection of tears of the lateral meniscus. The examiner supports the patient by holding his or her outstretched hands while the patient stands flatfooted on the floor on just the affected leg. The patient then rotates his or her knee and body, internally and externally, three times with the knee in slight flexion (5 degrees). The same procedure is carried out with the knee flexed 20 degrees. Patients with suspected meniscal tears experience medial or lateral joint-line discomfort and may have a sense of locking or catching. The test is always done on the normal knee first to teach the patient how to keep the knee in 5 and 20 degrees of flexion and how to recognize a possible positive result in the symptomatic knee. The Thessaly test at 20 degrees of knee flexion was suggested to be effective as a first-line clinical screening test for meniscal tears.

Two meta-analyses of the literature attempted to determine the relative accuracy of these clinical tests, but both found problems with methodology of studies and small sample sizes, as well as with differences in how the tests were defined, performed, and interpreted. One analysis determined that joint line tenderness is the best "common" test, while the other found sensitivities and specificities similar among the three tests: McMurray, 70% and 71%; Apley, 60% and 70%; and joint line tenderness, 63% and 77%. Combined testing will improve the accuracy.

IMAGING STUDIES
RADIOGRAPHY
Anteroposterior, lateral, and intercondylar notch views with a tangential view of the inferior surface of the patella should be routine. Ordinary radiographs will not confirm the diagnosis of a torn meniscus but are essential to exclude osteocartilaginous loose bodies, osteochondritis dissecans, and other pathologic processes that can mimic a torn meniscus. Occasionally, a relatively widened lateral joint space may suggest the presence of a discoid lateral meniscus.

ARTHROGRAPHY
The usefulness of arthrography in diagnosis of pathologic conditions of the meniscus usually is directly proportional to the interest and experience of the arthrographer (Fig. 1.30). To never use arthrography is to eliminate an extremely valuable diagnostic procedure, but to use it routinely on every injured knee is just as unfortunate. With the improvements in CT and MRI scanning, we rarely use arthrography for knee examination.

OTHER DIAGNOSTIC STUDIES
Other diagnostic studies, such as ultrasonography, bone scanning, CT, and MRI, have been shown to improve diagnostic accuracy in many knee disorders. Their principal attractiveness over arthrography or arthroscopy is that they are noninvasive procedures. Compared with arthroscopy, MRI has been shown to have 98% accuracy for medial meniscal tears and 90% for lateral meniscal tears. Others have reported that MRI had a positive predictive value of 75%, a negative predictive value of 90%, a sensitivity of 83%, and a specificity of 84% for pathologic changes in the menisci. More recently, a study of acute and chronic meniscal tears in 122 young adults found a sensitivity of 67%, specificity of 93%, and diagnostic accuracy of 88% in the detection of acute tears; sensitivity was 64%, specificity was 91%, and diagnostic accuracy was 86% for chronic tears. Menisco-capsular tears such as ramp lesions are not as easily detected by MRI and therefore should be evaluated at the time of arthroscopy. Although MRI appears to be efficient in detecting meniscal tears, it has not been shown to be effective in predicting the reparability of such tears. Motamedi reported that two experienced musculoskeletal radiologists, using established arthroscopic criteria to grade 119 meniscal tears, agreed on reparable or not reparable classifications 74% of the time but came to identical scores only 38% of the time.

High-resolution CT has been reported to have a sensitivity of 96%, specificity of 81%, and accuracy of 91%. We most often use CT for examining the patellofemoral joint because it allows evaluation of the normal and abnormal relation of the articulation at various degrees of knee flexion, with and without quadriceps contraction. CT arthrography is used when MRI is contra-indicated as in patients with pacemakers or other similar implants. It also is useful for delineating synovial cysts and other soft-tissue tumors around the knee.

ARTHROSCOPY
Details about equipment, principles, and diagnostic and surgical arthroscopic techniques are presented in other chapter.

NONOPERATIVE MANAGEMENT
Arthroscopy has made the diagnosis of acute meniscal injuries more precise, which aids in the treatment planning. Incomplete

tears or small peripheral tears (displaced <3 mm) are difficult to confirm without arthroscopy. An incomplete meniscal tear or a small (10 mm) stable peripheral tear with no other pathologic condition, such as a torn ACL, can be treated nonoperatively with predictably good results. Many incomplete tears will not progress to complete tears if the knee is stable. Small stable peripheral tears have been observed to heal after 3 to 6 weeks of protection. Many undiagnosed small peripheral tears probably occur with other knee injuries, such as sprains or patellar dislocations, and if they are in the vascularized zone (see section on surgical repair of torn menisci), these tears heal without surgical treatment. Weiss et al. reported healing of 17 of 26 vertical longitudinal tears with nonoperative treatment, compared with only four of 10 radial tears. Vertical longitudinal tears involving the body of the meniscus were classified as stable when the portion of the meniscus that was central to the tear could not be displaced more than 3 mm from the intact peripheral rim. Most tears were 1 cm long or less, and all partial-thickness tears were classified as stable. Duchman et al. from the Multicenter Orthopaedic Outcomes Network (MOON) Knee Group reported the results of meniscal tears left in situ at the time of ACL reconstruction. They identified 194 patients with 208 meniscal tears (71 medial and 137 lateral). At a minimum of 6 years of follow-up, 97.8% of lateral and 94.4% of medial tears did not require reoperation. Younger patient age and tear size of more than 10 mm were associated with reoperation. However, in a multicenter study of more than 400 patients aged 50 to 79 years, untreated meniscal tears, even minor radial tears, were strongly associated with the development of osteoarthritis: 63% of patients with untreated meniscal tears had evidence of osteoarthritis, compared with only 19% of those with no meniscal damage.

Nonoperative treatment is never appropriate in a patient with a locked knee caused by a bucket-handle tear of the meniscus. An attempt can be made to reduce the displaced meniscal fragment using gentle manipulation after intraarticular injection of a local anesthetic, but forceful repeated manipulations of such displaced tears is never justified, and most do not heal without surgery even if they are reduced.

Chronic tears even within the vascularized zone will not heal without surgery. However, chronic tears have been shown to heal when the synovial bed of the meniscus has been freshened and the torn edges have been apposed and sutured.

Tears associated with ligamentous instabilities can be treated nonoperatively if the patient defers ligament reconstruction or if reconstruction is contraindicated. Removal of the menisci, especially the medial meniscus, in such knees may make the instability even more severe. Nonoperative or delayed operative treatment of ligamentous injuries also increases the risk of medial meniscal tear; Yoo et al. found that further medial meniscal damage is common if surgery is delayed by 6 months or more.

Nonsurgical management for a meniscal tear with the potential to heal consists of a long leg motion-controlled brace worn for 4 to 6 weeks. Crutch walking with touch-down weight bearing is permitted when the patient gains active control of the extremity in the brace. The patient is instructed in a progressive isometric exercise program during the time the leg is in the brace to strengthen the quadriceps, the hamstrings, and the gastrocnemius and soleus muscles around the knee, as well as the flexors, abductors, adductors, and extensors around the hip. At 4 to 6 weeks, the immobilization is discontinued and the rehabilitative exercise program for the muscles around the hip and knee is intensified. The patient must be informed that any tear in the meniscus may not have healed despite this period of immobilization. If symptoms recur after a period of nonoperative treatment, surgical repair or removal of the damaged meniscus may be necessary.

Meniscal tears that cause infrequent and minimal symptoms can be treated with rehabilitation and restricted activity. Numerous studies have compared nonoperative treatment to arthroscopic partial meniscectomy in patients older than 40 years old. Lee et al. published a meta-analysis that found no difference in clinical outcomes, such as relief of pain and improved knee function, between the treatment methods. Another meta-analysis of randomized controlled trials by van de Graaf et al. found no significant difference between arthroscopic partial meniscectomy and conservative treatment for nonobstructive meniscal tears at 12 and 24 months after surgery. In a randomized controlled trial, Yim et al. compared outcomes of arthroscopic meniscectomy and nonoperative treatment in 102 patients with degenerative horizontal tears of the posterior horn of the medial meniscus and found no significant differences in pain relief, knee function, or patient satisfaction at 2-year follow-up. Monk et al. reviewed nine randomized controlled trials and eight systematic reviews and found no difference between arthroscopic meniscal debridement and nonoperative management as a first-line treatment strategy for patients with knee pain and a degenerative meniscal tear. Some evidence was found to indicate that patients with resistant mechanical symptoms in whom nonoperative management initially failed may benefit from meniscal debridement.

The most important aspect of nonoperative treatment, once the acute pain and effusion have subsided, is restoration of the power of the muscles around the injured knee to a level comparable to that of the opposite knee. As much motion of the joint as possible should be encouraged. This can be accomplished through a regular program of progressive exercises, not only for the quadriceps and hamstrings but also for the hip flexors and abductors.

■ OPERATIVE MANAGEMENT

Historically, the indications and surgical techniques for excision of torn menisci have been controversial; noted orthopaedic surgeons have advocated total excision of the torn meniscus, whereas others have proposed subtotal excision. Justification for total excision often was based on short-term, functional recovery criteria. With longer follow-up, increasing degenerative changes were noted, especially after total meniscectomy. Removal of even one third of the meniscus was shown to increase joint contact forces by up to 350%.

The greatest degenerative changes occur after total rather than subtotal meniscectomy. After subtotal excision of the meniscus, there is less articular cartilage degeneration, and it is localized principally to the area previously covered by the meniscus. The amount of degenerative change in the articular cartilage appears to be directly proportional to the amount of meniscus removed. In our experience, if the derangement produces almost daily symptoms, frequent locking, or repeated or chronic effusions, the pathologic portion of the meniscus, when determined to be irreparable, should be removed because the problems caused by the present disability far outweigh the probability or significance of future degenerative arthritis. If a significant portion of the peripheral rim can be retained by subtotal meniscal excision, the long-term result is improved. A study of 312 patients found that, despite joint space narrowing, decreases in meniscal thickness after partial meniscectomy with complete resection of the unstable leaf of horizontal tears had no additional adverse effect on functional and radiographic outcomes compared with conventional partial meniscectomy that preserved the whole meniscal thickness at 5-year follow-up.

Complete removal of the meniscus is justified only when it is irreparably torn, and the meniscal rim should be preserved if at all possible. Total meniscectomy is no longer considered the treatment of choice in young athletes or other people whose daily activities require vigorous use of the knee.

LATE CHANGES AFTER MENISCECTOMY

The knee can function well without the meniscus, but considerable evidence indicates that meniscectomy often is followed by degenerative changes within the joint; whether the injury, the damaged meniscus itself, or its excision led to the degenerative changes cannot be determined with certainty in most of these studies. More recent studies have found low percentages of joint narrowing of more than 50% 10 to 15 years after partial medial meniscectomy. One 12-year follow-up study showed that 88% of patients with partial medial meniscectomy had joint space narrowing of less than 2 mm and none had narrowing of more than 2 mm. Subjective results after partial medial meniscectomy generally are favorable, with 88% to 95% of patients reporting good to excellent results. A meta-analysis comparing meniscal repair with meniscectomy, however, found better long-term patient-reported outcomes and better activity levels with meniscal repair than with meniscectomy. In their systematic review of clinical outcomes of meniscectomy, Salata et al. identified several preoperative and intraoperative predictors of poor clinical or radiographic outcomes: total meniscectomy or removal of the peripheral meniscal rim, lateral meniscectomy, degenerative meniscal tears, chondral damage, hand osteoarthritis suggestive of genetic predisposition, and increased body mass index (BMI). Meniscal tear pattern, patient age or sex, mechanical alignment, activity level, and association with ACL reconstruction were not predictive of outcome, were inconclusive, or had mixed results.

Krych et al., in a retrospective study, compared nonoperative treatment to arthroscopic partial medial meniscectomy for isolated, complete degenerative medial meniscus posterior root tears. The patient cohorts were matched for age, sex, and BMI and followed for a minimum of 2 years. Partial meniscectomy provided no benefit in halting arthritic progression. Female sex, increased BMI, and meniscal extrusion were associated with worse outcomes. Conversely, Lee et al. reported 288 patients (24 male and 264 female) followed for at least 5 years after arthroscopic meniscectomy for degenerative medial meniscal posterior root tears. Well-aligned nonarthritic knees survived significantly longer before requiring total knee arthroplasty (TKA). The 5- and 10-year survival rates in these low-risk groups were 97.7% and 89.1%, respectively. Age, BMI, varus alignment, and Kellgren-Lawrence grade II or higher were significant risk factors for end-stage arthritis requiring TKA.

SURGICAL REPAIR OF TORN MENISCI

Clinical studies with long-term follow-up have shown that many acute or chronic tears in the periphery and in this outer vascularized zone heal when sutured and protected. Reports of repairs of chronic and acute tears, by either open or arthroscopically aided techniques, cited confirmation of healing by arthrography or arthroscopy in as many as 90% of patients. Healing rates

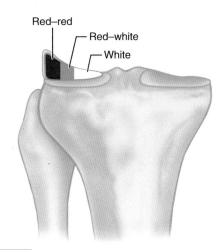

FIGURE 1.31 Zones of potential meniscal healing (see text). (From Miller MD, Warner JJP, Harner CD: Meniscal repair. In Fu FH, Harner CD, Vince KG, editors: *Knee surgery*, Baltimore, 1994, Williams & Wilkins.)

of 90% have been reported in conjunction with ACL reconstruction. Preserving the menisci, especially the medial meniscus, has been shown to improve knee stability when associated with ACL reconstruction. Cristiani et al. reported patients undergoing hamstring ACL reconstruction, comparing isolated ACL reconstruction or ACL reconstruction with medial meniscal meniscectomy, medial meniscal repair, lateral meniscectomy, lateral meniscal repair, or medial and lateral meniscectomy. Medial meniscectomy increased knee laxity, whereas medial meniscal repair preserved stability compared to ACL reconstruction with intact menisci. Isolated meniscal repairs have a reported healing rate of 50%. Hagmeijer et al. described 33 isolated meniscal repairs (without concomitant ACL reconstruction) at a mean follow-up of 17.6 years. At early follow-up, the overall failure rate was 14 of 33 (42%). Complex tears (80%) and bucket-handle tears (47%) had higher overall failure rates than simple tears (18.2%). No further failures occurred after mid-term follow-up with any tear type. The lower healing rate has been attributed to the release of growth factors and pluripotent cells after bone-tunnel drilling that results in biologic augmentation at the repair site. An alternative theory is that the meniscus is otherwise normal but tears as a result of the tibiofemoral subluxation in these traumatic cases, whereas menisci that tear in isolation are inherently susceptible or diseased. A 21-year follow-up of 18 patients with isolated open meniscal repair found good to excellent results in 17, with an average Lysholm score of 97.8 and International Knee Documentation Committee (IKDC) score of 93%. Degenerative joint changes in the operated knee were similar to those in the contralateral knee. A re-rupture rate of approximately 30%, however, is of concern. The ideal indication for meniscal repair is an acute, 1- to 2-cm, longitudinal, peripheral tear that is repaired in conjunction with ACL reconstruction in a young individual. Indications for repair in other situations are less clear-cut. Miller, Warner, and Harner categorized meniscal tears according to their location in three zones of vascularity (Fig. 1.31): red-red, fully within the vascular area; red-white, at the border of the vascular area; and white-white, within the avascular area. They recommended repair of red-red and red-white tears. The "reparability," or likelihood of healing, depends on several other factors in addition to vascularity, specifically, type of tear, chronicity, and size (Table 1.2). At an average 3-year follow-up, Choi et al. reported complete or partial healing of 93% of radial tears of the midbody of the lateral

TABLE 1.2

Reparability of Meniscal Tears

ZONE	TEAR TYPE	CHRONICITY	SIZE (CM)	REPARABILITY
Red-red	Longitudinal	Acute	1.5–4.0	
Red-red	Longitudinal	Chronic	1.5–4.0	
Red-white	Longitudinal	Acute	1.5–4.0	
Red-white	Longitudinal	Chronic	1.5–4.0	
Red-white	Radial/flap	Acute	1.5–4.0	
Red-white	Radial/flap	Chronic	1.5–4.0	
Red-white	Radial/flap	Damaged	1.5–4.0	
Red-white	Radial/flap	Damaged	1.0–4.0	
White-white	Longitudinal	Acute	1.5–4.0	
White-white	Radial/flap	Acute	1.5–4.0	
White-white	Longitudinal	Chronic	1.5–4.0	
White-white	Radial/flap	Chronic	1.5–4.0	
White-white	Radial/flap	Damaged	1.5–4.0	

From Miller MD, Warner JJP, Harner CD: Meniscal repair. In Fu FH, Harner CD, Vince KG, editors: *Knee surgery*, Baltimore, 1994, Williams & Wilkins.

meniscus after arthroscopic repair. Pujol et al. reported that clinical outcomes were slightly improved by the addition of platelet-rich plasma (PRP) to open repair of horizontal tears extending into the avascular zone. However, Griffin et al. found no difference in functional outcome measures with or without the use of PRP after arthroscopic meniscal repair. Extensive research currently is underway studying methods to improve healing rates using mechanical stimulation, marrow venting procedures, the use of fibrin clots, PRP injections, and stem-cell-based therapies.

Ramp lesions are unique variants of injuries of the peripheral posterior horn medial meniscus that are almost always seen in association with an ACL rupture. The term originally described a separation of the posterior meniscocapsular junction but has also been used to describe disruption of the meniscotibial ligament and tears in the red-red zone of the posterior horn. In most reports the incidence varies between 3% and 13%, although more recent studies have reported frequencies as high as 24% to 42%. DePhillipo et al. diagnosed medial meniscal ramp lesions in 17% of 301 patients undergoing ACL reconstruction and fewer than half were diagnosed on the preoperative MRI. A posteromedial tibial bone bruise was found to be a secondary sign of a ramp lesion in 72% of patients. The authors emphasized the need to carefully look for these lesions at the time of surgery. Most authors cite younger age as a possible risk factor; in one study those with ramp lesions were 7.5 years younger than those with meniscal body lesions.

Edgar et al. biomechanically tested eight cadaver knees to determine anterior tibial displacement and anteromedial bundle (AMB) ACL strain in the intact, posterior medial meniscocapsular junction (PMJC) lesion, and PMJC repair states at 0, 30, 60, and 90 degrees of flexion. Specimens with PMJC tears had statistically increased anterior tibial translation at 30 degrees (1.2 mm; $P < .01$) and statistically increased ACL strain at 30 degrees (24%; $P < .01$) and 90 degrees (50%; $P < .01$). With PMJC repair, translation was reduced ($P > .05$) by 12%, 18%, and 10% at 0, 30, and 90 degrees of flexion, respectively. PMJC repair reduced ($P < .05$) ACL strain by 40%, 39%, 43%, and 31% at 0, 30, 60, and 90 degrees of flexion, respectively. In a biomechanical study using 12 matched pairs of human cadaver knees, DePhillipo et al. evaluated the effects of meniscocapsular and meniscotibial lesions of the posterior medial meniscus in ACL-deficient and ACL-reconstructed knees and the effect of the repair of ramp lesions. Cutting the meniscocapsular and meniscotibial attachments of the posterior horn of the medial meniscus significantly increased anterior tibial translation in ACL-deficient knees at 30 degrees ($P < .020$) and 90 degrees ($P < .005$). Cutting both the meniscocapsular and meniscotibial attachments increased tibial internal (all $P > .004$) and external (all $P < .001$) rotation at all flexion angles in ACL-reconstructed knees. Reconstruction of the ACL in the presence of meniscocapsular and meniscotibial tears restored anterior tibial translation ($P > 0.053$) but did not restore internal rotation ($P < .002$), external rotation ($P < .002$), or the pivot shift ($P < .05$). To restore the pivot shift, an ACL reconstruction and a concurrent repair of the meniscocapsular and meniscotibial lesions were both necessary. Repairing the meniscocapsular and meniscotibial lesions after ACL reconstruction did not restore internal rotation and external rotation at angles of more than 30 degrees.

Research and understanding of meniscal root injuries have evolved since 2010. In cadaver studies, root tears of the medial meniscus have been shown to increase translational and rotational instability in both ACL-intact and ACL-deficient knees. Lateral root injury was found to reduce the stability of the ACL-deficient knee in rotational loading. Tang et al. studied 13 cadaver knees with a robotic testing system. In the ACL-reconstructed knee, a tear of the lateral meniscal posterior root significantly increased knee laxity under loading by as much as 1 mm. The transosseous pullout suture root repair improved knee stability under anterior tibial and simulated pivot shift loading. Root repair improved ACL graft force closer to that of the native ACL under anterior tibial loading. Another study by Allaire et al. analyzed loading and kinematics in intact knees, knees with a posterior root tear of the medial meniscus, knees with a repaired posterior root tear, and knees with a total meniscectomy. They found that a root tear resulted in increased tibiofemoral contact pressure equal to that following a total meniscectomy, whereas repair restored contact pressure to that of the uninjured knee. Repairs are recommended for active patients (typically younger than 50 years) following acute or chronic injury with no significant osteoarthritis (Outerbridge grade 3 or 4), joint-space narrowing, or malalignment. Repairs usually are done either by transtibial pullout or suture anchor and the results are reported to be equivalent. Reports of repair are somewhat controversial, with some showing inability to restore ultimate failure loads or prevent displacement of the root attachment, while others demonstrated improvements in clinical outcome scores compared to the preoperative baseline values. Lee et al. evaluated 56 patients who had pullout sutures for medial meniscal root repair using the Lysholm score, Hospital for Special Surgery score, IKDC subjective score, medial joint space height, and Kellgren-Lawrence grade. Thirty-three patients had second-look arthroscopy and were divided into a "stable healed group" (23 patients, 69.7%) and an "unhealed group" (10 patients, 30.3%). Medial joint space became significantly narrower ($P < .001$), and 23 patients showed progression of their Kellgren-Lawrence grade. All other clinical outcomes improved. The stable-healed group had higher HSS scores, IKDC subjective scores, and less progression of medial joint space narrowing. Two studies by Cho and Song and Seo et al. reported second-look arthroscopy in 24 patients; four were completely healed, nine healed in a lax position, eight healed with scar tissue, and three failed to heal. In spite of the controversy, given the known poor results of posterior root meniscal tears treated nonoperatively, an attempt at repair should be considered in appropriate patients.

Tears of the menisci can be sutured by open or arthroscopic techniques, which are described in other chapter. Open suturing of the meniscus has been successful in stable knees. In unstable knees, the sutured meniscus can tear again unless reconstruction stabilizes the knee or the patient alters physical activities. A cadaver study showed that anterior knee laxity significantly increased gapping of repaired and unrepaired posterior horn medial meniscal tears.

If the meniscal tear involves the periphery of the posterior horn, exposure through a posteromedial or posterolateral arthrotomy is relatively easy, the latter being more difficult. In such tears, the meniscal rim and the synoviocapsular junction can be prepared, and multiple sutures can be accurately placed. Because of the collagen arrangement within the meniscus, vertically oriented sutures can be used. We still prefer to repair posterior horn peripheral tears by open arthrotomy if posteromedial or posterolateral capsular reconstructions are being done concurrently. Arthroscopic techniques of suturing are necessary for tears at or near the junction of the vascular and avascular zones. A long tear at or near this junction is almost impossible to expose and to suture through a posteromedial or posterolateral arthrotomy. Medial tears that extend deep to the collateral ligament are difficult to expose by open techniques without risking injury to the ligament. Tears of the posterior horn of the lateral meniscus are difficult to expose and to suture because the posterolateral capsule is not nearly as well defined. These can be more easily repaired by arthroscopic techniques.

Meniscal repair sutures can approximate tissue and provide vascular access channels for ingrowth of healing tissue. The ideal suture material has not been determined. Most early reports of meniscal repair advocated the use of an absorbable suture, such as polyglycolic acid (Dexon), polyglactin-910 (Vicryl), or polydioxanone (PDS). The mechanical effects of normal joint motion probably cause failure of even nonabsorbable sutures over time. Because the human meniscus requires several months to heal completely, the suture selected for meniscal repair should be capable of providing adequate support for this period.

Significant instability adds tension to the meniscal repair, and the chance of another tear is greatly increased. We have repaired the meniscus without ligamentous stabilization but only when a patient is willing to seriously curtail activities and is fully aware that a second tear is more likely in an unstable joint. For younger, active patients, ligamentous stabilization should accompany meniscal suture because of the decreased likelihood of healing and increased risk of re-rupture in a knee with ligamentous laxity.

OPEN MENISCAL REPAIR
TECHNIQUE 1.1

- Systematically examine the entire knee arthroscopically to rule out additional pathologic conditions. The technique for repair is essentially the same for medial and lateral meniscal tears.
- Medial meniscal tears most commonly extend for 2 to 3 cm along the posterior horn anteriorly to the posterior edge of the MCL. The tear sometimes extends farther anteriorly, or a bucket-handle displacement occurs. Some bucket-handle tears and longitudinal tears in the outer third of the meniscus can be sutured.
- If the medial meniscus is torn, position the knee in 60 degrees of flexion.
- Then make a vertical posteromedial arthrotomy incision from the medial epicondylar area of the femur distally toward the semimembranosus tendon in line with the fibers of the POL.
- Use a right-angle retractor to retract the posterior capsule posteriorly and then explore the extent of the tear. Such tears usually are 2 to 3 mm from the periphery of the meniscus, well within the vascular zone. If the tear is 5 mm or more from the peripheral attachment, it can be difficult to see and to repair through the arthrotomy approach.
- Debride the edges of the tear with a small curet or scalpel. As a rule, do not remove any intact peripheral meniscal tissue. Removal of this tissue and pulling of the meniscal rim to the capsule with sutures narrow the meniscus and reduce its weight-bearing function.
- With a small rasp, abrade the debrided edges of the tear and also the parameniscal synovial tissue to evoke an increased inflammatory healing response.
- Once the tear has been prepared for suturing, identify the interval between the posterior capsule and the medial head of the gastrocnemius and retract the latter posteriorly.
- Free the posterior capsule from the overlying gastrocnemius head along the entire length of the meniscal tear to make accurate suture placement easier.
- Place interrupted sutures of Mersilene or other nonabsorbable surgical suture material every 3 to 4 mm. Beginning outside the posterior capsule, pass the sutures through the capsule, then vertically from inferior to superior through the meniscus, and then back out through the capsule, but do not tie them (Fig. 1.32). Each suture should be oriented vertically rather than horizontally to achieve maximal purchase on the meniscus.
- Before the arthrotomy incision is closed, gather the ends of the meniscal sutures and exert tension on them. Check to see that the approximation of the meniscal tear is accurate.

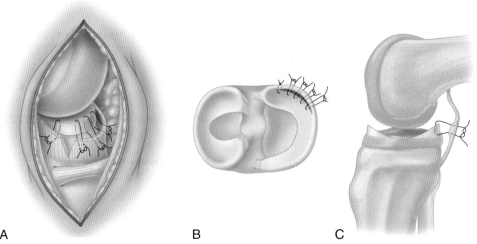

FIGURE 1.32 **A,** Through posteromedial arthrotomy, multiple interrupted sutures placed vertically through periphery of meniscus are spaced every few millimeters and tied outside joint capsule. **B,** Looking down on top of longitudinal tear of meniscus with multiple approximating sutures. **C,** Sutures tied outside capsule, approximating capsule or peripheral meniscal rim to body of meniscus. **SEE TECHNIQUE 1.1.**

- Maintain tension on the sutures, watch the tear, and slowly extend the knee to be sure the approximation is not pulled apart as the knee extends. If the sutures are placed too far superiorly in the posterior capsule, the edges of the tear will part as the knee extends. If the approximation involves a meniscal rim fragment, the fragment orients the proper placement of the sutures. If repair is of a peripheral attachment, pull the meniscus back to as near the original meniscocapsular junction as possible.
- If the medial meniscal tear extends anteriorly deep to the MCL and thus makes inspection and repair through the posteromedial arthrotomy difficult, the sutures are best placed with arthroscopic techniques (see other chapter). If one is not skilled in arthroscopic techniques, careful longitudinal incisions through the MCL and capsule may permit inspection and repair. Great care must be taken to avoid injury to the collateral ligament.
- If the arthrotomy has extended through the coronary ligament, be sure it is accurately approximated to restore peripheral stability. With the knee in 45 degrees of flexion, close the arthrotomy with multiple interrupted, nonabsorbable sutures, advancing and tightening the POL.
- Once the arthrotomy has been closed, tie the meniscal sutures individually, beginning with the most lateral suture and progressing to the most medial.

Tears of the lateral meniscus are treated by techniques similar to those described for medial meniscal tears, but lateral meniscal tears are more difficult to repair. The posterior horn of the lateral meniscus is exposed through a posterolateral capsular incision above the popliteal tendon, as described by Henderson. The coursing of the popliteal tendon through a hiatus in the periphery of the lateral meniscus adds to the difficulty. Because of this more difficult exposure and suturing, we prefer to repair all lateral meniscal tears by arthroscopic techniques.

POSTOPERATIVE CARE Postoperative care is determined by the size or extent of the tear, whether it is stable (not displaceable into the joint) or unstable (displaceable into the joint), and whether the repair is combined with a ligament reconstruction or other procedure. If the repair is not combined with another procedure and the tear is small and stable, the knee is placed in a hinged brace and immediate range of motion from 0 to 90 degrees is permitted. Touch-down weight bearing is permitted immediately, and full weight bearing is permitted at 6 weeks when the brace and crutches are discarded. No sports are allowed for 3 months. If the repair is not combined with other procedures but the tear is sufficiently large to allow displacement into the joint, the knee is placed in a hinged brace that is locked in full extension for 3 to 4 weeks. Only touch-down weight bearing with crutches is permitted. At 4 weeks, the hinge mechanism of the brace is adjusted and motion from 0 to 90 degrees is begun. The brace is worn for 6 weeks and then removed. Weight bearing to 50% is reached at this point. Crutches can be discontinued at 8 weeks. No sports are allowed for 6 months, depending on the success of rehabilitation. If the meniscal repair is combined with a reconstructive procedure, such as reconstruction of the ACL, motion, brace wear, and weight bearing are determined by the postoperative care required for the reconstructive procedure.

MENISCAL AUTOGRAFTS AND ALLOGRAFTS

Despite the best of efforts, not all meniscal tears can be repaired and arthritic changes may develop in the involved knee compartment. Perhaps one of the greatest dilemmas facing orthopaedists is the treatment of a young, active, healthy individual with an arthritic knee who is not a candidate for a total knee replacement. In response to this problem, investigators have studied the use of meniscal allografts, autograft fascial material, and synthetic menisci scaffolds. Reported results of meniscal allografts are mixed, and most studies report only short-term and medium-term follow-up (Fig. 1.33). Success usually is defined by pain relief, improved function, lack of meniscal symptoms, lack of rejection, and peripheral healing of the graft. True success will be

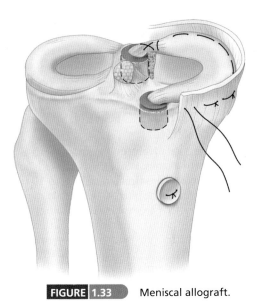

FIGURE 1.33   Meniscal allograft.

determined by the prevention of arthritis, which will be proved only with long-term follow-up. A systematic review of the literature found that meniscal extrusion was present in most patients with meniscal allografts but was not associated with clinical or radiographic outcomes. The authors concluded that there is some evidence to suggest that meniscal allograft transplantation reduces the progression of osteoarthritis; however, the quality of the studies was low, with a high risk for bias. A few studies have examined the histology and biochemistry of transplants, but this research needs further investigation. Long-term success requires that the meniscal allografts be histologically, biochemically, and biomechanically similar to the native meniscus.

Because of the difficulty in locating, harvesting, and distributing fresh donor allografts to a size-matched recipient, as well as the possibility of disease transmission, fresh menisci suitable for allograft implantation have given way to bank-preserved meniscal allografts. Currently, meniscal allografts are preserved in one of four ways: fresh, fresh frozen (deep-freezing), freeze-dried (lyophilization), and cryopreserved. Of these four methods, only cryopreservation has been shown to reproducibly maintain a substantially viable cell population (10% to 40%). The necessity of preserving viable cells in the allograft has been questioned because of animal studies showing that allograft is repopulated with host cells.

Preservation techniques also affect the immunogenicity of the allograft meniscus. Deep-freezing or freeze-drying of meniscal tissue tends to decrease immunogenicity. Cryopreservation maintains the content of donor human leukocyte antigen–encoded antigens and is more sensitizing to the host. Studies have demonstrated an immunologic response of the host to the transplant, but the clinical significance of this is unknown.

The potential for disease transmission also is affected by preservation techniques. Cryopreservation is not considered a process through which sterilization can be ensured, but freeze-drying and gamma irradiation have been shown to effectively eliminate the risk of viral transmission. Unfortunately, these techniques appear to have the deleterious effect of graft shrinkage. To eliminate human immunodeficiency virus DNA, allograft tissue must be irradiated with more than 3 Mrad of gamma irradiation, but exposure to more than 2.5 Mrad of irradiation negatively affects the mechanical

properties of collagen-containing tissues. Consequently, secondary sterilization with gamma irradiation is not currently recommended.

The appropriate candidate for meniscal allograft transplantation should be skeletally mature but too young for TKA and have significant knee pain and limited function. All other options for medical management of pain, including a thorough trial of conservative therapy and bracing techniques, should be exhausted. The cause of meniscal damage must be mechanical, not degenerative, and the meniscal damage must not be caused by synovial disease. If a nonmechanical disease state exists, the allograft will fail. The ideal candidate is a patient younger than 40 years with an absent or nonfunctioning meniscus. On occasion, patients up to 50 years old may benefit from transplantation if they are highly active with only limited arthritis and are not good candidates for arthroplasty. The pain should be localized to the affected compartment with activities of daily living or sports. In addition, the patient should have normal mechanical alignment, a stable knee, and only Outerbridge grade I or grade II articular cartilage changes. Contraindications include knee instability or varus-valgus malalignment, unless these can be corrected. Varus-valgus malalignment is defined as asymmetry of 2 to 4 degrees or more compared with the contralateral knee. Malalignment also exists if the weight-bearing line on long-leg alignment radiographs falls into the affected meniscus-deficient compartment. ACL reconstructions and osteotomies can be performed simultaneously or as staged procedures. Most investigators believe that advanced osteoarthritis is an absolute contraindication because of questionable graft survival. Poorer results have been reported when meniscal allografts have been used in association with osteochondral allograft transplantations, ACL reconstructions, and realignment procedures.

Because mostly short-term and medium-term results of transplantation of meniscal allografts are available, questions remain about their survivorship and function. In one study the beneficial effects of pain relief and improved function remained in approximately 70% of the patients at 10 years after surgery; another study with follow-up of 14 years found deterioration of clinical results during follow-up. Bin et al. reported a meta-analysis that assessed survival rates in patients who had medial or lateral meniscal allograft transplantation with more than 5 years of follow-up. They found that 85.8% of medial and 89.2% of lateral meniscal allograft transplants survived at midterm (5 to 10 years), while 52.6% of medial and 56.6% of lateral transplants survived long term (>10 years). Patients with lateral meniscal allograft transplantation demonstrated greater pain relief and functional improvement than patients with medial transplantation. A more recent meta-analysis found that, regardless of the follow-up period and the scoring system used, patients showed continuous clinical improvement, and a systematic review of the literature reported patient satisfaction ranging from 62% to 100% at follow-ups ranging from 3 to almost 12 years. Extrusion of the meniscal transplant has been a concern, but Lee et al. found no significant differences in clinical outcomes in 45 medial and lateral meniscal transplants at a minimum of 8 years of follow-up. They divided the patients into two groups: extrusion (≥3 mm) and nonextrusion (<3 mm) and compared loss of joint space width. They found a greater decrease in joint space width in the extrusion group than in the nonextrusion group. In a meta-analysis analyzing fixation methods

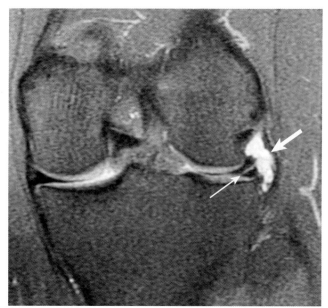

FIGURE 1.34 Meniscal cyst. Fat-suppressed coronal T2-weighted MR sequence shows high-signal intensity meniscal cyst *(large white arrow)* with an associated oblique tear *(small white arrow)* in the body of the lateral meniscus. (From Miller TT: Magnetic resonance imaging of the knee. In Scott WN, editor: *Insall & Scott surgery of the knee*, ed 4, Philadelphia, 2006, Churchill Livingstone.)

for the meniscal allograft root, Jauregui et al. compared two groups: fixation that preserved the graft's root insertions on the allograft bone (bone fixation) and suture fixation of the root soft tissue without the allograft bone (soft-tissue suture group). No significant differences were found between the groups in terms of meniscal allograft tear rates, failure rates, Lysholm scores, meniscal extrusion, and visual analogue scale pain scores. Van Der Straeten et al. reported 276 meniscal allograft transplants done between 1989 and 2013 in patients with a mean age of 33 years, 60% of whom were male. Absent to mild cartilage damage was found in 156 cases and moderate to severe in 130. Simultaneous procedures were done in 118 patients, including cartilage procedures, osteotomy, or ACL reconstruction. At a mean follow-up of 6.8 years, 56.5% were in situ, while 27.4% had been removed, including 19.2% converted to TKA. At 24.0 years, cumulative allograft survival was 15.1%. In patients younger than 35 years at surgery, survival was significantly better (24.1%) than in those older than 35 years (8.0%) (p=0.017). Consecutive radiographs showed significant osteoarthritis progression at a mean of 3.8 years (p<0.0001). Incremental Kellgren-Lawrence grade was +1.1 grade per 1000 days (2.7 years). Noyes and Barber-Westin reported long-term function and survival rates of 69 consecutive medial and lateral bone-meniscus-bone transplants. For all transplants, the estimated probability of survival was 85% at 2 years, 77% at 5 years, 69% at 7 years, 45% at 10 years, and 19% at 15 years. Knees that had a concurrent osteochondral autograft transfer had significantly lower survival rates beginning at the seventh year. The factors of articular cartilage damage (grade 2B/3 vs. none), patient age (<30 years vs. 39 to 49 years), and tibiofemoral compartment (medial vs. lateral) had no significant effect on the survival, symptom, or functional analyses.

Meniscal allografts have not been shown to have a significant long-term effect on progressive joint destruction, and the patient should have realistic expectations. However, pain relief and improvement in function, even if only temporary, are reasonable expectations. The technique for meniscal transplantation is described in other chapter.

OTHER CONDITIONS OF MENISCI
■ CYSTS OF MENISCI

Meniscal cysts are relatively uncommon, with a reported frequency of approximately 1.5%. Cysts of the lateral meniscus (Fig. 1.34) have been estimated to be 3 to 10 times more common than cysts of the medial meniscus. Several theories have been advanced to explain the etiology of meniscal cysts, including (1) trauma, which results in contusion and hemorrhage within the substance of the meniscus, leading to mucoid degeneration; (2) degeneration with age, which results in local necrosis and mucoid degeneration into a cyst; (3) developmental inclusion of synovial cells within the substance of the meniscus, or a metaplastic event in which the cells secrete mucin and result in cyst formation; and (4) displacement of synovial cells into the substance of the meniscus through microscopic tears in the fibrocartilage, which results in secretion of acid mucopolysaccharides to form the contents of meniscal cysts. More recently, formation of meniscal cysts has been suggested to be related to the influx of synovial fluid through microscopic and macroscopic tears in the substance of the meniscus. A number of authors have noted a close correlation (nearly 100%) between cyst formation and meniscal pathologic conditions, most commonly tears of the peripheral portion of the middle third of the lateral meniscus. An analysis of 1571 menisci identified 112 with meniscal cysts, all of which were associated with a horizontal or bucket-handle tear with a peripheral horizontal component.

When located laterally, meniscal cysts usually are palpable immediately anterior and proximal to the head of the fibula and anterior to the LCL. They usually are firm and apparently fixed to the capsular tissue. They contain a clear, gelatinous material and usually are multilocular. When of average size, they are characteristically more prominent when the knee is extended and less prominent when the knee is flexed; small cysts may disappear within the joint on flexion (Pisani sign). A large, untreated cyst of the lateral meniscus may erode the tibial condyle just inferior to the lateral margin of the articular cartilage and produce a defect visible both radiographically and at surgery. MRI most clearly defines the cyst and any associated meniscal pathologic conditions.

Pain usually is the most prominent symptom and is accentuated by activity. The patient may note a mass along the lateral joint line, and the mass can vary in size according to the degree of activity. If the cyst is associated with a meniscal tear, the classic signs are present, such as catching, popping, snapping, and giving way. In rare cases, larger cysts that manifest posteriorly into the popliteal space can be confused with popliteal (Baker) cysts.

Treatment of cysts of the meniscus usually requires surgery. Rarely will conservative measures—consisting of injections or antiinflammatory medications—result in more than temporary relief of symptoms. Currently, the recommended treatment is arthroscopic partial meniscectomy and decompression of the cyst. As such a tear is resected, the cyst often is decompressed, which can

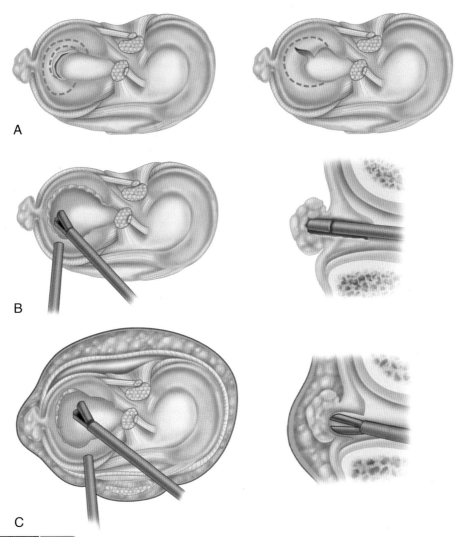

FIGURE **1.35**   **A** and **B,** Excision of tears associated with meniscal cysts (see text). **C,** Decompression of meniscal cyst with basket-punch forceps. (**A** and **B** from Parisien JS: *Techniques in therapeutic arthroscopy*, New York, 1993, Lippincott-Raven.) **SEE TECHNIQUE 1.2.**

be noted by exudation of a gelatinous material into the arthroscopic field. If the cyst does not spontaneously decompress, the shaver can be passed through the body of the meniscus (often through the mid-portion of a horizontal cleavage tear) into the cyst decompressing the cyst internally.

ARTHROSCOPIC PARTIAL MENISCECTOMY AND DECOMPRESSION OF MENISCAL CYST

TECHNIQUE 1.2

- General or regional anesthesia is used, and standard arthroscopy portals are established, with inflow through a superomedial parapatellar portal. Inferomedial and inferolateral portals are used to pass instruments.

- Carefully probe the meniscus to identify the extent of the meniscal tear.
- If a radial tear is found, trim it to a stable peripheral rim (Fig. 1.35A,B).
- If the tear is a stable horizontal tear, resect only the inferior leaf after gently trimming the superior leaf.
- Palpate the cyst externally; this may push the cyst material into the joint and decompress the cyst, allowing identification of the cyst communication.
- If this is not successful, introduce a spinal needle percutaneously through the cystic mass to help locate the track between the cyst and the meniscus. Punch forceps passed through the tear and track into the cyst may widen the track enough for the contents of the cyst to be evacuated into the joint (Fig. 1.35C, *inset*).
- If necessary, insert a small, motorized shaver into the cyst to break up loculations, to assist in cystic decompression, and to stimulate inflammation and scarring of the cyst and its track (Fig. 1.35B, *inset*). Tesner et al. recommended suturing the remnants of the track within the meniscus, but Lonner and Parisien did not find this necessary.

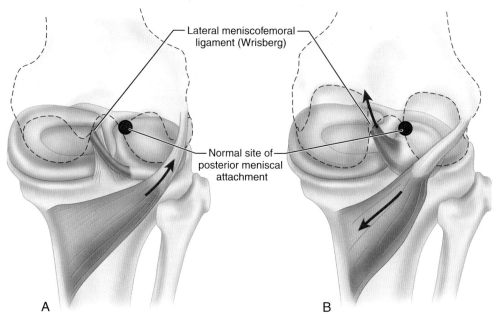

Lateral meniscofemoral ligament (Wrisberg)

Normal site of posterior meniscal attachment

A

B

FIGURE 1.36 **A,** Wrisberg ligament-type discoid lateral meniscus with knee in flexion. Posterior meniscal tibial attachment is absent. Meniscus is not subluxated. **B,** With knee in extension, meniscus is displaced into intercondylar notch by its attached Wrisberg ligament.

- If a peripheral margin of meniscus is left that appears unstable, the meniscus can be repaired to the joint capsule with an arthroscopically aided technique. The knee is irrigated, and the arthroscopy portals are sutured.

POSTOPERATIVE CARE Immediate full weight bearing is allowed, with crutches if necessary, and early isometric quadriceps exercises are encouraged.

EXCISION OF MENISCAL CYST

TECHNIQUE 1.3

- Examine the knee arthroscopically and carefully inspect the meniscus for a tear and the extent of the degeneration.
- If the symptoms are of relatively short duration, the surfaces of the meniscus and the capsular attachment may appear fairly normal. If so, make a small lateral incision directly over the cyst and excise the peripheral cyst by careful dissection.
- A pedicle of the cyst can occasionally be traced into the periphery of the degenerated area of the meniscus. Excise and freshen the peripheral bed of the meniscus, expose the degenerated area to a vascular access channel, and suture the peripheral edge of the meniscus carefully to the meniscosynovial junction of the capsule with multiple interrupted, absorbable sutures.
- Immobilize the knee in extension for 4 weeks.

POSTOPERATIVE CARE Postoperative care is as described in the section on meniscal suturing (see Technique 1.1).

■ DISCOID MENISCUS

Discoid meniscus is an uncommon meniscal anomaly that occurs more frequently laterally than medially. The reported incidence of discoid lateral meniscus has ranged from 26% in Japanese and Korean patients to less than 1% in other populations of patients; the incidence of discoid medial meniscus has varied from 0% to 0.3%.

Discoid lateral menisci generally are categorized, according to the system of Watanabe et al., as complete, incomplete, and Wrisberg type, on the basis of the degree of coverage of the lateral tibial plateau and the presence or absence of the normal posterior meniscotibial attachment. Complete and incomplete types are more common, are disc shaped, and have a posterior meniscal attachment. These types usually are asymptomatic, with no abnormal motion of the meniscus during knee flexion or extension. If an incomplete or complete discoid meniscus is torn, symptoms are similar to those of any other meniscal tear: lateral joint line tenderness, clicking, and effusion. Wrisberg-type discoid menisci can be nearly normal in size and shape and have no posterior attachment except the ligament of Wrisberg (Fig. 1.36). When this type is not disc shaped, Neuschwander et al. described it as a "lateral meniscal variant with absence of the posterior coronary ligament" to distinguish it from a truly discoid meniscus. Wrisberg-type discoid menisci often occur at a younger age than complete or incomplete types and are unassociated with trauma. Abnormal motion of this type of discoid meniscus results in a popping sound during knee flexion and extension ("snapping knee syndrome"). Instability patterns in discoid menisci have recently been recognized in the anterior and middle sections.

Discoid medial menisci are much less common than discoid lateral menisci, are disc shaped, and are more often associated with trauma, usually meniscal tears. Most patients with discoid medial menisci have symptoms consistent with a medial meniscal tear. Radiographic evidence of discoid meniscus usually is absent unless suggested by squaring of the lateral femoral condyle, cupping of the lateral tibial plateau, widening of the lateral joint space up to 11 mm, and a hypoplastic lateral tibial spine. The diagnosis may not be made before surgery unless MRI is used.

▌ TREATMENT

An intact, complete or incomplete discoid meniscus seen as an incidental finding at arthroscopy or arthrotomy does not necessarily require treatment. However, it is unknown how many patients left untreated eventually develop tears or degeneration within the meniscus. The proper treatment must be selected for each patient, and unless a stable, complete or incomplete discoid meniscus has caused grooving, chondromalacia changes, or other pathologic conditions within the compartment, treatment probably should be deferred.

Tears of complete or incomplete discoid menisci that cause pain, popping, and snapping within the knee and that show a hypermobile medial segment but intact peripheral attachments are best treated by subtotal meniscectomy or a so-called saucerization of the mobile fragment. This can be done either by arthroscopic techniques or through an arthrotomy. If a symptomatic meniscus is saucerized in a young child, the increased vascularity in the immature meniscus has been suggested to result in adaptive changes within the remaining peripheral rim as growth and joint function continue, and a stable, healthy, and useful meniscal rim may develop. Attempts should be made to preserve intact a 6- to 8-mm rim of meniscal tissue. Short-term results are favorable, but Ahn et al. reported that in 38 children (48 knees) with a mean age of 9.9 years, degenerative changes had occurred in 23% of those managed with saucerization alone, in 39% of those managed with partial meniscectomy with repair, and in 88% of those managed with subtotal meniscectomy at 10-year follow-up. Patient age has been shown to be an important prognostic factor; patient-oriented outcomes worsen with increasing age.

For a Wrisberg-type discoid meniscus, which lacks an adequate posterior tibial attachment, the treatment generally is total meniscectomy, either open or arthroscopic. With this lesion, subtotal meniscectomy alone leaves an unstable rim of meniscus that is certain to cause future problems. Although total meniscectomy of a nondiscoid lateral meniscus may lead to progressive osteoarthrosis in children and adults, children with discoid menisci seem less prone to these degenerative changes.

ACUTE TRAUMATIC LESIONS OF LIGAMENTS
GENERAL CONSIDERATIONS

Biomechanical loading, scanning electron microscopy, and high-speed photography have shown that ligaments fail by a progressive, serial, and sequential mechanism of microfiber failure. Single collagen fibers are not extensible and begin to fail at 7% to 8% elongation. The number of disrupted collagen fibers in the ligament determines whether it is functionally or morphologically disrupted. Investigators have shown that gross morphologic continuity may exist in a ligament after the yield point, the indicator of complete failure, has occurred. Complete disruption with loss of continuity requires extreme joint displacement. Visual observation of ligament integrity at the time of surgery is an inadequate indicator of (1) extent of the failure, (2) damage to the blood supply to the ligament, (3) residual elongation, or (4) future functional capabilities. Complete rupture of isolated ligaments is rare without damage to other structures because the extreme joint displacement required to disrupt a ligament completely must produce at least some disruption in the other supporting structures.

ETIOLOGY

Knee ligaments often are injured in athletic activities, especially those involving contact, such as American football. Skiing, ice hockey, gymnastics, and other sports also can produce enough sudden stress to disrupt knee ligaments. Motor vehicle accidents, especially those involving motorcycles, are common causes of knee ligament disruptions (e.g., a passenger's flexed knee strikes the automobile dashboard on impact, tearing the PCL). Ligament disruption can occur without a fall or direct contact when sudden, severe loading or tension is placed on the ligaments, such as when a running athlete plants a foot to suddenly decelerate or change directions.

MECHANISM

Four mechanisms have been described as capable of disrupting the ligamentous structures around the knee: (1) abduction, flexion, and internal rotation of the femur on the tibia; (2) adduction, flexion, and external rotation of the femur on the tibia; (3) hyperextension; and (4) anteroposterior displacement.

By far the most common mechanism is abduction, flexion, and internal rotation of the femur on the tibia when the weight-bearing leg of an athlete is struck from the lateral aspect by an opponent. This mechanism results in an abduction and flexion force on the knee, and the femur is rotated internally by the shift of the body weight on the fixed tibia. This mechanism produces injury on the medial side of the knee, the severity of which depends on the magnitude and dissipation of the applied force. When abduction, flexion, and internal rotation of the femur on the tibia occur, the medial supporting structures—the MCL and the medial capsular ligament—are the initial structures injured. If the force is of sufficient magnitude, the ACL also can be torn. The medial meniscus may be trapped between the condyles of the femur and the tibia, and it may be torn at its periphery as the medial structures tear, thus producing "the unhappy triad" of O'Donoghue. The mechanism of adduction, flexion, and external rotation of the femur on the tibia is much less common and produces the primary disruption laterally. Again, the severity of the disruption depends on the magnitude and dissipation of the force applied. The LCL usually is disrupted initially, and, depending on the magnitude of the trauma and displacement, the capsular ligaments, the arcuate ligament complex, the popliteus, the iliotibial band, the biceps femoris, the common peroneal nerve, and one or both cruciate ligaments may be disrupted. Force directed to the anterior aspect of the extended knee, a hyperextension mechanism, usually injures the ACL, and if the force continues or is severe, stretching and disruption of the posterior capsule and PCL may result. Anteroposterior forces applied to either the femur or the tibia, such as the tibia striking a car dashboard, can cause injuries to either the ACL or the PCL, depending on the direction of the tibial displacement.

The incidence and mechanism of so-called isolated ligament disruption continue to be debated. As previously stated, all the supporting structures around the knee function in concert, and probably no single ligament can be disrupted without some degree of injury being sustained to other supporting structures. Injury to the other structures may be minimal and thus may heal with conservative measures, leaving what is apparently an isolated injury to clinical examination. This is most common with the ACL. Mechanisms reported as possibly able to disrupt the ACL with minimal injury of other supporting structures are hyperextension, marked internal rotation of the tibia on the femur, and pure deceleration. Isolated posterior cruciate disruption can result from a direct blow to the front of the tibia with the knee flexed.

LIGAMENT HEALING

The ability of a torn ligament to heal depends on a variety of factors, including anatomic location, presence of associated injuries, and selected treatment modality, as well as various systemic and local factors. Clinically, a grade I or grade II MCL injury will heal within 11 to 20 days, but a grade III MCL tear may take years to heal.

The healing process can be roughly divided into four overlapping phases: hemorrhage, inflammation, repair, and remodeling. The process can be described on the basis of histologic, biochemical, and biomechanical events. After a midsubstance tear of the MCL, the hemorrhage phase begins with blood flowing into the space created by the retracting ligament ends, forming a hematoma. The inflammatory phase follows when inflammatory and monocytic cells migrate into the injury site, converting the clot into granulation tissue and phagocytosing the necrotic tissue. Within 2 weeks, a network of immature, parallel collagen fibers replaces the granulation tissue. The inflammatory phase ends with the reparative phase and begins with the formation of extracellular matrix in a random pattern. This phase begins within 5 to 7 days after injury and lasts for several weeks. New blood vessels begin to form, and fibroblasts continue to produce extracellular matrix. The final phase, remodeling, overlaps the reparative phase; it begins several weeks after injury and lasts months or even years. Collagen fibers align along the long axis of the ligament, resulting in increased maturation of the collagen matrix. The progressive alignment of the fibers has been shown to correlate directly with an improvement in the biomechanical properties of the ligament. Although the healing ligament appears to grossly resemble the normal original ligament, long-term animal studies have demonstrated that the histologic and morphologic appearance is different. Compared with the noninjured ligament, the healing tissue has an increased number of collagen fibrils, and their diameter and masses are smaller. Furthermore, the "crimping" patterns within the healing ligament remain abnormal for up to 1 year, and the collagen alignment remains poor.

Biochemical analysis of the healing process reveals changes in collagen fiber type and distribution. Early in the process there is a greater proportion of type III fibers, but the ratio returns to normal after 1 year. Although the healing ligament shows an increased number of collagen fibers, the number of mature collagen crosslinks is only 45% of the normal value after 1 year. Ligament healing also can be studied biomechanically. Functional testing determines the contribution of the ligament to knee kinematics, as well as the in situ forces in the ligament in response to external loads. Tensile testing assesses the structural and mechanical properties of the ligament. Weiss et al. showed that the biomechanical properties of a healing MCL remain inferior to those of an intact ligament for as long as 1 year after injury. Although the stiffness approaches normal levels, the ultimate load to failure is still significantly lower than normal.

CLASSIFICATION

According to the American Medical Association handbook, *Standard Nomenclature of Athletic Injuries,* a *sprain* is defined as an injury limited to ligaments (connective tissue attaching bone to bone) and a *strain* as a stretching injury of muscle or its tendinous attachment to bone. Sprains are classified into three degrees of severity. A first-degree sprain of a ligament is defined as a tear of a minimal number of fibers of the ligament with localized tenderness but no instability; a second-degree sprain, as a disruption of more ligamentous fibers with more loss of function and more joint reaction with mild-to-moderate instability; and a third-degree sprain, as a complete disruption of the ligament with resultant marked instability. These often are classified as mild, moderate, and severe for first-, second-, and third-degree sprains, respectively. Third-degree sprains, that is, those demonstrating marked instability, can be further graded by the degree of instability demonstrated during stress testing. With 1+ instability, the joint surfaces separate 5 mm or less; with 2+ instability, they separate 5 to 10 mm; and with 3+ instability, they separate 10 mm or more. A standardized classification is important for accurate communication, and although it obviously is not always precise, it does provide a workable scale for clinical purposes.

The treatment of first-degree sprains is symptomatic only; a person with a first-degree sprain usually can return to full activity within a few days. Second-degree sprains with moderate local injury and joint reaction but without pronounced instability can be treated conservatively, but the ligament needs protection. A return to vigorous activity must be delayed until the inflammatory reaction has subsided and rehabilitation has been completed. A functional brace that restricts motion through certain arcs can provide protection. Third-degree sprains with complete disruption of the ligament may require surgical repair unless there is a specific contraindication. The restoration of both anatomic structure and normal tension should be the goal of ligament repair. Surgical results, as a rule, are superior to conservative results in third-degree sprains, especially on the lateral side. Isolated third-degree sprains of collateral ligaments can be treated nonsurgically in specific circumstances with results comparable to those of surgical repair. These indications are discussed in the section on treatment of acute MCL injuries.

DIAGNOSIS
■ HISTORY AND PHYSICAL EXAMINATION

With a careful history and physical examination, an acute injury to a knee ligament usually can be localized and classified and graded according to its severity. The history of the mechanism of injury is always important and usually can be obtained through careful questioning. Information about previous difficulty or injury assists in the evaluation. The position of the knee at the time of the injury, the weight-supporting status, the force applied (either direct and external or indirect and generated by the patient's momentum), and the position of the extremity after the injury are all important. The patient's description of the experience at the time of injury may be valuable as the following are described: the knee's buckling or jumping out of place; an audible pop; the location, severity, and relative time at onset of pain; the ability to walk after the injury occurred; the sensation of stability or instability once walking was attempted; the freedom of motion, both active and passive, of the knee after the injury; and the rapidity and localization of swelling. In regard to the last point, intraarticular swelling or effusion within the first 2 hours after trauma suggests hemarthrosis, whereas swelling that occurs overnight usually is an indication of acute traumatic synovitis.

The physical examination should be complete, precise, systematic, and carried out as soon after the injury as possible to minimize problems of severe swelling, tense effusion, and involuntary muscle spasm.

Both lower extremities should be undressed completely for examination to allow comparison of the position or attitude assumed by the injured extremity and to detect deformity, including a variation in the position of the patella. Areas of ecchymosis and large effusions are readily noted, although smaller effusions may require careful palpation. Hemarthrosis suggests rupture of a cruciate ligament, an osteochondral fracture, a peripheral tear in the vascular portion of a meniscus, or a tear in the deep portion of the joint capsule. A nonbloody effusion suggests an irritative synovitis that may be caused by a degenerative meniscus or a chronic process with no superimposed acute injury. The absence of a hemarthrosis does not necessarily indicate a less severe ligament injury because severe disruptions often cause only minimal joint distention. The disruption may be so complete that the blood escapes into the soft tissues of the popliteal space rather than distending the joint. The presence of muscle atrophy is especially important when the examination is done several days after injury. The circumference of the distal thigh near the middle of the vastus medialis should be compared with the normal thigh, because the musculature, especially the quadriceps, undergoes a rapid reflex atrophy after a significant disorder around the knee. The range of motion of the joint, especially full extension, should be compared with that of the opposite, uninjured knee. A tense hemarthrosis or effusion can prevent full extension and should be evacuated; this leaves an entrapped meniscus as the most common cause of incomplete extension after injury.

Palpation of the collateral ligaments and their bony attachments should locate tenderness at the point of ligament injury. A defect in the ligament occasionally is palpable if the examination is carried out immediately after the injury. A palpable defect is most likely when the tibial insertion of the MCL or the LCL is torn. On occasion, an area of crepitation can be palpated from localized hematoma at the site of ligament disruption. Finally, after the neurovascular status has been assessed, stability should be determined by stress testing.

Evaluation for stability of the knee usually is easy when the examination is done immediately after the injury and before the onset of the protective involuntary muscle spasm. When it is performed at a much later time, evaluation is much more difficult and under some circumstances may require anesthesia. When anesthesia is required to evaluate joint stability, we prefer general anesthesia unless it is contraindicated. Other investigators have infiltrated the areas of injury with a local anesthetic or used the Bier intravenous block technique, but we have had little experience with these methods. Successful stress testing sometimes is possible even several hours or several days after

injury if the examiner explains the test and reassures the patient that the pain will be minimal so that the patient can at least partially relax and cooperate. The uninjured knee is best examined first to evaluate the normal laxity for a baseline. Beginning with the nonpainful, normal knee also tends to instill confidence in the patient if the examination is unhurried and gentle but firm. If adequate evaluation of stability is not possible, it is preferable to proceed with MRI rather than further traumatizing the patient. We believe that an MRI should be obtained with all suspected ligamentous injuries or hemarthroses. Examination under anesthesia also should be performed at the time of surgery to establish the degree of instability and guide the repair or reconstruction.

Commercially available stress-testing arthrometers are available and can measure the varus or valgus opening of the joint or its anterior or posterior translation. These devices are no substitute for careful clinical examination but are useful in measuring the degree of instability. They are most helpful in a chronically unstable joint. Muscle spasm and guarding in an acutely injured knee can mask instability the same as during clinical examination.

▌ STANDARD STRESS TESTS

In stress testing for disruptions of ligaments around the knee, the quality of the "end point" of the test varies from "hard," implying a firm, definite stop, to "soft or mushy," a less distinct and less sudden stop. This aspect of stress testing is subjective, and its usefulness depends on the experience and knowledge of the examiner.

Abduction (Valgus) Stress Test. The abduction, or valgus, stress test is done with the patient supine on the examining table. Again, the opposite, normal extremity should be examined initially to gain the patient's confidence and to establish a baseline of the patient's normal ligamentous tightness. The knee to be examined is placed on the side of the table next to the examiner. The extremity is abducted off the side of the table, and the knee flexed approximately 30 degrees (Fig. 1.37A). One of the examiner's hands is placed around the lateral aspect of the knee, with the other hand supporting the ankle. Gentle abduction or valgus stress is applied to the knee while the hand at the ankle externally rotates the leg slightly. Stability with the knee flexed to 30 degrees is observed. The test is repeated several times in this position up to the point of producing mild pain. The knee is brought into full extension, and the gentle rocking or valgus stressing is repeated with a gentle swinging motion. It is a mistake to grasp the leg and forcibly abduct it enough to be markedly painful; rarely will the patient cooperate or relax for subsequent examinations. As an alternative, the patient's ankle can be placed in the examiner's axilla, with the examiner then placing one hand on each side of the knee near the joint line and gently producing a rocking motion as described previously; the available hand is used to palpate the medial ligaments and joint line to help assess the degree of instability. Opening on valgus stress at full extension suggests concomitant injury to the POL and either the ACL or PCL.

Adduction (Varus) Stress Test. The adduction, or varus, stress test is performed in a manner similar to the valgus stress test, and this test also is done after the normal knee has been examined. Adduction stress is applied by changing the hand to the medial side of the knee and applying an adduction force (Fig. 1.37B). The examination should be done with the knee both in full extension and in 30 degrees of flexion. In addition, with

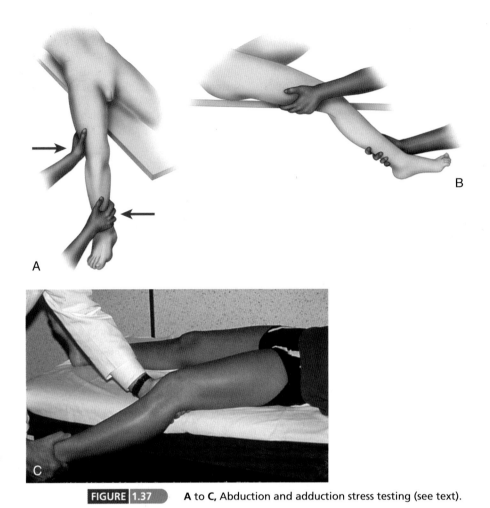

FIGURE 1.37   **A** to **C,** Abduction and adduction stress testing (see text).

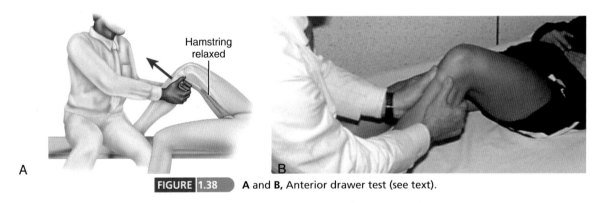

FIGURE 1.38   **A** and **B,** Anterior drawer test (see text).

the patient's hip abducted and externally rotated and the knee flexed, the heel of the injured leg is placed on the opposite knee in a figure 4 position and the lateral aspect of the knee is palpated for a taut, narrow band consisting of the LCL. When the LCL is torn, this band is not as prominent as on the uninjured side.

The degree of instability depends on the structure or structures torn, the severity of the tears, and whether the knee is stressed in flexion or extension. When a collateral ligament is torn and the knee is tested in extension, the intact cruciate ligaments and posterior capsule are taut and little abduction or adduction instability is detectable. When the knee is tested in flexion, which relaxes the posterior capsule, the same ligamentous laxity results in a much greater degree of instability. Abduction or adduction stress testing in extension that reveals significant varus and valgus instability suggests cruciate ligament disruption in addition to collateral ligament disruption (Fig. 1.37C).

Anterior Drawer Test. With the patient supine on the examining table, the hip is flexed to 45 degrees and the knee to 90 degrees, with the foot placed on the tabletop. The dorsum of the patient's foot is sat on to stabilize it, and both hands are placed behind the knee to feel for relaxation of the hamstring muscles (Fig. 1.38). The proximal part of the leg then is gently and repeatedly pulled and pushed anteriorly and

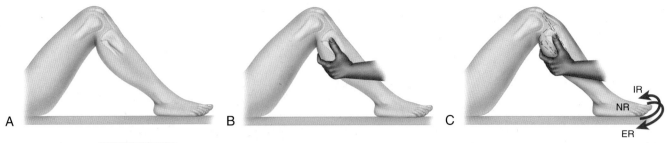

A B C

IR
NR
ER

FIGURE 1.39 Anterior drawer test. **A,** In resting position, tibial plateau is held in normal position by intact posterior cruciate ligament. **B** and **C,** With anterior cruciate insufficiency, tibia can be pulled forward against force of gravity and tone of flexors. ER, external rotation; IR, internal rotation; NR, neutral rotation.

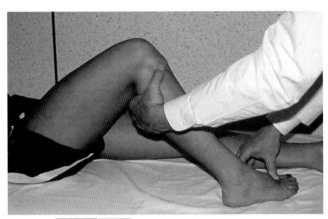

FIGURE 1.40 Anterior drawer test.

posteriorly, noting the movement of the tibia on the femur. The test is done in three positions of rotation, initially with the tibia in neutral rotation and then in 30 degrees of external rotation and finally 30 degrees of internal rotation. The examiner should be aware that internal rotation to 30 degrees may tighten the posterior cruciate enough to obliterate an otherwise positive anterior drawer test result (Figs. 1.39 and 1.40). The degree of displacement in each position of rotation is recorded and compared with the normal knee.

An anterior drawer sign 6 to 8 mm greater than that of the opposite knee indicates a torn ACL. However, before applying anterior drawer stress, the examiner must make sure that the tibia is not sagging posteriorly as a result of laxity of the PCL. In such knees, an apparent sign of anterior drawer instability simply may be the return of the tibia to the neutral starting point; posterior instability frequently is misdiagnosed because of this fact. Perceived anterior translation may be the movement of the tibia from a posteriorly subluxated position back to neutral rather than true anterior displacement. The relationship of the anterior medial femoral condyle to the anterior medial tibia should be noted. When the PCL is intact, the medial tibia should extend 5 to 10 mm anterior to the medial femoral condyle. Even if an anterior drawer sign is not accompanied by a pivot shift phenomenon, a PCL insufficiency exists until proved otherwise. Any tendency of one tibial plateau to rotate abnormally should be noted as the test is carried out.

In an acutely painful knee, it may not be possible to carry out the anterior drawer test in the conventional 90-degree flexed position. Small degrees of anterior translation of the tibia on the femur may be detected better in the relatively extended position, in which the "doorstop" effect of the posterior horn of the menisci is negated (Fig. 1.41).

Lachman Test. The Lachman test can be useful if the knee is swollen and painful and is the preferred test for ACL injury. The patient is placed supine on the examining table with the involved extremity to the examiner's side (Fig. 1.42). The involved extremity is positioned in slight external rotation with the knee between 15 and 20 degrees of flexion; the femur is stabilized with one hand, and firm pressure is applied to the posterior aspect of the proximal tibia, which is lifted forward in an attempt to translate it anteriorly. A positive grade 1 Lachman test produces 1 to 5 mm of anterior translation compared to the uninjured knee. A grade 2 moves 6 to 10 mm, and grade 3 is more than 10 mm of displacement compared to the opposite knee. Further subclassification adds an "A" for a firm or hard endpoint and a "B" for soft endpoint. The position of the examiner's hands is important in doing the test properly. One hand should firmly stabilize the femur while the other grips the proximal tibia in such a manner that the thumb lies on the anteromedial joint margin. When an anteriorly directed lifting force is applied by the palm and the fingers, anterior translation of the tibia in relation to the femur can be palpated by the thumb. Anterior translation of the tibia associated with a soft or a mushy end point indicates a positive test result.

The hamstrings must be relaxed (any tension in them will prevent anterior translation of the tibia). The patient must be supine and relaxed because the sitting position rotates the pelvis and places the hamstrings on stretch. The fingers of the examiner's hand on the femur should palpate the tension in the hamstrings so that he or she can feel when the hamstrings relax and the fingers "sink" into the posterior thigh. The hand on the tibia should rapidly accelerate the tibia anteriorly and feel for the ACL snapping tight much like a short 30-mm section of rope might feel when snapped tight with rapid distraction. This is a short, rapid acceleration. The examiner should feel for the firm, hard endpoint rather than looking only for excursion. The displacement may be only 5 mm, which is difficult to appreciate visually in a large knee.

When viewed from the lateral aspect, a silhouette of the inferior pole of the patella, patellar tendon, and proximal tibia shows slight concavity. With disruption of the ACL, anterior translation of the tibia obliterates the patellar tendon slope.

Other tests for anterior instability combined with a rotary element are discussed later.

Posterior Drawer Test. The posterior drawer test is done with the patient supine and the knee flexed to 90 degrees; the foot is secured to the table by sitting on it. A posterior force is applied on the proximal tibia, which is opposite but similar to the force applied in the anterior drawer test. Posterior movement of the tibia on the femur shows posterior

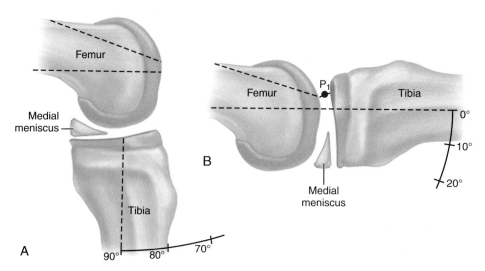

Femur

Medial
meniscus

Tibia

A

90°   80°   70°

Femur   P₁   Tibia

Medial
meniscus

B

0°

10°

20°

FIGURE **1.41**   **A,** With knee flexed to 90 degrees for classic anterior drawer sign, medial meniscus, being attached to tibia, abuts against acutely convexed surface of medial femoral condyle and has "doorstop" effect, preventing or hindering anterior translation of tibia. **B,** With knee extended, relationships are changed. Comparatively flat weight-bearing surface of femur does not obstruct forward motion of meniscus and tibia when anterior stress is applied.

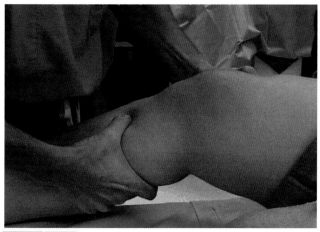

FIGURE **1.42**   Lachman test for anterior cruciate instability.

instability compared with the normal tibia. It is sometimes difficult to interpret whether the tibia is abnormally moving too far anteriorly or too far posteriorly. Careful attention to the neutral position or unstressed reduction point prevents misinterpretation. Both knees are placed in the position to perform a posterior drawer test, and a thumb is placed on each anteromedial joint line (Fig. 1.43). Loss of the normal 1-cm anterior stepoff of the medial tibial plateau with respect to the medial femoral condyle indicates a torn PCL. As with the anterior drawer test, any abnormal rotation of the tibial condyles is noted as the posterior drawer is tested (Fig. 1.44). To further evaluate stability, the patient's hips are positioned 90 degrees in the supine position and the knees are flexed to 90 degrees while the heels of each extremity are supported in the examiner's hands. If posterior instability is present, the examiner, by sighting across the horizon of the flexed knees, will note that the tibia sags visibly posteriorly from the effects of gravity (Fig. 1.45). This test also should be done with the patient prone and the knee flexed to 90 degrees. The examiner should observe for presence of the posterior drawer sign and

for rotation of the foot, which would indicate a rotary component as well.

Frequently, when an anterior or a posterior drawer test is performed, increased excursion in the anteroposterior direction is misinterpreted as presence of the anterior drawer sign when in fact the PCL has been torn. The examiner does not recognize that the anterior movement arises from a position of posterior subluxation to neutral instead of from neutral to anterior displacement. This misinterpretation can be prevented by careful palpation of the relationship between the femur and tibia of both knees simultaneously. Both knees are placed in the position for a posterior drawer test, with the patient supine, the hips flexed 45 degrees, and the knees flexed 90 degrees. A thumb is placed on the anteromedial joint line of each knee. Normally, the anterior aspect of the tibia can be palpated as a 10-mm anterior stepoff in relation to the anterior aspect of the medial femoral condyle. A posterior drop back with decreased prominence of the tibial margin compared with the opposite knee indicates injury to the PCL. When the anteromedial tibia is flush with the medial femoral condyle, there is approximately 10 mm of posterior drop back, indicating a grade II laxity.

The presence of a relatively hard endpoint on both the anterior and posterior drawer tests may be a result of the posterior capsule snapping tight, and the examiner should always consider the amount of excursion that has occurred relative to the normal knee. Some clinicians believe that the posterior horn of the medial meniscus also may be responsible for an endpoint on the anterior drawer acting much like a chock block.

Quadriceps Active Test. With the patient supine, the relaxed limb is supported with the knee flexed to 90 degrees in the drawer test position (Fig. 1.46). Adequate support of the thigh is important so that the patient's muscles are completely relaxed. The patient makes a gentle quadriceps contraction to shift the tibia without extending the knee. At this 90-degree angle, the patellar ligament in the normal knee is oriented slightly posterior and contraction of the quadriceps

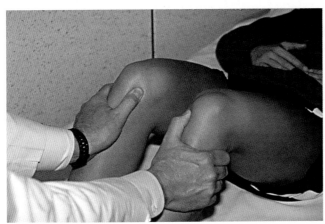

FIGURE 1.43 Posterior drawer testing (see text).

does not result in an anterior shift. If the PCL has ruptured, the tibia sags into posterior subluxation and the patellar ligament is then directed anteriorly. Contraction of the quadriceps muscle in a knee with a PCL deficiency results in an anterior shift of the tibia of 2 mm or more.

ROTARY TESTS

Slocum Anterior Rotary Drawer Test. As described in the discussion of the anterior drawer test, Slocum demonstrated that varying the rotation of the tibia on the femur as the anterior drawer test is done is valuable in determining rotational instability of the knee. The degree of anterior displacement of the tibia on the femur is noted and recorded as the test is done in 15 degrees of internal rotation, 30 degrees of external rotation, and neutral rotation (see Fig. 1.40). A positive anterior drawer test result in neutral tibial rotation that is accentuated when the test is repeated in 30 degrees of external tibial rotation and reduced when it is performed with the tibia in 15 degrees of internal rotation indicates anteromedial rotary instability. The opposite indicates anterolateral rotary instability.

Jerk Test of Hughston and Losee. Several methods of this test have been described. In Hughston's method, with the patient supine, the lower extremity is supported by the examiner while the knee is flexed to 90 degrees and the tibia is rotated internally. When the right knee is being examined, the foot is grasped with the right hand and the tibia is internally rotated while valgus stress is exerted with the left hand over the proximal end of the tibia and fibula. The knee is then extended gradually, maintaining the internal rotation and valgus stress (Fig. 1.47). When the test result is positive, the lateral tibia spontaneously subluxes forward in the form of a sudden jerk at approximately 30 degrees of flexion.

Lateral Pivot Shift Test of Macintosh. With the knee extended, the foot is lifted and the leg internally rotated, and a valgus stress is applied to the lateral side of the leg in the region of the fibular neck with the opposite hand. The knee is flexed slowly while valgus and internal rotations are maintained. With the knee extended and internally rotated, the tibia is subluxed anteriorly. As the knee is flexed past approximately 30 degrees, the iliotibial band passes posterior to the center of rotation of the knee and provides the force that reduces the lateral tibial plateau on the lateral femoral condyle.

An isolated tear of the ACL produces only a small subluxation; greater subluxation occurs when the lateral capsular complex or semimembranosus corner also is deficient. Severe

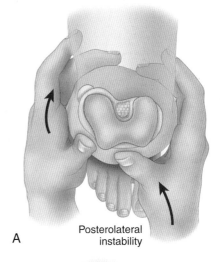

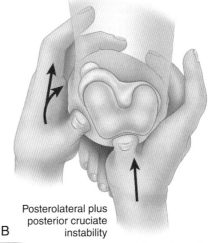

FIGURE 1.44 Transverse section of knee joint showing rotational movement of tibia on femur during posterolateral and posterior drawer tests. **A,** With posterolateral instability, tibia rotates posteriorly and laterally around axis in intact posterior cruciate ligament. **B,** With combined posterior cruciate and posterolateral instability, tibia subluxates posteriorly and knee joint shows increase in posterolateral subluxation.

valgus instability may make this test difficult to do because of lack of medial support.

The pivot shift is tested while the knee is moved from extension to flexion, and the jerk test is elicited while the knee is moved from flexion to extension.

All of the forces applied to the knee by the examiner's hands should be gentle but firm. Forceful gripping of an acutely injured knee and application of vigorous stress usually causes apprehension and guarding on the part of the patient, negating the exam. If one successful subluxation is accomplished in this scenario, it usually is painful, and the patient will not relax for a second attempt.

Slocum reported that more subtle degrees of rotary instability can be detected if the test is carried out as follows. The patient is placed in a lateral decubitus position with the affected side up (Fig. 1.48). The patient's pelvis is placed 30 degrees posteriorly, and the medial side of the foot is placed on the firm examining table with the knee in full extension. This position eliminates the rotational effects of the hip, allows the knee to fall into a valgus position, and internally rotates the tibia on the femur.

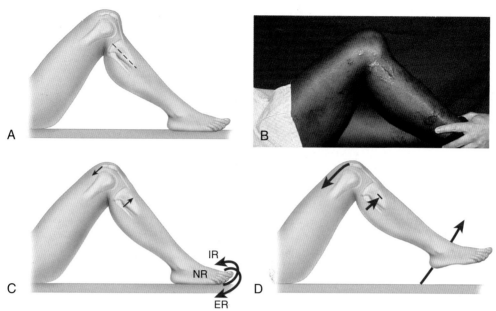

FIGURE 1.45 "Posterior drawer" often is mistaken for "anterior drawer" because tibia sags posteriorly and appears to move abnormal distance forward when examiner tests for anterior drawer phenomenon. **A,** "Posterior sag" of right tibia is obvious compared with normal silhouette of healthy knee joint. **B,** Tibial sag in resting position. If patient starts to raise the foot from this position, pull of quadriceps first displaces tibia anteriorly into neutral position until anterior cruciate ligament is tight **(C)**. Only then is foot raised from table **(D)**. *ER,* External rotation; *IR,* internal rotation; *NR,* neutral rotation. (**A, C,** and **D** from Müller W: *The knee: form, function, and ligamentous reconstruction,* New York, 1983, Springer-Verlag.)

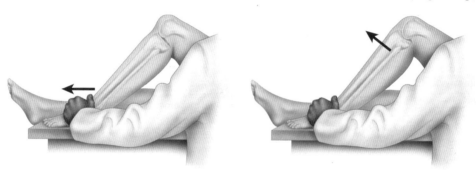

FIGURE 1.46 Quadriceps active test for posterior cruciate ligament deficiency (see text). (From Veltri DM, Warren RF: Isolated and combined posterior cruciate ligament injuries, *J Am Acad Orthop Surg* 1:67, 1993.)

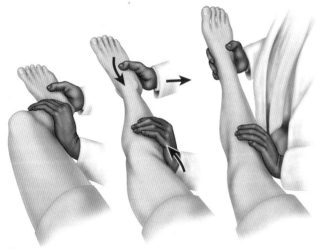

FIGURE 1.47 Jerk test, or lateral pivot shift test. (Courtesy J. C. Hughston, MD; redrawn.)

A thumb is placed on each of the femoral and tibial sides of the joint posteriorly, and an index finger is placed across the joint anteriorly. The knee is then pressed gently forward into flexion. A test result is positive if reduction occurs as the knee passes the 25- to 45-degree range of flexion. This may occur smoothly or as a sudden palpable and occasionally audible repositioning. In our experience, lesser degrees of instability are detected by Slocum's method, which also is not as likely to be painful.

Flexion-Rotation Drawer Test. Noyes described a flexion-rotation drawer test that in his opinion is more reliable than the anterior drawer test in detecting anterior cruciate insufficiency. It tests anterior cruciate function in two planes, the anteroposterior and femoral rotation, and the result is positive when other test results for anterior cruciate function are negative (e.g., pivot shift). It combines the features of the Lachman test and the Hughston pivot shift test.

The test is carried out in the following manner (Fig. 1.49). With the patient supine and the knee at 0 degrees (not hyperextended), the leg is lifted upward, with the femur allowed to

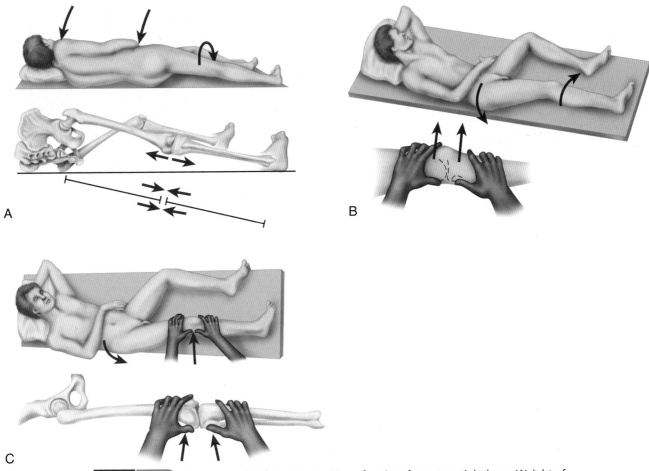

FIGURE 1.48 Lateral pivot shift test. **A,** Position of patient for test on right knee. Weight of right lower extremity is borne on right heel. **B,** Same position viewed from above. Right thumb of examiner is placed behind fibular head, and index finger palpates anterior aspect of subluxated lateral tibial plateau. Left thumb is placed behind lateral femoral condyle (see text). **C,** With knee unsupported in valgus and tibia internally rotated on femur, knee is flexed by pushing anteriorly with both thumbs. Tibia is reduced from its anteriorly subluxated position by tension of iliotibial band as knee reaches 25 to 45 degrees of flexion. Reduction should be readily palpable.

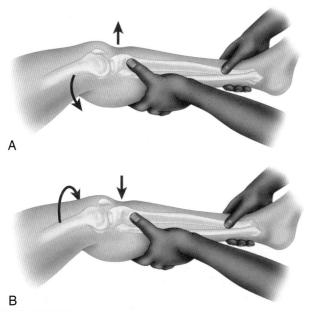

FIGURE 1.49 **A** and **B,** Flexion-rotation drawer test for anterior cruciate ligament insufficiency (see text). (Courtesy F. R. Noyes, MD.)

fall back and to rotate externally. This results in anterolateral tibial subluxation as the starting position for the test. While the knee is flexed, the tibia moves backward and the femur rotates internally, causing the joint to reduce when the test result is positive. Mild valgus stress and anterior pressure on the upper calf applied by the examiner's hand can be done to elicit a positive test result. This test often can be performed gently without significant pain and subsequent guarding.

External Rotation-Recurvatum Test. In addition to the ordinary evaluation of recurvatum in an injured and uninjured knee, the external rotation-recurvatum test can be done as follows to detect abnormal external rotation of the tibia on the femur associated with or in combination with excessive recurvatum. This test is done with the patient supine, and the result is compared with the normal knee. The knee is moved from about 10 degrees of flexion to maximal extension while external rotation of the proximal end of the tibia, as well as the amount of recurvatum, is observed and palpated. The test result is positive if excessive rotation and recurvatum with a subtle apparent varus deformity occur. A markedly positive test result indicates that the PCL, posterolateral corner, and LCL are torn. Hughston described doing this test by simultaneously lifting

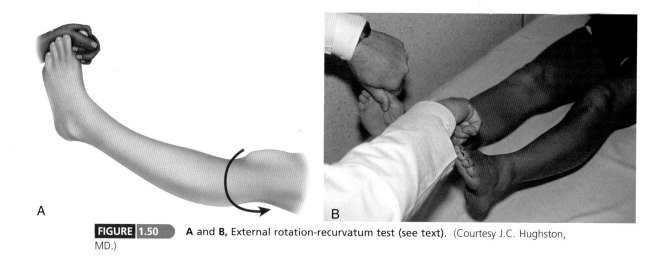

FIGURE 1.50 **A** and **B,** External rotation-recurvatum test (see text). (Courtesy J.C. Hughston, MD.)

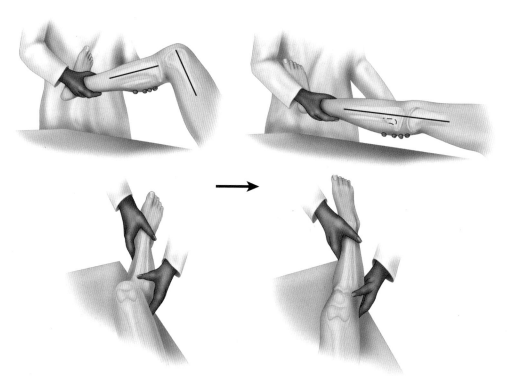

FIGURE 1.51 Reverse pivot shift sign (see text). (From Jakob RP, Hassler H, Stäubli HU: Observations on rotatory instability of the lateral compartment of the knee: experimental studies on the functional anatomy and the pathomechanism of the true and the reversed pivot shift sign, *Acta Orthop Scand Suppl* 191:1, 1981.)

each extremity by the great toe and noting the degree of recurvatum and rotation of the tibia that occur on the normal and the abnormal side as the maneuver is performed (Fig. 1.50).

Reverse Pivot Shift Sign of Jakob, Hassler, and Stäubli. This sign is present in patients with acute or chronic posterolateral instability of the knee. The lateral tibial plateau shifts from a position of posterior subluxation to a position of reduction as the flexed knee is extended under valgus stress and with the foot held in external rotation. The plateau subluxates again as the knee is flexed in the opposite manner. The maneuver produces discomfort and simulates the feeling of giving way to the patient. Although similar to the true pivot shift on first inspection, it can be clearly distinguished from

it by the position of the foot (external rotation) and by other definite signs of posterolateral instability. Because it describes a shift of the lateral tibial plateau in the opposite direction from the true joint shift, it is called the reverse pivot shift. A significantly positive reverse pivot shift suggests that the PCL, the arcuate complex, and the LCL are all torn. In the position of tibial internal rotation, the sign disappears.

The patient is positioned supine on the examining table. To test the right knee, with the examiner facing the patient, the foot and ankle are lifted with the right hand and allowed to rest on the right side of the examiner's pelvis (Fig. 1.51). The lateral side of the calf is supported with the palm of the left hand on the proximal fibula. The knee is moved several

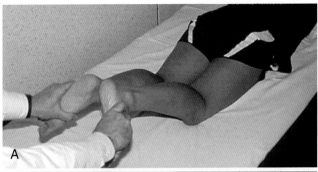

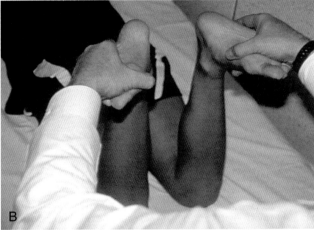

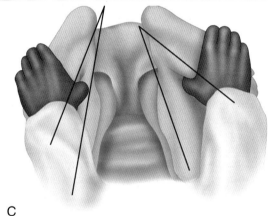

FIGURE 1.52   A–C, Prone external rotation test. Increased external rotation at 30 degrees that decreases at 90 degrees indicates isolated injury to posterolateral corner; increased external rotation at both 30 and 90 degrees indicates injury to both posterior cruciate ligament and posterolateral corner.

times through a full range of motion to reduce muscle resistance. Then the knee is bent to 70 to 80 degrees of flexion. At this position, the foot and the leg are externally rotated to cause the lateral tibial plateau to subluxate posteriorly in relation to the lateral femoral condyle. This is seen as a posterior sag of the proximal tibia. The knee is allowed to straighten through nothing more than the weight of the leg. An axial load is transmitted through the leg while the foot is leaned on slightly. A valgus stress is applied to the knee, with the examiner's iliac crest used as a fulcrum. As the knee approaches 20 degrees short of full extension, the lateral tibial plateau is felt and is observed moving anteriorly in a jerklike shift from a position of posterior subluxation and external rotation into a position of reduction and neutral rotation.

Reverse pivot shift also can be tested with the tibia initially in the reduced position of full extension. In neutral rotation, the knee is quickly bent under continuous valgus stress, and the foot is allowed to rotate externally. At about 10 degrees of flexion, the same jolt will occur as the tibia falls into posterior subluxation. In this way, the two phases, posterior subluxation and reduction, can be repeated from flexion to extension and back to flexion. The test is even more pertinent if it reproduces the patient's symptoms. The intensity of the findings of subluxation and reduction and the patient's reaction to it depend on the degree of instability, the skill with which the examiner performs the test, and the patient's ability to relax the muscles.

Tibial External Rotation (Dial) Test. When an injured knee is tested for posterolateral instability, external rotation of the tibia on the femur is measured at both 30 and 90 degrees of knee flexion. The test can be done with the patient supine or prone (Fig. 1.52A,B). The medial border of the foot in its neutral position is used as a reference point for external rotation. At the chosen knee flexion angle, the foot is externally rotated with force. The degree of external rotation of the foot is measured relative to the axis of the femur and is compared with the opposite leg. External rotation is measured by noting the foot–thigh angle (Fig. 1.52C). In addition, the tibial plateaus are palpated to determine their relative positions compared with the femoral condyles. This determines whether the external rotation is caused by the lateral tibial plateau moving posteriorly (posterolateral instability) or by the medial plateau moving anteriorly (anteromedial instability). A 10-degree difference between knees in the amount of external rotation is considered pathologic. More than a 10-degree increase in external rotation compared with that of the contralateral side at 30 degrees of knee flexion, but not at 90 degrees, indicates an isolated injury to the posterolateral corner. If pathologic external rotation exists at 30 degrees of knee flexion and the external rotation increases when the knee is flexed to 90 degrees, this test indicates injury to both the posterior cruciate as well as the posterior lateral cornet. A cadaver study found that after transection of the MCL the results of the dial test were similar to those from a solitary injury to the posterolateral corner; the authors suggested that the dial test probably is not reliable in the presence of medial instability. Jung et al. reported that reducing the tibia with an anterior force increased the ability of the examiner to detect posterolateral rotary instability combined with PCL injuries.

Posterolateral Drawer Test. The posterolateral drawer test is done with the patient supine and the hip flexed 45 degrees, the knee flexed 90 degrees, and the tibia in 15 degrees of external rotation. With the foot fixed, a posterior drawer test is done. The test result is positive for posterolateral instability if the lateral tibial condyle externally rotates relative to the lateral femoral condyle. The sensitivity of this test for detecting isolated injury to the posterolateral structures of the knee is questionable. The quality of the end point felt during external rotation in normal knees can vary considerably. Because external rotation is coupled with posterior translation, a grossly positive result of the posterolateral drawer test may indicate injury to the PCL and the posterolateral corner.

■ RADIOGRAPHIC EXAMINATION

Standard anteroposterior and lateral radiographs, as well as a tangential view of the patella as described by Hughston, are routine. The tangential view is necessary because of the frequent association of acute patelloquadriceps instability with

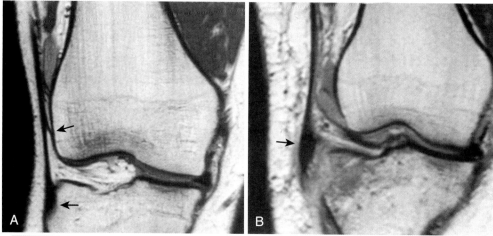

FIGURE 1.53   MR images demonstrating superficial and deep layers of iliotibial band *(arrows)*. **A,** Normal superficial and deep layers (coronal view, right knee). **B,** Tear of superficial layer off Gerdy's tubercle (coronal view, left knee). (From LaPrade RF, Gilbert TJ, Bollom TS, et al: The magnetic resonance imaging appearance of individual structures of the posterolateral knee: a prospective study of normal knees and knees with surgically verified grade III injuries, *Am J Sports Med* 28:191, 2000.)

acute medial ligamentous disruptions. Tunnel views through the intercondylar notch and weight-bearing views are desirable if the patient can tolerate the positioning. In children, avulsions of osteocartilaginous portions of the intercondylar eminences are more common than cruciate ligament disruptions. In adults, pieces of bone occasionally are avulsed from the femoral condyle or from the tip of the fibula where the collateral ligament inserts. Routine radiographs in an acutely traumatized adult knee more often are normal, and rarely is the anterior intercondylar eminence avulsed as an isolated finding. On occasion, a fragment off the back of the tibia can be seen in a PCL disruption. Small fragments along the medial or lateral tibial joint line suggest avulsion of the capsular ligament at that location. On the lateral side, a small avulsion fragment off the lateral tibial plateau joint line is called a Segond fracture or lateral capsular sign and is pathognomonic for an ACL injury. Also on the lateral side, a bony impaction fracture of the lateral femoral condyle at the sulcus terminalis (also called the lateral femoral notch sign) has been associated with ACL injuries. Recently, interest has focused on the anterior and posterior slopes of the tibial articular surface along, with the depth of the medial tibial plateau, as risk factors for ACL and PCL injuries.

Stress radiographs rarely should be required if stress tests are gently performed; exceptions are injuries to children before physeal closure and in tibial plateau fractures, in which apparent instability may instead be caused by the bony rather than ligamentous disruption. As a rule, stress radiographs should be obtained in all apparent ligamentous disruptions of the knee in patients whose distal femoral and proximal tibial physes are still open. In these patients, the instability frequently is from a physeal separation rather than from ligamentous disruption. The relationship of the tibial spine with the intercondylar notch of the femur should be noted. On abduction stress radiographs showing opening of the joint medially, a lateral shift of the tibial spine in the intercondylar notch suggests PCL disruption, and a medial shift suggests ACL disruption. LaPrade et al., in a cadaver study, determined that an isolated LCL injury should be suspected if lateral compartment opening with varus stress increases by

approximately 2.7 mm and a grade III posterolateral corner injury is suggested if values increase by approximately 4 mm.

Remarkably clear images of the soft tissues can be obtained with MRI, and with increasing experience with this noninvasive method, investigators have advocated its use in patients instead of diagnostic arthroscopy (Fig. 1.53). A high degree of accuracy has been reported for detection of ACL and PCL injuries. The course of the PCL is more vertical and more in the midline plane than that of the ACL, making it easier to include the entire PCL in the MRI cut. MRI cuts obtained with the tibia externally rotated 15 degrees (so-called nonorthogonal) usually provide a complete image of the ACL in at least one frame. MRI may be useful in acute collateral ligament disruptions combined with ACL tears. Some authors suggest surgical repair or reconstruction of the ACL combined with a limited incision to expose the collateral ligament disruption if it is precisely localized on preoperative MRI.

CLASSIFICATION OF KNEE INSTABILITY

In the past, instability from ligamentous injury was classified as medial, lateral, posterior, anterior, and rotary on the basis of the direction in which the tibia was displaced. Although useful, this classification was an oversimplification and did not include multiplane instabilities, which commonly occur. Traumatic disruption of knee ligaments often results in complex, multiplane instabilities; if these instabilities are not corrected, normal mechanics cannot be restored to the knee. There is some confusion over terminology, pathomechanics, and the principal pathologic condition responsible for producing each type of instability.

The vertical axis of the knee joint normally passes near the center of the joint. The tibial plateau is divided into four quadrants that serve as the reference points in the definition of knee instability. Any disruption of the complex of supporting structures around the knee can permit a shift in this vertical axis away from the center of the tibia into one of the lateral quadrants as the tibia shifts excessively and abnormally in relation to the femur. The specific classification of each instability depends on the movement of the tibia in relation to the femur

Normal position of left knee, no rotation

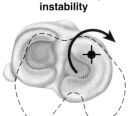

Tibia
(proximal aspect)

Lateral　　　　　　　　　**Medial**

Axis and
direction of rotation

Femur
(distal aspect)

**Anterolateral complex
instability**

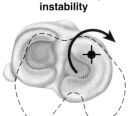

**Anteromedial complex
instability**

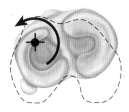

**Posterolateral complex
instability**

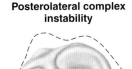

**Posteromedial complex
instability**

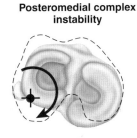

FIGURE 1.54 Demonstration of shift in vertical axis away from center of tibia as tibia shifts excessively and abnormally in relation to femur. Position of femur is designated by *shaded area*.

during stress testing (Fig. 1.54). This may not be precise and completely accurate for acute injuries unless the examination is done with the patient under general anesthesia. The classification probably has its greatest usefulness in chronic instabilities.

Box 1.1 outlines the classification of knee instability proposed by the Committee on Research and Education of the American Orthopaedic Society for Sports Medicine. It was developed by pooling resources from major knee centers throughout North America. This classification attempts to describe the instability by the direction of the tibial displacement and, when possible, by structural deficits. It refers to instability occurring from joint trauma or to acute instability progressing to a chronic state and ignores congenital and acquired instability from other causes, such as tibial plateau fractures and congenital hyperextension. This is an anatomic classification in that one-plane medial instability means that the tibia moves abnormally away from the femur on the medial side and that anteromedial rotary instability means that the tibia rotates anteriorly and externally and moves away from the femur on the medial side. It is understandable that the classification becomes more complex as attempts are made to include anatomic or structural deficits.

■ ONE-PLANE INSTABILITY

One-plane medial instability with the knee in full extension is apparent, as the abduction or valgus stress test is performed,

---

when the knee joint opens on the medial side; that is, the tibia moves away from the femur. This is a major instability and indicates disruption of the MCL, the medial capsular ligament, the ACL, the POL, and the medial portion of the posterior capsule. It strongly suggests disruption of the PCL, but it is not totally confirmatory in most investigators' opinion. One-plane medial instability detected only when the knee is tested in 30 degrees of flexion indicates a tear limited to the medial compartment ligaments.

One-plane lateral instability with the knee in extension is apparent on adduction or varus stress testing when the knee opens on the lateral side; that is, the tibia moves away from the femur. This indicates disruption of the lateral capsular ligament, the LCL, the biceps tendon, the iliotibial band, the arcuate-popliteus complex, the popliteofibular ligament, the ACL, and, often, the PCL. One-plane lateral instability detected only with the knee in 30 degrees of flexion may be present in minor lateral complex tears or may be normal compared with the opposite knee.

One-plane posterior instability is apparent when the tibia moves posteriorly on the femur during the posterior drawer test. This indicates disruption of the PCL, the arcuate ligament complex (partial or complete), and the POL complex (partial or complete). A grade 1 or 2 posterior drawer suggests an isolated PCL injury. Most clinicians believe that a grade 3 or greater posterior drawer indicates additional injury to either the posterolateral or posteromedial corner.

One-plane anterior instability is present when the tibia moves forward on the femur during the anterior drawer test in neutral rotation. This instability is difficult to comprehend fully. It indicates that disrupted structures include the ACL, the lateral capsular ligament (partial or complete), and the medial capsular ligament (partial or complete). The anterior drawer sign is present in neutral rotation when the ACL is disrupted with immediate or subsequent stretching of the medial and lateral capsular ligaments. Although laboratory studies suggest that loss of only a portion of the ACL can produce an anterior drawer sign, the instability clinically suggests loss of functional integrity of the entire ligament. In this type of instability, the test result becomes negative as the tibia is internally rotated because the PCL becomes taut in this position. When the anterior drawer test with the tibia in neutral rotation shows equal displacement of both condyles and this displacement is eliminated by internal rotation of the tibia, both anteromedial and anterolateral rotary instability may be present. This can be confirmed by the jerk test (see Fig. 1.49).

Severe grades of instability (i.e., severe varus, valgus, anterior, or posterior instability) are accompanied by additional central or peripheral ligamentous deficiencies, and therefore most are accompanied by rotary instabilities as well.

■ ROTARY INSTABILITY

Anteromedial rotary instability is apparent with stress testing when the medial plateau of the tibia rotates anteriorly and externally as the joint opens on the medial side. This implies disruption of the medial capsular ligament, the MCL, the POL, and the ACL.

Anterolateral rotary instability detected at 90 degrees of flexion has little relation to the anterior drawer sign or major anterior displacement of the tibia. The lateral tibial plateau rotates forward in relation to the femur at 90 degrees of flexion with excessive lateral opening of the joint. There is then excessive internal rotation of the tibia on the femur with the knee in flexion. This implies disruption of the lateral capsular ligament, the arcuate ligament complex (partial), and the ACL (partial or complete). Anterolateral rotary instability detected as full extension of the knee is approached is more common. With a specific test (jerk test, anterolateral rotary instability test of Slocum, or lateral pivot shift test of MacIntosh), the lateral tibial plateau subluxates forward on the femur as the knee approaches extension. This implies disruption of the ACL and possible involvement of the lateral capsular ligament. Clinically, as the knee comes into extension while weight bearing, the anterior subluxation of the lateral tibial plateau is dramatic.

Posterolateral rotary instability is apparent, with stress testing, when the lateral tibial plateau rotates posteriorly in relation to the femur, with lateral opening of the joint. This implies disruption of the popliteal tendon, the arcuate ligament complex (partial or complete), and the lateral capsular ligament and at times stretching or loss of integrity of the PCL. It is important to distinguish this type of instability from one-plane posterior instability resulting from a tear of the PCL. In posterolateral rotary instability, the posterolateral corner of the tibia drops off the back of the femur and the lateral opening of the joint is detected when the external rotation-recurvatum and reverse pivot shift tests are performed.

Posteromedial rotary instability is apparent with stress testing when the medial tibial plateau rotates posteriorly in reference to the femur, with medial opening of the joint. This implies disruption of the MCL, the medial capsular ligament, the POL, the PCL, and the medial portion of the posterior capsule, plus stretching or major injury to the semimembranosus insertions. The ACL also may be injured.

■ COMBINED INSTABILITIES

One-plane and rotary instabilities usually are understandable, although some of the implied structural deficits are still debatable. However, combined instabilities rarely are either clearly defined or consensual, and each orthopaedic surgeon will have to satisfy personal suspicions as to which structures are specifically damaged and their relative degree of involvement in the instability. When a severe rotary instability is noted in one quadrant, rotary, varus, or valgus instability in another quadrant must be sought. Most severe rotary instabilities are accompanied by some degree of varus or valgus instability as well.

Combined anterolateral-anteromedial rotary instability is the most common combined instability. The result of the anterior drawer test with the tibia in neutral rotation is markedly positive, with both tibial condyles being displaced anteriorly. The displacement is exaggerated when the tibia is externally rotated and diminished but usually not obliterated when the test is done with the tibia internally rotated. The test results for anterolateral rotary instability are positive. Varus and valgus stress tests often show instability of varying degrees.

Combined anterolateral-posterolateral rotary instability is apparent when the lateral tibial plateau rotates in a posterior direction as the external rotation-recurvatum test is performed, and there is excessive forward displacement of the lateral tibial plateau on the femur when the anterolateral rotary instability tests are performed. Lateral (varus) instability is great with disruption of most of the structures on the lateral side of the knee, as well as the ACL, and with occasional stretching of the PCL.

Combined anteromedial-posteromedial rotary instability is apparent when medial and posteromedial structures are severely disrupted. The knee opens on the medial side, and the tibia may rotate anteriorly when tested; in addition, with further testing, the tibia rotates posteriorly, dropping off the posteromedial corner of the joint. All medial structures, including the semimembranosus complex, are disrupted in combination with the anterior and most likely the PCLs.

TREATMENT CONSIDERATIONS

Treatment of first-degree sprains is entirely symptomatic, and the patient usually can return to normal function and activities within a few days. Rest, ice, and a compression bandage are usually all that are required. Second-degree sprains require protection. In these injuries, a part of the ligament has been torn, and although the remaining untorn portion may stabilize the knee to routine stress testing, the strength of the ligament has been significantly impaired. If these patients are permitted to return promptly to full activity, especially in sports, complete disruption of the ligament is a real possibility. These patients are best treated with a controlled motion brace, allowing full, protected motion for 4 to 6 weeks. Recovery usually can be expected with no residual laxity once the rehabilitation program has been completed. Third-degree sprains may require operative treatment, depending on factors such as age, general health, associated injuries, and activity demands.

■ NONOPERATIVE TREATMENT

Isolated third-degree sprains of the MCL can be treated successfully by nonoperative means. MRI or stress testing with the patient under general anesthesia and an arthroscopic examination usually are required to rule out any associated articular surface, meniscus, or cruciate ligament injury. Nonoperative treatment of third-degree sprains of the MCL is more predictable and successful if the tear is at the proximal attachment and there is no evidence of other ligamentous damage. Equally severe tears of the distal end of the MCL do not heal as well as those at the proximal end. The distal end of the ligament may be pulled proximally and occasionally is displaced superficial to the pes anserinus insertion; therefore, with conservative treatment, healing at the distal end is not as predictable as it is at the proximal end. Furthermore, elderly patients who do not expect to return to vigorous activities or to place great demands on the knee can be treated adequately without surgery, but they often have mild residual laxity.

Nonoperative treatment is reasonable for all second-degree sprains and for some third-degree collateral ligament sprains. Third-degree sprains of 2+ to 3+ severity that occur in conjunction with meniscal injury are best treated by surgical repair. After stress testing has been performed and the grade and severity of the injury have been determined, the extremity is placed in a hinged knee brace for 4 to 6 weeks. We may lock the brace for the first 2 weeks in 30 degrees of flexion. Crutch walking is permitted with toe-touch weight bearing as soon as the leg can be controlled. After 2 weeks, as the inflammation subsides and the healing begins, the brace is adjusted to provide full flexion and the extension block is reduced by 15 degrees. Full extension is obtained by 6 weeks. Numerous investigators have documented the deleterious effects of immobilization on the muscles, ligaments, and articular surfaces.

Because the biomechanical and biochemical properties of the healing ligament fail to return to normal, researchers are exploring new modalities to improve the quality of healing tissues and to accelerate the rate of healing. Tissue engineering with use of growth factors, gene transfer, and cell therapies are being studied. The results with growth factors may be species, dosage, and treatment specific, demonstrating the complex nature of ligament healing. Growth factors have half-life periods of a few days in vivo, and their use would require repetitive applications to maintain potency, which is inconvenient and perhaps unfeasible in the clinical setting. Gene transfer has the potential to overcome this problem by providing the ability to control expression and regulation of proteins in a host cell. Transplantation of genetically altered tissues through a retroviral vector has resulted in the expression of the *lacZ* marker gene for as long as 6 weeks in the anterior cruciate and MCLs of animals. Studies of gene transfer have shown positive effects on collagen fibril diameter and distribution, as well as significant increases in mechanical properties. Cell therapy involves the implantation of genetically manipulated cells to enhance the repair of ligaments as those cells become constituents of the healing tissue. Nucleated cells, including mesenchymal stem cells, from bone marrow have been transplanted into a pocket around the transected MCL of inbred rats; donor cells could be identified in the midsubstance of the ligament after 7 days, demonstrating the potential for migration of transplanted cells.

Many investigators recommend nonoperative treatment of the MCL in combined injuries of the ACL and MCLs. The medial side is treated with a motion-control brace for 2 to 3 weeks while motion in the knee is regained. Once the inflammatory process has diminished, the ACL is reconstructed arthroscopically. The delay allows initiation of the healing process in the MCL, which also seals the capsular rent and prevents extravasation of fluid. Fewer problems with postoperative arthrofibrosis occur when motion is restored preoperatively. However, Nakamura et al., in a study of the use of MRI in determining a treatment regimen for acute grade III MCL injuries associated with ACL tears, found that restoration of valgus stability was significantly correlated with the location of superficial MCL fiber damage. When damage was evident over the whole length of the superficial layer and not confined to either the proximal or distal attachment sites, preoperative bracing did not restore valgus stability, and those patients required surgery for the MCL injury along with ACL reconstruction. Narvani et al. identified a subgroup of deep MCL injuries at the femoral origin that caused persistent symptoms after conservative treatment in high-level athletes. After operative repair, all athletes returned to their sports and remained asymptomatic 1 year later.

Reconstruction of the ACL appears to be important for adequate healing of the MCL when there are combined injuries. Biomechanical evaluation of the effects of ACL deficiency on the healing of the injured MCL in rabbit and canine models demonstrated that knees with untreated combined anterior cruciate and MCL injuries showed significantly increased valgus laxity and a reduction in tissue quality of the healed MCL. In addition, considerable joint degeneration was observed.

Several studies have reported good results with nonoperative treatment of MCL injuries combined with reconstruction of the ACL. A randomized, controlled trial comparing operative with nonoperative treatment of MCL injuries in 47 patients with combined ACL and grade III MCL injuries found no statistically significant differences between the two groups. Subjective outcomes and Lysholm scores were good and anteroposterior knee stability was excellent in both. A later study comparing outcomes in patients with isolated ACL injuries and those with combined ACL and chronic grade II MCL injuries found that residual valgus laxity did not significantly affect anteroposterior laxity at minimum follow-up of 3 years, suggesting that no additional surgical procedure is needed for the MCL in combined lesions. Not all medial-sided knee injuries heal with nonoperative treatment. As Tibor et al. emphasized, injury to the posteromedial corner of the knee differs anatomically and biomechanically from isolated injury of the MCL. Valgus instability places additional strain on a reconstructed ACL or PCL, which can contribute to late graft failure, and in patients with multiligament injuries, operative reconstruction of the posteromedial corner, including the MCL, may be indicated.

The rehabilitation protocol must be individualized on the basis of the patient's age, the degree of instability, and other factors. The patient is prescribed a program of quadriceps and hamstring isometric exercises and leg lifts for the hip flexors and hip abductors while in the brace. When the brace is removed, motion in the knee is advanced, and a vigorous rehabilitative exercise program is instituted. A reinforced elastic knee support usually is applied, and the patient is not permitted to return to normal activities, especially sports, until the range of motion is normal and the strength in all muscle groups has returned to 90% of that in the uninjured extremity. When the patient returns to athletics, the injured ligament usually is protected by a functional brace for 3 or 4 months. This is the minimal time necessary for stress orientation of the collagen fibers to be regained in the healing ligament.

Healing of the LCL has not been as well researched as that of the MCL, but reports in the literature indicate that grade

I and II LCL injuries can be successfully treated nonoperatively, whereas good results seldom are obtained with nonoperative treatment of grade III injuries.

■ OPERATIVE TREATMENT

Although most authors recommend nonoperative treatment of isolated MCL injuries, some prefer to repair the medial side when the injury is associated with an ACL disruption. Indelicato recommended reconstruction of the ACL and reassessment of the medial laxity. If the knee continues to be unstable in full extension or slight flexion (grade II or grade III), the MCL and the POL are repaired.

By definition, *repair* of ligaments of the knee refers to surgical treatment of acute injuries, and *reconstruction* usually refers to surgical treatment of ligamentous laxity several months after injury. Skillful repair or reconstruction depends on a thorough knowledge of anatomy. The best possible repair restores the anatomic integrity and tension of a torn ligament and should be done without unnecessary delay. Optimal surgical dissection and repair become increasingly difficult beyond 10 to 14 days after injury.

Absolute rules as to when it is too late to repair a ligament cannot be given. In addition to the time since injury, the severity of the disruption, the location of the principal pathologic condition, and the patient's age and activity needs must all be considered. Although surgical repair should proceed as soon as possible, conditions for surgery must be optimal. Surgery should proceed only after a definite diagnosis has been made and a specific plan of repair has been formulated. The type of repair selected must depend on the experience and skill of the surgeon, the location of the injury, and the condition of the tissues. The search for additional abnormality must be diligent before a diagnosis of isolated injury is accepted.

Major tears indicate a marked initial displacement of the joint surfaces and the probability of injury to other supporting structures. Incisions must be planned properly, and exposure usually must be extensive, often from the midline of the limb anteriorly to the midline posteriorly, because the principal pathologic condition usually is in the posterior two thirds of the medial and lateral compartments. Without sufficient exposure to reach these areas, incomplete repair is likely. Repairs always are performed with use of a pneumatic tourniquet for hemostasis. The tourniquet is removed before closure to control bleeding and to prevent severe hemarthrosis or hematoma. Joint stability may be impaired by a few millimeters of capsular stretching from a tense hemarthrosis. Although the anatomic integrity of the ligament is restored under proper tension, the repair procedure must not destroy the blood supply of the ligament. Dissection should be limited to only that necessary to identify and to correct the pathologic condition. Skin flaps developed during the approach should be deep to the fascia, when possible, to reduce the vascular and cutaneous nerve injury inherent in superficial subcutaneous dissection.

Whenever possible, ligaments should be anchored into freshened bone with nonabsorbable sutures, suture anchors, screws with toothed or spiked washers (Fig. 1.55), or staples. This can be accomplished by passing sutures through multiple holes drilled in cortical bone at the site of attachment or preferably through parallel holes drilled through to the opposite side of the bone. Staples, preferably with barbs to prevent extrusion, must be placed a sufficient distance from the articular margin so that joint function is unimpaired. Suture anchors, staples, and screws with toothed washers are intended for use at sites of ligamentous attachments to bone, and again at a sufficient distance from the joint not to interfere with joint or ligament function. Neither the screw with toothed washer nor the staple should be overly tightened or countersunk because of the possibility of pressure necrosis of the ligamentous tissue beneath the crown of the staple or beneath the toothed washer. Staples,

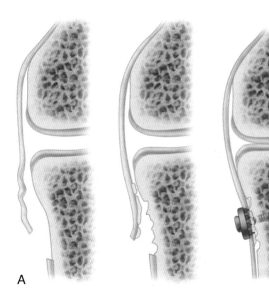
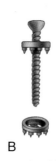
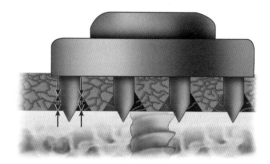

A   B

FIGURE 1.55 Reattachment of avulsed ligaments with AO screw and toothed washer. **A,** Fixation of avulsed ligament, with or without bony fragment. **B,** Washer is designed so that it grips ligament and bone over broad area with its peripherally arranged teeth, compressing and fixing them within limits designed by a stop on each tooth. Little pressure is exerted on tissue next to and between teeth. Microcirculation in these areas of ligament is normal; it is compromised only in compressed area represented by *solid trapezoids*. (From Müller W: *The knee: form, function, and ligamentous reconstruction*, New York, 1983, Springer-Verlag.)

screws, or other forms of internal fixation should not be used in areas where normal gliding of the ligament is required during flexion and extension. If they are placed in these areas, such as near the articular margin of the medial femoral or tibial condyle, anteroposterior excursion of the tibial collateral ligament will be limited during flexion and extension movements. Thus, either it will be difficult to regain joint motion or the ligament will have to tear or stretch to permit motion.

Numerous studies have identified radiographic landmarks of ligament attachment sites, and these landmarks are being used more frequently for ligament reconstructions. Nonabsorbable sutures should be used for strength where tension is the greatest. Absorbable sutures can be used where approximation without appreciable tension is required. Approximating sutures apposing the dissected torn edges of the ligament should be reinforced with tension sutures of nonabsorbable material. A square or rectangular pattern is used in the manner of a mattress suture to secure the tension sutures. These sutures restore the normal length of the ligament while protecting the area of repair. Careful alignment of the tension sutures along the course of the ligament fibers is necessary if they are to perform their intended function. Tension sutures can be tested for functional placement and isometry during flexion and extension of the knee before being tied definitively. Sutures properly placed will not pull out or interfere with normal joint motion.

The menisci should be salvaged if at all possible, and peripheral tears should be repaired. However, multiple tears within the substance of the meniscus may require that the meniscus be excised. If so, attempts should be made to leave a peripheral meniscus cuff or rim. Fragile areas of the ligament repair should be reinforced with fascia or other local tissue or supported by a muscle-tendon unit.

After ligamentous repair, the knee should be briefly immobilized initially in a hinged brace in 30 degrees of flexion. The length of immobilization, if any, should be selected for each patient; it depends on the severity of the tear, the structures torn, the accuracy of repair, the method of ligament fixation, the age of the patient, and the health of the articular surfaces. At least theoretically, early motion is feasible if the ligamentous repair and attachment sites are truly isometric. Under such circumstances, normal unstressed motion of the knee should not place undue tension on the fixation points. Full extension should be achieved as soon as possible to prevent the development of a flexion contracture.

The success of repair depends on the proper analysis of the instability by clinical examination; during surgery, it depends on the quality of the tissue involved directly by injury and the quality of the tissue available to reinforce lax or ruptured structures, the exacting performance of the surgical procedure, the postoperative care, the motivation of the patient, and the thoroughness of rehabilitation. The long-range prognosis for function depends on the amount of initial laxity and the presence of any associated internal derangement or posttraumatic degenerative arthritis. The objective of treatment is to attain maximal function and to minimize or prevent degenerative changes within the joint. Hanley et al. compared their long-term patient-reported outcomes in 34 patients with multiligamentous knee injuries after MCL repair or MCL reconstruction. They identified time to surgery, patient age, and MCL reconstruction as risk factors for poorer results. At a mean 6-year follow-up, patients with repair generally had higher patient-reported outcomes than those with reconstruction.

MEDIAL COMPARTMENT (COLLATERAL) DISRUPTIONS
■ REPAIR

If surgical repair of the torn medial support of the knee is planned, arthroscopic examination of the knee to rule out other intraarticular pathologic conditions is done before open surgical exploration. The surgeon must be aware of the capsular disruption that may allow significant extravasation of irrigation fluid during arthroscopy of an acutely unstable knee. A synovial or capsular rent ordinarily will seal sufficiently to prevent dangerous extravasation of irrigation fluid if the arthroscopic examination is delayed for 5 to 7 days and the surgeon is skilled and expedites the examination. The arthroscopic pump pressure should be low or only gravity pressure and valgus stress on the knee should be avoided. A lengthy examination of an acutely injured knee is not justified, and massive extravasation of irrigation fluid may occur in such instances. Once arthroscopic examination has been completed, or if such examination is not carried out, the following open technique is used.

REPAIR OF MEDIAL COMPARTMENT DISRUPTIONS

TECHNIQUE 1.4

- Place the patient supine on the operating table with a pneumatic tourniquet inflated on the upper thigh.
- Flex the hip approximately 45 degrees, flex the knee approximately 60 degrees, and allow the lower extremity to lie with gravity in abduction at the hip.
- For positioning of the extremity, a special bolster posterior to the midthigh that permits the knee to flex to 90 degrees may be preferred.
- Begin a midmedial incision 2 cm proximal to the adductor tubercle, curving it gently distally over the adductor tubercle parallel to the medial aspect of the patella and patellar tendon and approximately 3 cm medial to these structures. Carry it distally along the anteromedial aspect of the tibia to end 5 to 6 cm below the joint line.
- Dissect the skin, subcutaneous tissues, and superficial fascia as a single layer from the midline anteriorly to the posteromedial corner. Wide exposure is necessary to identify and to correct all of the pathologic conditions.
- Take care during the dissection and retraction not to injure the large saphenous vein, which is in the subcutaneous tissue at the posteromedial aspect of the dissection.
- The infrapatellar branches of the saphenous nerve cannot always be preserved with this incision, although the sartorial branch of the saphenous nerve should be identified and protected as it exits between the sartorius and gracilis to supply sensation over the entire medial aspect of the leg to the ankle.
- A hematoma in the posteromedial area of the exposure may identify the site of principal damage.
- Stress test the knee again for ligamentous and patellar instability.

- Incise the medial longitudinal extensor retinaculum along the anterior edge of the sartorius from its tibial insertion posteriorly to the posteromedial corner. Take care not to incise the tibial insertion of the tibial collateral ligament immediately beneath.
- With the knee in the flexed position, retract the sartorius and other components of the pes anserinus to allow inspection of the tibial insertion of the tibial collateral ligament, which is deep and distal to the anterior edge of the sartorius.
- An alternative to incising the longitudinal extensor retinaculum along the anterior border of the sartorius is to detach the bony insertion of the pes anserinus from the tibia and reflect these tendons upward. This uncovers the MCL, the POL area, and the semimembranosus complex at the posteromedial corner of the knee. The first step in surgical identification of the pathologic condition should be the assessment of the integrity of this tibial insertion. We do not release the pes anserinus tendon.
- Make a medial parapatellar fascial incision extending from the edge of the vastus medialis muscle distally to join the incision along the anterior edge of the pes anserinus.
- Dissect this medial longitudinal patellar retinaculum off the anteromedial capsule and the MCL and reflect it proximally and posteriorly to the margin of the vastus medialis. This can be done without undue difficulty when surgery is performed within a few days after injury. This exposes the MCL and the medial capsular structures.
- Deepen the medial parapatellar capsular incision into the joint and thoroughly inspect it.
- If arthroscopy has not been done to evaluate the intraarticular structures, systematically inspect the undersurface of the patella, the articular surfaces of the femur and the tibia, the medial and lateral menisci, and the ACL and PCL.
- With the knee flexed, place the heel on the opposite knee and retract the patellar fat pad to see the entire lateral meniscus through the medial parapatellar capsular incision.
- Inspect the cruciate ligaments and palpate them with the finger and with ligament hooks.
- If the menisci are torn within their substance, excise areas that cannot be repaired. Attempt to preserve a meniscus rim or cuff even if most of the meniscus must be excised.
- When a cruciate ligament is torn, it should be reconstructed (see Techniques 1.19 and 1.20).
- Again, stress test the joint to better identify the area of medial ligament injury. Throughout the dissection, take care not to make the ligamentous pathologic condition unidentifiable.
- If the MCL is avulsed from the tibia beneath the pes, reflect it proximally, exposing the underlying midcapsular portion of the medial capsular ligament. A definite interval is present between the MCL and the midcapsular portion of the medial capsular ligament anteriorly so that proximal retraction of the MCL is possible and the anteromedial, the midmedial, and the posteromedial capsular structures can be readily identified and inspected.
- Expose the posterior capsule by locating the interval between the medial head of the gastrocnemius and the semimembranosus and incising the sheath of the semimembranosus. Dissect the posterior capsule off the medial head of the gastrocnemius muscle. With the knee maintained in flexion, the posterior capsule can be easily exposed to the midline. Carefully retract the popliteal vessels during this exposure.

- Expose the medial capsular ligament further by using an intraarticular retractor deep to the medial capsular ligament. This may reveal a bare area on the femoral condyle from which the capsular ligament and synovium have been avulsed.
- When the capsular tear cannot be identified easily, a vertical incision splitting the fibers of the MCL often will reveal tears in its meniscofemoral portion. Medial capsular tears often begin near the medial condylar origin and proceed in an L- or Z-shaped path toward the posteromedial corner. Tears in the meniscofemoral portion of the deep capsular ligament may leave the peripheral attachment of the medial meniscus undisturbed, and the medial meniscus can be retained. Tears of the weaker meniscotibial portion of the medial capsular ligament frequently accompany tears of the meniscus or its peripheral attachment.
- Repair all tears in the peripheral attachment as the capsular ligament is repaired; tears within the outer 25% of the substance of the meniscus should be repaired.
- Tears of the midmedial capsular ligament and that portion designated by Hughston as the POL often extend for variable distances into the posterior capsule, and the extent must be determined. The posteromedial capsular tear often extends well around the posteromedial corner to involve the posterior capsule and its tibial insertion.
- If a major tear is not present in the posteromedial capsular structures, incise in line with the fibers of the POL, creating an arthrotomy for examination of the posterior horn of the medial meniscus.
- Do not remove an untorn medial meniscus or one that can be repaired to make reattachment of the posterior capsule easier. This is not necessary, and sacrifice of the meniscus with its protective and stabilizing function should be avoided.
- Begin the procedures of repair with the intraarticular abnormality (meniscectomy, meniscal suture, or cruciate reconstruction) as indicated.
- Place multiple interrupted sutures in the meniscus if repair is needed and pass them out through appropriate capsular sites. Do not tie these sutures until the medial repair is complete. Manipulation of the knee in the course of medial repair may disrupt such sutures if they are tied initially.
- Proceed with repair of other ligaments as follows. Repair first the posteromedial capsule if it is torn, maintaining the knee at 60 to 90 degrees of flexion at all times. If the posterior capsule has been torn from its tibial attachment, pull it down to the back of the tibia (see later).
- If the posteromedial capsule has been torn in its midportion, approximate it with multiple interrupted, nonabsorbable sutures, placing the knots extraarticularly as the medial head of the gastrocnemius is retracted and the knee is maintained in 90 degrees of flexion.
- If the posteromedial capsule has been torn from its femoral attachment, reattach the capsule to the femur with suture anchors.
- Alternatively, drill holes from the anteromedial epicondylar area to exit posteriorly in the area of insertion of the medial head of the gastrocnemius muscle. Use sutures to bring the upper edge of the posterior capsule to its normal insertion, pass the sutures through the bone, and tie them over the bone anteromedially.
- If the posterior capsule has been torn from its tibial attachment, reattach the freshened edge to the posterior surface of the tibia using suture anchors.

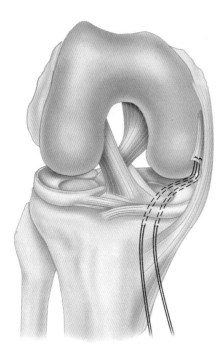

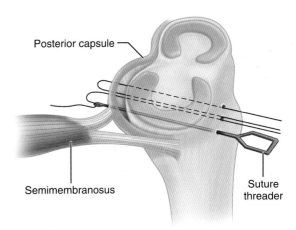

FIGURE 1.56 Repair or reconstruction of posteromedial corner of knee; sutures are placed in periphery but not tied. (Redrawn from Dohrmann [copyright 1988]. In Feagin JA Jr, editor: *The crucial ligaments: diagnosis and treatment of ligamentous injuries about the knee*, New York, 1988, Churchill Livingstone.) **SEE TECHNIQUE 1.4.**

FIGURE 1.57 Reattachment of capsule to posterior tibia. **SEE TECHNIQUE 1.4.**

- Roughen or freshen the posterior rim of the tibia with an osteotome to aid in reattachment of the posterior capsule.
- Alternatively, drill three parallel holes beginning on the anteromedial surface of the tibial condyle and exiting just below its posterior articular margin.
- Place sutures through the freshened edge of the capsule and pass the ends of the sutures through these holes to the anterior aspect of the tibia with a suture passer, passing two sutures through the center hole.
- With the knee in 60 degrees of flexion, bring the edge of the posterior capsule to its insertion by tying the sutures anteriorly (technique of O'Donoghue) (Figs. 1.56 and 1.57).
- If the posterior horn of the medial meniscus is salvageable, do not advance the tibial attachment too far distally or the meniscus will be displaced off the back of the tibial plateau. With the knee held in a flexed position as the advancement is made, anchoring the attachment too far distally is a possibility. Before the sutures are tied, extend the knee to be sure that the reattachment is in the correct location.
- When the posterior capsule has been reattached, return to the anteromedial aspect of the exposure.
- Repair the medial extensor retinaculum and the vastus medialis muscle if they are torn and then close the anterior arthrotomy incision with multiple interrupted sutures. Failure to close the anteromedial arthrotomy incision before repairing the other medial and posteromedial structures may result in inability to close this anterior incision once those structures have been shortened and tightened.
- Close the synovium with a continuous 3-0 absorbable suture and the anteromedial capsular incision with multiple interrupted no. 0 absorbable sutures.
- Return to the posteromedial corner.

- Repair of the tear in the medial capsular ligament complex and the POL or semimembranosus complex is determined mainly by the pattern of the tear. The objective is to anatomically approximate the torn ligament ends with multiple interrupted sutures and then to reinforce it with tension sutures in the manner of mattress sutures. These suture patterns should be square or rectangular in orientation. The purposes of the tension sutures are to restore normal length and tension to the collagen fibers and to prevent stress on the suture line. The placement and direction of pull of the tension sutures must be precise and in line with the ligament fibers. Similar to other sutures, they must be tested for correct functional placement and isometry during flexion and extension of the knee before they are tied definitively. The approximating sutures are usually absorbable (0 Vicryl), and the tension sutures are nonabsorbable (0 Mersilene) (Fig. 1.58).
- If the posteromedial corner (POL complex) has been pulled from its femoral attachment, Hughston recommended placing two or three nonabsorbable mattress sutures well anchored distally in the ligament at the posterior corner of the tibia (Fig. 1.59A) and anchoring them proximally at the attachment of the ligament to the adductor tubercle of the femur (Fig. 1.59A-C).
- If the capsular arm of the POL has been torn from its femoral attachment, it produces a fold in the posterior part of the capsule that is continuous with the OPL. If such a tear is found, draw the torn end of the capsular arm forward and suture it to the portion of the ligament still attached to the adductor tubercle (Fig. 1.59A-D); when the attachment of the ligament to bone has been avulsed, leaving a bare bony surface, drill holes in the bone, elevate a small bone flap near the adductor tubercle, and attach the ligament with sutures, a screw with a toothed washer, or a staple (Fig. 1.60A,B). Suture anchors also can be used to attach the ligament to a roughened bone surface.
- When this POL portion of the medial capsular complex has been secured, a gentle abduction stress should show medial stability.
- If the tibial arm of the posterior oblique portion of the medial capsular complex has been torn from the tibia and insufficient stump of the ligament or periosteum remains on the tibia to hold sutures, repair with sutures anchors. Alternatively, drill holes through the tibia as shown in Figure 1.61A, B. With a suture passer, pass long sutures from the ligament

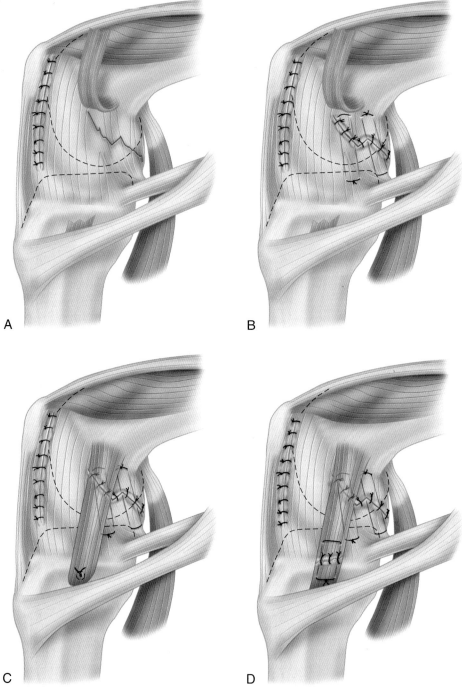

FIGURE **1.58**   **A,** Common tear pattern, medial compartment, superficial or medial collateral ligament torn distally near its tibial attachment with oblique tear in midmedial and posteromedial capsular ligament. **B,** Repair of midmedial and posteromedial deep ligament with interrupted approximating sutures; nonabsorbable tensioning sutures inserted to relieve tension on suture line. **C,** Superficial medial collateral ligament fixed to tibial metaphysis. **D,** If tear in superficial medial collateral ligament is near or just below joint line, it is repaired with interrupted sutures, with tensioning suture bridging tear to relieve tension along suture line. **SEE TECHNIQUE 1.4.**

through anteriorly directed holes and tie them over the bone anteriorly to approximate the ligament to the posteromedial corner of the tibia. Additional sutures to secure the tibial arm to the direct and deep heads of the semimembranosus provide reinforcement of this important structure.

■ When the posterior oblique portion of the medial capsular complex has been reattached, repair the medial capsular ligament anterior to the point already repaired. Reattach the avulsed ligament to bone or approximate torn ligament ends with multiple interrupted, nonabsorbable

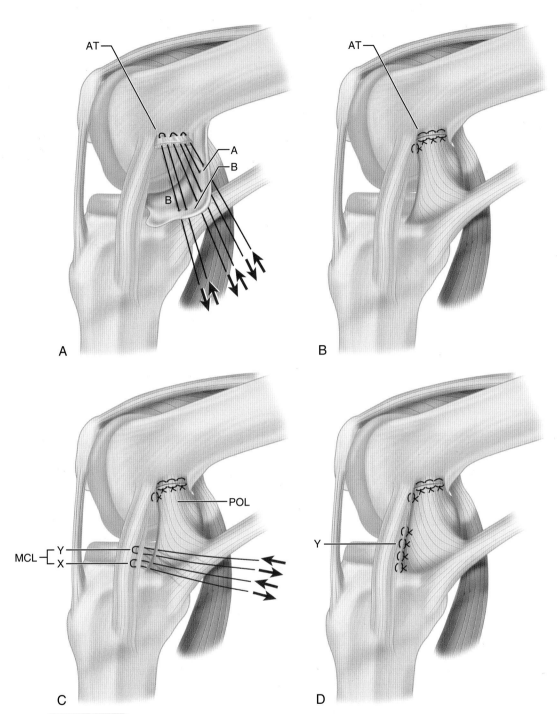

FIGURE 1.59 Repair of ligaments of medial compartment of knee. **A,** Sutures are inserted into stump at original attachment of posterior oblique ligament (POL) and periosteum on adductor tubercle *(AT)* and through capsule *(A)* and tibial portions *(B)* of posterior oblique ligament (see text). **B,** Posterior oblique ligament is pulled forward and fixed and tied as tightly as possible to adductor tubercle with knee at 60 degrees of flexion when sutures are tied (see text). **C,** Advancement of tibial end of *POL,* with suturing to periosteum of tibia and to repaired medial collateral ligament *(MCL)* (see text). **D,** Anterior border of POL advanced and sutured over posterior border of MCL. X and Y, Sutures attaching POL to repaired medial collateral ligament. (Redrawn from Hughston JC, Eilers AF: The role of the posterior oblique ligament in repairs of acute medial [collateral] ligament tears of the knee, *J Bone Joint Surg* 55A:923, 1973.) **SEE TECHNIQUE 1.4.**

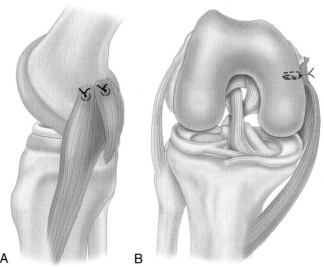

FIGURE 1.60 Repair of ligaments of medial compartment of knee. **A,** Isometric fixation of medial ligaments secured with screw and washer. **B,** Medial collateral and posterior oblique ligaments are repaired individually with AO screws and washers. **SEE TECHNIQUE 1.4.**

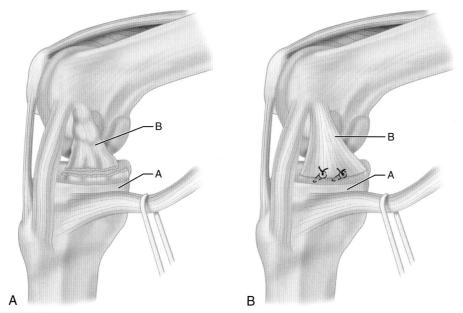

FIGURE 1.61 **A,** Repair of posterior oblique ligament torn from tibia. **B,** Sutures tied and ligament reattached. *A,* Point of original ligament attachment; *B,* torn ligament; attachment of ligament. (Redrawn from Hughston JC, Eilers AF: The role of the posterior oblique ligament in repairs of acute medial [collateral] ligament tears of the knee, *J Bone Joint Surg* 55A:923, 1973.) **SEE TECHNIQUE 1.4.**

sutures (Fig. 1.62A,B). This should complete the repair of the medial capsular structures.

- If the MCL, the midportion of the medial capsular ligament, and the femoral attachment of the POL are avulsed with a piece of bone from the femur, a relatively rare occurrence, all can be reattached in continuity with a staple or screw with a toothed washer. This is an optimal tear pattern to encounter.
- Repair any vertical or oblique tears with multiple interrupted sutures (Fig. 1.63). Then repair the superficial portion of the MCL. Krackow et al. designed a locking stitch that is ideal for grasping flat structures such as this liga-

ment (Fig. 1.64). It allows tension to be applied to the ligament without causing it to bunch up.

- If the femoral attachment has been torn, reattach it to the adductor tubercle area with a staple, a screw with a toothed washer, suture anchors, or interrupted sutures.
- If the midportion is torn, use interrupted absorbable sutures to approximate the ends. Supplement the repair with tension, box, or mattress nonabsorbable sutures.
- If the ligament has avulsed from its tibial insertion, reattach it distal to the joint line with interrupted sutures through holes drilled in the bone, by a staple or suture

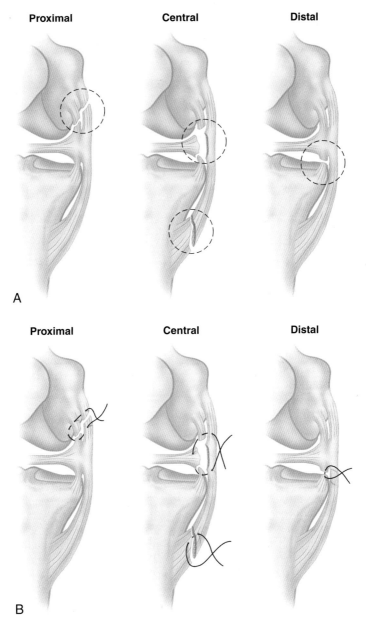

FIGURE 1.62 Primary repairs of tears within medial capsular ligament. **A,** Tears. **B,** Repairs.
SEE TECHNIQUE 1.4.

anchors to roughened bone, or by elevation of a bone flap, placing the ligament beneath it and securing the flap with a table staple. Then pull the tibial portion of the POL anteriorly and suture it to the periosteum of the tibia and the meniscotibial ligament distally and to the repaired posterior edge of the MCL proximally (see Fig. 1.59C). Advance the entire anterior border of the POL and suture it in a pants-over-vest fashion to the posterior border of the MCL (Fig. 1.59D).

■ If the medial capsular ligament has been torn through the meniscotibial portion, the coronary ligament attachment of the medial meniscus also may be torn. If so, carefully repair it. In such tear patterns, the undersurface of the meniscus is visible as the tear is retracted superiorly. Determine the method of repair for this type of tear by the length of the meniscotibial stumps.

■ If the tear is in the midsubstance of the meniscotibial ligament, use multiple approximating, interrupted nonabsorbable sutures. Two box-shaped tension sutures also are usually inserted (Fig. 1.65A).

■ If the meniscotibial attachment of the medial capsular complex has been pulled off the tibia near its bony insertion, we prefer to reattach it using suture anchors after freshening the side of the tibia near its articular margin to cancellous bone with a burr or osteotome. Alternatively, insert multiple interrupted nonabsorbable no. 0 sutures through the torn meniscotibial capsular edge and test for good purchase. Drill multiple holes horizontally across the tibia. Expose the exit of the drill through the lateral tibia via a lateral incision and clear the soft tissues. Pass the sutures through the transosseous tunnels with suture passers to the lateral side, beginning with the most pos-

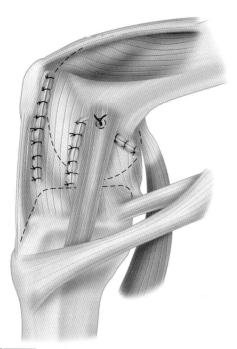

FIGURE 1.63 Superficial and deep medial ligaments avulsed from femoral attachment reattached and vertical and oblique tears closed with interrupted sutures. **SEE TECHNIQUE 1.4.**

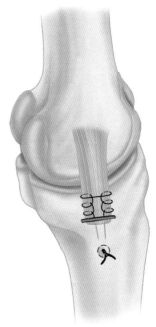

FIGURE 1.64 Krackow locking stitch allows application of tension to ligament without bunching up. (Redrawn from Krackow KA, Thomas SC, Jones LC: Ligament-tendon fixation: analysis of a new stitch and comparison with standard techniques, *Orthopedics* 11:909, 1988.) **SEE TECHNIQUE 1.4.**

terior suture. Tie each suture, proceeding from the most posterior to the most anterior. Be careful not to pull the meniscus down over the medial articular rim as shown in Figure 1.65B.

- If the tears have been extensive and support is fragile, after repair has been completed, special procedures can be added to provide reinforcement or dynamic support. For example, suturing of the semimembranosus tendon to the posteromedial corner reinforces the POL. Other procedures include suturing of the semimembranosus into the posterior aspect of the MCL, advancement of the sartorius and gracilis, a pes plasty, and advancement of the vastus medialis muscle. These and other procedures are described in subsequent sections of this chapter.
- Bring the medial longitudinal patellar retinacular flap to its normal position and reattach it to the anterior border of the sartorius. Close the anteromedial capsular incision with multiple interrupted sutures.
- Release the tourniquet and obtain hemostasis.
- Close the wound over suction drainage tubes.
- Place the leg in a long-leg cast or controlled motion brace from groin to toes with the knee flexed 45 to 60 degrees and the tibia internally rotated but not forcibly.

POSTOPERATIVE CARE We have found that the addition of a preoperative adductor canal or saphenous nerve block aids in pain control for the first 24 hours, often allowing these procedures to be done in the out-patient setting. We no longer use femoral nerve blocks, which might give somewhat better pain relief but sometimes result in significantly delayed recovery of quadriceps function. The extremity is elevated to reduce swelling. The patient is instructed in active quadriceps and hamstring

exercises beginning the day after surgery. Ideally, these exercises are practiced before surgery. Quadriceps and hamstring isometric exercises are performed on a regular basis each hour, and leg lifts for strengthening of the hip flexors and abductors are instituted as soon as possible. In selected patients, epidural analgesia and a continuous passive motion machine can be used. Crutch walking with touch-down weight bearing is begun as soon as possible. Drainage tubes are removed at 12 to 24 hours. The patient usually is released from the surgical facility ambulatory with crutches the day of or the day after surgery. The patient is encouraged to continue quadriceps- and hamstring-setting exercises on a regular basis in addition to leg lifts. Transcutaneous muscle stimulation has not been proved to reduce atrophy or to aid in rehabilitation. If a motion brace is used, motion between 30 and 90 degrees is encouraged. The sutures are removed at 2 weeks. If a cast is used, it is changed at 2 weeks, maintaining the 30-degree flexed position. The protective cast or brace is changed every 2 weeks and is worn for a total of 4 to 6 weeks. Usually 4 weeks of complete immobilization is the maximum. A long-leg, restricted motion brace or a femoral cast brace that will permit freedom of flexion but will block extension, usually at 30 degrees, is worn. Total immobilization usually is unnecessary for acute MCL repairs, and immobilization often has deleterious effects on the articular surfaces, especially of the patellofemoral joint. The flexible brace usually is worn until 6 to 8 weeks after surgery. If the brace has an adjustable dial lock mechanism in the knee hinge, the amount of extension can be increased (e.g., from 30 to 15 to 0 degrees) during the 6 to 8 weeks after surgery.

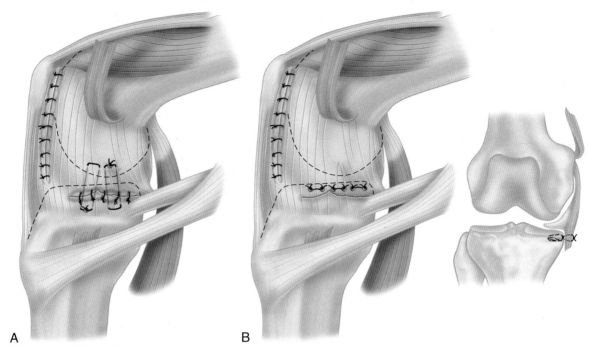

A   B

FIGURE **1.65**   **A,** Horizontal tear in meniscotibial ligament approximated with multiple interrupted sutures. Two tensioning sutures to relieve tension on approximated tear are placed vertically.
B, Horizontal tear in meniscotibial ligament near its insertion on tibia. Repair is accomplished by
multiple interrupted sutures through transosseous tunnels *(inset)*. **SEE TECHNIQUE 1.4.**

On removal of the cast or other appliance, a reinforced knee
brace is applied. Partial weight bearing on crutches continues until at least 60 degrees of motion is present in the knee
and the patient is lifting 7 kg, 50 repetitions, with the quadriceps. Agility and proprioceptive retraining are emphasized as
late components of the rehabilitation program. Rehabilitation
proceeds similarly to that prescribed after meniscectomy, but
it is more intense and more prolonged. Also, extension to
within 5 degrees of the opposite extremity must be present
before the crutches can be discontinued. With early motion
in a controlled motion brace, the patient often has full extension by 8 weeks, and full weight bearing can be permitted. The
patient should understand that maximal strength and function in the repaired ligaments probably are not attained for 12
months after surgery.

■ RECONSTRUCTION

Chronic medial compartment instability is rarely a single-
plane valgus laxity. Medial instabilities sufficient to justify
reconstruction are more often combined with other instabilities, such as anterior cruciate insufficiency, that also must be
taken into consideration. However, for simplification, reconstructions in the following sections are described as medial
reconstruction, lateral reconstruction, and so on, but the
reader must realize that combinations of procedures and frequent modifications often are necessary. Simultaneous reconstruction of chronic ACL and MCL lesions has been shown to
be effective in improving medial, sagittal, and rotatory stability of the knee.

The principles of reconstruction of the medial side are (1)
repair and retention of the medial meniscus, if possible; (2)
reconstruction of the capsular structures, especially the posterior capsule; (3) restoration of the meniscotibial connection

of the semimembranosus complex; (4) reconstruction of the
POL at the deep posterior corner; (5) reestablishment of the
influence of the semimembranosus unit to the POL, medial
meniscus, and posterior capsule; and (6) reconstruction of
the MCL. Severe valgus laxity generally requires tightening
of the MCL in addition to the posterior capsule, the posterior
oblique area of the posteromedial capsule, and the midmedial
capsular ligament.

RECONSTRUCTION OF MEDIAL COMPARTMENT

TECHNIQUE 1.5

(SLOCUM)

- Place the patient on the operating table supine so that
  the lower end of the table can be dropped beyond a right
  angle to flex the knee. A bolster can be used to support
  the distal aspect of the thigh and to flex the knee with
  the table flat. Most of the surgical exposure, exploration,
  and reconstruction is carried out with the knee flexed;
  the method is the choice of the surgeon. We prefer the
  bolster and leave the foot on the table, but either method
  permits the knee to flex to 90 degrees and allows access
  to the posterior joint.
- Carefully prepare the skin, drape the extremity, and inflate
  a pneumatic tourniquet. If arthroscopic examination immediately precedes the planned reconstruction, it should
  be done without inflation of the tourniquet.

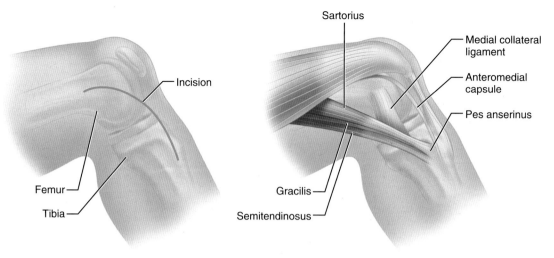

FIGURE 1.66 Exposure for repair of posteromedial capsule. Medial skin incision is represented by *green line*. **SEE TECHNIQUE 1.5.**

- Begin a medial skin incision 4 to 5 cm proximal to the medial femoral epicondyle and curve it forward and downward, paralleling the lower fibers of the vastus medialis muscle, to the midpoint of the medial edge of the patella.
- Continue the incision distally, paralleling the patellar tendon across the joint line to the level of the lower border of the pes anserinus, as with the standard medial parapatellar incision.
- Reflect the skin and subcutaneous fat flap posteriorly to the medial popliteal space to expose the deep fascia covering the medial compartment and anteriorly to expose the musculotendinous structures around the medial side of the patella, patellar tendon, and tibial tuberosity (Fig. 1.66).
- With the extensor retinaculum and deep fascia still overlying the medial ligaments and with the posteromedial corner of the knee exposed, check the knee for stability by the abduction stress test and Slocum's anteromedial rotary test. Note points of greatest laxity and scarring during the testing to determine which will require special reinforcement during the surgical repair.
- Check the lateral stability of the patella by attempting to force it laterally over the lateral femoral condyle with the knee in several different degrees of flexion. When the patella can be subluxated or dislocated from the patellofemoral groove, laxity of the extensor retinaculum and the vastus medialis muscle insertion is present and requires repair. Patellar stability must be tested at this stage because it is extremely difficult to evaluate after capsular arthrotomy incisions have been made.
- Make a medial parapatellar arthrotomy incision and explore the joint by a definite routine as follows.
- Inspect the medial meniscus for tears or tears of its attachment. If the medial meniscus and the synovium over the peripheral attachment are both intact on the upper surface and the meniscus is held tightly to the femur by the meniscofemoral portion of the medial capsule while abduction stress is applied, the meniscotibial portion of the ligament is lax; when the meniscus remains fixed to the tibia during abduction stress testing, the meniscofemoral portion of the capsule is the principal site of laxity. Use a

meniscus hook or a blunt ligament hook to detect posterior peripheral or inferior surface tears not detectable by inspection from above.
- Then inspect the lateral meniscus by placing the foot on the opposite knee and allowing the flexed knee to be stressed into varus as the hip falls into external rotation.
- Retract the ligamentum mucosum and the patellar fat pad to see most of the lateral meniscus.
- Inspect the articular surfaces of the patella, the femoral condyles, and the tibial plateaus for chondral or osteochondral defects (treat them appropriately by chondroplasty or excision of loose fragments).
- Test the anterior and PCLs for laxity by inspection, palpation with a gloved finger, and tension testing with a ligament hook.
- If a cruciate ligament feels "soft" as it is stressed with a finger or a ligament hook but the overlying synovium appears intact, carefully incise the synovium to determine whether an intrasynovial rupture of the cruciate ligament has occurred.
- When reconstruction of medial compartment structures is necessary and the laxity seems to be principally meniscofemoral rather than meniscotibial, tightening of the medial capsular ligament by proximal advancement with an intact meniscotibial portion or medial and anterior advancement of the posterior capsule sufficient to correct mild-to-moderate posterior capsular laxity will not sufficiently disturb an intact medial meniscus to justify its excision.
- If the meniscotibial (coronary) ligament portion of the capsule is markedly lax and the peripheral attachment of the meniscus is intact, distal advancement of the posterior and medial capsule may be more difficult. In such instances, instead of excising the meniscus, we prefer to detach the posterior and posteromedial attachment of the meniscus along its meniscocapsular attachment, advance the capsule distally, and suture the meniscus to the tightened capsule.
- If the posterior periphery of the meniscus is already detached, the capsule is advanced distally and the periphery of the meniscus is sutured.

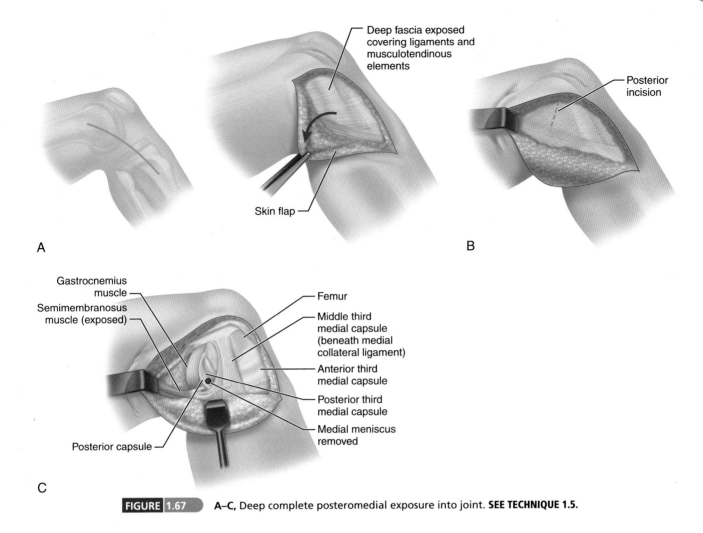

A

B

C

FIGURE 1.67 A–C, Deep complete posteromedial exposure into joint. **SEE TECHNIQUE 1.5.**

- Incise the deep fascia overlying the posteromedial corner of the knee from the level of the vastus medialis anteriorly to the sartorius posteriorly to expose the posterior part of the medial capsule and the semimembranosus tendon (Fig. 1.67A-C). We prefer to join the anterior parapatellar incision and the incision in the deep fascia of the posteromedial corner with an incision along the anterior border of the sartorius, thus reflecting a deep fascial flap proximally to the origin of the vastus medialis. This allows inspection of the tibial insertion of the MCL in addition to better defining areas of maximal laxity of the medial supporting structures. Reflection of this deep fascial flap proximally may be difficult because of scarring, but with care it usually can be accomplished.
- Now enter the posterior joint through the relatively thin part of the capsule lying between the medial and posterior capsular ligaments. This capsular incision lies just posterior and parallel to the strong ligamentous band forming the posterior margin of the medial capsule that extends from the medial femoral epicondyle to the posterior capsule and direct tendon of the semimembranosus.
- Expose the semimembranosus complex at the posteromedial corner of the knee by incising its tendon sheath from the posterior edge of the tibial collateral ligament to its muscle fibers proximally.
- Locate the interval between the posterior capsule and the medial head of the gastrocnemius muscle and retract the gastrocnemius off the posterior capsule over to the midline of the tibia.
- Because the tendon of the semimembranosus is lax with the knee in flexion, release it from its sheath and retract it distally from the groove on the tibia to provide easy access to the interval between the semimembranosus and the posteromedial aspect of the joint where the fibers of the posterior capsule, the oblique fibers of the posteromedial capsule, and the direct head of the semimembranosus and the OPL intermingle.
- Release the ligamentous band between the semimembranosus and the gastrocnemius tendon sheath to further mobilize the semimembranosus complex; however, do not incise the popliteal oblique ligament from the semimembranosus.
- Expose the posterior joint, excise remnants of the medial meniscus or loose bodies, and correct other joint disorders, such as a torn meniscus, as indicated.
- Grasp the conjoined tendons of the semimembranosus with a heavy clamp and draw them forward, upward, and medially.
- Expose the interval between the medial head of the gastrocnemius and the semimembranosus tendon with finger dissection posteriorly to the point where the OPL inserts into the back of the femur and the posterior capsule of the lateral compartment of the knee.

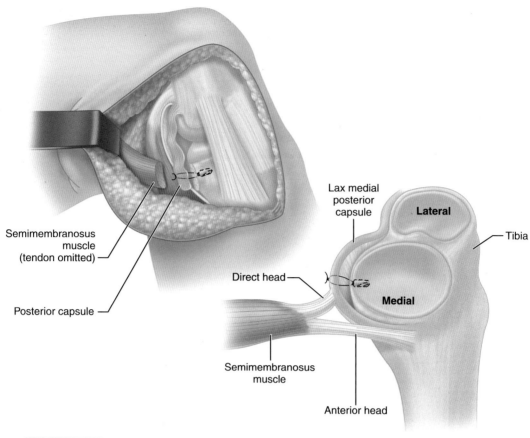

Semimembranosus muscle (tendon omitted)

Posterior capsule

Lax medial posterior capsule

Lateral

Tibia

Direct head

Medial

Semimembranosus muscle

Anterior head

FIGURE 1.68 Repair of posterior capsule torn from posterior tibia. **SEE TECHNIQUE 1.5.**

- Palpate the direct insertion of the semimembranosus at its tibial attachment.
- Protect the popliteal vessels while exposing the posterior capsule.
- The objectives of repair at the posteromedial corner of the knee are to reattach the posterior capsule to the tibia, to suture the meniscus if possible, to restore tension in the posterior and medial capsular structures, and to reestablish the semimembranosus tendon complex, restoring its dynamic influence, especially on the OPL. Slocum carried this out in the following manner.
- If the medial meniscus has previously been removed and when significant laxity exists, dissect the posterior capsule off the back of the tibia to unscarred ligamentous tissue. Use an osteotome to freshen or roughen the bone on the posterior aspect of the tibia for distal advancement of the edge of the posterior capsule using suture anchors to secure the capsule to the tibia (Fig. 1.68).
- Alternatively, drill two or three holes from the anterior to the posterior aspect of the tibia into the freshened area, place sutures in the distal edge of the posterior capsule, and pass them through these drill holes to reattach the capsule to the posterior tibia from the intercondylar area to the medial edge of the insertion of the direct head of the semimembranosus.
- In advancing the tibial attachment of the posterior capsule, place the sutures in the distal posterior capsule so that when the sutures are passed anteriorly through the

parallel drill holes the posterior capsule is pulled downward (Fig. 1.69).
- Extend the knee with the capsule pulled downward before the sutures are tied to be sure that extension is not markedly limited. The joint should begin to feel "tight" as the last 15 or 20 degrees of extension is reached. This restores the tension to the lateral half of the posterior capsule. Posterior capsular advancement obviously is not necessary when avulsion of this portion of the capsule has not occurred.
- If the medial meniscus has not been removed previously, it should be retained, if possible, as already described. The technique for open meniscal suturing is described in Technique 1.1.
- Now close the anteromedial arthrotomy incision; failure to do so at this point may result in difficulty in approximating the edges once the posteromedial capsular and medial collateral ligamentous reconstructions have been completed.
- Next, pull the heavy oblique band at the posterior margin of the medial capsule distally and posteriorly to reattach it to the posterior capsule, the posterior margin of the tibia, the direct head of the semimembranosus, and the OPL while at the same time pulling the inferior medial margin of the posterior capsule forward.
- Finally, advance medially and anteriorly the anteromedial edge of the direct head of the semimembranosus tendon.

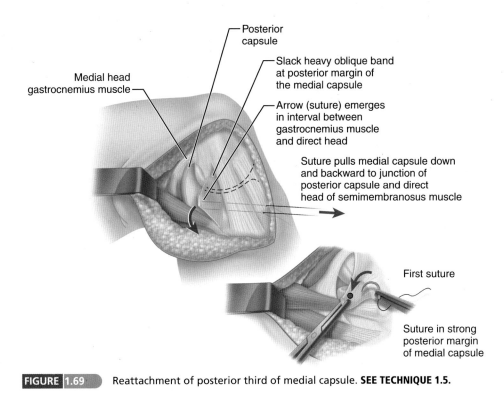

Posterior capsule

Slack heavy oblique band at posterior margin of the medial capsule

Arrow (suture) emerges in interval between gastrocnemius muscle and direct head

Medial head gastrocnemius muscle

Suture pulls medial capsule down and backward to junction of posterior capsule and direct head of semimembranosus muscle

First suture

Suture in strong posterior margin of medial capsule

FIGURE 1.69   Reattachment of posterior third of medial capsule. **SEE TECHNIQUE 1.5.**

REPAIR OF POSTEROMEDIAL CORNER

TECHNIQUE 1.6

- The insertion of the direct head of the semimembranosus tendon into the posterior tubercle of the tibia is the strongest soft-tissue anchor point at the posteromedial corner (Fig. 1.70). Place a mattress suture through the direct tendon near the bone to emerge at the confluence of the direct tendon, the posterior capsule, and the medial capsule.
- Then return anteriorly to the posteromedial capsule for the posteromedial capsular ligament, or that portion referred to by Hughston as the POL.
- Place a suture through the inferior corner of this capsular ligament near the tibial articular margin and then back through the direct tendon of the semimembranosus and tie it securely. Placement of this suture is crucial to restoration of tension within the POL or medial capsule. The posterior fibers of the ligament should lie in juxtaposition with the direct head of the semimembranosus and the tibial insertion of the posterior capsule. This should eliminate valgus and rotary instability.
- The posteroinferior corner of the medial capsule can be attached to a prepared site at the posteromedial tibial margin with suture anchors; or sutures can be passed through holes drilled through the bone when the direct head of the semimembranosus appears to be of insufficient strength.
- Advance the posterior capsule medially and anteriorly around the corner so that it overlies the posterior portion of the medial capsule.

- With the knee flexed, imbricate the medial capsular and posterior capsular edges 1 to 2 cm if possible and secure them with multiple interrupted sutures. Secure also the inferior aspect of the medial edge of the posterior capsule to the direct head of the semimembranosus and then to the medial capsule so that any remaining laxity of the posteromedial capsule is eliminated as the posterior joint is closed. Thus a double-thickness imbricated layer of capsular tissue fixed either to bone or to the direct head of the semimembranosus distally and to the medial epicondyle proximally restores ligamentous tension with good-quality tissue at this most vulnerable point.
- Reinforce the repair by advancement of the semimembranosus tendon, using the direct head as a pivot point.
- Draw the conjoined tendon anteriorly, medially, and proximally to snugly cover the repaired medial and posterior capsule. With two or three interrupted sutures, secure this serpentine course of the semimembranosus complex.
- Slocum released the anteromedial tendon of the semimembranosus from its tibial insertion beneath the longitudinal fibers of the MCL and freed it from its distal attachment to its tendon sheath and the tibial metaphysis. He fixed this freed tendon to the posterior edge of the MCL without disturbing its overlying fascia. Securing it to the posterior edge of the MCL as well as to the reefed posterior capsular ligament above the joint line provides dynamic tightening of the important posterior oblique portion of the medial capsular ligament and of the MCL. We prefer not to detach the anteromedial head of the semimembranosus because significant stabilizing function is lost if the suture line pulls loose. We recognize that bringing it in a serpentine manner over the posteromedial corner may not direct its pull in the line of its fibers, but we prefer this to detachment.

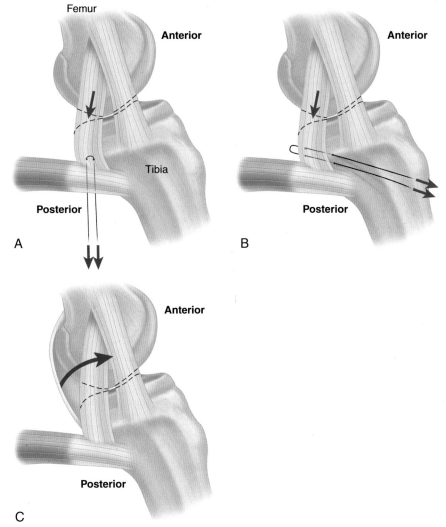

RECONSTRUCTION OF POSTEROMEDIAL CORNER

TECHNIQUE 1.7

(HUGHSTON)

- Use a standard medial incision with the knee held in 60 degrees of flexion, the thigh resting on the operating table, and the hip in external rotation.
- Incise the capsule in the soft spot interval behind the MCL and anterior to the POL. This interval provides access to the posteromedial aspect of the joint and exposure of the medial meniscus.
- Determine the site of the original injury by use of a probe to assess the laxity of the femoral and tibial attachments.
- If the MCL is markedly unstable, especially off the femoral attachment, advance it superiorly and reattach it at the end of the tubercle with suture anchors or sutures to the perios-

teum. Avoid reattaching it below the femoral epicondyle, which would shorten the ligament and restrict flexion.
- Next, advance the POL anteriorly and superiorly onto the femur in the region of the adductor tubercle and the medial epicondyle (Fig. 1.71A). Suture it to the periosteum under moderate tension.
- Then advance the POL inferiorly and distally, anchoring it through holes drilled in the tibia, or through the use of suture anchors, or to adequate soft tissue. Reinforce the midportion of the POL by advancing it over the MCL with mattress sutures in a vest-over-pants fashion (Fig. 1.71B).
- In the final step of the reconstruction, determine the status of the capsular arm of the semimembranosus tendon. If it is lax, advance the tendon distally and superiorly onto the site of reconstruction of the POL with mattress sutures (Fig. 1.71C). This restores the direct line and pull of the semimembranosus muscle and contributes to the dynamic stability.

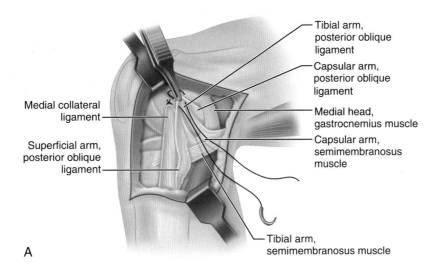

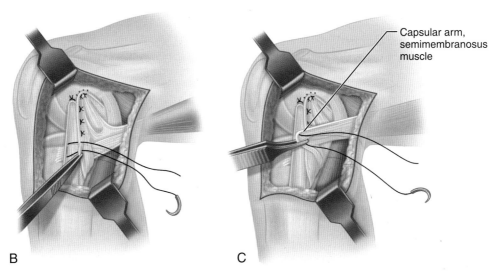

FIGURE 1.71 Repair of posterior oblique ligament. **A,** Medial collateral ligament is sutured to medial femoral epicondyle; loose posterior oblique ligament is pulled anteriorly and proximally onto femur, where it is sutured to periosteum. **B,** Proximal part of torn posterior oblique ligament is sutured to medial collateral ligament, and two ligaments are sutured together in pants-over-vest fashion. **C,** Lax capsular arm of semimembranosus tendon is pulled anteriorly onto site of repair of posterior oblique ligament and sutured in position. **SEE TECHNIQUE 1.7.**

- If the anteromedial capsule is lax or of poor quality, two procedures have been described for reinforcing this area: shifting the patellar tendon medially (Elmslie-Trillat technique) and using the medial half of the patellar tendon to reinforce the repair of the anteromedial capsule. We have not found these necessary. For descriptions of these techniques, the reader is referred to earlier editions of this text.

POSTOPERATIVE CARE The knee is protected for a total of 3 to 6 weeks, depending on the type of reconstruction, the age of the patient, and other factors. As soon as full extension is achieved, partial weight bearing is begun. The rate of progression to full weight bearing depends on quadriceps strength and the integrity of the reconstruction. Isometric exercises are instituted as soon after surgery as tolerated and are progressed with increasing weights during the protected mobilization. When the brace is discontinued, at about 6 weeks, isotonic and isokinetic exercises are begun, along with active full range of motion.

■ RECONSTRUCTION WITH ALLOGRAFT TENDONS

An alternative method for reconstruction of the MCL involves the use of allograft tendons. Commonly used graft sources are the semitendinosus tendon, the posterior tibial tendon, and the anterior tibial tendon. These tissues can be doubled on themselves to provide sufficient strength and yet still maintain adequate length to span the distance required. The tendon is placed in a drill hole at the femoral epicondyle and secured there with a biodegradable interference screw. The graft is attached on the tibial side at the distal end of the tibial insertion site beneath the pes anserinus tendons. It is secured to roughened bone with a screw and spiked soft-tissue washer or staple. The knee can be taken through a range of motion to determine proper isometric placement of this graft before final fixation. Alternatively, the graft can be placed into a drill hole at the tibial site with this technique. Sutures are placed in the free ends of the graft and brought through the tibial drill hole and across the knee to the lateral surface of the tibia to apply tension. The graft is fixed in the tibial tunnel with a biodegradable interference screw. Zhang et al. described a tibial inlay reconstruction of the MCL using Achilles tendon allograft. The bone block was fixed with a cancellous screw and washer into a cancellous trough created on the medial surface of the tibia, and the tendinous portion was fixed with a bioabsorbable interference screw into the femoral insertion site of the superficial MCL. According to the authors, this technique reproduces the native anatomy and orientation of the MCL.

Although fascia lata and the semitendinosus tendon have been recommended as a graft, we prefer allograft tissue to the use of the autogenous tissue from the medial side of the knee when chronic medial instability is present. We believe that the intact medial structures may provide some stability to the medial side of the knee and that their integrity should be maintained. Sacrifice of the semitendinosus or other medial structure may contribute to medial instability.

LATERAL COMPARTMENT (COLLATERAL) DISRUPTIONS

On the lateral side of the knee, a distinction should be made between isolated LCL injuries and posterolateral corner injuries, which include the LCL, the popliteus complex, and the posterolateral capsule. As with medial-side injuries, isolated grade I and II tears of the LCL can be managed with nonsurgical treatment and early rehabilitation. This was demonstrated in clinical studies by Krukhaug et al. and Kannus, but nonsurgical management of grade III injuries produced poor results. However, Bushnell et al. reported on nonsurgically treated isolated grade III LCL injuries in a cohort of National Football League players. They found that those managed nonoperatively were as likely to return to play as those managed surgically and they did so more quickly. In spite of their controversial results, the authors still recommended surgical treatment for most grade III injuries.

For acute lateral compartment disruptions, as for medial tears, the knee is examined for instability classification and grading after the patient has been anesthetized, and systematic arthroscopic examination is usually carried out to assess and rule out other intraarticular pathologic conditions before proceeding with open repair of the lateral complex. Investigators have demonstrated that failure to repair or to reconstruct the posterolateral corner can lead to increased forces and subsequent failure of reconstructed ACL and PCL. Biomechanical studies have shown a significantly higher graft force during varus loading at 0 and 30 degrees of knee flexion after transection of the LCL than with intact posterolateral structures, leading to recommendations that in knees with grade III posterolateral injuries and evidence of varus or coupled posterior-external rotation instability, repair or reconstruction of the posterolateral structures should be performed at the time of PCL reconstruction to decrease the chance of later graft failure. Posteromedial corner injuries also have been implicated in anteromedial rotary instability and failed ACL reconstructions.

In recent years, as a result of residual laxity experienced in some ACL reconstructions, researchers have shown a renewed interest in the ALL of the knee. Its existence is still somewhat debated because it has been identified as a distinct structure in 12% to 100% of human specimens. The ALL is not an isometric ligament; its length increases with knee flexion as well as internal rotation. It usually is reported as originating on the femur, posterior and proximal to the lateral femoral epicondyle, although some have located it either directly on the lateral epicondyle or anterior and distal to the attachment site of the LCL. The tibial attachment site has more agreement, residing halfway between the center of Gerdy's tubercle and the anterior margin of the fibular head and 1 cm distal to the joint line. Biomechanically, the ALL has a mean ultimate load to failure between 50N and 205N, a mean stiffness of 20 to 42 N/mm, and a mean ultimate strain of 36%. Cadaver and biomechanical studies have shown the importance of the ALL as a restraint to internal tibial rotation and anterior tibial translation and in preventing the knee pivot shift phenomenon. Experimental sectioning of the ALL was found to invariably induce high-grade pivot shifts in ACL-deficient cadaver knees, unlike isolated ACL injury, suggesting that reconstruction of the ALL may play a major role in improving results of isolated ACL reconstruction by providing better rotational control of the knee. Several studies have shown that the ALL has an effect of rotational stability when its reconstruction is done in conjunction with a standard intraarticular reconstruction of the ACL.

Currently, there is no consensus regarding the proper angle of knee flexion at which fixation of ALL reconstruction should occur. All flexion angles have been described, but the ligament is not isometric and lengthens with flexion. In a cadaver study, Schon et al. assessed the effect of ALL reconstruction graft fixation angle on knee joint kinematics in the setting of concomitant ACL reconstruction to determine the optimal ALL reconstruction graft fixation angle. They found that anatomic ALL reconstruction at all graft fixation angles significantly overconstrained internal rotation of the knee joint beyond 30 degrees of flexion and at 45 and 60 degrees during the pivot shift test. Furthermore, there were no significant kinematic differences between any tested graft fixation angles during anterior drawer, pivot shift, and internal rotation tests. Consequently, most authors report fixing the graft at 30 degrees of flexion to avoid overconstraint. Sonnery-Cottet et al. reported full range of motion in 83 patients at a minimum 2-year follow-up after combined reconstructions of the ACL and ALL; 76 patients had a negative pivot shift and seven had a grade 1. They also reported significant improvements in Lysholm scores, subjective IKDC scores, and objective IKDC scores. In another study, Sonnery-Cottet et al. found that ALL reconstruction protected the repaired medial meniscus. Their indications for combined reconstructions were an associated Segond fracture, a chronic ACL lesion, grade 3 pivot shift, high level of sports activity, participation in pivoting sports, and lateral femoral notch sign on radiographs. Other surgeons have included revision ACL reconstruction as an indication for ALL reconstruction. Conversely, in a study of 552 patients who had primary ACL reconstruction, Gaunder et al. identified 47 patients who required revision ACL reconstruction. The incidence of Segond fractures was 6% in the primary reconstruction group. After ACL reconstruction, the Segond fracture healed in 90% of patients. No patient with revision surgery had a Segond fracture, and no patient with a Segond fracture had graft failure. Lee et al. reviewed 87 patients who had revision ACL reconstruction and divided them into two groups: isolated revision ACL reconstruction group (group I, $n = 45$) and revision ACL reconstruction in combination with ALL reconstruction (group C,

$n = 42$). The IKDC subjective score, the Tegner score, and the ACL-return to sport after injury (RSI) score were significantly better in group C. Pivot shift test and return to the same level of sports activity were significantly better in group C, but there were no significant differences between the groups for KT-2000 arthrometer, isokinetic extensor strength, single-legged hop for distance, co-contraction test, or carioca test. In a meta-analysis of clinical outcomes after combined ACL and ALL reconstruction compared to isolated ACL reconstruction, Delaloye et al. found that the overall graft failure rate was less than 3% at 2 years after surgery. Comparison analysis in a high-risk population demonstrated that the graft failure rate in combined ACL and ALL reconstruction was 2.5 times lower than with isolated bone–patellar tendon–bone graft and 3.1 times lower than with isolated hamstring graft. The medial meniscal repair failure rate was also two times lower in the combined ACL and ALL reconstructions group compared to isolated ACL reconstruction group. However, return to sport and functional outcomes did not show any significant difference between groups. Further research with long-term follow-up is needed to determine if ALL reconstruction impacts the natural history of ACL reconstruction.

RECONSTRUCTION OF THE ANTEROLATERAL LIGAMENT

TECHNIQUE 1.8

- Harvest a gracilis tendon autograft with a tendon stripper as described in Technique 1.23, and whipstitch the end of the graft.
- Make a femoral stab incision slightly proximal and posterior to the lateral epicondyle and a tibial stab incision 22 mm posterior to Gerdy's tubercle (approximately halfway between the tubercle and the center of the fibular head) (Fig. 1.72A).
- Through the femoral stab wound, insert a 2.4-mm guide pin 8 mm proximal and 4.3 mm posterior to the lateral epicondyle. When drilling this guide pin, aim slightly anterior and proximal to avoid drilling into the femoral socket of the ACL reconstruction.
- After the pin is drilled, split the iliotibial band around it with a scalpel to facilitate insertion of a suture anchor (Fig. 1.72B).
- Through the fibular stab wound, drill a 2.4-mm guide pin 22 mm posterior to Gerdy's tubercle and 10 mm distal to the joint line (Fig. 1.72C).
- Test the isometry of the graft by wrapping a Fiber-Wire (Arthrex, Naples, FL) around the pins and moving the knee through a range of motion (Fig. 1.72D). When the FiberWire is held taut at extension, the graft should be isometric or become slightly shorter by no more than 5 mm as it moves to 90 degrees of flexion. If it becomes shorter by more than 5 mm, adjust the femoral pin.
- Overdrill the femoral guide pin with a 4.5-mm cannulated drill to a depth of 20 mm.
- Load the whipstitched sutures of the gracilis graft through the eyelet of a 4.75-mm SwiveLock anchor (Arthrex, Naples, FL).

- Insert the SwiveLock into the drilled hole. Make sure the eyelet is fully seated so that the threads of the anchor have started to touch the bone. Hold the paddle of the SwiveLock and turn the knob to insert the anchor (Fig. 1.72E). The SwiveLock sutures can be removed.
- Overdrill the tibial guide pin with a 7-mm cannulated drill to a depth of 20 mm.
- Use a curved hemostat to dissect underneath the iliotibial band to create a plane from the femoral incision to the tibial incision (Fig. 1.72F). Place a passing suture from distal to proximal with the hemostat. Use the passing suture to pass the graft to the tibial side (Fig. 1.72G).
- Hold the graft to the drilled hole and mark it at that location. Whipstitch 20 mm of the graft distally from the mark, using a no. 2 FiberLoop suture (Arthrex, Naples, FL) (Fig. 1.72H). This allows the whipstitched section to enter the drilled socket with the SwiveLock and increases the pull-out strength of the graft.
- Place the 7-mm forked Tenodesis SwiveLock anchor over the graft. Push the forked end into the tunnel and adjust tension by pulling on the graft (Fig. 1.72I). It is important not to overconstrain the ALL.
- Fix the anchor with the knee in extension and neutral rotation. Once the anchor is in place, the sutures can be removed. Cut the end of the graft exiting the tibial socket (Fig. 1.72J).

POSTOPERATIVE CARE Patients are allowed to begin a standard ACL rehabilitation program, with full weight bearing, without a brace, and progressive range-of-motion exercises. A gradual return to sports activities is allowed starting at 4 months for nonpivoting sports, at 6 months for pivoting noncontact sports, and at 8 to 9 months for pivoting contact sports.

If repair of acute lateral side injuries is anticipated, the surgery should be done within 2 to 3 weeks of the injury before tissue quality deteriorates and loses the ability to hold sutures and identification of structures becomes difficult. The surgeon should also be prepared to augment the repairs because many of them may be tenuous.

REPAIR OF LATERAL COMPARTMENT DISRUPTIONS

TECHNIQUE 1.9

- Place the patient supine with a sandbag beneath the ipsilateral hip to slightly tilt the patient to the opposite side. A bolster beneath the thigh to hold the knee near 90 degrees of flexion may be preferred. Apply a pneumatic tourniquet and inflate it. Keep the knee flexed for the skin incision, surgical approach, exposure, and repair.
- Begin a midlateral incision 2 cm proximal to the level of the patella, directly over and in line with the fibers of the iliotibial band (Fig. 1.73A), 3 cm lateral to the patella and

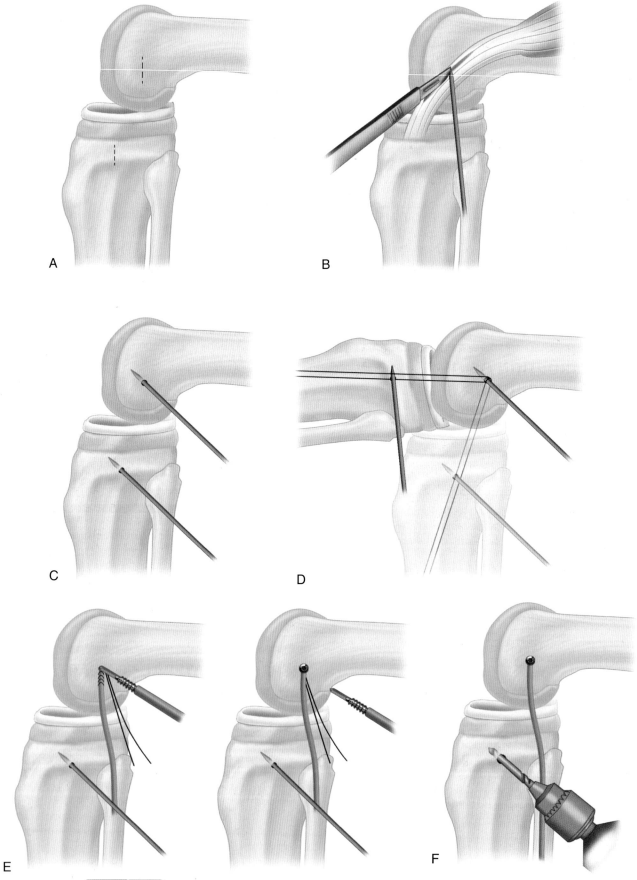

FIGURE 1.72   Reconstruction of the anterolateral ligament. **A,** Incisions. **B,** Splitting of the iliotibial band. **C,** Guide pin inserted 22 mm posterior to Gerdy's tubercle and 10 mm distal to joint line. **D,** Testing of graft isometry. **E,** Insertion of the SwiveLock. **F,** Overdrilling of the tibial guide pin with a 7-mm cannulated drill to a depth of 20 mm.

Continued

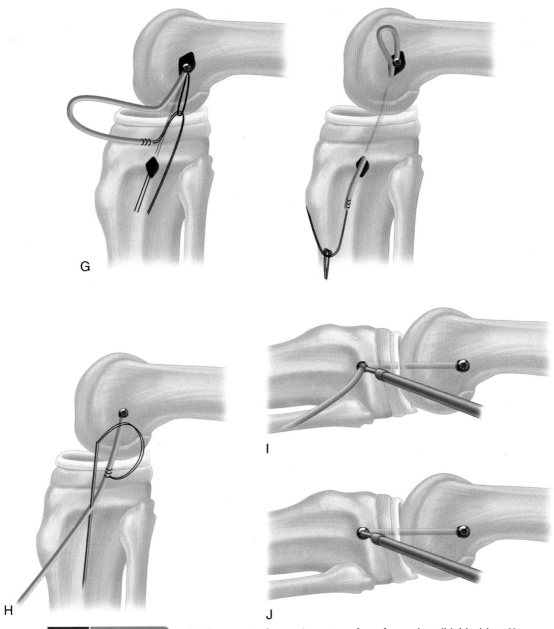

FIGURE 1.72 Cont'd   **G,** Placement of a passing suture from femoral to tibial incision. **H,** Whipstitching of the graft. **I,** Placement of a SwiveLock anchor over graft. **J,** Fixation of the anchor. (Redrawn from Arthrex Surgical Technique Guide, Arthrex Inc., Naples, FL, 2016.) **SEE TECHNIQUE 1.8.**

patellar tendon and parallel to these structures. Proceed with the incision distally over the region of the tubercle of insertion of the iliotibial band (Gerdy's tubercle), ending it approximately 4 cm distal to the joint.

- Dissect the skin, subcutaneous tissue, and superficial fascia as a single layer off the deep fascia to expose the entire lateral aspect of the knee from the midpatella anteriorly to the posterolateral corner.
- Inspect the deep structures for hematoma that may indicate the site of significant pathologic changes.
- Identify the common peroneal nerve deep to the biceps tendon and around the neck of the fibula and carefully protect it. With severe lateral compartment disruptions, stretching or disruption of the common peroneal nerve may occur. The preoperative functional status of the nerve should have

been noted and recorded. Towne et al. and Novich and Newark recommended early exploration of a nonfunctioning peroneal nerve with definitive repair as indicated. We advocate tagging the ends of the nerve when complete disruption exists to make them easy to locate for later repair.

- The nerve occasionally sustains a stretching type of injury with intrafascicular disruption at numerous levels and therefore is not suitable for a successful repair. Even then, when repair is indicated, microscopic technique at a later, more optimal time is preferred.
- With severe lateral disruptions, the biceps femoris insertion into the fibula may be avulsed with a small piece of bone and the iliotibial band also may be torn.
- Once wide exposure has been achieved and the iliotibial band, biceps femoris, and common peroneal nerve have

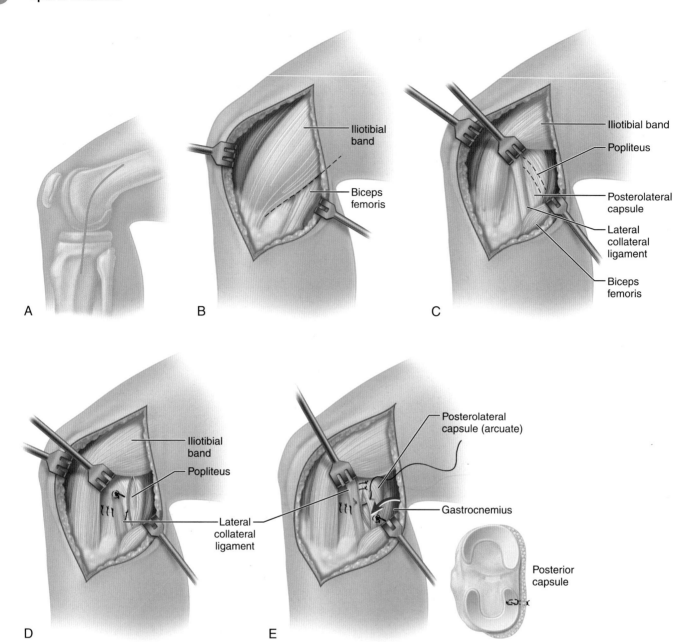

FIGURE 1.73 Repair of acute lateral compartment (collateral ligament) disruption. **A,** Skin incision (see text). **B,** Entering between posterior edge of iliotibial band and anterior edge of biceps femoris. **C,** Exposure of midlateral and posterolateral capsular structures and lateral collateral ligament. **D,** Reattachment of lateral collateral ligament and popliteal tendon to femur after repair of lateral capsule. **E,** Advancing lateral edge of posterolateral capsule anteriorly and suturing to midlateral capsule and posterior edge of lateral collateral ligament. Lateral edge of lateral head of gastrocnemius muscle is sutured as far anteriorly as possible over reconstructed ligament complex. **SEE TECHNIQUE 1.9.**

been inspected, stress test the knee for localization of ligamentous and capsular instability. This usually will correspond with the areas of hemorrhage.

- Make an anterolateral parapatellar capsular incision and explore the interior of the joint.
- If arthroscopy has not been carried out, carefully inspect and palpate the lateral meniscus, the cruciate ligaments, and the anterior two thirds of the medial meniscus. Placement of the knee in the figure-four position (hip flexed and externally rotated and the heel on the opposite knee)

often permits sufficient varus opening of the joint to allow complete visibility of the lateral meniscus and lateral compartment.

- If the lateral meniscus is irreparably torn, excise it completely or subtotally at this time. Retain as much of its peripheral rim as possible.
- If the periphery of the meniscus can be sutured, delay this until further lateral and posterolateral exposure is accomplished.
- If the ACL is torn, it should be reconstructed.

- If the ACL is avulsed from its tibial attachment and no medial compartment abnormality is noted, sutures can be placed in the ligament through the lateral arthrotomy incision.
- Treat any PCL tears in a similar manner, usually through an additional medial approach.
- If the iliotibial band and biceps femoris are intact, locate the interval between the posterior edge of the iliotibial band and the anterior edge of the biceps femoris (Fig. 1.73B). Separate them sharply and retract the iliotibial band anteriorly and the biceps with the common peroneal nerve posteriorly. This exposes the midlateral and posterolateral capsular structures and the LCL (Fig. 1.73C).
- It is often impossible to achieve adequate exposure of the area of the tears through this interval between the anterior edge of the biceps and the posterior edge of the iliotibial tract.
- If exposure of this deeper layer (layer II in the classification of Warren and Marshall) of the lateral compartment is not adequate, reflect the insertion of the iliotibial tract and its anterior expansion from Gerdy's tubercle with a button of bone; be careful not to cut into the articular surface of the tibia as the osteotomy detaches it. Reflect this layer proximally to the level of the lateral femoral epicondyle and the lateral intermuscular septum.
- If the posterior third of the iliotibial tract is released from its attachment at the epicondyle, or if it is torn as is commonly found, it must be anchored to this site at the completion of the repair when the insertion is secured to Gerdy's tubercle. This proximal reflection of the iliotibial tract and the lateral patellar extensor retinaculum uncovers the deepest layer (layer III) of the lateral compartment and allows careful identification of the important stabilizing structures of the posterolateral corner. Dissection and identification of these structures are critical in the repair.
- The posterolateral corner often sustains the most severe injury in lateral compartment disruptions. The interior of the posterior compartment can be explored through tears of the posterolateral capsule, but an anterolateral arthrotomy is usually needed for thorough exploration of the joint.
- If the capsular tear is not large enough to allow thorough inspection of the posterior horn of the lateral meniscus and the tibial insertion of the PCL, make a vertical incision in the capsule between the LCL and the popliteal tendon. Take care not to cut the popliteal tendon as it courses from its posterior origin through the capsular hiatus and attaches deep to and anterior to the LCL.
- With the knee flexed to 90 degrees to relax the posterior capsule for retraction, inspect the posterior horn of the lateral meniscus and the tibial insertion of the PCL. This incision also permits determination of the extent of tear in the posterolateral capsule. As with tears in the posteromedial corner, they may extend from the corner all the way to the midline posteriorly.
- The posterior capsule is not as distinctly identifiable laterally as it is medially because of the passage of the popliteus from its attachment to the back of the tibia through a hiatus in the coronary ligament to its attachment on the lateral femoral condyle just anterior to the LCL. Repair of this posterior capsule medial to the posterolateral corner is therefore difficult and probably not required. Far more important is the careful repair of the arcuate and fabellofibular complexes, the midlateral capsule, the LCL, the popliteus, the popliteofibular ligament, and the iliotibial tract.
- If the posterolateral capsule requires repair, it should be repaired in a manner similar to that described for the pos-

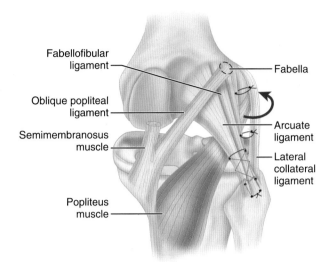

FIGURE 1.74 Posterolateral structures of knee and arcuate and fabellofibular ligament complexes. **SEE TECHNIQUE 1.9.**

(Labels in figure: Fabellofibular ligament; Oblique popliteal ligament; Semimembranosus muscle; Popliteus muscle; Fabella; Arcuate ligament; Lateral collateral ligament)

teromedial capsule, preferably pulling it below the articular surface of the tibia and securing it to the tibia with suture anchors or sutures placed through the edge of the capsule and passed to the anterior surface of the tibia through holes drilled from anterior to posterior (Fig. 1.73E). Freshen or roughen the back of the tibia at the site of reattachment with an osteotome before securing the capsule in place.

- Identify the LCL and determine where it is torn. It may be avulsed from its femoral origin, torn in its midportion, or avulsed from its fibular attachment (Fig. 1.73D). If the tip of the fibula has been avulsed, often the biceps tendon, the fibular attachment of the LCL, and the fibular styloid attachment of the arcuate ligament, popliteofibular ligament, and fabellofibular ligament have come off together. This is the optimal situation for repair of the posterolateral structures.
- Next determine whether the popliteal tendon and the popliteofibular ligament have been torn. The popliteal tendon comes through the hiatus in the coronary ligament at the posterolateral aspect of the meniscus, runs deep to the LCL, and inserts onto the femoral condyle anterior to the LCL insertion. The popliteofibular ligament arises from the posterior part of the fibula and joins the popliteal tendon just above the musculotendinous junction. Warren et al. demonstrated the importance of this ligament for posterolateral stability.
- The midlateral capsule (lateral capsular ligament) is a strong thickening in the capsule just anterior to the LCL, and it may avulse a fragment of metaphyseal bone from the tibial articular margin in severe lateral disruptions (the lateral capsular sign, or Segond fracture). Careful inspection of and traction on the popliteal tendon with a ligament hook will generally determine if it is torn. It can escape injury in posterolateral disruptions of the static ligaments because it is dynamic and can stretch to some extent.
- If the tendon appears intact but tension is soft when traction is applied with the ligament hook, suspect a tear at the musculotendinous junction just posteroinferior to the popliteal hiatus. These tears often are missed and can result in significant posterolateral instability. Such tears are difficult to repair but must be sought.
- Now identify the arcuate, popliteofibular, and fabellofibular ligament complexes (Fig. 1.74). The arcuate and fabellofibular ligaments insert onto the fibular styloid and ascend

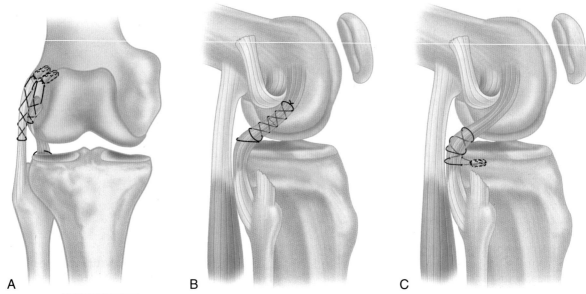

FIGURE 1.75 **A,** Repair of femoral attachment avulsion of lateral collateral ligament and popliteal tendon with use of transosseous drill holes. **B,** Repair of midsubstance tear of popliteal tendon with Bunnell-type suture. **C,** Repair of musculotendinous avulsion of popliteus by tenodesis of tendon to posterior aspect of tibia with Bunnell-type transosseous sutures. **SEE TECHNIQUE 1.9.**

vertically to their femoral attachments with the lateral head of the gastrocnemius. The popliteofibular ligament ascends to blend with the popliteal tendon. No severe posterolateral instability will exist without tears in these structures. Locate the area of tear in preparation for a systematic repair.

- Now close the anterolateral capsular incision with continuous 3-0 absorbable sutures for the synovium and multiple interrupted nonabsorbable sutures for the capsule and retinaculum.
- If the popliteus is torn, repair it first. If it is avulsed from its femoral attachment and the LCL also is avulsed from the femur, using suture anchors reattach the two structures to a raw bony bed with Bunnell-type sutures in each, or place the sutures and pull them through holes drilled across the femur and tied over a bony bridge over the medial femoral epicondylar area (Fig. 1.75A).
- If the popliteal tendon is torn within its substance, approximate its ends with a Bunnell-type suture of nonabsorbable material (Fig. 1.75B).
- If it is torn distal to the popliteal hiatus near its musculotendinous junction, repair is difficult at best. Mobilize the arcuate and fabellofibular complexes and the lateral head of the gastrocnemius for exposure and then insert approximating sutures.
- If the tear is within the muscle or is so near the musculotendinous junction that suture purchase is impossible, attach the tendon to the back of the tibia using suture anchors or by inserting a Bunnell-type suture in the tendon (no. 2 Polydek) and passing the sutures through holes drilled to exit on the anterolateral surface of the tibia near Gerdy's tubercle (Fig. 1.75C).
- If the repair of the popliteus is tenuous, it can be augmented with a strip of iliotibial band. Harvest and tube a strip of iliotibial band 2 cm wide, leaving it attached to Gerdy's tubercle. Using a standard ACL drill guide, create a tunnel the size of the graft from anterior to posterior in

the proximal lateral tibia, 2 cm below and parallel to the joint line and exiting where the popliteal tendon crosses the tibia. Pass the graft anterior to posterior through the tunnel and secure it to the popliteal tendon from the tibia to the femur with sutures.
- If the popliteofibular ligament is torn, repair it with sutures.
- If the ligament has been avulsed from the fibular styloid, it may be repaired back to the styloid with suture anchors or sutures may be placed in the ligament, passed through holes drilled in the fibula from posterior to anterior, and tied over a bony bridge.
- When augmentation is required for the popliteofibular ligament, harvest the central third of the biceps tendon by dissecting the tendon free of its muscle belly.
- Leave this strip of tendon attached to the fibula, extend it proximally 12 cm, and transect it. Because the biceps tendon insertion on the fibula is anterior to the normal posterior insertion of the popliteofibular ligament, the graft must be passed posterior and beneath the remaining posterior third of the biceps tendon.
- Place the graft under tension and suture it to the posterior fibula to re-create the fibular origin of the popliteofibular ligament.
- Then pass the graft under the remaining biceps tendon and the posterior half of the iliotibial band to the lateral femur.
- Free the peroneal nerve from the biceps tendon to prevent tension on the nerve when the graft is advanced.
- Determine the isometric point for femoral fixation by drilling a Kirschner wire near the femoral attachment of the LCL. Bring the graft over the Kirschner wire and mark with methylene blue where it touches the wire. Move the knee through a range of motion and observe the relationship between the mark and the wire. Reposition the Kirschner wire until there is minimal movement of the mark with respect to the wire.
- Once this isometric position has been determined, secure the graft to the femur with a 6.5-mm cancellous screw

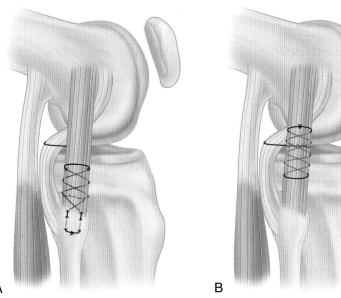

FIGURE 1.76 **A,** Repair of avulsion of fibular attachment of lateral collateral ligament with Bunnell-type suture. **B,** Repair of midsubstance tear of lateral collateral ligament with Bunnell-type suture. **SEE TECHNIQUE 1.9.**

and ligament washer and to the remaining popliteal tendon with interrupted sutures.

- Now begin repair of the LCL. The technique chosen depends on the level of the tear.
- Secure avulsions from the femoral or fibular attachments to bone with suture anchors or place Bunnell-type nonabsorbable sutures and pass through bone tunnels (Fig. 1.76A). Rarely will the LCL avulse a sufficient fragment of bone to allow reattachment with a screw or staple.
- If it is torn within its substance, approximate the ends with nonabsorbable sutures (Fig. 1.76B). Reinforce this tenuous repair by fashioning a strip of biceps tendon (6 to 8 cm long), leaving a distal attachment to the fibula. Place this strip lengthwise over the LCL, suture it to the ligament, and secure it at the femoral attachment of the ligament with multiple nonabsorbable sutures or a 6.5-mm cancellous screw and ligament washer.
- If the midlateral capsular ligament has been avulsed, reattach it with suture anchors or nonabsorbable sutures pulled through holes drilled across the tibial plateaus and tied over a bony bridge medially.
- Now direct attention to the arcuate, popliteofibular, and fabellofibular ligament complexes.
- If they have been torn from their fibular styloid attachment, secure them with nonabsorbable sutures.
- If they have been torn at the upper end, secure them to the periosteum beneath the lateral head of the gastrocnemius.
- If they have been torn within their substance, approximate them under tension with multiple interrupted, nonabsorbable sutures.
- Increase tension by advancing their lateral edge anteriorly around the posterolateral corner and suturing it to the posterior edge of the midlateral capsule and posterior edge of the LCL (see Fig. 1.73E).
- It is necessary to secure this arcuate ligament complex around the posterolateral corner to restore lateral compartment stability.

- Then bring the lateral edge of the lateral head of the gastrocnemius as far anteriorly as possible and secure it over the reconstructed arcuate ligament complex.
- Close the interval between the posterior edge of the iliotibial band and the biceps femoris with interrupted sutures.
- If the iliotibial tract and lateral patellar retinaculum have been released from Gerdy's tubercle and reflected proximally for exposure, secure the button of bone back in its bed on the anterolateral tibia with a staple or a screw with a toothed washer.
- If the posterior third of the iliotibial tract was torn or detached from the lateral epicondylar area near the lateral intermuscular septum, secure it to a bony bed. We prefer to do this with suture anchors. Alternatively, it can be repaired by placing a crisscrossing, Bunnell fashion, large no. 2 nonabsorbable suture, passing it through holes drilled across the femur to the opposite side, and tying it over a bony bridge. Failure to restore this epicondylar attachment of the iliotibial tract may result in varus instability and permit excessive internal rotation, especially if the ACL is also deficient.
- If stability remains precarious because of the quality of the tissues repaired or the pathologic condition, transfers of the biceps tendon, gastrocnemius muscle, and iliotibial band can be done to reinforce the repair. These procedures are described in a subsequent section on reconstruction.
- Close the incision over suction drainage tubes after the tourniquet has been deflated and hemostasis is obtained.

POSTOPERATIVE CARE The repair can be protected by applying a long-leg cast with the knee flexed 30 degrees, but we prefer to allow immediate protected motion by placing the knee in a controlled motion brace, which initially is locked in full extension. The leg is removed from the brace several times each day for range-of-motion exercises.

■ RECONSTRUCTION OF LATERAL COMPARTMENT

Similar to medial compartment reconstruction, lateral reconstruction should be done to correct functional deficiencies and not simply for anatomic restoration. Lateral instabilities usually are complex and include rotary as well as varus and anteroposterior components. The first requisite is an accurate classification of the instability. This knowledge permits a rational surgical technique. When the lateral side injury is associated with a cruciate injury, there is a debate about staging the repairs or reconstructions or treating them simultaneously.

The basic surgical principles are the same as those for the medial side: (1) restoration of normal tension of the capsular and collateral ligamentous structures from the midlateral axis of the tibia to the midline posteriorly, (2) reinforcement of the structures by fascial suture when tissue quality is poor, (3) meniscal retention if it can be repaired, (4) reinforcement of the reconstructed tissues with dynamic transfers, and (5) proper postoperative care and rehabilitative measures. Most lateral compartment reconstructions are required for complex combined rotary instabilities. Thus the techniques described usually are combined with anterior or posterior cruciate reconstruction.

The most common types of lateral instability are anterolateral rotary instability, posterolateral rotary instability, and combined anterolateral-anteromedial rotary instability. Obviously not every lateral compartment instability requires all of the procedures described here. The surgeon must determine during the operation which procedure is required alone or which combination of procedures is required on the basis of the location and degree of laxity, the severity of scarring, and the quality of tissue available for reconstruction.

During the preoperative evaluation, the knee should be inspected carefully for any signs of bony varus alignment and varus thrust during ambulation. Noyes described a triple varus knee that had genu varum alignment, soft-tissue varus instability, and lateral or varus thrust in the stance phase of ambulation. Soft-tissue reconstructions alone in such knees will fail because varus forces will stretch out the repair; valgus osteotomy should be done before or at the time of posterolateral stabilization. Correction of bony malalignment will protect the reconstruction and may eliminate the symptoms of instability without the need for soft-tissue reconstruction. A cadaver study showed that a proximal tibial medial opening wedge osteotomy decreased varus and external rotation laxity in posterolateral corner–deficient knees, owing in part to tightening of the superficial MCL. The long-term consequences of the increased force on the superficial MCL are unknown.

Anterior and posterior translation of the tibia on the femur, as well as rotary instability, can be controlled by extraarticular procedures, by an intraarticular substitution for the anterior cruciate or PCL, or by a combination of intraarticular and extraarticular reconstruction. Intraarticular cruciate substitution is described in the sections on anterior cruciate and posterior cruciate reconstruction. Common extraarticular procedures use the iliotibial band, the biceps, and the gastrocnemius as a part of or a supplement to capsular and collateral ligamentous reconstruction.

■ POSTEROLATERAL ROTARY INSTABILITY

Patients with isolated PCL deficiencies frequently do not have major symptoms of knee instability; however, if the PCL disruption is associated with other deficiencies, severe, disabling instability is common. One of the most common and disabling types is posterolateral rotatory instability. In addition to the posterior tibial translation, the tibia is excessively externally rotated, causing a severe reverse pivot shift phenomenon. Because selective sectioning of the PCL alone does not increase external rotation, increased external rotation associated with PCL tears indicates posterolateral instability. In such instability, reconstruction of the PCL alone, with persistent excessive external rotation of the tibia, may cause medial rotation of the tibial insertion of the PCL graft and laxity of the graft because of the shortened distance to its medial femoral condylar attachment. Furthermore, failure to treat laxity in the posterolateral corner leads to increased stress and higher failure rates after ACL and PCL reconstructions.

Numerous techniques for reconstruction of the posterolateral structures have been suggested, but none has had universal success. We usually attempt to correct this difficult instability by PCL reconstruction combined with posterolateral corner reconstruction, attempting to reestablish the LCL along with the arcuate and popliteus complexes as described earlier in this chapter (see Technique 1.9). Although Hughston and Jacobson reported excellent results with their technique for lateral and posterolateral instability, critics argue that this reconstruction is not isometric and consequently stretches out over time. In our experience, this technique is adequate for mild-to-moderate posterolateral instability but is not sufficient for severe instability associated with PCL disruption. The procedure should not be performed if posterolateral tissues are inadequate, thinned, or scarred (these knees require graft reconstruction) or in varus-aligned knees. In this instance, PCL reconstruction (intraarticular) should be combined with posterolateral reconstruction by the technique described by Müller, Clancy, Warren, Noyes, LaPrade, Yang, or Larson (Video 1.1).

RECONSTRUCTION OF THE POSTEROLATERAL STRUCTURES FOR MILD-TO-MODERATE POSTEROLATERAL INSTABILITY

TECHNIQUE 1.10

(HUGHSTON AND JACOBSON)

- After the induction of general anesthesia, do another complete examination of the knee ligaments and compare the findings with the preoperative evaluation.
- After the lower limb has been prepared and draped, make an anteromedial incision (described later) that will permit examination of the menisci, patella, anterior and PCLs, femoral condyles, tibial plateaus, and suprapatellar pouch.
- With the knee joint open, repeat the examination of the ligaments; use a ruler to measure the amounts of tibiofemoral displacement.
- Flex the knee to 90 degrees with the knee upright and the foot in a weight-bearing position on the operating table.
- Make a lateral hockey-stick incision beginning over the anterolateral aspect of the leg at a point between Gerdy's tubercle and the tibial tuberosity. Extend the incision proximally

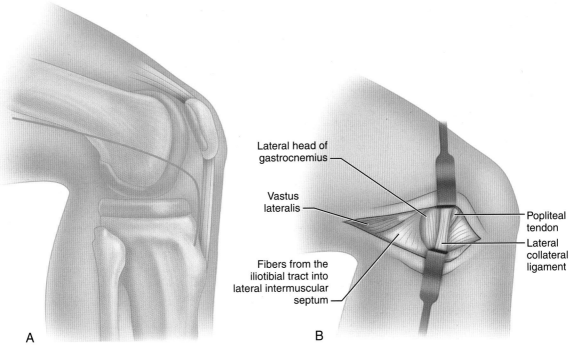

Lateral head of gastrocnemius

Vastus lateralis

Popliteal tendon

Lateral collateral ligament

Fibers from the iliotibial tract into lateral intermuscular septum

A   B

FIGURE 1.77   **A,** Initial incision for lateral reconstruction. **B,** Retraction of iliotibial band reveals superficial surface of lateral capsular ligament, popliteal tendon, and lateral collateral ligament. (Redrawn from Hughston JC, Jacobson KE: Chronic posterolateral rotatory instability of the knee, *J Bone Joint Surg* 67A:351, 1985.) **SEE TECHNIQUE 1.10.**

about 2 cm anterior and parallel to the posterior margin of the iliotibial tract for approximately 20 cm (Fig. 1.77A).

- Develop a posterior flap between the superficial and deep fascial planes to maintain the blood and nerve supplies and to minimize scarring.
- Incise the deep fascia posterior to the biceps tendon and identify and mobilize the common peroneal and lateral sural nerves from their surrounding fascia. If the common peroneal nerve is not mobilized, it may become displaced into a tortuous course by the advancement of the muscle-tendon units and ligaments during the reconstruction.
- Then identify the tendon of the lateral head of the gastrocnemius distally and mobilize it proximally as it passes deep to the biceps tendon and the iliotibial tract.
- Next, longitudinally incise the iliotibial band in line with its fibers, approximately 2 cm anterior to its palpable posterior border, thereby separating the band anteriorly from the tract posteriorly.
- Extend this incision from the midpoint of Gerdy's tubercle to approximately 5 cm proximal to the lateral femoral condyle. Retraction of this fascial incision reveals the superficial surface of the lateral capsular ligament, with an outline of the deep structures, the popliteal tendon, the LCL, and the mobilized lateral tendon of the gastrocnemius (Fig. 1.77B).
- Palpate the origin of the popliteal tendon in the groove just anterior to the lateral epicondyle of the femur and make a lateral capsular incision beginning superiorly approximately 2 mm anterior to this tendon (Fig. 1.78A). The incision remains anterior to the LCL and extends distally to the level of the lateral meniscus. Avoid the popliteal recess with this oblique incision and continue the incision in a vertical direction distally through the meniscotibial portion of the capsule.

- With the retractors in place, perform a posterolateral drawer test to confirm and to measure the amount of posterolateral displacement by observing the external rotation and posterior subluxation of the lateral tibial plateau. Again examine the lateral meniscus. If it is torn, remove it or repair it as described in Technique 1.1.
- Next, incise the iliotibial band at its anterior border in line with its fibers that separate it from the fascia lata, free it from the underlying synovial tissues and vastus lateralis, and retract it posteriorly to expose the area of the lateral femoral condyle.
- In the posterolateral area of the exposure, make an incision along the lateral border of the lateral gastrocnemius tendon through the posterior part of the capsule (arcuate ligament fibers) distally to the level of the popliteal tendon and its aponeurosis (Fig. 1.78B, *line AB*).
- Then, with an osteotome, outline the lateral femoral epicondyle anterior and proximal to the attachments of the popliteus, the LCL, and the lateral gastrocnemius tendon and posterior to the gastrocnemius tendon attachment to create a bony flap with these structures attached (Fig. 1.78B, *line BC*). The bone mass should be 0.6 to 0.9 cm thick and should incorporate the underlying cancellous bone.
- Then remove the epicondyle with the osteotome by connecting the osteotomy cuts in the direction of the longitudinal axis of the femur.
- Retract this flap of bone and arcuate complex attachment posteriorly, bringing into view the intraarticular surfaces and courses of the structures of the arcuate complex (Fig. 1.78C).
- Elevate the periosteum of the lateral femoral condyle with an osteotome and retract it anteriorly at the edge of the osteotomy site in preparation for receiving the bony portion of the arcuate complex flap.

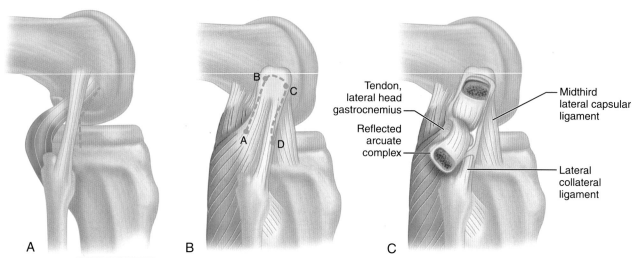

FIGURE 1.78 **A,** Lateral capsular incision just anterior to lateral collateral ligament and popliteal tendon insertion. **B,** Line AB is incision along lateral border of lateral gastrocnemius tendon. Line BC is edge of osteotomized area. Line CD is lateral capsular incision. **C,** Intraarticular structures exposed when arcuate ligament complex is folded back. Area prepared to receive bone mass also is shown. **SEE TECHNIQUE 1.10.**

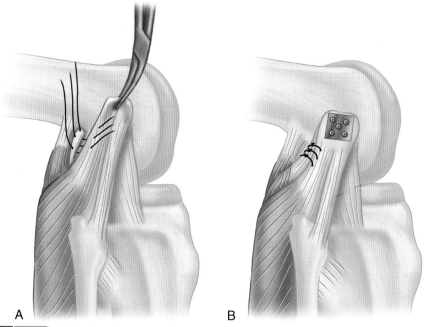

FIGURE 1.79 **A,** Most anterior sutures. **B,** Stone staple in place and advancement of arcuate ligament complex. Lateral part of capsule is advanced when there is an associated anterolateral rotary instability. **SEE TECHNIQUE 1.10.**

- However, before restoration is begun, remove the tourniquet, secure hemostasis, and irrigate the knee joint. Close the deep layers of the anteromedial incision.
- Keep the hip in approximately 45 degrees of flexion, flex the knee approximately 90 degrees, and hold the foot firmly on the operating table. Have an assistant hold the tibia in mild internal rotation while gently maintaining an anterior pull on the tibia to ensure a reduced and internally rotated posture of the tibiofemoral joint.
- Advance the arcuate complex flap and hold it at the point of its anticipated fixation to the lateral femoral condyle; place

mattress sutures in the posterior incision along the gastrocnemius tendon and the posterior part of the capsule, thus approximating the arcuate ligament at a point farther proximal than its original position. The most anterior sutures fix the arcuate ligament and the lateral gastrocnemius tendon to the periosteum at approximately the point of attachment of the lateral intermuscular septum (Fig. 1.79A). Posterolateral advancement and closure of the arcuate ligament are necessary for achieving and maintaining stability.
- Advance the bone plug with its attached arcuate ligament complex as tautly as possible anteriorly and proximally

and secure it to the previously prepared raw surface of the lateral femoral condyle with a table staple (Fig. 1.79B). Be sure that the staple fits flush against the soft-tissue attachments to the bone plug.

- Now perform the posterolateral drawer test again to determine if the instability has been corrected. If the drawer test result is still positive, take the reconstruction down and correct it. Lack of correction usually indicates that the arcuate complex has been insufficiently advanced, that the distal attachment has not been secured, or that the sutures have been incorrectly placed. If the knee has been stabilized, tie the previously placed sutures in the arcuate ligament.
- Next, close the anterolateral capsular incision.
- If anterolateral instability also is present, advance the lateral capsular ligament anteriorly and distally and suture it to the tibia.
- Under tension, suture the iliotibial tract to the lateral intermuscular septum.
- The biceps tendon may or may not be advanced onto the iliotibial tract fibers while an associated extraarticular anterolateral reconstructive procedure is performed.
- Then close the incisions in the iliotibial band and iliotibial tract.
- Reexamine the common peroneal nerve to make sure that the movement of tissues by the reconstruction has not placed it under tension.
- Obtain final hemostasis, close the subcutaneous tissues and skin, and apply a compressive dressing.
- Originally, Hughston and Jacobson recommended cast immobilization with the knee flexed to approximately 45 degrees and the tibia in slight internal rotation. More recently, a controlled motion brace has been used with the knee in 45 degrees of flexion.

POSTOPERATIVE CARE Range of motion is permitted in flexion, but extension is blocked in the terminal 45 degrees. Moving in flexion will not stretch the reconstructed lateral and posterolateral structures if the attachment sites are reasonably isometric. Any motion in flexion moves the articular surfaces, especially the patellofemoral joint. Failure to move the patellofemoral joint often results in troublesome and symptomatic chondromalacia. The brace is adjusted periodically to allow increasing extension beginning the third or fourth week. Partial weight bearing is permitted from the beginning, with the objective of full weight bearing when the brace is discontinued at 8 weeks, provided extension is within 5 degrees of full.

RECONSTRUCTION OF THE POPLITEAL TENDON USING THE ILIOTIBIAL BAND FOR POSTEROLATERAL INSTABILITY

TECHNIQUE 1.11

(MÜLLER)
- Müller stated that the key structures in the posterolateral corner of the knee in posterolateral rotary instability are the popliteus and its tendon.
- After obtaining lateral exposure as previously described, carefully determine the status of the popliteal tendon.

In many posterolateral rotary instabilities, the popliteal tendon will have been injured and is thin in the area just below its femoral insertion. Inspect the tendon from its femoral condylar insertion down through the hiatus in the lateral capsule to its musculotendinous junction.

- If the tendon is sound from the hiatus distally to the musculotendinous junction, advance its femoral attachment with a small block of bone as follows.
- Remove the insertion of the popliteus with a 1- × 1-cm plug of bone and, if sufficient laxity is present, wrap the tendon around the block by flipping the block over 180 degrees, pulling the tendon taut, and then reattaching the block in its original bed with a staple, a screw with a toothed washer, or transosseous sutures. With this technique, the tendon will advance by 1 to 1.5 cm.
- If the tendon is not lax enough to permit this technique, advance the bone plug proximally and anteriorly to place the popliteal tendon under adequate tension and secure it to a bony bed in a similar manner. According to Müller, it is important to advance and to adjust the tension on the popliteus and the LCL separately because these two critically important structures course in different directions. Advancing them together alters this normal anatomic arrangement.
- If the popliteal tendon has been stretched and thinned by a severe initial injury, create a substitution for the tendon and its function. This can be accomplished by several techniques.
- If the initial injury has occurred at the musculotendinous junction and sufficient distal tendon is present, attach the musculotendinous junction to the posterolateral tibia by means of a transosseous suture or suture anchor, as previously described in repairs of the lateral compartment.
- If this is impossible or if the tendon is absent, use a strip of tissue fashioned from the iliotibial band or biceps tendon to serve as a suitable replacement.
- If the iliotibial band is to be the donor, fashion a strip 1.0 to 1.5 cm wide from the midportion of the band long enough to pass from Gerdy's tubercle to the posterolateral corner of the knee and then diagonally back to the anatomic insertion of the popliteal tendon. Use a suture to estimate the desired length, which usually is 16 to 20 cm. Leave the strip of iliotibial band attached to Gerdy's tubercle and reflect it distally (Fig. 1.80A).
- Then use a 4.5-mm drill to create a tunnel through the lateral tibial plateau from anterior to posterior. The posterior hole should emerge just below the articular cartilage of the lateral tibial plateau adjacent to the normal groove for the popliteal tendon.
- Place a suture in the end of the strip of iliotibial band and pass the strip through the tunnel in the lateral tibial plateau from anterior to posterior with a suture passer. Pull it firmly through the opening in the bony tunnel at the posterolateral corner of the knee.
- Then weave it into the lateral capsule parallel to the normal course of the popliteal tendon and pull it up anteriorly and superiorly to the area of insertion of the popliteal tendon on the femur. Here, with the knee flexed 90 degrees and the tibia internally rotated, secure it under tension with a transosseous suture, a suture anchor, a staple, or a screw with a toothed washer (Fig. 1.80B). The passageway in the posterior capsule and arcuate complex is best developed with a curved clamp.

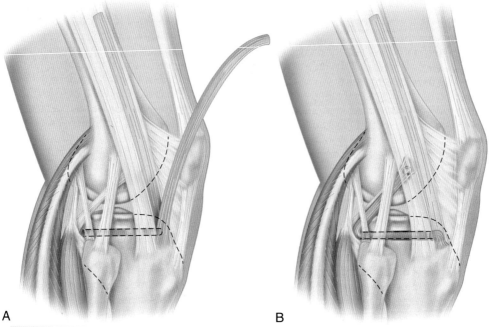

A   B

FIGURE 1.80   Popliteal bypass with use of graft from anterior portion of iliotibial tract. Graft is passed through transosseous tunnel from area of Gerdy's tubercle to posterolateral corner of knee **(A)**, grasping the popliteofibular ligament structures, and then diagonally **(B)**, replicating course of popliteal tendon. It is then attached near popliteus attachment on femur just anterior to lateral collateral ligament attachment. (From Müller W: *The knee: form, function, and ligamentous reconstruction*, New York, 1983, Springer-Verlag.) **SEE TECHNIQUE 1.11.**

- To aid in revascularization and recollagenization, cover the transplanted strip with synovium or other soft tissue throughout its course and do not let it communicate with the intraarticular structures.
- If the iliotibial band is not suitable as a donor, mobilize a strip of biceps tendon left attached to the fibula, with its length determined as previously described (Fig. 1.81A). The thickness of the strip should be approximately one third that of the biceps tendon.
- Then create a soft-tissue channel from the fibular head to the posterolateral corner of the tibia in the region of the groove for the popliteal tendon.
- Next, pass the tendon strip from the fibular head through this passageway in the tibia.
- At a site just below the articular cartilage adjacent to the groove for the popliteal tendon on the back of the tibia, freshen the bone with an osteotome. Anchor the biceps tendon strip here with a transosseous suture, suture anchor, or screw with a toothed washer so that its free portion can be pulled anteriorly and superiorly through the posterolateral capsule up to its attachment near the anatomic insertion of the popliteal tendon.
- Secure the end of the tendon strip to the femur with a transosseous suture, a suture anchor, a staple, or a screw with a toothed washer (Fig. 1.81B).
- Close the posterior arthrotomy incision with multiple absorbable sutures.
- Before further closure is undertaken, inspect the posterior capsule to be sure that it is not too lax; if it is, secure the posterior capsule and coronary ligament attachment of the posterior horn of the lateral meniscus to a freshened bony surface on the posterior tibia by transosseous sutures

or suture anchors (Fig. 1.82). If the midlateral capsule is lax just anterior to the LCL, pull it snugly down to a freshened bony bed by transosseous sutures or suture anchors.
- Once the reconstruction of the popliteal tendon and the coronary and capsular ligaments has been completed, reconstruct the arcuate ligament complex. It is often difficult to locate the site of an old tear in the arcuate ligament complex because of extensive posterolateral scarring.
- If the complex has been detached from its posterolateral attachment to the tibia, reattach it to a freshened bony surface by transosseous sutures or suture anchors just below the posterolateral tibial articular cartilage (Fig. 1.83).
- If it has been detached from the femur superiorly, advance it by transosseous sutures or suture anchors to a raw bony surface on the back of the lateral femoral condyle superior to the lateral articular margin.
- If the old tear has been in the midportion of the arcuate complex, it usually is necessary to advance this arcuate ligament complex anteriorly by pulling it around the posterolateral corner and suturing it to the posterior edge of the LCL.
- Again, posterolateral reconstructions generally are not for isolated injuries and often involve reconstructions of the anterior and PCLs. If these ligaments are to be reconstructed by intraarticular techniques, this should be done before the previously described techniques.
- Once the LCL has been reconstructed (Fig. 1.84), the popliteal tendon has been tightened or reconstructed by means of an iliotibial band or a biceps tendon strip, and the arcuate ligament complex has been advanced, close the posterolateral capsular structures with multiple interrupted sutures.

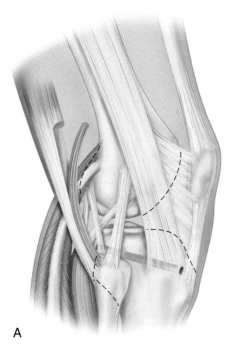
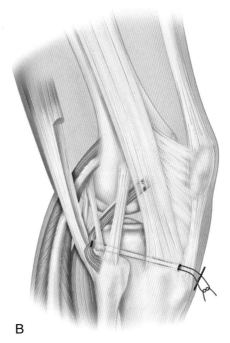

A   B

FIGURE 1.81   **A,** Popliteal bypass with use of pedicle graft from biceps tendon. **B,** This has effect of restoring portion of arcuate ligament attachment by reattaching arcuate ligament to back of tibia while simultaneously closing abnormal meniscal tibial recess that forms posterolaterally. (From Müller W: *The knee: form, function, and ligamentous reconstruction*, New York, 1983, Springer-Verlag.) **SEE TECHNIQUE 1.11.**

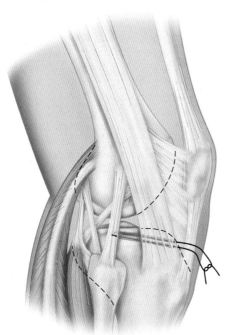

FIGURE 1.82   Repair of lateral coronary meniscal ligament. If Segond-type avulsion is present, suture should include arcuate expansions directly below coronary ligament, as well as posterior iliotibial fibers that course to posterior part of upper tibia. (From Müller W: *The knee: form, function, and ligamentous reconstruction*, New York, 1983, Springer-Verlag.) **SEE TECHNIQUE 1.11.**

- Then close the incision or defect in the iliotibial band with multiple interrupted sutures, with particular emphasis on reestablishing the posterior third of the iliotibial tract coursing from Gerdy's tubercle to its attachment over the lateral femoral epicondyle and lateral intermuscular septum area. This is most commonly done by use of transosseous sutures or suture anchors at the level of the femoral epicondyle, reestablishing the lateral static tibiofemoral ligamentous attachment.
- If the tissues are extensively scarred or attenuated, obtain a strip of fascia 15 to 20 cm long from the iliotibial band and use it, attached to a Gallie needle, to reinforce and snug up the posterolateral corner.
- For fascial reinforcement, the procedure up to this point is identical to that just described. Start the fascial suture inferiorly in the posterior edge of the lateral capsule and LCL (posterolateral arthrotomy incision) and run it posteriorly through the distal portion of the posterior capsule and the lateral edge of the arcuate ligament. Place several turns of fascia, proceeding from distal to proximal until the posterior capsular incision has been tightly closed. In addition to adding strength to the attenuated tissues, the fascial repair is designed to advance and to tighten the distal portion of the posterior capsule and arcuate ligament. Place the fascial sutures so that they do not penetrate the synovium.

We have used Müller's technique in a number of knees with severe posterolateral rotary instability, usually in combination with a PCL reconstruction with a portion of the patellar tendon. We have been concerned with the strength of the thin strip of iliotibial band fashioned as described by Müller. The

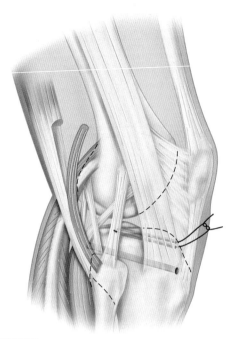

FIGURE **1.83**   In all peripheral repairs and reconstructions, deep layer also must be repaired. This includes reattachment of capsule and arcuate ligament to posterior tibia, fixation of lateral meniscus, and fixation of avulsed ligamentous fibers. Proximal attachment of arcuate ligament also must be restored where it passes to femur together with lateral gastrocnemius tendon. (From Müller W: *The knee: form, function, and ligamentous reconstruction*, New York, 1983, Springer-Verlag.) **SEE TECHNIQUE 1.11.**

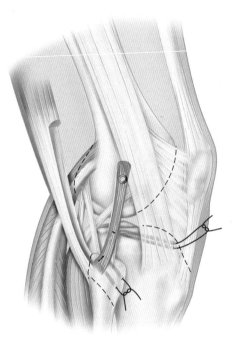

FIGURE **1.84**   Reconstruction of lateral collateral ligament with graft from biceps tendon. (From Müller W: *The knee: form, function, and ligamentous reconstruction*, New York, 1983, Springer-Verlag.) **SEE TECHNIQUE 1.11.**

anterior part of the band, especially proximally, is its weakest part, and this is the part of the strip that often traverses the posterolateral aspect of the tibia to the popliteal tendon insertion on the lateral femoral condyle. The biceps tendon strip is much stronger and is a better structure to transfer when the popliteal tendon must be replaced. We believe that allografts have provided us with more latitude and flexibility in replacing deficiencies at the posterolateral corner of the knee. Allograft materials, such as wide expanses of iliotibial band and semitendinosus, posterior tibial, and peroneus longus tendons, have provided a much stronger replacement for the popliteal tendon, and early results indicate that these are superior to thin strips of iliotibial band as described by Müller.

REROUTING OF THE BICEPS TENDON TO THE FEMORAL EPICONDYLE FOR POSTEROLATERAL INSTABILITY

TECHNIQUE 1.12

(CLANCY)
- Begin a lateral skin incision just at Gerdy's tubercle and carry it superiorly in a curvilinear fashion, ending approximately 15 cm proximally.

- Locate the lateral femoral epicondyle and incise the iliotibial band longitudinally where it overlies the lateral femoral epicondyle.
- Dissect the biceps tendon free of the surrounding soft tissues. Free the biceps muscle and tendon from their attachments to the lateral gastrocnemius muscle.
- Expose the peroneal nerve at the inferior portion of the biceps tendon and carefully dissect it free and protect it.
- Retract the biceps muscle anteriorly, exposing the peroneal nerve as it courses proximally. Free it from any attachments to the biceps muscle (Fig. 1.85A).
- Free the inferior portion of the iliotibial band from its attachments to the intermuscular septum. Bring the biceps tendon and muscle up underneath this inferior portion of the iliotibial band so that the tendon can be fixed to the lateral femoral epicondyle.
- Then dissect the epicondyle free of the surrounding soft tissues, exposing the superior insertional fibers of the FCL (Fig. 1.85B,C).
- Create a trough ½ inch wide × 1 inch long at the upper portion of the lateral femoral epicondyle, dissecting it proximally to the flare of the lateral condyle (Fig. 1.85D).
- Drill a 3.2-mm hole in the trough just superior to the lateral femoral epicondyle and slightly cephalad to the medial femoral condyle, avoiding the tunnel for the PCL graft in the condyle.
- Place a 6.5-mm screw with a spiked washer in the hole.
- Resect the distal 2 inches of the biceps muscle away from the tendon; otherwise, fixation of the tendon to the lateral femoral epicondylar trough is impossible because of interposition of the muscle.
- Bring the biceps tendon with its arcuate ligament attachments proximally, loop them over the screw, and fix them in place (Fig. 1.85E,F).

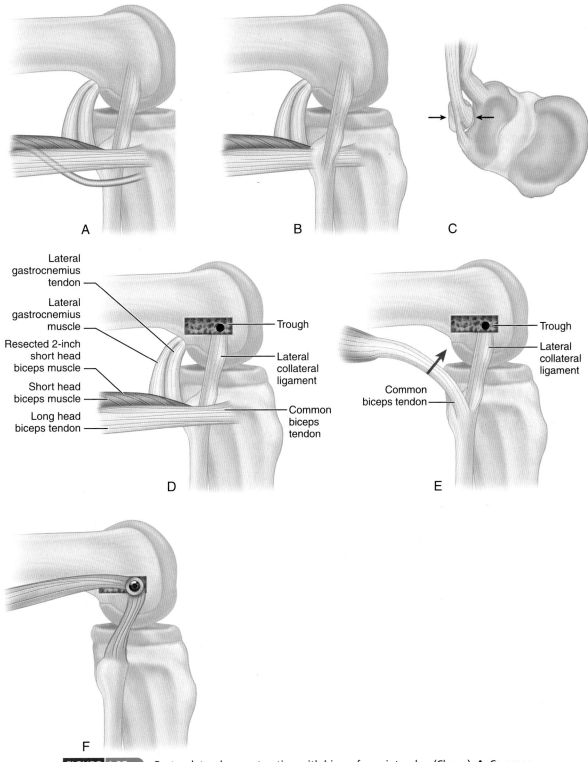

FIGURE 1.85   Posterolateral reconstruction with biceps femoris tendon (Clancy). **A,** Common peroneal nerve must be carefully dissected free; biceps muscle is freed from attachments to lateral gastrocnemius muscle and tendon. **B,** Superior insertion of lateral collateral ligament on lateral epicondyle. **C,** Insertions of common biceps tendon into arcuate complex posteriorly and horseshoe insertion around lateral collateral ligament. **D,** Trough is made in upper third of the lateral femoral epicondyle. Distal 5 cm of biceps muscle is removed to allow fixation of tendon to epicondyle. **E,** Tendon is brought anteriorly to trough in epicondyle. **F,** AO cancellous screw and washer are placed inferior to tendon and tightened to hold tendon in place. **SEE TECHNIQUE 1.12.**

- Move the knee through a full range of motion and again test varus laxity and external rotation. If static stability is satisfactory, place drains and close the wound.

POSTOPERATIVE CARE If the PCL has been reconstructed, the knee is held in full extension for about 6 weeks. If no other procedures have been performed or if the ACL has been reconstructed, the knee is held in approximately 30 degrees of flexion for 6 weeks.

LaPrade et al. described an anatomic posterolateral knee reconstruction based on the quantitative attachment anatomy of the LCL, the popliteus tendon, and the popliteofibular ligament. They reported improved clinical outcomes and objective stability in 64 patients with grade III chronic posterolateral instability at 4-year follow-up. Eighteen of their patients had isolated posterolateral knee reconstruction, and 46 had a single-stage multiple-ligament reconstruction that included one or both cruciate ligaments.

ANATOMIC POSTEROLATERAL KNEE RECONSTRUCTION FOR GRADE III POSTEROLATERAL INJURY

TECHNIQUE 1.13

(LAPRADE ET AL.)

- Make a hockey-stick incision to gain access to the posterolateral knee structures. Identify the attachment sites of the LCL on the lateral aspect of the fibular head and the popliteofibular ligament on the posteromedial aspect of the fibular styloid.
- With the help of a cannulated cruciate ligament reconstruction aiming device, drill a guide pin through the LCL attachment in a posteromedial direction toward the popliteofibular ligament attachment. Ream a 7-mm tunnel over the guide pin.
- Identify the posterior tibial popliteal sulcus, which marks the location of the musculotendinous junction of the popliteus muscle, by palpation through the interval between the lateral head of the gastrocnemius and the soleus.
- Drill a transtibial guide pin from anterior, at the flat spot just distal and medial to Gerdy's tubercle, to posterior at this sulcus. Use a large Chandler retractor to protect the neurovascular bundle.
- Ream a 9-mm tunnel over this guide pin and smooth the entry and exit sites with a rasp.
- Identify the femoral attachments of the LCL and the popliteus tendon. The midpoints of these two structures have been reported to be 18.5 mm apart.
- Drill two eyelet-tipped guide pins from lateral to anteromedial through the femur at these attachment sites. Use a 9-mm reamer to ream over these guide pins to a depth of 20 mm to prepare the femoral tunnels.
- If there is any intraarticular pathologic process to be treated, remove the guide pins and perform any arthroscopic intraarticular or cruciate ligament reconstruction procedures as needed.

- Once articular cartilage and meniscal abnormalities have been treated, pass the cruciate ligament grafts into their respective femoral tunnels and fix them there. The order for final graft fixation is (1) secure the PCL graft to the tibia, (2) secure the posterolateral grafts to the fibula and tibia, and (3) secure the ACL graft to the tibia.
- Prepare the grafts from an allogenic Achilles tendon, split lengthwise, and two 9 × 20 mm bone plugs prepared for the femoral tunnels. Tubularize the tendons and size them to fit through the fibular and tibial tunnels.
- Place the passing sutures in the bone plugs into the eyelet pins and pull the bone plugs into the femoral tunnels. Anchor the bone plugs in the superior aspect of the femoral tunnels with 7-mm cannulated interference screws.
- The graft anchored in the popliteal sulcus is used to reconstruct the static function of the popliteus tendon. Pass it distally through the popliteal hiatus.
- The second graft, anchored proximally and posterior to the lateral femoral epicondyle, is used to reconstruct both the lateral collateral and popliteofibular ligaments. Pass it medial (deep) to the superficial layer of the iliotibial band and the anterior arm of the long head of the biceps femoris, following the normal path of the LCL. Then pass the graft through the fibular tunnel in a posteromedial direction.
- Anchor the posterolateral graft passed through the fibular tunnel with a 7-mm cannulated screw with the knee in 30 degrees of flexion, the tibial in neutral rotation, and a slight valgus force applied to reduce any potential lateral compartment gapping.
- Use the remaining portion of the graft, which is now medial to the fibula, to reconstruct the popliteofibular ligament.
- Pass both the popliteofibular ligament graft and the popliteus tendon graft from posterior to anterior through the tibial tunnel and tighten them by applying an anterior force with the knee flexed 60 degrees and the tibia in neutral rotation.
- Fix the grafts in the tibial tunnel with a 9-mm cannulated interference screw (Fig. 1.86).

POSTOPERATIVE CARE Patients are kept non–weight bearing for the first 6 weeks after surgery. For the first 2 weeks, quadriceps sets and straight-leg raises are done in a knee immobilizer and range-of-motion exercises are done without the immobilizer, with a goal of at least 90 degrees of flexion by the end of the second week. These are continued for the next 4 weeks, during which time range of motion is increased as tolerated. Weight bearing is allowed at 7 weeks, and crutches are discontinued when the patient can walk without a limp or other subtle gait abnormalities or compensation patterns. Stationary bicycling is allowed once 105 to 110 degrees of knee flexion has been obtained. No active, isolated hamstring exercises are allowed for the first 4 months after surgery. Limited-resistance weight training is begun with one-quarter body weight and progressing to half of body weight as tolerated, but patients are instructed not to exceed 70 degrees of flexion while performing leg presses or minisquat exercises. Other weight-bearing exercises to restore joint proprioception and balance also are begun. From 4 to 6 months postoperatively, patients work on increasing endurance, strength, and proprioception. At 7 months (or 9 months for combined reconstructions), if cleared by their surgeon, patients are allowed to return to full competitive and pivot activities.

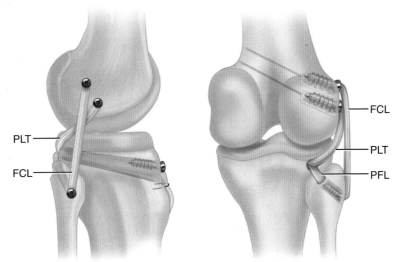

FIGURE 1.86 Graft and tunnel locations for anatomic posterolateral knee reconstruction. *FCL*, Fibular collateral ligament; *PLT*, popliteus tendon; *PFL*, popliteofibular ligament. (Redrawn from LaPrade RF, Johansen S, Wentorf FA, et al: An analysis of an anatomic posterolateral knee reconstruction: an in vitro biomechanical study and development of a surgical technique, *Am J Sports Med* 32:1405, 2004.) **SEE TECHNIQUE 1.13.**

Although described by LaPrade et al. as an anatomic reconstruction, tibial-fibular double-sling reconstruction is not completely anatomic and requires an extensive lateral approach. Several authors have described success with a single fibular or tibial sling technique, reporting restoration of varus and rotational stability. Yang et al. reported good clinical outcomes, with decreased external rotation, in 60 patients with fibular-sling reconstructions as described by Kim et al.

POSTEROLATERAL CORNER RECONSTRUCTION WITH A SINGLE ALLOGRAFT FIBULAR SLING

TECHNIQUE 1.14

(YANG ET AL.)
- After careful arthroscopic examination of the knee, make a curvilinear skin incision in the lateral aspect of the knee, extending from the lateral femoral epicondyle to the anterior aspect of the fibular head. Make the incision between the retinaculum and iliotibial band to expose the biceps tendon and the posterolateral corner of the knee.
- Identify the peroneal nerve and retract it with the biceps tendon.
- Identify the LCL, popliteal tendon, and patellofemoral ligament, and make two femoral tunnels just proximal to these anatomic locations.
- Place two guide pins just proximal to the lateral epicondyle and just distal to the popliteal tendon, followed by a 6-mm diameter cannulated reamer with a 30-mm depth.
- Direct the fibular head tunnel from the anteroinferior superficial aspect to the posterosuperior deep location,

making it 6 mm in diameter at the distal portion of the anatomic insertion site.
- Prepare a fresh-frozen anterior tibial tendon allograft with a diameter of 6 mm and a length of 24 to 27 mm. Place an interlocking Krackow suture in each end of the graft.
- Pull one end of the graft into the femoral socket for the popliteus tendon and tension it from the medial side of the knee by pulling on the passing suture. Fix the graft to the femur with a 7-mm bioabsorbable screw.
- Pass the free end of the graft under the iliotibial band and the original LCL to the posterosuperior portion of the fibular head through the soft spot between the LCL and the superior border of the biceps tendon.
- Pull the graft into the previously drilled 6-mm fibular tunnel and tension it from the anteroinferior side of the fibular head by pulling on the passing suture. Fix the graft to the fibula with a 7-mm bioabsorbable screw (Fig. 1.87).
- Pass the free end of the graft anteriorly under the iliotibial band again, pull it into the other femoral socket for the LCL, tension it, and fix it in the same manner.
- If the popliteus tendon is ruptured, expose its femoral attachment and repair it in a pull-out manner to the femoral socket of the graft.

POSTOPERATIVE CARE Postoperative rehabilitation protocol depends on the concomitant ligamentous reconstruction.

Noyes reported his results with use of allograft tissue to reconstruct the LCL in 21 patients. The success rate for the operative procedure was 76% as judged by knee stability examination and stress radiographs. The grafts used for the LCL reconstruction included a tendinous portion of the Achilles tendon, fascia lata, and bone–patellar tendon–bone. More recently, Noyes and Barber-Westin reported long-term (mean of 6 years) evaluation of 13 of the original patients: 9

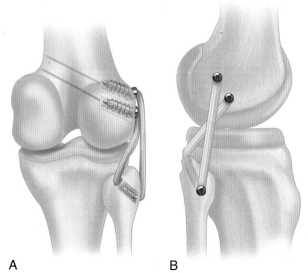

A   B

FIGURE 1.87   Posteroanterior **(A)** and lateral **(B)** views of single fibular sling procedure for posterolateral corner reconstruction. (Redrawn from Kim JG, Ha JG, Lee YS, et al: Posterolateral corner anatomy and its anatomical reconstruction with single fibula and double femoral sling method: anatomical study and surgical technique, *Arch Orthop Trauma Surg* 129:381, 2009.) **SEE TECHNIQUE 1.14.**

had no symptoms with low-impact sports; however, 2 with concurrent arthritis had symptoms with sports but not with daily activities, and 2 had symptoms with daily activities. Cited advantages of their technique include simplicity of graft placement and the ability to place a large doubled graft at the lateral side of the knee joint. They recommended the procedure for LCL replacement in acute posterolateral disruptions because repair of other disrupted posterolateral tissues usually is possible. They cited as a contraindication a knee with 5 degrees or more of varus recurvatum for which a popliteal-tibial graft is required to restore this portion of the posterolateral structures.

ALLOGRAFT RECONSTRUCTION OF THE LATERAL COLLATERAL LIGAMENT

TECHNIQUE 1.15

(NOYES)
- Make a straight lateral incision approximately 15 cm long centered over the lateral joint line; extend it distally to expose the fibular head and peroneal nerve and proximally to expose the attachment of the posterior collateral ligament to the femur.
- Identify the attachment of the iliotibial band and incise it along the anterior border proximally. Preserve the attachment of the iliotibial band to the lateral intermuscular septum.
- Make a second parallel inferior incision along the posterior aspect of the iliotibial band and the attachments overlying the biceps muscle. This creates a central portion

of the iliotibial band that can be reflected either anteriorly or posteriorly to expose the posterolateral aspect of the knee.
- If there is stretching of the iliotibial band and gross lateral joint opening, advance the iliotibial band at Gerdy's tubercle distally.
- Identify the peroneal nerve proximally and dissect it distally around the fibular neck until it enters the anterior tibial muscle compartment. Protect the nerve throughout the procedure, especially when holes are drilled through the head-neck junction of the fibula for placement of the posterior collateral ligament allograft.
- Expose the fibular head and neck region anteriorly and posteriorly by subperiosteal dissection. This should require only 12 to 15 mm of proximal fibular exposure.
- Drill a 6-mm hole from anterior to posterior at the head-neck junction in the center of the fibula. Enlarge this hole with a curet. Do not disturb the proximal tibiofibular joint.
- Drill two 6-mm holes, one anterior and one posterior to the femoral attachment of the LCL. The holes should be 10 mm deep and should be separated by 8 mm of intervening bone corresponding to the posterior collateral ligament attachment site. Carefully use a curved curet to connect the two drill holes, establishing a bony tunnel beneath the ligament insertion site.
- Prepare the Achilles tendon allograft. Usually, the allograft measures 6 to 7 mm in diameter and 19 to 20 cm in length. This length allows the proximal and distal posterior arms of the circle graft to overlap, adding additional tissue to the posterolateral aspect of the joint. Place no. 2 Dacron, interlocking, closed-loop (baseball) sutures into both ends of the allograft, and pretension the allograft for 15 minutes under an 8-N or 9-N load.
- Make a vertical incision into the posterolateral capsule just behind the posterior collateral ligament and anterior to the arcuate complex.
- Inspect the tissues of the posterolateral capsule, arcuate ligament complex, popliteal tendon, and posterior collateral ligament.
- If the posterolateral structures are not excessively redundant, plicate the posterolateral capsule to the posterior collateral ligament allograft reconstruction in a simple vest-over-pants fashion (Fig. 1.88).
- However, if the posterolateral structures are markedly redundant, advance the posterolateral capsule with half of the gastrocnemius tendon proximally on the femur, using the Hughston and Jacobson technique (see Technique 1.10).
- Reconstruct the posterior collateral ligament by passing the allograft through the bony tunnels in the femur and fibula in a circular fashion with the two free ends overlapping each other on the posterior aspect. The graft should lie next to the stretched and slack posterior collateral ligament.
- Tension the graft with the knee at 30 degrees of flexion and neutral tibial rotation and with the lateral side of the joint closed.
- Suture the two free ends of the graft to each other with multiple interrupted sutures. Then suture both the anterior and posterior limbs of the allograft to the intervening LCL with horizontal sutures.

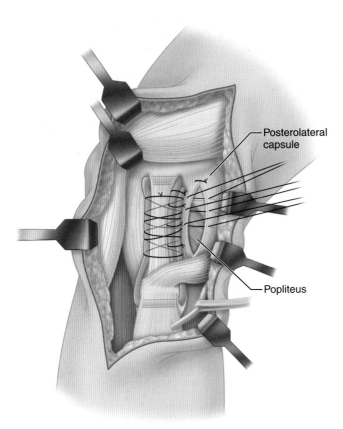

FIGURE 1.88 Vest-over-pants plication of posterolateral complex to lateral collateral ligament reconstruction. (From Noyes FR, Barber-Westin SD: Surgical reconstruction of severe chronic posterolateral complex injuries of the knee using allograft tissues, *Am J Sports Med* 23:2, 1995.) **SEE TECHNIQUE 1.15.**

- If the posterior collateral ligament is markedly lax (allowing more than 15 mm of lateral joint opening), incise the ligament in its midportion and repair the overlapping ends with multiple interrupted, nonabsorbable sutures. Then secure the allograft to the shortened posterior collateral ligament as previously described.
- Check the knee motion from 0 to 90 degrees of flexion to confirm normal internal and external rotation and to avoid over constraining the joint.
- Plicate the posterolateral capsule to the allograft reconstruction under sufficient tension to allow 0 degrees of extension without any hyperextension.

POSTOPERATIVE CARE A dial-locked hinged brace or bivalved cylinder cast is worn for 4 weeks. Muscle-strengthening exercises are begun the day after surgery. The cast is removed for immediate intermittent, protected active-assisted range-of-motion exercises, six to eight times daily, in the range of 10 to 90 degrees. Periodically, the knee should be gently moved to 5 degrees to make sure excessive posterior capsular scarring does not occur. Hyperextension should be avoided. The motion is increased gradually until full motion is achieved by the 12th postoperative week. Hyperextension is avoided for 6 months after surgery. After 4 weeks, the cast is removed and a full lower extremity, hinged, double-upright brace is used. The patient is kept non–weight bearing during the

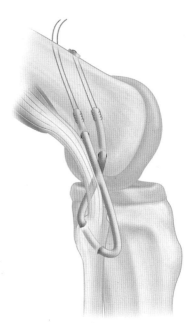

FIGURE 1.89 Modification of Larson procedure with two graft limbs secured independently for the lateral collateral and popliteofibular ligaments; this configuration is suggested to result in a more physiologic load—sharing pattern. (Redrawn from Niki Y, Matsumoto H, Otani T, et al: A modified Larson's method of posterolateral corner reconstruction of the knee reproducing the physiological tensioning pattern of the lateral collateral and popliteofibular ligaments, *Sports Med Arthrosc Rehabil Ther Technol* 4:21, 2012.)

first 4 weeks, and then weight bearing of 25 pounds is allowed for the next 2 weeks. Patients are taught to walk with normal knee flexion to avoid knee hyperextension or varus position of the lower extremity. Weight bearing is slowly advanced until the 16th week, when the patient is weaned from crutch support. The brace is used for the first 9 months after surgery to prevent abnormal hyperextension, varus angulation, rotation, and external tibial rotation.

Swimming is encouraged at the third postoperative month, and a progressive resistive exercise program in a protected range of 30 to 90 degrees of flexion is begun. No hamstring exercises are allowed until the 12th week. A running program is delayed until at least the 12th month in patients in whom articular cartilage changes do not contraindicate strenuous activity.

Larson's procedure was one of the first fibular-based techniques and reconstructs the LCL and popliteofibular ligament with distal insertion sites on the fibula. The technique is less technically demanding than combined tibial-fibular-based procedures and has good reported clinical results. Niki et al. modified the Larson technique to reproduce the physiologic load-sharing pattern of the lateral collateral and popliteofibular ligaments. Two graft limbs are secured independently for the lateral collateral and popliteofibular ligaments to achieve differential, more anatomic tension patterns (Fig. 1.89). The authors cite technical simplicity as an advantage of their modification, in addition to a more physiologic load-sharing pattern.

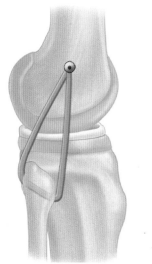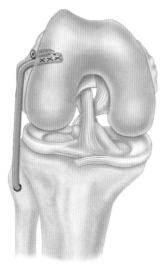

FIGURE 1.90   Reconstruction of posterolateral structures with use of semitendinosus tendon. Fixation is accomplished by placement of interference screw 1 to 2 mm larger than drilled tunnel. (Redrawn from Fanelli GC, Larson RV: Practical management of posterolateral instability of the knee, *Arthroscopy* 18[Suppl 1]:1, 2002.) **SEE TECHNIQUE 1.16.**

RECONSTRUCTION OF POSTEROLATERAL STRUCTURES WITH SEMITENDINOSUS TENDON

TECHNIQUE 1.16

(LARSON)

- Drill a hole into the fibular head from anterior to posterior, angling it slightly superiorly from anteroinferior to posterosuperior in the head to pass deep to the insertion of the biceps tendon onto the fibular head.
- Place the semitendinosus in a figure-of-eight position from the lateral femoral epicondyle deep to the iliotibial band and through the head of the fibula.
- Make a small transverse incision in the iliotibial band over the lateral femoral epicondyle.
- Make another incision at the lower border of the iliotibial band between the iliotibial band and the biceps femoris tendon.
- Insert a Kirschner wire as a temporary anchoring point in the lateral femoral epicondyle. It can be used to help determine the isometric point and can be moved when needed.
- Pass the semitendinosus tendon through the fibular head, bringing it out posteriorly deep to the biceps tendon, and then pass it through an opening in the lateral intermuscular septum and deep to the iliotibial band.
- Pass the graft to the anterior aspect of the lateral femoral epicondyle and loop it over the Kirschner wire, bringing it beneath the iliotibial band to the anterior aspect of the fibular head.
- With tension on the graft, place the knee through a range of motion. Mark the graft with indelible ink to determine if its placement is isometric. Any change in the length of

the graft can be identified by a movement of this mark. The Kirschner wire in the lateral epicondyle can be moved until the isometric point is identified.

- Make a blind-end tunnel in the lateral femoral epicondyle at this isometric point and insert the looped end of the semitendinosus into the tunnel. It can be pulled with a looped suture that has been passed through the tunnel and knee and brought out on the medial side. This suture can be removed later.
- Secure the graft in the femoral tunnel with a biodegradable interference screw.
- Tension the graft and then suture it on itself distally (Fig. 1.90).
- Biomechanical tests have indicated that the posterior limb of this construct reproduces the function of the popliteofibular ligament and the anterior limb reproduces the function of the LCL.

POSTOPERATIVE CARE   Postoperative care is the same as that described after Technique 1.15.

▥ POSTEROLATERAL INSTABILITY WITH VARUS KNEE

Biomechanical selective cutting studies have demonstrated that the LCL and the popliteal tendon are the major restraints to posterolateral instability. Attention has focused on the anatomy of the posterolateral corner, where a consistently strong attachment of the popliteal tendon to the fibula has been found—the popliteofibular ligament. The popliteofibular ligament is an important component of the popliteal muscle-tendon unit, and its anatomic orientation performs a static stabilizing function to resist varus and external rotation moments and posterior forces. In cutting studies, section of the LCL and popliteus attachment to the tibia resulted in limited increases in primary varus rotation and primary external rotation because of the remaining intact popliteofibular ligament. Therefore, for both acute and chronic posterolateral injuries, repair or reconstruction of the LCL, the popliteal tendon and its attachment to the tibia, and the popliteofibular ligament is recommended.

In patients with chronic posterolateral instability, limb alignment must be evaluated before posterolateral reconstruction is considered. If the patient has varus knee alignment and a lateral thrust in the stance phase of gait, simple soft-tissue posterolateral reconstructions fail because of chronic repetitive stretching. A valgus proximal tibial osteotomy may be performed before or simultaneously with the reconstruction to correct the alignment and to protect the repair. In some patients, osteotomy alone may alleviate the symptoms of posterolateral instability. The osteotomy may be a closing lateral or an opening medial osteotomy, but most osteotomies end up biplanar, with a resulting impact on ACL- and PCL-deficient knees. With a closing lateral wedge tibial osteotomy, more bone often is removed anteriorly, which results in leveling of the slope of the tibial plateau. This reduction in the normal posterior slope of the tibia benefits the ACL-deficient knee. Conversely, the opening medial wedge osteotomy typically is wider anteriorly than posteriorly, which increases the posterior tibial slope, aiding the PCL-deficient knee.

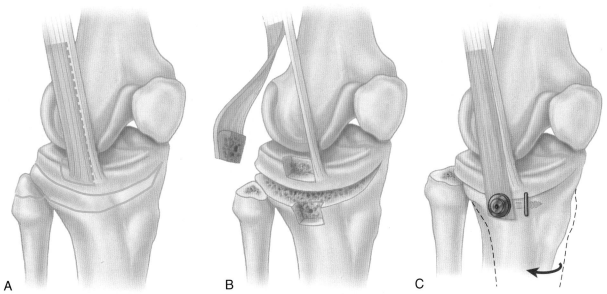

A   B   C

FIGURE 1.91 Valgus high tibial osteotomy for chronic posterolateral instability and varus alignment. **A** and **B,** Iliotibial band is removed with bone block and advanced across osteotomy. **C,** Bone block is secured with cancellous screw distal to osteotomy. (From Veltri DM, Warren RF: Treatment of acute and chronic injuries to the posterolateral and lateral knee, *Oper Tech Sports Med* 4:174, 1996.) **SEE TECHNIQUE 1.17.**

VALGUS TIBIAL OSTEOTOMY AND POSTEROLATERAL RECONSTRUCTION

TECHNIQUE 1.17

VALGUS TIBIAL OSTEOTOMY
- Make a long lateral longitudinal incision midway between the tibial tubercle and the fibula, extending proximally for 15 to 20 cm.
- Isolate the iliotibial band along its anterior and posterior borders to its insertion at Gerdy's tubercle.
- Develop, drill, and pretap a 2-cm-square bone block for a 6.5-mm cancellous screw.
- Use an oscillating saw to remove the bone block with its attached iliotibial band (Fig. 1.91A,B).
- Unlike proximal tibial osteotomy for osteoarthritis, the fibular osteotomy is performed at the midshaft level. The proximal tibiofibular joint is not released because this would allow proximal migration of the fibula, with subsequent shortening of the posterolateral structures and exacerbation of the posterolateral instability.
- Perform the proximal valgus tibial osteotomy, and once it has been closed, make a trough distal to the osteotomy site to accept the bone block with its attached iliotibial band.
- Secure the block in the trough with a 6.5-mm cancellous screw (Fig. 1.91C). Angle the screw distally to avoid the osteotomy site. Advancement of the iliotibial band increases tension on the lateral side of the knee and helps stabilize the osteotomy. If necessary, additional fixation is achieved with staples.

- After the osteotomy, posterolateral reconstruction can be performed concurrently or delayed until the clinical results of the osteotomy have been determined.

POSTEROLATERAL RECONSTRUCTION (FIG. 1.92)
- If the bony alignment is acceptable or has been corrected, attention can be turned to the pathologic condition of the posterolateral corner.
- If chronic cruciate deficiency is present, reconstruct the ligament, preferably by arthroscopically assisted techniques.
- Through these same lateral skin incisions, release the attachments between the biceps tendon and iliotibial band to allow the iliotibial band to be retracted anteriorly.
- Split the iliotibial band anteriorly at the level of the lateral femoral epicondyle to leave a 5-cm strip composed of a posterior iliotibial band. This can be retracted as needed to further expose the posterolateral corner.
- Next, make a vertical incision in the posterior capsule just posterior to the LCL, exposing the posterior aspect of the joint in the area of the popliteal tendon.
- Examine the LCL and the popliteal tendon to determine the site of injury and the quality of the tissues.
- Follow the popliteus from its femoral insertion proximally to its tibial insertion distally and to its fibular insertion (the popliteofibular ligament). (Options for treatment of the chronic popliteal injury include those discussed in Technique 1.9.)
- If an ipsilateral patellar tendon autograft has been used for cruciate ligament reconstruction, a contralateral patellar tendon autograft or an allograft can be used for reconstruction of the popliteus. The length of a patellar tendon graft is a major consideration for posterolateral reconstruction. The patellar tendon graft rarely exceeds 5 cm and may not be long enough to pass from the tibial

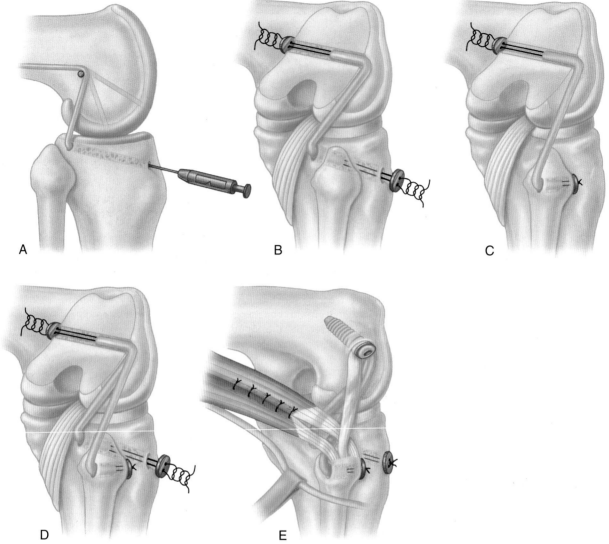

A

B

C

D

E

FIGURE **1.92** For reconstruction of popliteus, placement of femoral tunnel is determined with isometer **(A)**, and graft is passed through femoral and tibial tunnels and secured with sutures tied over ligament buttons **(B)** or with interference screws. Patellar tendon graft used for reconstruction of popliteofibular ligament **(C)** can be split to reconstruct both components **(D)**. **E,** Lateral collateral ligament is reconstructed with central third of biceps tendon. (From Veltri DM, Warren RF: Treatment of acute and chronic injuries to the posterolateral and lateral knee, *Oper Tech Sports Med* 4:174, 1996.) **SEE TECHNIQUE 1.17.**

or fibular tunnels posterolaterally to the femur, especially in larger knees. In these circumstances, an Achilles tendon allograft may be required. In the reconstruction of a popliteal tendon, both the tibial and fibular attachments should be treated with a single split patellar tendon or a split Achilles tendon allograft.

- Reconstruct the tibial component of the popliteus by creating a tibial tunnel from anterior to posterior in the lateral proximal tibia, using a standard ACL drill guide.
- Begin the tunnel 2 cm below and parallel to the joint line, exiting where the popliteal tendon crosses the tibia. Before creating the tibial attachment, identify the peroneal nerve and dissect it off the fibular neck.
- Create a tunnel of appropriate size from posterior to anterior in the fibula, beginning distal and posterior to the fibular styloid.

- The femoral tunnel site for reconstruction is determined by an isometer. Drill a Kirschner wire through the center of rotation on the knee, which is a point proximal and posterior to the femoral attachment of the popliteus. Tie a suture to the Kirschner wire and then pass this from posterior to anterior through the tibial tunnel and the fibular tunnel. Attach the free end of the suture to an isometer and move the knee through a full range of motion, noting the change in the length of the suture. Adjust the Kirschner wire until the least change in length is determined. Then drill the Kirschner wire from lateral to medial through the femur and overream it with the appropriate-size reamer to create a femoral tunnel.
- In placing a graft, anchor it first in the fibular head, tension one limb by securing the graft in the femoral tunnel, and then secure the graft in the tibial tunnel under tension with the tibia in neutral rotation.

- If a split patellar tendon graft is used, the bone plugs can be secured in their respective tunnels with interference screws or with bone block sutures tied over a button on the opposite cortex.
- When a split Achilles tendon allograft is used, the bone plug is anchored in the femoral tunnel with either an interference screw or bone block sutures tied over a button on the medial femoral condyle. The tibial portion of the tendon graft is fixed to the proximal tibia with a 6.5-mm cancellous screw and ligament washer. The fibular portion can be secured within the fibular tunnel with sutures tied over a button or a 6.5-mm cancellous screw and ligament washer over the anterior fibula.
- If only one component of the popliteus is reconstructed, the popliteal fibular ligament should be reestablished because this has a greater moment arm in preventing rotational instability. In reconstructing only one of the distal attachments, simply forgo the unnecessary tunnel and do not split the graft.
- Chronic posterolateral instability that occurs secondary to deficiency of the LCL usually requires reconstruction. The central third of the biceps tendon can be used as previously described under augmentation techniques for the LCL. In rare cases, the biceps tendon will not be available, and reconstruction of the LCL should proceed with a patellar tendon autograft or allograft. The peroneal nerve should have been previously isolated and protected.
- Make a blind-end tunnel at the top of the fibula to receive one bone plug.
- Drill two holes to intersect this blind tunnel for the bone block sutures.
- Use a Kirschner wire to determine the isometric point for the femoral tunnel and create the tunnel as previously described.
- Place the graft into the fibula and secure it by tying the bone block sutures distally over the fibular bone bridge.
- Place the proximal end of the graft in the femoral tunnel, tension it, and secure it with an interference screw.

POSTOPERATIVE CARE The patient is placed in a controlled motion brace and is allowed immediate postoperative knee motion. Posterior forces in varus and external rotation moments that would stress the posterolateral reconstruction are avoided. The patient is kept to toe-touch weight bearing for 6 weeks with the brace locked in extension. Quadriceps-setting and isometric exercises are performed immediately. Passive and active-assisted knee flexion and passive knee extension exercises are emphasized. Stationary bicycling is started at 4 weeks after surgery. At 6 weeks, a standard closed kinetic chain exercise program is begun. Jogging is allowed at 4 months. Open kinetic chain knee flexion and extension exercises are not done until 3 to 4 months. A hinged brace is worn for 6 months. Return to sports generally is allowed at 6 to 9 months after surgery.

◼ ANTEROLATERAL ROTARY INSTABILITY

When the indication for lateral reconstruction is anterolateral rotary instability, numerous procedures have been used to control the anterior displacement or internal rotational tendencies of the tibia, in addition to the basic reconstruction previously described. These procedures are of three general types: intraarticular procedures, extraarticular procedures, and combinations of the two. Intraarticular procedures for anterior cruciate substitution are described in the section on ACL reconstruction (see subsequent section). Intraarticular procedures include use of a strip of iliotibial band, tenodesis with use of the gracilis or semitendinosus, an "over-the-top" procedure with a strip of the lateral patelloquadriceps tendon, the iliotibial band transferred through the intercondylar notch to the anterior tibia, and other procedures that use portions of the patellar tendon. Extraarticular procedures include biceps-plasty, iliotibial band tenodesis and various modifications, and anterolateral femorotibial ligament tenodesis. Extraarticular procedures combined with lateral compartment reconstruction to control anterolateral rotary instability mainly involve variations in the use of the iliotibial band. The two basic types of extraarticular procedures using the iliotibial band are (1) creation of a static checkrein and (2) creation of a dynamic force on the tibia to prevent its displacement forward by the powerful quadriceps muscle as full extension approaches.

We have had some success with each of these types of procedures. Mild grades of anterolateral rotary instability where the pivot shift phenomenon is only mild may benefit from an extraarticular procedure alone, especially if the activity demands of the patient are not great. We suspect that when these procedures are analyzed after 10 years, the results will not be as good and degenerative changes will be apparent within the joint. We rarely use an extraarticular procedure alone for anterolateral rotary instability. For moderate and severe instability of this type, we use an intraarticular replacement for the ACL to correct the anteroposterior instability and correct the abnormal rotational component with a lateral extraarticular checkrein procedure if the rotatory component is great.

Techniques using allografts are described in the section on intraarticular replacement of the ACL.

ANTERIOR CRUCIATE LIGAMENT INJURIES
INCIDENCE

The exact incidence of ACL injuries is unknown; however, it has been estimated that more than 400,000 are torn each year, and at least 200,000 ACL reconstructions are done each year in the United States. The controversy for managing this injury now centers more on the choice of graft selection, the precise tunnel location, transtibial tunnel versus tibial inlay, and the use of single or double bundle grafts for reconstruction instead of whether surgery is necessary. In the past 2 decades alone, more than 2000 scientific articles on the ACL have been published, as well as a number of textbooks, making a detailed review of the literature beyond the scope of this section. MOON and Multicenter ACL Revision Study (MARS) are National Institutes of Health (NIH)-funded consortia of orthopaedic surgeons from multiple sites who seek to identify modifiable predictors of poor outcomes after ACL reconstruction. These groups have generated multiple studies with large volumes of patients and increasing lengths of follow-up.

ANATOMY

The ACL is composed of longitudinally oriented bundles of collagen tissue arranged in fascicular subunits within larger functional bands. The ligament is surrounded by synovium, thus making it extrasynovial. Functionally, the ligament has been described as two bundles, the anteromedial bundle (AMB) and the posterolateral bundle (PLB), which are named for their insertion sites on the tibia. Relative to the anterior insertion of the lateral meniscus, the AMB inserts approximately 2.7 mm posterior and 5.2 mm medial, while the PLB inserts 11.2 mm posterior and 4.1 mm medial. The tibial ACL insertion has a coronal width of 10 mm and a sagittal length of 14 mm. The AMB is slightly larger (12%) than the PLB. On the femoral side, the AMB inserts more proximally and slightly anterior on the femur, whereas the PLB inserts more distal and slightly posterior. The AMB occupies slightly more of the ACL insertion area (52%) than does the PLB (48%). The ovoid femoral insertion measures 8 by 15 mm. The anterior border of the femoral insertions of the AMB and PLB is the lateral intercondylar ridge, also called the resident's ridge. The bifurcate ridge separates the AMB and PLB anatomically from proximal to distal in the sagittal plane.

The ligament is 31 to 35 mm in length and 31.3 mm^2 in cross section. The primary blood supply to the ligament is from the middle geniculate artery, which pierces the posterior capsule and enters the intercondylar notch near the femoral attachment. Additional supply comes from the retropatellar fat pad via the inferior medial and lateral geniculate arteries. This source plays a more important role when the ligament is injured. The osseous attachments of the ACL contribute little to its vascularity. The posterior articular nerve, a branch of the tibial nerve, innervates the ACL. Histologic study has revealed nerve fibers of the size most consistent with transmitting pain in the intrafascicular spaces. Mechanoreceptors also have been identified on the surface of the ligament, mostly at the insertions of the ligament (especially femoral), well beneath the external synovial sheath.

BIOMECHANICS

The ACL is the primary restraint to anterior tibial displacement, accounting for approximately 85% of the resistance to the anterior drawer test when the knee is at 90 degrees of flexion and neutral rotation. Selective sectioning of the ACL has shown that the anteromedial band is tight in flexion, providing the primary restraint, whereas the posterolateral bulky portion of this ligament is tight in extension. The PLB provides the principal resistance to hyperextension. Tension in the ACL is least at 30 to 40 degrees of knee flexion. The ACL also functions as a secondary restraint on tibial rotation and varus-valgus angulation at full extension.

In vivo, it is an oversimplification to limit the description of ACL function to the function of its two fiber bundles. In fact, similar to the fibers in all ligaments, those in the ACL are recruited differently on the basis of every subtle three-dimensional change in the position of the joint. The normal ACL has been shown to carry loads throughout the entire range of flexion and extension of the knee. Consequently, the ACL can fail differently at different loads, depending on the position of the bones and the direction in which the loads are applied at the time of injury. The complexity of the arrangement of the ligament fibers and their response to load have important implications regarding the results of tensile tests. Tensile testing of the ACL depends on the age of the specimen, angle of knee flexion, direction of tensile loading with respect to the ACL, and rate of the applied load. In other words, the maximal strength of the ACL should not be assumed to have one fixed value.

Notwithstanding this qualification, investigators have studied the biomechanical properties of the ACL. A comprehensive biomechanical study determined the ultimate load to be 1725 ± 269 N; the stiffness, 182 ± 33 N/mm; and the energy absorbed to failure, 12.8 ± 2.2 N/mm. In younger specimens the ultimate load was found to be 2160 ± 157 N and the stiffness 242 ± 28 N/mm.

In addition to the function as a mechanical restraint to translation, the ACL has proprioceptive function, as evidenced by the presence of mechanoreceptors in the ligament. These nerve endings may provide the afferent arc for postural changes of the knee through deformations within the ligament. The exact contributions of the receptors have not been clearly defined.

HISTORY AND PHYSICAL EXAMINATION

The classic history of an ACL injury begins with a noncontact deceleration, jumping, or cutting action. Obviously, other mechanisms of injury include external forces applied to the knee. The patient often describes the knee as having been hyperextended or popping out of joint and then reducing. A pop is frequently heard or felt. The patient usually has fallen to the ground and is not immediately able to get up. Resumption of activity usually is not possible, and walking is often difficult. Within a few hours, the knee swells, and aspiration of the joint reveals hemarthrosis. In this scenario, the likelihood of an ACL injury is greater than 70%. Before the development of a hemarthrosis, the physical examination is easier and more revealing; conversely, the examination is more difficult once pain and muscle guarding appear. The Lachman test (see Fig. 1.42) is the most sensitive test for anterior tibial displacement (95% sensitivity). Increased excursion relative to the opposite knee and absence of a firm end point suggest an injury to the ACL.

The pivot shift test requires a relaxed patient and an intact MCL (see Fig. 1.48). When the result is positive, this test reproduces the pathologic motion in an ACL–deficient knee and is easier to elicit in a chronic ACL disruption or in an anesthetized patient with an acute ACL injury.

Knee ligament arthrometers such as the KT-1000/2000 can assist in the diagnosis but are more effective in evaluating patients with chronic ACL disruption when pain and associated muscle guarding are absent. These devices also are useful for documentation of surgical results both intraoperatively and postoperatively. With a manual maximal anterior displacement, the right-left difference is less than 3 mm in 95% of normal knees. The right-left difference is 3 mm or more in 90% of knees with an acute ACL injury.

Radiographic studies also are useful in diagnosis of ACL injuries. Plain radiographs often are normal; however, a tibial eminence fracture indicates an avulsion of the tibial attachment of the ACL. The Segond fracture, or avulsion fracture of the lateral capsule, is pathognomonic of an ACL tear (Fig. 1.93). A depressed impaction fracture of the lateral femoral condyle (the lateral femoral notch sign) at the sulcus terminalis where the MRI demonstrates the lateral femoral condylar bone bruise suggests an ACL tear. MRI is the most helpful diagnostic radiographic technique. The reported accuracy for detecting tears of the ACL has ranged from 70% to 100%. Because the ACL crosses the knee joint at a slightly oblique angle, the complete ligament rarely is captured in its entirety by a single MRI in the true sagittal plane. Vellet introduced the

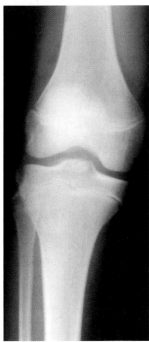

FIGURE 1.93 Avulsion fracture of tibia (Segond fracture) with anterior cruciate ligament tear.

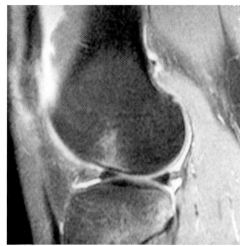

FIGURE 1.94 MRI shows bone bruise after anterior cruciate ligament tear.

concept of a nonorthogonal plane, which usually shows the entire ACL in one frame. The nonorthogonal plane is achieved by externally rotating the knee approximately 15 degrees. More recently, investigators have reported that the accuracy of MRI in evaluating injuries to the ACL approaches 95% to 100%.

Bone bruises, which are apparent on MRI in 80% of patients with ACL tears, occur primarily in the lateral femoral condyle and lateral tibial plateau and have been suggested to predict pain and other symptoms after ACL reconstruction (Fig. 1.94). In a study of 525 patients, however, Dunn et al. found that bone bruises on MRI were not associated with pain or symptoms after reconstruction. The only demographic or injury-related factors associated with bone bruises were younger age and not jumping at the time of injury.

Stress radiographs have been advocated to document both ACL and PCL injuries. With the availability and accuracy of MRI, we rarely use stress radiographs except to evaluate chronic PCL injuries when the PCL appears healed on MRI.

NATURAL HISTORY

The method chosen for treating an ACL tear is influenced by the natural history of the injury. Controversy still exists regarding the course that an ACL–deficient knee will follow because the studies to date have been biased toward symptomatic patients who seek care. Furthermore, not all knee injuries are reported and accurately diagnosed as ACL injuries. Additional confusion arises because of the variability in previous studies in patients' ages and activity levels, extent of injury, resultant instability, type of nonoperative management, and follow-up duration and evaluation. It has been well documented that an individual with an ACL–deficient knee who resumes athletic activities and has repeated episodes of instability will sustain meniscal tears and osteochondral injuries that eventually lead to arthrosis. Furthermore, patients exhibit varying degrees of instability after ACL rupture because of their inherent knee laxity and associated injuries. Joint laxity has been identified as a risk factor for ACL injury, as well as contributing to poor results and late failure of ACL reconstructions. Musahl et al. determined that concomitant injury to the anterolateral capsule, medial meniscus, or lateral meniscus was associated with increased knee rotatory laxity, and Song et al. found the best set of predictors of grade 3 pivot shift were participating in pivoting sports at the time of injury, increased lateral posterior-inferior tibial slope, anterolateral capsular ligament disruptions, and combined lateral meniscal lesions. Conversely, at midterm follow-up, Malugin et al. saw no difference in pivot shift test results, graft failure rates, and activity levels in patients undergoing ACL reconstruction with or without a Segond fracture.

Results of nonoperative treatment of ACL tears have been discouraging and can be attributed partially to the associated injuries that occur at the time of the ACL rupture. A controlled laboratory study using MRI and dual orthogonal fluoroscopic imaging techniques determined that ACL injury caused a significant elongation of the fiber bundles of the superficial and deep MCL at every flexion angle, whereas the LLC fiber bundles shortened. These alterations in the collateral ligaments demonstrate that abnormal tibiofemoral joint kinematics after ACL injury disrupts normal joint function. Several investigators reported the incidence of meniscal tears with acute ACL injuries to range from 50% to 70%.

The lateral meniscus is more commonly injured with the initial incident than is the medial meniscus. As a result of abnormal loading and shear stresses in the ACL-deficient knee, the risk of late meniscal injury is high and appears to increase with time from the initial injury. Most late meniscal tears occur in the medial meniscus because of its firm attachment to the capsule. Stone et al. reported that delay in ACL reconstruction of more than 1 year in patients 40 years of age or older was associated with increased risk of medial meniscal tear. The same risk of further meniscal injury and articular cartilage damage with delay in treatment has been reported in children and adolescents by Anderson et al. and Newman et al. Sanders et al. presented a cohort of 964 patients with new-onset, isolated ACL tears and an age- and sex-matched cohort of 964 patients without ACL tears. A total of 509 patients were treated with early ACL reconstruction, 91 with delayed ACL reconstruction, and 363 nonoperatively. At a mean follow-up of 13.7 years, patients with nonoperative treatment or delayed reconstruction had a significantly higher likelihood of developing secondary meniscal tear and being diagnosed with arthritis. The nonoperative group also had a higher risk of undergoing TKA. Conversely, van Yperen et al. reported 50 patients, 25 treated nonoperatively, who responded well to a 3-month structured rehabilitation program and lifestyle adjustments, and 25 treated surgically, who had persistent instability after 3 months of nonoperative treatment. At 20-year follow-up, there was no difference in knee osteoarthritis between groups when treatment was allocated on the basis of a patient's response to 3 months of nonoperative treatment. Although knee stability was better in the operative group, it did not result in better subjective and objective functional outcomes.

Osteochondral damage also influences prognosis. The reported incidence ranges from 21% to 31% in patients examined after the initial injury. MRI provides a sensitive technique for detecting bone injury in patients with acute and even chronic ACL-deficient knees (see Fig. 1.94). These MRI lesions are classified as geographic, reticular, or linear on the basis of their architectural appearance, relationship to cortical bone, and short-term osteochondral sequelae. Geographic lesions are associated with the cortical margin and have increased density. Reticular lesions are not associated with the cortical bone, and most resolve between 6 and 12 months. Osteochondral abnormalities identified on MRI may be precursors of osteoarthritis. However, a long-term (15 years) follow-up study by Neuman et al. found no relationship between an osteochondral injury diagnosed at primary arthroscopy after an ACL injury and subsequent knee osteoarthritis. They did find meniscectomy to be a potent risk factor for the development of osteoarthritis. Of the 79 patients treated in their study, radiographic tibiofemoral osteoarthritis was present in 13 (16%), all of whom had meniscectomies for a major meniscal tear. The frequency of osteoarthritis also was higher in patients who had ACL reconstruction than in those treated nonoperatively.

Much current research is focused on the biochemical environment of the knee after ACL injury. Cameron et al. found that in chronic ACL–deficient knees, the levels of proinflammatory cytokines such as interleukin-1 and tumor necrosis factor-alpha are markedly elevated, whereas protective, antiinflammatory proteins, such as the interleukin receptor antagonist protein, are significantly decreased. Lohmander et al. reported elevated levels of stromelysin-1 and tissue inhibitor of metalloproteinases-1 in synovial fluid samples 6 months to 18 years after trauma. They speculated that the increased release may be associated with the frequent development of posttraumatic osteoarthritis.

A number of investigators have studied the epidemiology of ACL–deficient knees and have implicated sex and femoral intercondylar notch width as factors contributing to injury of the ACL. Numerous investigators have reported that athletes sustaining noncontact ACL tears have statistically significant intercondylar notch stenosis. Souryal and Freeman formulated the notch width index, which is the ratio of the width of the intercondylar notch to the width of the distal femur at the level of the popliteal groove measured on a tunnel view radiograph of the knee (Fig. 1.95). The normal intercondylar notch ratio was 0.231 ± 0.044. The intercondylar notch width

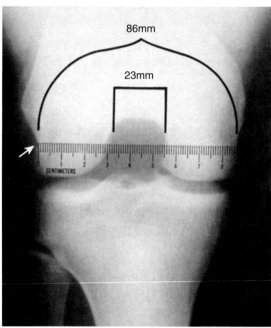

FIGURE 1.95   Notch width index is ratio of width of intercondylar notch to width of distal femur at level of popliteal groove *(arrow)*. Must be parallel to joint line. Narrowest portion of notch at level of ruler is to be measured. (From Souryal TO, Moore HA, Evans JP: Bilaterality in anterior cruciate ligament injuries: associated intercondylar notch stenosis, *Am J Sports Med* 16:449, 1998.)

index for men was larger than that for women. They found noncontact ACL injuries to be more frequent in athletes who had a notch width index that was at least 1 standard deviation below the mean. Shelbourne et al. studied a group of patients who had ACL reconstruction and found that women had statistically significantly narrower notches than men did, but the frequency of tearing of the autograft was the same between groups, presumably because a notchplasty had been performed. Data from the National College Athletic Association Injury Surveillance System as well as several studies have shown significantly higher ACL injury rates in female soccer, basketball, and rugby players than in male players (two to eight times). Possible causative factors for the increased incidence in women may be extrinsic (body movement, muscle strength, shoe-surface interface, and skill level) or intrinsic (joint laxity, hormonal influences, limb alignment, notch dimensions, and ligament size). Female sex hormones (i.e., estrogen, progesterone, and relaxin) fluctuate radically during the menstrual cycle and are reported to increase ligamentous laxity and to decrease neuromuscular performance.

Herman et al. demonstrated that healthy athletes with lower baseline neurocognitive performance generate knee kinematic and kinetic patterns in an unanticipated jump-landing task that are linked to ACL injury. Johnson et al. studied the gene expression differences between ruptured ACLs in young male and female patients. Microarray analysis of the RNA isolated from the ruptured ACL tissue identified 32 genes with significant differential expression. Fourteen of these genes were not linked to the X or Y chromosome. Further analysis grouped these genes into pathways involving development and function of skeletal muscle and growth, maintenance, and proliferation of cells. Reverse transcription-quantitative polymerase chain reaction confirmed significant differences in expression of three selected genes: *ACAN* (aggrecan) and *FMOT* (fibromodulin), which regulate the matrix, were upregulated in females compared to males and *WISP2* (WNT 1 inducible signaling pathway protein 2), which is involved in collagen turnover and production, was downregulated. The authors proposed that this may contribute to the weaker ACLs in females compared to males.

An increased posterior tibial slope also has been identified as a possible risk factor for ACL injury in both men and women. Increased posterior tibial slope has been reported to alter the kinematics of the knee joint by anteriorly shifting the resting position of the tibia and subsequently increasing the in situ forces on the ACL. Furthermore, increased posterior tibial slope was directly correlated to higher anterior tibial translation, predisposing patients to ACL injury. Hashemi et al. and Sonnery-Cottet et al. identified a steep posterior tibial slope as a significant risk factor for ACL injuries, as well as for anterior knee instability after reconstruction. Christensen et al. compared 35 patients with early failure of ACL reconstructions (within 2 years) with 35 matched controls who had undergone primary ACL reconstructions with at least 4 years of follow-up. The mean time to failure in the study group was 1 year (range, 0.6 to 1.4 years). The mean lateral tibial plateau slope in the early ACL failure group was 8.4 degrees, which was significantly larger than that in the control group at 6.5 degrees (p= .012). The odds ratio for graft failure considering a 2-degree increase in the lateral tibial plateau slope was 1.6 and continued to increase to 2.4 and 3.8 with 4-degree and 6-degree increases in lateral tibial plateau slope, respectively. Li et al. found that patients with a steeper medial or lateral posterior tibial slope had a higher risk of anterior tibial translation of 5 mm or more at thresholds of 5.6 and 3.8 degrees, respectively. Other authors have determined that a 5-degree increase in posterior tibial slope produces a 2-mm increase in anterior tibial translation during stance, and a 10-degree increase results in a 3-mm increase on radiographic Lachman testing.

Pfeiffer et al. evaluated the lateral femoral condyle ratio as a risk factor for ACL injury in 200 patients who were stratified into four groups: (1) a control group of patients without ACL injury, (2) patients with primary ACL injury, (3) patients with failed ACL reconstructions, and (4) patients with previous ACL injury and subsequent contralateral ACL injury. With the use of lateral radiographs, the ratio of posterior femoral condylar depth to total condylar length was defined as the lateral femoral condylar ratio. The main lateral femoral condylar ratios (and standard deviations) were 61.2% ± 2.4% for the control group, 64.2% ± 3.8% for the primary ACL injury group, 64.4% ± 3.6% for the failed ACL reconstruction group, and 66.9% ± 4.3% for the contralateral injury group. The ratios for the latter three groups were significantly higher than the control group ($P < .008$). The receiver operating characteristic curve analysis demonstrated that a lateral femoral condylar ratio of more than 63% was associated with an increased risk for ACL injury, with a sensitivity of 77% and a specificity of 72%.

Hewett et al. prospectively measured 205 female athletes in the high-risk sports of soccer, basketball, and volleyball for neuromuscular control by three-dimensional kinematics (joint angles) and for joint loads by kinetics (joint moments) during a jump-landing task. The nine athletes in whom ACL tears occurred had significantly different knee posture and loading compared with the 196 who did not have an ACL injury. The knee abduction angle at landing was 8 degrees greater in the ACL–injured athletes than in the uninjured athletes. ACL–injured athletes had a 2.5 times greater knee abduction moment and 20% higher ground reaction force, whereas stance time was 16% shorter; hence, increased motion, force, and moments occurred more quickly. Knee abduction moment predicted ACL injury status with 73% specificity and 78% sensitivity; dynamic valgus measures showed a predictive r^2 of 0.88. In an analysis of three-dimensional knee kinematics, Koga et al. suggested that valgus loading coupled with internal tibial rotation is a contributing factor in the ACL injury mechanism in female athletes. Less strength and smaller size of the ACL in females have also been postulated to contribute to the frequency of injuries. However, Mahajan et al. used static and dynamic ultrasound to measure the diameter of the ACL in normal contralateral knees of 25 individuals with noncontact ACL injuries and in 25 matched control subjects. Although the diameter near the tibial insertion site was significantly smaller in those with ACL injuries, the diameter was proportional to body weight and not significantly associated with height, sex, or age.

The efficacy of injury prevention programs for female athletes remains controversial. Pfeiffer et al. reported that a 20-minute plyometric-based exercise program focusing on the mechanics of landing from a jump and deceleration when running performed twice a week throughout the season did not reduce the rate of noncontact ACL injuries in high-school female athletes. In a meta-analysis of six studies, Hewett et al. found that four reported significant decreases in the number of ACL injuries after training, whereas two reported no differences between trained and untrained female athletes. They concluded that neuromuscular training may reduce the frequency of ACL injuries in female athletes if (1) plyometrics, balance, and strengthening exercises are incorporated into a comprehensive training protocol; (2) the training sessions are performed more than once a week; and (3) the duration of the training program is a minimum of 6 weeks.

TREATMENT

With the natural history in mind, the surgeon must determine which therapy is most appropriate for a specific patient. The treatment options available include nonoperative management, repair of the ACL (either isolated or with augmentation), and reconstruction with either autograft or allograft tissues or synthetics. Nonoperative treatment is a viable option for a patient who is willing to make lifestyle changes and avoid the activities that cause recurrent instability. In one of the most comprehensive series, Daniel et al. observed 236 patients with unstable knees by KT-1000 measurement. The patients were assessed by physical examination, KT-1000 measurements, and activity and frequency of sports participation. A total of 19% elected early ACL reconstruction, 20% required late reconstruction, and 61% were able to deal with their injury, although many were symptomatic. The authors found three factors known at the time of the initial examination that correlated with the need for surgery: younger age, preinjury hours of sports participation, and amount of anterior instability as measured by the KT-1000 arthrometer. If a nonoperative approach is chosen, it should include an aggressive rehabilitation program and counseling about activity level. The use of a functional knee brace is controversial and has not been shown to reduce the incidence of reinjury significantly if a patient returns to high-level sports.

Recently, ACL repair techniques have garnered renewed interest. This resurgence is likely due to a combination of the improved results seen in preclinical studies and the availability of biologic augmentation and internal bracing techniques. In a systematic review, van Eck et al. found that proximal ACL tear patterns showed a better healing potential with primary repair than did distal or midsubstance tears. Some form of internal bracing increased the success rate of ACL repair. Improvement in the biologic characteristics of the repair were obtained by bone marrow access by drilling tunnels or microfracture. Augmentation with PRP was beneficial only in combination with a structural scaffold. Skeletally immature patients had the best outcomes. Acute repairs (within 3 weeks of injury) were better than delayed repairs and produced improved outcomes with regard to load, stiffness, laxity, and rerupture. Jonkergouw et al. compared 28 patients with primary suture repair to 28 patients with primary suture repair and additional suture augmentation; all patients had isolated proximal ACL tears (type I). At a mean follow-up of 2.3 years (range, 1.0 to 2.9), the total failure rate was 10.7% and was lower with additional suture augmentation (7.1%) than primary repair alone (14.3%). Murray et al. reported their preliminary results with the bridge-enhanced ACL repair (BEAR) procedure, which augments a suture repair with a proprietary scaffold—the BEAR scaffold—placed between the torn ends of the ACL at the time of suture repair; 10 mL of autologous blood is added to the scaffold before wound closure. They compared 10 patients nonrandomly allocated to the BEAR procedure to 10 patients who had hamstring autograft ACL reconstructions. There were no differences between groups with respect to pain or effusion and no failures by Lachman examination criteria. There were no joint infections or signs of significant inflammation in either group. A larger study is planned. Conversely, Gagliardi et al. compared 22 consecutive adolescent patients treated with ACL repair and suture ligament augmentation to 157 adolescent patients with quadriceps–patellar bone autograft reconstruction. The frequency of graft failure in the repair group was 10.66 times higher than in the reconstruction group. The cumulative incidence of graft failure in the first 3 years after surgery was 48.8% in the repair group compared to 4.7% in the reconstruction group. Other studies have reported failure rates as high as 27%. Numerous studies from Europe have described ACL repair using a dynamic intraligamentary stabilization device (Ligamys, Mathys Ltd, Bettlach, Switzerland). Henle et al. reported revision ACL surgery in 7.9% of 381 patients at a 2.5-year follow-up after ACL repair with dynamic intraligamentary stabilization. Younger age, higher Tegner activity score, and increased knee laxity were significantly associated with revision ACL surgery. Mid-substance ACL rupture location also has been identified as a risk factor for failure. Many studies have reported high rates of additional surgery for scar and implant removal and manipulations. The long-term viability of ACL repair is still unknown.

The use of orthobiologics is under intense investigation. To date, no studies have definitively shown an enhanced healing response or improved results when orthobiologics are added to intraarticular ACL reconstructions. However, Setiawati et al. did show improved graft tunnel healing with increased collagen type III fibers and better outcomes on MRI and biomechanical analysis with intratunnel injections of bone marrow mesenchymal stem cells and vascular endothelial growth factor.

The techniques for augmentation of a primary repair use the same tissues and approaches as those for reconstruction with the exception that the augmenting tissue is passed through the posterior capsule high in the intercondylar notch and over the lateral femoral condyle. This over-the-top orientation preserves the femoral attachment of the ACL, and the tissue is secured to the lateral aspect of the distal femur with the staples or a screw and spiked soft-tissue washer. The tibial tunnel should be placed at the anteromedial edge of the tibial footprint of the ACL to minimize disruption of the tibial attachment. Further details are available in the techniques for intraarticular reconstruction of the ACL.

All of the preceding discussion has dealt with primary repair of a midsubstance ACL tear. Acute repair is appropriate when a bony avulsion occurs with the ACL attached. The avulsed bone fragment often can be replaced and fixed with sutures passed through transosseous drill holes or screws placed through the fragment into the bed. A clinical comparison of screw and suture fixation of ACL tibial avulsion fractures found no significant differences in Lysholm knee scores or return to preinjury activities; some patients in both groups had residual laxity or flexion contractures. ACL avulsions usually occur from the tibial insertion. Rarely does a disruption from its femoral origin avulse a piece of bone. Steadman reported a high frequency of avulsions of the femoral attachment of the ACL in skiers sustaining low-velocity injuries. He advocated repair of the ligament back to a freshened femoral bed and reported early success. Long-term results of this procedure are not available, and we have no experience with this technique. With repair of bony tibial avulsions of the ACL, the literature reports residual objective anterior laxity in 50% to 90% of patients, but subjective or functional instability is rare. Loss of fixation and knee stiffness are reported complications. Instituting range-of-motion exercises by 4 weeks postoperatively has been shown to lessen the incidence of arthrofibrosis.

REPAROF BONY TIBIAL AVULSIONS OF ANTERIOR CRUCIATE LIGAMENT

TECHNIQUE 1.18

- If the ACL has been avulsed with a fragment of bone from its tibial insertion, make an anteromedial incision, clear the crater in the tibia of clots and debris, and reduce the fragment.
- The method of fixation of the fragment depends on its size; occasionally a screw can be used, but more often the fragment is too small, so nonabsorbable sutures are best.
- For this, place a Bunnell suture in the base of the cruciate ligament, pass the two ends through holes drilled in the attached fragment, if it is large enough, and lay the sutures aside.
- Loop a second suture over the bone fragment through the base of the ACL and pass it through the holes in the fragment with the previous Bunnell suture. The two sutures are required so that not only is the ligament reattached under tension, but the second suture also pulls the bone fragment securely into place (Fig. 1.96).
- Beginning on the anteromedial surface of the tibia approximately 4 cm below the joint margin, drill two parallel

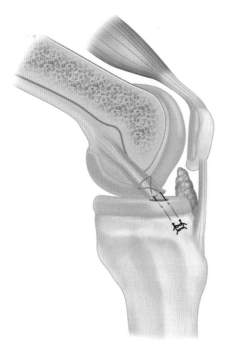

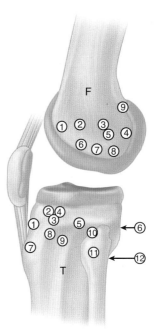

FIGURE 1.96 Repair of avulsion of tibial attachment of anterior cruciate ligament with fragment of bone. Crater in tibia should be deepened, and bone fragment on end of ligament is pulled into crater depth to restore tension in avulsed ligament. **SEE TECHNIQUE 1.18.**

FIGURE 1.97 Network of points selected on lateral femur, lateral tibia, and proximal fibula. *F*, Femur; *T*, tibia. *F-5*, Origin of lateral collateral ligament at lateral epicondyle; *T-10*, insertion of lateral collateral ligament; *T-3*, Gerdy's tubercle (slightly more proximal than in specimen); *T-7*, superior lateral aspect of tibial tuberosity; *F-1*, proximal to joint line; *F-7*, closer to joint line.

holes obliquely and superiorly to emerge in the base of the crater near the intercondylar eminence.

- With suture passers, pull the previously placed sutures through the holes and tie them over the bone anteriorly, making sure that the fragment in the base of the cruciate has been anatomically reduced and that tension in the cruciate ligament has been restored.
- If blood clot and debris are left within the depths of the crater before reduction, the repaired cruciate will be lax and normal tension will not be regained.
- Note at what degree of knee flexion the fragment is best reduced and apply a controlled motion brace in this position.

POSTOPERATIVE CARE At 3 weeks, flexion from 0 to 90 degrees is allowed in the brace and isometric quadriceps and hamstring exercises are begun. Crutches are discontinued at 6 weeks, and full active and passive range of motion should be obtained by 8 weeks. Progressive resistance exercises are continued for at least 3 months.

■ RECONSTRUCTION FOR ANTERIOR CRUCIATE LIGAMENT INSUFFICIENCY

As evidence mounted that primary repair of midsubstance ACL tears routinely failed, interest turned to reconstruction of the ligament. Previous experience with intraarticular reconstruction procedures was discouraging because of the frequent postoperative stiffness and persistent anterior laxity. Extraarticular procedures were developed to obviate these problems. These procedures generally create a restraining band on the lateral side of the knee, extending from the lateral femoral epicondyle to Gerdy's tubercle

in a line parallel with the ACL. They avoid the problem of a lack of blood supply to the intraarticular reconstructions. Most lateral extraarticular procedures use the iliotibial band or tract connecting the lateral femoral epicondyle to Gerdy's tubercle. Krackow and Brooks, in a kinematic study to determine the optimal attachment points for extraarticular lateral reconstructions for anterolateral rotary instability, found the best attachments to be at or in front of Gerdy's tubercle on the anterolateral aspect of the tibia and proximal to the origin of the LCL on the femur (Fig. 1.97). The stress exerted on the reconstructions depended primarily on changes in the femoral fixation point and much less so on changes in the tibial fixation point. Thus, regardless of which extraarticular procedure is chosen, the transfer should be anchored high on the femur, proximal to the attachment of the LCL.

These procedures may diminish the anterolateral rotary subluxation by virtue of their lateral placement, but they do not re-create the normal anatomy or function of the ACL. When used alone, extraarticular techniques have been associated with high failure rates. The Ellison procedure reportedly led to an unsatisfactory result in 16 (76%) of 21 patients, and the MacIntosh procedure yielded an unsatisfactory result in 13 (48%) of 27 patients. Currently, extraarticular procedures are used primarily in conjunction with an intraarticular reconstruction when severe anterior instability as a result of injury or late stretching of the secondary stabilizing capsular structures on the lateral side of the knee. For most grades of anterolateral instability, we prefer an intraarticular ACL replacement and do not attempt to correct the laxity of the secondary stabilizer.

Extraarticular techniques described are those of MacIntosh, Losee, Andrews (iliotibial band tenodesis and bicepsplasty), and LaPrade.

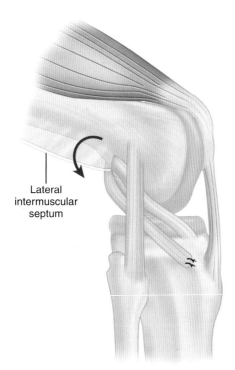

Lateral intermuscular septum

MacIntosh technique of lateral reconstruction with strip of iliotibial band. **SEE TECHNIQUE 1.19.**

EXTRAARTICULAR PROCEDURES (ILIOTIBIAL BAND TENODESIS)

TECHNIQUE 1.19

(MACINTOSH)

- Perform lateral reconstruction as previously described for lateral and posterolateral capsular structures (see Technique 1.10).
- Dissect a 1.5-cm-wide strip of iliotibial band from its midportion beginning approximately 16 cm from its distal insertion and turn it down to its attachment at Gerdy's tubercle.
- Pass this strip of iliotibial band to the posterolateral corner of the knee through a tunnel deep to the LCL (Fig. 1.98).
- At the distal insertion of the lateral intermuscular septum at the lateral femoral epicondyle, use a right-angle clamp to create a hiatus of sufficient size to receive the strip of iliotibial band.
- Loop it back to retrace its course deep to the LCL and secure it near its insertion into Gerdy's tubercle.
- Pull it taut before securing it with a staple or sutures while the knee is flexed to 90 degrees and the tibia is externally rotated.
- Suture the defect in the iliotibial band with multiple interrupted sutures and close the interval between the posterior part of the iliotibial band and the biceps femoris in a similar manner.

EXTRAARTICULAR PROCEDURES (ILIOTIBIAL BAND TENODESIS)

TECHNIQUE 1.20

(MACINTOSH, MODIFIED BY LOSEE)

Losee modified Mackintosh's iliotibial band technique in the following manner:

- After reconstruction of the posterior capsule, posterolateral corner, and midlateral capsular area as described in the section on reconstruction of the posterolateral compartment, fashion a strip of iliotibial band 18 cm long and 1.5 cm wide, beginning near the midportion and leaving it attached distally to Gerdy's tubercle (Fig. 1.99A).
- Make a superficial osseous tunnel beginning on the anterolateral aspect of the femoral condyle, passing deep to the femoral attachment of the LCL and popliteal tendon, and emerging posterolaterally where the superior part of the posterior capsule, the lateral head of the gastrocnemius muscle, and the iliotibial band insert into the femoral epicondylar region.
- Pass the strip of iliotibial band through this osseous tunnel from anterior to posterior and pull it taut with the knee flexed 90 degrees and the tibia externally rotated.
- Then pass the strip through the femoral attachment of the lateral intermuscular septum and the lateral head of the gastrocnemius muscle and weave it through the lateral-most portion of the arcuate complex at the reconstructed posterolateral corner of the knee (Fig. 1.99B).
- Again pull it taut inferiorly and anteriorly. This further tenses the posterior capsular structures and arcuate ligament complex.
- Pass the strip of iliotibial band anteriorly through a soft-tissue tunnel deep to the LCL, distal to the level of the joint surface, and back to the area of Gerdy's tubercle and secure it to bone with sutures or a staple while the knee is flexed 90 degrees and the tibia is maximally externally rotated (Fig. 1.99C). Besides supplying an anterior and internal rotary checkrein, this iliotibial strip should supply reinforcement to the anterolateral capsule, the posterolateral capsule, and the arcuate complex.
- Close the defect in the iliotibial band with multiple interrupted sutures.
- Then roll the posterior part of the biceps femoris and suture it to the posterior edge of the iliotibial band in a similar manner.

We have used this technique combined with an intraarticular ACL reconstruction for severe anterolateral rotary instability, especially if some varus laxity also is present. Used alone, it has effectively reduced the pivot shift phenomenon, but on critical evaluation beyond a 2-year follow-up, it has not stopped the anteroposterior translation of the tibia on the femur.

Andrews reported success with a "minireconstruction" technique for treating anterior cruciate insufficiency primarily of the anterolateral rotary type by an iliotibial band tenodesing procedure. Because it is an extraarticular procedure, the blood supply and healing potential are good, with the

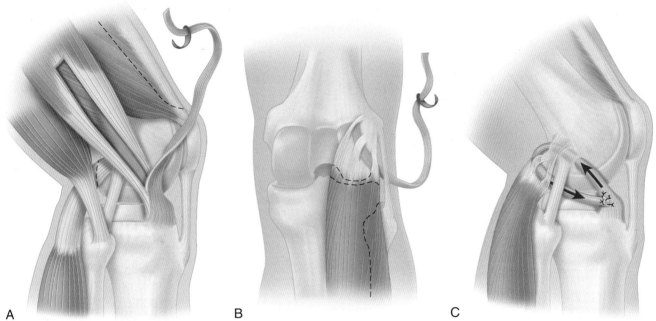

A B C

FIGURE 1.99 Losee modification of MacIntosh technique of lateral reconstruction with iliotibial band. **A,** Fascial strip (18 cm long × 1.5 cm wide) of iliotibial tract attached to Gerdy's tubercle. **B,** Imbrication through lateral head of gastrocnemius plus posterolateral corner. **C,** Rerouting of fascial strip deep to lateral collateral ligament, with reattachment to Gerdy's tubercle. **SEE TECHNIQUE 1.20.**

tensile strength in the reconstruction reaching a maximum early in the recovery period. It functions mainly to stabilize the lateral compartment against the anterior translation and excessive internal rotation of the tibia on the femur seen in anterolateral rotary instability. The two tenodesing bands created by the technique are roughly parallel with the course of the ACL, and by being firmly attached to Gerdy's tubercle and the lateral femoral epicondyle, they can replace some of the functions of the lost ACL and the deficient lateral capsular structures.

EXTRAARTICULAR PROCEDURES (ILIOTIBIAL BAND TENODESIS)

TECHNIQUE 1.21

(ANDREWS)
- Place the anesthetized patient supine on the operating table with the affected extremity draped to allow free hip and knee motion.
- Perform full ligament and arthroscopic examinations to obtain an accurate diagnosis of the instability and any meniscal lesions.
- With a pneumatic tourniquet ensuring a bloodless field, perform any necessary medial repairs or reconstructions for other instabilities, along with a lateral reconstruction. Repair meniscal tears, if possible; otherwise, do a partial meniscectomy, arthroscopically, when feasible.

- With the foot resting on the operating table and the knee flexed approximately 90 degrees, make an initial anterolateral 10-cm hockey-stick incision, exposing the iliotibial band and iliotibial tract.
- Longitudinally divide the iliotibial tract with a 10-cm fiber-splitting incision placed 3 to 4 cm anterior to its posterior margin.
- Retract the anterior edge of the tract and the vastus lateralis from the lateral side of the distal femur.
- With a periosteal elevator, elevate the fatty tissue and periosteum and expose the linea aspera and the distal insertion of the lateral intermuscular septum.
- Use an osteotome to "fish scale" the lateral femoral cortex in this area to promote a proliferative healing response of bone to the iliotibial tract.
- Hold the iliotibial tract against the distal femur by sutures passed through the tract and through two parallel holes in the distal femur and tied to each other on the medial side of the femur, beneath the vastus medialis as described later. By fixing the tract to the distal femur, a ligament is created that closely approximates the biomechanical function of the ACL, extending from the distal femur to Gerdy's tubercle and preventing anterolateral subluxation of the lateral tibial plateau on the lateral femoral condyle (Fig. 1.100).
- On the lateral side of the femur at the linea aspera, select two points that correspond closely to the two major femoral intraarticular attachments of the ACL.
- Drill the first hole at or slightly distal to the insertion of the lateral intermuscular septum on the linea aspera (Fig. 1.101A). Just anterior to the posterior cortex, it corresponds to the intraarticular attachment of the AMB of the ACL.
- Drill the second hole parallel to the first and 0.5 to 1 cm distal and anterior to it, corresponding to the femoral attachment of the PLB of the ligament.

- With the foot externally rotated, locate a point on the posterior edge of the iliotibial tract that will align with the posterior hole on the femur when the tract is pulled against the femur. At this point, separate the iliotibial tract into two bundles with no. 5 Bunnell sutures; the anterior bundle will be tight in flexion and the posterior bundle tight in extension, creating an isometric repair (Fig. 1.101B,C). Begin the suture creating the lower bundle proximally and inside the iliotibial tract, running distally 4 to 5 cm. Begin the upper, or anterior, bundle approximately 1 cm anterior and 0.5 cm distal to the lower bundle. These bundles are approximately 0.5 cm apart.

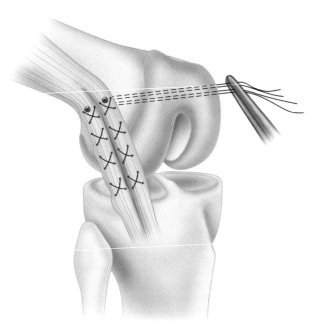

FIGURE 1.100 Attachment of two bundles to lateral femoral condylar area through transosseous drill holes to medial side of femur. (Redrawn from original illustration by Beverly Kessler; courtesy LTI Medica and The Upjohn Company, Learning Technology, 1981.) **SEE TECHNIQUE 1.21.**

- Pass the two Bunnell sutures through the two drill holes, from the lateral to the medial side of the femur, and test stability and range of motion. Constant tension is essential to prevent anterolateral subluxation of the tibia. If tibial subluxation is possible, the repair is too loose. Conversely, if the iliotibial tract cannot be pulled against the lateral femur or if the range of motion is excessively limited, the repair is too tight.
- Adjust tension and range of motion by repositioning either of the fixation sutures or the holes in the femur. Correct tension is crucial to the success of the procedure, which is determined by an isometric reconstruction and full range of motion. Perform the jerk, Lachman, and anterior drawer tests at this time; the results of all should be negative. Because it is a static repair without dynamic muscle support, the reconstruction will not increase in strength after surgery. Make certain, therefore, that the knee is absolutely stable at the end of the procedure, without laxity in either flexion or extension.
- With stability attained, tie the sutures together medially over the adductor tubercle and again test stability.
- Before the wound is closed, release the tourniquet and obtain hemostasis.
- After placing a large suction drainage tube intraarticularly and a second tube subcutaneously in the lateral wound, close the incisions.
- Place the knee in a well-padded cylinder cast in 30 to 40 degrees of flexion for pure anterolateral rotary instability and in 60 degrees of flexion for combined anteromedial and anterolateral rotary instability.

POSTOPERATIVE CARE At 5 days after surgery, the wound is inspected and the cast changed. The cast is removed at 6 weeks. We prefer not to rigidly immobilize the knee in flexion for several weeks because of the deterioration of the articular cartilage surfaces associated with the absence of motion, especially in the patellofemoral joint. If extension beyond 30 degrees is detrimental to the reconstruction early, we prefer to use a controlled motion brace locked at 30 degrees of extension but allowing flexion.

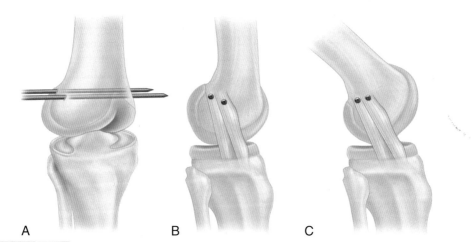

FIGURE 1.101 **A,** Two points on lateral femoral condyle corresponding to major femoral intraarticular attachments of anterior cruciate ligament. **B,** Posterior band tight in extension. **C,** Anterior band tight in flexion. **SEE TECHNIQUE 1.21.**

▌INTRAARTICULAR RECONSTRUCTION

The advances made in arthroscopy have led to the development of arthroscopic techniques for ACL reconstruction. Simultaneously, our increased understanding of technical issues of graft selection, placement, tensioning, and fixation, as well as of postoperative rehabilitation, led to dramatically improved results compared with previous intraarticular reconstructions. These same principles can be applied to open intraarticular reconstruction of the ACL through a small arthrotomy incision, which preserves attachment of the vastus medialis obliquus muscle to the patella, or through the patellar tendon defect when the central third is used as a graft source. Arthroscopic techniques have minor advantages compared with miniarthrotomy, mainly, earlier resolution of postoperative pain. With either technique, we prefer to delay the reconstruction until after the patient has recovered from the initial injury or reinjury. Resolution of inflammation around the knee and return of full motion reduce the incidence of postoperative knee stiffness.

Graft Selection. Once the decision is made to reconstruct the ACL, the surgeon must select a graft. Autograft tissue is used most commonly, but allografts and synthetics also are available and are discussed later in this chapter. Autografts have the advantages of low risk of adverse inflammatory reaction and virtually no risk of disease transmission. As a biologic graft, an autograft undergoes revascularization and recollagenization, but initially a 50% loss of graft strength occurs after implantation. Therefore, it is desirable to begin with a graft stronger than the tissue to be replaced. Virtually every structure around the knee has been used as a substitute. The most common current graft choices are bone–patellar tendon–bone graft, the quadrupled hamstring tendon graft, and the quadriceps tendon with or without bone from the patella. The bone–patellar tendon–bone graft usually is an 8- to 11-mm-wide graft taken from the central third of the patellar tendon, with its adjacent patella and tibial bone blocks. This graft's attractive features include its high ultimate tensile load (approximately 2300 N), its stiffness (approximately 620 N/mm), and the possibility for rigid fixation with its attached bony ends.

The use of the hamstring tendon graft has increased in recent years because of its relatively low donor site morbidity. Use of a single strand of the semitendinosus or gracilis tendon is inadequate because the semitendinosus tendon has only 75% and the gracilis tendon only 49% the strength of the ACL. Now, surgeons are using either a triple- or quadruple-stranded semitendinosus graft or a quadruple-stranded semitendinosus-gracilis tendon graft with both ends folded in half and combined. This latter graft has an ultimate tensile load reported to be as high as 4108 N. This quadruple-stranded graft also provides a multiple-bundle replacement graft that may better approximate the function of the two-bundle ACL. Disadvantages of this soft-tissue graft include the concern over tendon healing within the osseous tunnels and the lack of rigid bony fixation.

The quadriceps tendon graft also has attracted interest recently. It can be harvested with a portion of patellar bone or entirely as a soft-tissue graft. Biomechanical studies have shown the ultimate tensile load of this graft to be as high as 2352 N. This graft has become an alternative replacement graft, especially for revision ACL surgeries and for knees with multiple ligament injuries.

Most investigators have reported comparable results with the use of either a bone-patella tendon-bone graft or a quadrupled hamstring graft. Spindler et al., in a systematic review of randomized, controlled trials comparing patellar tendon with hamstring tendon autografts, identified nine studies that met their criteria. Slight increased laxity on arthrometer testing was reported in the hamstring group in three of seven studies, pain with kneeling was greater for the patellar tendon group in all of the four studies in which it was evaluated, and only one of nine studies showed increased anterior knee pain in the patellar tendon group. Frequency of additional surgery seemed to be related to the fixation method and not the graft type. No study reported a significant difference in graft failure between patellar tendon and hamstring tendon autografts; graft failure rates for the combined populations of the nine studies were 3.1% for patellar tendon grafts and 4.1% for hamstring grafts. Objective differences (range of motion, isokinetic strength, arthrometer testing) were not detected between groups in most of the studies, suggesting that their sensitivity to detect clinical outcomes may be limited.

Selection of either graft results in some residual morbidity to the patient. Using ultrasonographic and power Doppler evaluation, Jarvela et al. studied the morphologic changes in the patellar tendon of 31 patients 10 years after harvest of its central third and closure of the defect. They found intratendinous calcification in nine patients, hypoechoic lesions in 20 patients, a hyperechoic lesion in one patient, and peritendinous changes in one patient. Only three of the 31 patients had no changes in the harvested patellar tendon. In most patients, the harvested patellar tendon was significantly thicker than the contralateral tendon. Harvest of the hamstring tendons has raised concerns about potential weakness of knee flexion. Most studies have reported no significant difference in hamstring muscle torque between the surgical extremity and the control extremity at 2 years after surgery, possibly because of regeneration of these tendons, as shown in MRI studies by Rispoli et al. However, Tashiro et al. reported significant weakness of hamstring muscle strength with both isokinetic and isometric measurements when subjects' knees were at positions of 70 degrees or more of flexion.

Graft Placement. The next important decision is graft placement. Extensive research has been devoted to identification of the ideal position for graft placement to reproduce the anatomy and function of an intact ACL.

Numerous authors have shown that, although both the tibial and femoral attachment sites are important, errors in the femoral site are more critical because of the proximity to the center of axis of knee motion. A femoral tunnel that is too anterior will result in lengthening of the intraarticular distance between tunnels with knee flexion. The practical implications of this anterior location are "capturing" of the knee and loss of flexion or stretching and perhaps clinical failure of the graft as flexion is achieved. Posterior placement of the femoral tunnel or placement of the graft over the top of the lateral femoral condyle produces a graft that is taut in extension but loosens with flexion. This location produces an acceptable result because the instability from an ACL deficiency occurs near terminal extension. The clinical examination yields a negative Lachman test result and a 1+ anterior drawer. If this location is chosen, the surgeon must secure the graft with the knee in extension because securing the posteriorly located graft with the knee in flexion may result in loss of extension. If an over-the-top

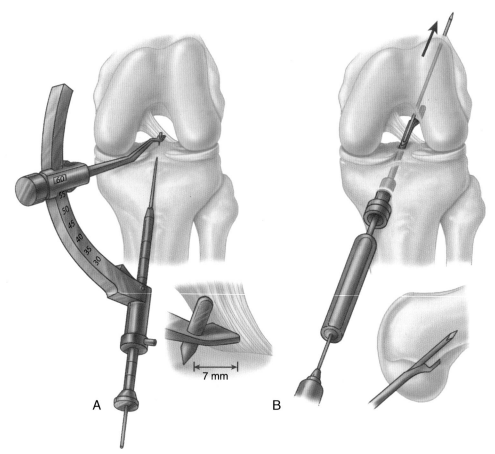

FIGURE 1.102   **A,** Tibial drill guide for anterior cruciate ligament referencing off posterior cruciate ligament. **B,** Anterior cruciate ligament femoral guide.

position is chosen, the route may be deeply grooved to approximate the "isometric" femoral position. The preferred location has been isometric placement of the graft that limits changes in graft length and tension during knee flexion and extension, which possibly may lead to overstretching or failure of the graft. Currently, however, the concept of isometry is considered oversimplified because basic science studies have shown that the normal ACL is not isometric. The fiber bundles of the ACL are under variable stress during knee motion. The AMB undergoes higher stress during flexion, and the PLB undergoes higher stress during extension. Robotic technology has been used to study the in situ force in the ACL in response to an anterior tibial load. The PLB shows a trend similar to the intact ACL, in which the in situ force in the AMB remains relatively unchanged throughout the range of knee motion.

After more than 30 years of experience with reconstruction of the ACL, controversy remains over the location of both the tibial and femoral graft attachment sites. A growing number of surgeons advocate placing the tibial tunnel more anterior in a more anatomic site in the center of the tibial attachment site, accepting the fact that it is not isometric. This position will produce a negative Lachman test but slight excursion on the anterior drawer. Other surgeons advocate placement of the graft at the posterior portion of the ACL tibial insertion site near the PLB position for best reproduction of the function of the intact ACL. This location also decreases graft impingement against the roof of the intercondylar notch with knee extension that can occur with anterior placement.

Various tools have been developed to assist the surgeon with placement of the tunnels (Fig. 1.102). These include devices in which the key point of reference is the over-the-top position, the roof of the intercondylar notch, or the anterior surface of the PCL. Isometers also have been proposed as a means of confirming proper location of the tunnels. Although helpful in locating anatomic areas for insertion, isometers have not proved useful for accurate prediction of the relationship between the tension and the length of the graft. Earlier techniques often included widening of the intercondylar notch or notchplasty to prevent impingement, which is more likely with anterior placement of the graft. The posterior tibial location requires a minimal notchplasty, if at all, unless the ACL deficiency is chronic and the intercondylar notch has become stenotic with osteophytes. On occasion, the surgeon encounters a narrow intercondylar notch, which has been shown to contribute to ACL injury, and notchplasty will protect the graft. In routine cases, we prefer a limited notchplasty that improves visualization in the posterior aspect of the intercondylar notch and assists in the proper placement of the femoral tunnel. The anterior aspect of the notch is deepened by 2 to 3 mm, depending on the size of the graft. The notchplasty is tapered posteriorly so that no bone is removed at the femoral insertion site. A bony ridge ("resident's ridge") anterior to the femoral attachment of the ACL should be removed, if present, because it impairs the proper identification of the femoral attachment site and also hinders the proper placement of the over-the-top guides used to drill the femoral tunnel. An excessive notchplasty may move the femoral attachment site, creating abnormal knee kinematics. The long-term results of notchplasty remain unknown.

Whereas past research has focused on the anteroposterior location of the femoral tunnel in the intercondylar notch, more recent study has investigated the appropriate position of the tunnel along the side wall of the lateral femoral condyle. This location frequently has been referred to in terms of a clock face. A vertical tunnel position high in the intercondylar notch near the 12 o'clock position has been shown to provide stability in the anteroposterior plane but does not restore stability in the rotational direction. With this tunnel placement, the Lachman test result is normal but the pivot shift test result is positive. Consequently, surgeons are beginning to place the femoral tunnel lower on the lateral wall toward the 10- or 2-o'clock position or even lower, which more accurately reproduces the femoral attachment site of the ACL and provides rotational stability. For single-bundle ACL reconstruction, the center of the femoral tunnel should be placed 1.7 mm proximal to the bifurcate ridge and approximately 8 mm anterior to the posterior articular margin of the lateral femoral condyle. Use of transtibial femoral guide systems tends to place the femoral tunnel in a more vertical position. With effort, the surgeon can get the guidewire to approximate the 10 or 2 o'clock position. Two cadaver studies have pointed out limitations of the transtibial technique. Strauss et al. found that the constraints imposed by a coupled drilling technique resulted in nonanatomic femoral tunnels that were superior and posterior to the native femoral insertion, and Heming et al. reported that if tunnels are to be centered in the ACL attachment site, a short tibial tunnel is necessary, which may compromise graft fixation and incorporation or result in tunnel length/graft length mismatch. However, studies by a number of investigators have suggested that tibial and femoral tunnels can be positioned in a highly anatomic manner with the transtibial technique, but this requires meticulous positioning of the tibial tunnel with little margin for error and some degree of tunnel length/graft length mismatch.

Alternatively, the femoral guide can be placed through a low anteromedial portal hugging the patellar tendon to reach the lower spot on the lateral femoral condylar wall. Advocates of this technique argue that independent drilling of the tunnels allows the surgeon to place the tunnels within the native ACL footprints for single-bundle reconstructions or create an accurate AMB and PLB for double-bundle reconstruction. When the two-incision technique is used, the femoral guide is not restricted in its placement by the native knee anatomy or previous tunnel placement and can be directed to the lower position on the lateral wall. A survey of National Basketball Association team physicians indicated that nearly half now use an anteromedial portal for femoral tunnel drilling, compared with only 13% reported in a survey 4 years earlier.

Numerous studies comparing transtibial versus anteromedial portal technique have not found any substantial differences between the two groups in subjective outcome measures, such as subjective IKDC, Lysholm, Knee Injury and Osteoarthritis Outcome Score (KOOS), and Tegner scores. Knee laxity scores have been equivocal. Using the Kaiser Permanente ACL registry, Tejwani et al. evaluated isolated ACL reconstruction (19,059 patients) and compared the transtibial femoral tunnel technique with the tibial-independent techniques, which include the anteromedial portal and lateral (outside-in, retro-drill) methods. They found that the tibial-independent techniques carried a higher risk of aseptic revision compared to the transtibial technique. A study from the Danish Knee Ligament Registry by Rahr-Wagner et al. compared anteromedial and

transtibial tunnel drilling and found a higher overall rate of revision surgery (5.16%) for the anteromedial portal technique than the transtibial drilling (3.2%). Some have speculated that the anteromedial portal puts the graft in a more anatomic position and consequently subjects the graft to higher forces.

Tashiro et al. studied the MRI signal intensity in relation to graft bending angle of an autograft quadriceps tendon with a bone plug used in ACL reconstructions. Anatomic single-bundle reconstructions were performed on 24 patients using the transportal technique. Lower signal intensity suggests improved healing, and they found significantly higher signals in the proximal region of the graft at 6 months postoperatively and a steep graft bending angle was significantly correlated with high signal intensities in the early postoperative period. The authors speculated that a steep graft bending angle may negatively affect proximal graft healing after ACL reconstruction. Most authors assert that they are now placing their tunnels in the "anatomic" position. However, Hart et al. reported 41 patients with unilateral ACL reconstruction done by four experienced sports orthopaedic surgeons who had 3D MRI imaging of the reconstructed knee and the contralateral knee to define their native footprint. The location and percentage overlap of the reconstructed femoral footprint were compared with the patient's native footprint. Despite contemporary techniques and a concerted effort to perform anatomic ACL reconstruction by these four surgeons, the position of the femoral footprint was significantly different between the native and reconstructed ACLs. Furthermore, each surgeon used a different technique, but all had comparable errors in tunnel placements.

Although the reported clinical results of ACL reconstruction are very good (90% to 95% good and excellent), biomechanical studies have revealed persistent deficiencies in our attempts to replicate the function of the ACL. The single-bundle technique traditionally used re-creates the AMB and ignores the PLB. Considering the two-bundle anatomy of the native ACL, some investigators have suggested a two-tunnel ACL reconstruction. The technique usually involves making two femoral tunnels with one tibial tunnel, but some also use two tibial tunnels. A biomechanical comparison of one-tibial-tunnel and two-tibial-tunnel techniques determined that anatomic reconstruction with two tibial tunnels may produce a better biomechanical outcome, especially close to extension. Although double-bundle and single-bundle reconstructions were equally effective in controlling anterior translation during Lachman testing in a cadaver study by Bedi et al., the double-bundle reconstruction was significantly better in limiting anterior translation of the lateral compartment during a pivot shift maneuver. The authors suggested that the double-bundle technique may be more effective in restoring knee kinematics in at-risk knees with associated meniscal injuries or significant preoperative pivot shift. Biomechanical testing has demonstrated improved ability to restore ACL function with reconstruction by two femoral tunnels, but improved clinical results have not yet been confirmed. In three randomized controlled trials comprising 375 patients and comparing double-bundle with single-bundle ACL reconstruction, no differences were seen in clinical or subjective outcomes and all three trials found no advantage to double-bundle ACL reconstruction. Caution should be exercised before embracing a two-tunnel technique because the added complexity may negate the theoretical advantages. Furthermore, the presence of two femoral tunnels may significantly complicate a revision procedure.

Graft Tension. The application of tension to the graft at the time of initial fixation can significantly alter joint

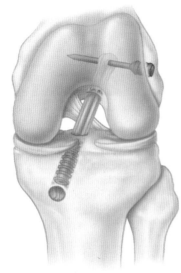

FIGURE 1.103   Cross-pin fixation.

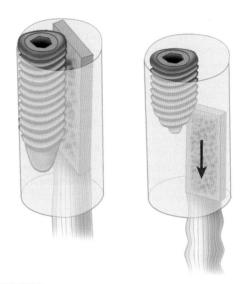

FIGURE 1.104   Appropriate graft fixation by interference screw *(left)* and inappropriate graft advancement by screw *(right)*.

kinematics and in situ forces in the graft during knee motion. Theoretically, the desired tension in the graft should be sufficient to obliterate the instability (Lachman test). Too much tension may "capture" the joint, resulting in difficulty in regaining motion, or it may lead to articular degeneration from altered joint kinematics. The tension in the graft necessary to restore stability has been shown to be tissue specific and to depend on the length and stiffness of the graft; less tension is required for a bone–patellar tendon–bone graft than for a semitendinosus graft because the tendon portion of the former is shorter and stiffer. The results of applying tension to the graft also depend on the position of the knee when tension is applied and the direction of tension. Studies have suggested that if tensioning is performed at 30 degrees, hamstring tendons may require 80 N of tension but do not benefit from further tension. Bone–patellar tendon–bone grafts fixed at 30 degrees of flexion are unlikely to require more than 20 N of tension, but if fixed at full extension, tensioning to 90 N is recommended. The force in the graft may decrease by as much as 30% after fixation of the graft unless the graft has been cyclically preconditioned. Nicholas et al. studied 49 patients who had ACL reconstruction with bone–patellar tendon–bone grafts and were randomized into high-tension (90 N) or low-tension (45 N) groups at initial fixation. At an average 20 months after surgery, anterior tibial displacement was significantly greater in the patients in the low-tension group as measured by KT-1000 arthrometer and manual maximal force.

Initial graft tension remains controversial because the in situ forces in the ACL during daily activities are unknown. In addition, the significance of the viscoelastic behavior of the ACL replacement grafts has not been entirely characterized. To date, an optimal protocol for applying tension to a graft has not been defined, but overtensioning should be avoided. Supraphysiologic tendon tension has been shown to lead to focal degeneration, increased vacuolization, coarser and less oriented collagen fibers, and a significant decrease in tensile strength.

Graft Fixation. In the early weeks after surgery, the weakest links in reconstruction are the fixation sites, not graft tissue itself. Fixation of replacement grafts can be classified into direct and indirect methods. Direct fixation devices include interference screws, staples, washers, and cross pins (Fig. 1.103). Indirect fixation devices include polyester tape/

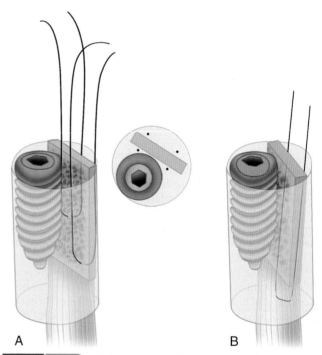

A   B

FIGURE 1.105   **A,** Improper passing suture position at screw-bone interface increases risk of suture laceration and loss of graft tension. **B,** Placement of passing suture opposite bone-screw interface decreases risk of suture laceration.

titanium button and suture-post. Significant research has been undertaken to determine the stiffness and ultimate tensile load of these devices, which has been found to range from 200 to 1600 N. Each of the techniques has advantages and pitfalls. Interference screw fixation is the most popular fixation method for bone–patellar tendon–bone grafts. Potential complications of the interference screw fixation technique include (1) inadvertent graft advancement can occur unless constant tension is applied to the bone plug as the screw is inserted (Fig. 1.104); (2) screw laceration of the passing suture can occur unless at least one of the sutures is placed opposite the side of the bone plug that contacts the screw threads (Fig. 1.105); and (3) the screw thread can lacerate the

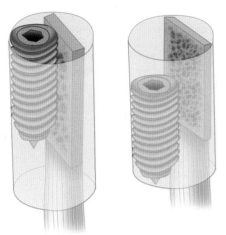

FIGURE 1.106 Proper relationship of interference screw to bone graft *(left)* and improper advancement of screw leading to potential tendon injury *(right)*.

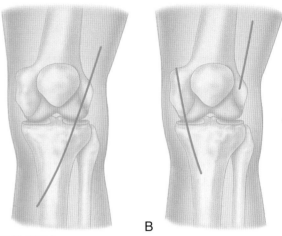

A   B

FIGURE 1.107 Modified Clancy technique. **A,** Single skin incision. **B,** Anteromedial and lateral incisions. **SEE TECHNIQUE 1.22.**

tendon if the tip of the screw protrudes beyond the end of the bone plug (Fig. 1.106). The screw must parallel the side of the bone plug and the tunnel wall. This is ensured by the use of a cannulated screw system over a guidewire inserted down the tunnel over which the screw is inserted. Screw divergence or lack of parallel placement of the screw to the bone plug can significantly affect the ultimate failure load. In a porcine study, screw divergence of more than 15 degrees lowered the ultimate tensile load up to 50%. Interference screw size must be determined by the size of the bone plug and the tunnel. A small bone plug in a large tunnel requires a larger-diameter screw than a larger bone plug. Interference screw fixation in osteopenic bone may need to be supplemented by tying the passing sutures around a screw for added security. It also is possible to "explode" a tunnel in soft bone (most often the tibia) if the tunnel begins too near the tibial articular surface and the screw size is too large for the tunnel and bone peg. Larger-diameter screws are necessary in tibial metaphyseal bone.

Bioabsorbable screws have been introduced as an alternative to metal screws. With improvements made in the material properties and in screw design, the pull-out strength of bioabsorbable screws is comparable to that of their metal counterparts.

Soft-tissue grafts can be secured to bone with soft-tissue interference screws, screws and spiked washers, screws and fixation plates, or staples. Studies comparing sutures, staples, screws with spiked washers, and plates have shown that spiked washers and plates have the greatest holding power. Interwoven heavy suture through the soft-tissue graft can be tied to bony bridges or around screws or staples. The screw is seated, and care is taken not to twist the washer in the soft tissue. The spacing and peripheral location of the spikes on the washer allow microcirculation to the graft. The limbs of the graft are sutured to each other with interrupted nonabsorbable sutures. Using the Danish ACL Reconstruction Registry, Eysturoy et al. found that cortical suspensory fixation of hamstring tendon grafts had a significantly increased risk of revision, while intratunnel transfixation had a lower risk. Conversely, Browning et al. in a meta-analysis demonstrated improved overall arthrometric stability and fewer graft ruptures using suspensory fixation compared to aperture fixation

of a quadrupled hamstring tendon autograft. There were no differences in IKDC, Lysholm, Lachman, and pivot shift outcomes between the techniques.

ANTERIOR CRUCIATE LIGAMENT RECONSTRUCTION WITH BONE– PATELLAR TENDON–BONE GRAFT

TECHNIQUE 1.22

(CLANCY, MODIFIED)

- A rear-entry commercial drill guide system (Acufex, Smith & Nephew, Memphis, TN) is used for the femoral tunnel, and the bone plugs of the bone-tendon-bone composite free patellar tendon graft are secured in the tunnels with interference screws. This technique can be used with entirely open or arthroscopically aided approaches. However, even if entirely open surgical techniques are used, thorough diagnostic arthroscopy is carried out.
- Correct any intraarticular pathologic condition with chondroplasty, meniscal repair, or partial meniscectomy, and examine the contents of the intercondylar notch.
- Harvest of the graft and the reconstruction can be done through two incisions or a single incision. The necessity of posteromedial or posterolateral incisions (as for meniscal repair), previous incisional scars, or surgical preference influences the choice of incision placement.
- The single skin incision begins 8 cm superolateral to the patella and courses distally to cross the tibial tuberosity to the anteromedial tibia (Fig. 1.107A).
- The two separate incisions are (1) an anteromedial incision beginning just medial to the superomedial border of the patella and paralleling the patellar tendon to 2 cm distal to the tibial tuberosity, and (2) a lateral incision 8 to 10 cm long, beginning at the lateral epicondyle of the femur and extending proximally over the midlateral aspect of the iliotibial band (Fig. 1.107B).

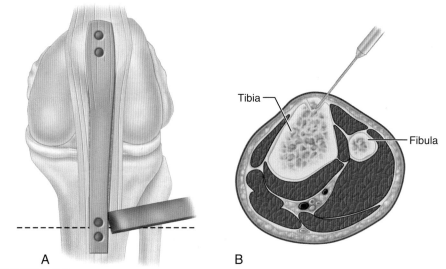

FIGURE 1.108   **A,** Release of graft with patellar and tibial tuberosity bony attachments. **B,** Removal of segment of tibial tuberosity. **SEE TECHNIQUE 1.22.**

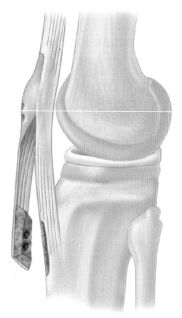

FIGURE 1.109   Graft freed from tibial tuberosity. **SEE TECHNIQUE 1.22.**

- Expose the patella and patellar tendon through the plane of the prepatellar bursa.
- Measure the width of the patellar tendon.
- Make two parallel incisions through the full thickness of the tendon, 10 mm apart, from the inferior pole of the patella to the attachment of the tibial tuberosity if the patellar tendon is at least 30 mm wide. If the patellar tendon is not this wide, use only the central third.
- Continue the parallel incisions through the aponeurosis, over the anterior surface of the patella from its inferior pole to the quadriceps tendon insertion, and distally through the periosteum over the tibial tuberosity, extending 2 to 3 cm inferior to the tendon insertion. The inci-

sions mark the line for releasing the graft with its patellar and tibial tuberosity bony attachments (Fig. 1.108A).
- With an oscillating saw, remove a 2- to 3-cm-long segment of tibial tuberosity bone by sawing along the previously made periosteal incisions, directing the saw from each side of the bone at a 45-degree angle (Fig. 1.108B).
- After both sides of the tibial tuberosity bone have been sawed, release the proximal and distal bony extents with a 1-cm osteotome and then "pop up" and free the graft (Fig. 1.109).
- Now attend to the patellar end of the graft.
- Using the oscillating saw along the previously made parallel incisions in the anterior patellar aponeurosis, make parallel cuts through the outer cortex of the patella from the inferior pole 20 to 25 mm. Connect these cuts with a transverse cut at the proximal extent. The depth of these cuts is crucial; too deep a cut risks osteotomy or subsequent fracture of the patella, and too shallow a cut risks fashioning a graft too thin for satisfactory fixation in the femoral tunnel.
- Extend the knee fully and have an assistant pull the distally released graft superiorly while depressing the superior pole of the patella to expose the inferior pole.
- With a 1-cm osteotome, release the full thickness of the outer cortex of the patella from inferior to superior, determined by the depth of the two previously made parallel saw cuts. Take care not to damage or to weaken the patellar tendon graft insertion on the bone at the inferior pole of the patella.
- Smooth any sharp edges or corners of the bony defect in the patella with a rongeur or rasp to eliminate a stress riser effect.
- When it is completed, the free, nonvascularized, bone-tendon-bone graft should consist of a piece of patellar bone 5 mm thick, 10 mm wide, and 2 to 2.5 cm long connected to a 10-mm-wide, full-thickness patellar tendon attached to a piece of tibial tuberosity bone 8 mm thick, 10 mm wide, and 2 to 3 cm long (Fig. 1.110A).
- Size the bone–tendon–bone graft so that it passes snugly but easily through a 10-mm cylindrical sizer.

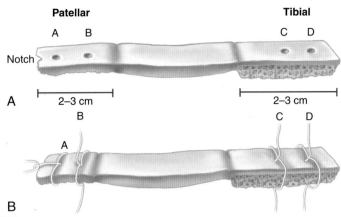

Patellar **Tibial**

A, Free, nonvascularized, bone-tendon-bone graft; patellar bone is 5 mm thick, 10 mm wide, and 2-3 cm long and is connected to 10-mm-wide full-thickness patellar tendon attached to piece of tibial tuberosity 8 mm thick, 10 mm wide, and 2-3 cm long. **B,** Sutures are placed through holes in bony portions of graft. **SEE TECHNIQUE 1.22.**

FIGURE 1.110

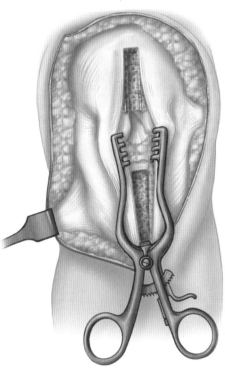

FIGURE 1.111 Intercondylar notch can be explored through defect in patellar tendon created by harvesting of graft. **SEE TECH-NIQUE 1.22.**

- Drill two holes through the patellar bone fragment and two through the tibial tuberosity bone.
- Place no. 5 Tevdek sutures through holes A, B, C, and D (Fig. 1.110B).
- Place the bone-tendon-bone graft in lactated Ringer solution with antibiotics.
- Explore the intercondylar notch; this can be done with an arthroscopically aided technique, through an anteromedial arthrotomy, or through the defect in the patellar tendon created by harvesting of the bone-tendon-bone graft (Fig. 1.111).
- Excise the femoral and tibial stump remnants of the torn ACL, carefully protecting the PCL.

- Remove all soft tissue from the lateral wall of the intercondylar notch all the way posteriorly to the posterolateral capsule and the over-the-top site. Figure-four positioning of the knee (hip flexed and externally rotated, knee flexed, and foot on the opposite knee) may be helpful at this stage.
- Perform a notchplasty if needed, using osteotomes, curets, or arthroscopic motorized burrs.
- A bony ridge anterior to the over-the-top site can be confused with the proper over-the-top location (referred to as "resident's ridge"). If this ridge is used as a reference for placement of the femoral tunnel, the femoral attachment site will be too far anterior.
- With a probe or angled curet, explore the posterior limits of the intercondylar notch to determine precisely the drop-off point where the instrument goes over the top of the posterolateral femoral condyle (Fig. 1.112). Repeat this probing several times to confirm the posterior location. By observation of the probe or curet as it drops over the posterior edge of the femoral condyle, the over-the-top route can be hooked with the curet or probe.
- Bring the tip of the curved curet back into the posterior intercondylar notch and create a pilot hole for the tip of the rear-entry guide 5 to 6 mm anterior to the drop-off point over the top of the femoral condyle. With the posterosuperior apex of the intercondylar notch representing the 12 o'clock position, this pilot hole should be at the 11 o'clock position in a right knee (Fig. 1.113A) and at the 1 o'clock position in a left knee (Fig. 1.113B).
- Now direct attention to the lateral side of the knee.
- Make a longitudinal midlateral incision, beginning 4 to 5 cm proximal to the patella and ending at the lateral femoral epicondyle.
- Incise the iliotibial band longitudinally at its anterior two thirds/posterior one third junction, extending from the lateral epicondylar level proximally for 4 to 5 cm.
- Retract the vastus lateralis anteriorly to expose the lateral femoral epicondyle and the metaphyseal cortex of the distal femur. Incise the periosteum and strip it off the posterior femur into the posterior intercondylar notch. Take care not to detach the lateral intermuscular septum or the posterior third of the iliotibial band from their important attachments to the lateral femoral epicondyle.

- The exit site for the femoral tunnel is 3 to 4 cm proximal to the lateral femoral epicondyle (Fig. 1.114).
- Pass the blunt-end, curved passer through the intercondylar notch and pierce the posterolateral capsule at the over-the-top location, just posterior to the previously fashioned pilot hole for the rear-entry guide. Keep the knee flexed during passage to minimize risk of injury to the popliteal structures.
- Insert a double-gloved fingertip through the lateral epicondylar incision and palpate for the tip of the curved passer. Keep the tip of the passer against the bone at all times as it is maneuvered to the gloved fingertip. Bring the tip of the passer through the lateral intermuscular septum and into view.
- Affix the appropriate rear-entry guide (right or left) into the eye of the passer (Fig. 1.115).
- Pull the tip of the rear-entry guide into the posterior intercondylar notch with the passer. As the passer is pulled back into the intercondylar notch, maintain a gentle pull on the rear-entry guide to prevent disengagement of the guide from the passer as it is pulled through the posterior capsule.
- Then remove the curved passer from the joint.
- View the tip of the rear-entry guide in the posterior intercondylar notch and engage it in the pilot hole at the anatomic femoral attachment site.
- Insert the bullet-shaped attachment to the rear-entry guide and slide it down to engage the midlateral femoral metaphysis 3 to 4 cm proximal to the lateral femoral epicondyle. This site can be marked and a hole drilled through the cortex.
- Secure the tip of the bullet-shaped guide in the hole in the femoral cortex and tighten the screw to secure the guide into the rear-entry guide system and then lock the guide (Fig. 1.116).
- Drill a Kirschner wire through the bullet-shaped guide from outside inward to enter the intercondylar notch at the tip of the rear-entry guide.
- Fashion the tibial tunnel by drilling a guide pin through the medial tibial condyle, entering the joint at the posterior half of the tibial attachment of the ACL.
- Direct the Kirschner wire at an approximately 30-degree angle with the tibia, beginning just medial to the tibial tuberosity and 25 to 30 mm below the joint surface. The guidewire can be inserted by a commercial drill guide system or with freehand technique.

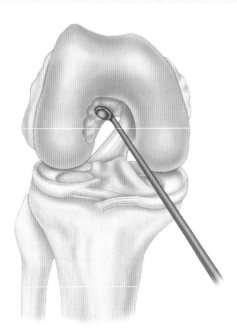

FIGURE 1.112 Small curet marks femoral anatomic attachment site. **SEE TECHNIQUE 1.22.**

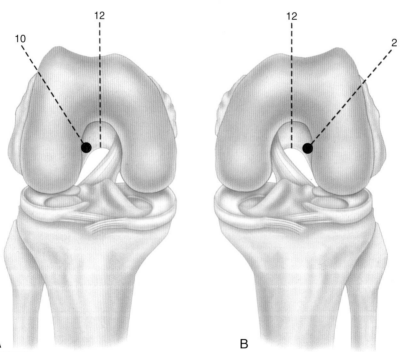

A

B

FIGURE 1.113 Correct positioning of pilot holes for right knee **(A)** and left knee **(B)**. **SEE TECHNIQUE 1.22.**

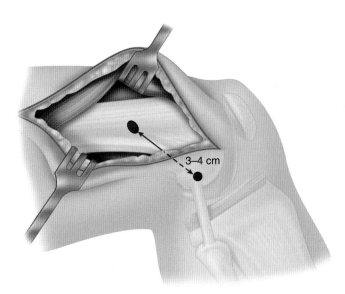

FIGURE 1.114 Exit site for femoral tunnel 3 to 4 cm proximal to lateral femoral epicondyle. **SEE TECHNIQUE 1.22.**

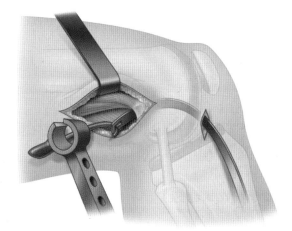

FIGURE 1.115 Rear entry guide is affixed into eye of passer. **SEE TECHNIQUE 1.22.**

- Advance the Kirschner wire 2 to 3 mm into the intercondylar notch to be sure it clears the PCL and does not encroach on the lateral edge of the notch. Advancement of the Kirschner wire farther into the intercondylar notch should bring the tip of the wire near the tip of the femoral guide pin, ensuring a straight-line course of the graft through each tunnel and through the notch.
- Extend the knee fully and observe the tibial guide pin to ensure adequate clearance between the graft and the roof of the notch. Redirect the tibial guide pin if necessary.
- Remove the femoral and tibial guide pins, pass a wire or strong suture through the drill holes, attach an isometer or tensiometer, and carry the knee through a range of motion. Excursion or length change of 2 mm or less indicates acceptable isometric sites of the femoral and tibial tunnels. If the length changes more than 2 mm, adjust the tunnel sites by drilling different guide pins into the notch and retesting.
- Once isometric sites have been confirmed, ream 10-mm tunnels over the guide pins.
- Smooth each internal and external tunnel aperture with chamfering rasps.
- Pass a suture passer from proximal to distal through the femoral tunnel, the intercondylar notch, and the tibial tunnel.
- Place the sutures through the patellar-bone component of the graft and through the suture passer and pull the sutures and graft through the tibial tunnel, the intercondylar notch, and the femoral tunnel. If the tunnels have been fashioned in a straight line, the graft should pass easily. Tying the proximal suture tightly over a notch in the leading end of the patellar bone plug guides the plug directly into the femoral tunnel.
- Position the bone-tendon junction of the graft at the internal aperture of the femoral tunnel; marking the bone-tendon junction with a colored suture or marking pen before graft insertion makes accurate positioning possible. The bone plug should not be placed too far into the tunnel to avoid exposure of the tendinous part of the graft to potential attrition on the tunnel edge (Fig. 1.117); the bone plug also should not protrude from the tunnel's internal aperture.

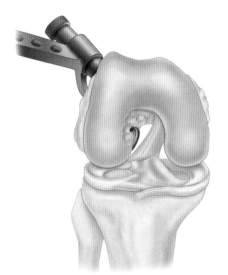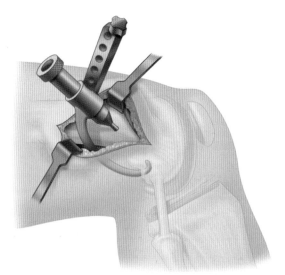

FIGURE 1.116 With tip of guide engaged at anatomic site, bullet is positioned so that two of three teeth engage lateral cortex and guide is locked. **SEE TECHNIQUE 1.22.**

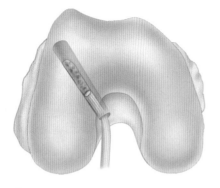
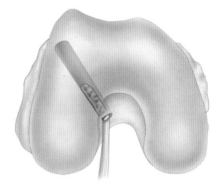

A   Incorrect   B   Correct

FIGURE 1.117   Incorrect **(A)** and correct **(B)** positioning of graft. Bone plug should not be too far into tunnel to avoid wear on tendinous part of graft. **SEE TECHNIQUE 1.22.**

- Once the graft has been properly positioned in the tunnel, insert an appropriate-size Kirschner wire down the femoral tunnel parallel with the bone plug.
- Insert a cannulated interference screw over the guide pin.
- While holding tension on the sutures in the distal end of the graft, move the knee through several ranges of motion.
- Then secure the distal bone plug in the tibial tunnel with an interference screw while the knee is held in full extension and moderate tension is maintained on the graft by way of the previously placed sutures.
- Carefully probe the secured graft to confirm proper tension and to ensure that neither interference screw exits at the internal apertures of either tunnel and that articular fragments of bone and cartilage have not been pulled into the joint.
- Thoroughly lavage the joint and close the incisions in a standard manner.
- Others have preferred an over-the-top route for the femoral attachment.
- Harvest the graft as previously described and thin the piece of patellar bone with a dental bur so that it is malleable.
- With osteotomes and curved rasps, fashion a deep slot or trough in the over-the-top location and into the posterior intercondylar notch.
- Pull the proximal end of the composite graft through the posterolateral capsule and wrap it around the lateral femoral condyle in the previously fashioned trough.
- Secure the patellar bone in the trough with a table staple, screws, or bone block sutures tied around the shank of a screw as an anchoring post.

See also Videos 1.2 and 1.3.

▌RECONSTRUCTION WITH HAMSTRING TENDONS

The use of hamstring tendon grafts for ACL reconstructions has increased in popularity. Initially, the semitendinosus tendon and gracilis tendon were used together as two single strands. Their initial combined strength according to Noyes' research exceeded that of the ACL. The tendons could be released proximally and left attached to the tibia, allowing a firm site of anchorage distally. Otherwise, they could be released both proximally and distally and used as a free graft.

The tendons can be released proximally by using a commercially available tendon stripper or by making a second, more proximal incision.

Surgeons more recently have chosen to fold the semitendinosus and gracilis tendons on themselves, creating four strands and theoretically doubling the strength of the graft construct. Others have chosen to use only the semitendinosus tendon, folding it on itself to create either three or four strands.

ANTERIOR CRUCIATE LIGAMENT RECONSTRUCTION WITH HAMSTRINGS (WITH PROXIMAL RELEASE OF HAMSTRINGS)

TECHNIQUE 1.23

- Make a medial parapatellar incision beginning just above the level of the superior pole of the patella and extending approximately 8 cm distal to the joint line near the tibial insertion of the pes anserinus tendon.
- Perform an anteromedial arthrotomy and treat any intraarticular abnormalities, such as a torn meniscus.
- Identify the semitendinosus tendon at the posteromedial part of the pes anserinus (this tendon is the lowermost component of the pes anserinus). The gracilis tendon is just proximal to the semitendinosus tendon. The insertion of the semitendinosus can be identified by its Y-shaped insertion onto the anteromedial tibia and the tibial crest, frequently blending into the fascia of the calf. Take care to avoid injury to the sartorial branch of the saphenous nerve into the saphenous vein.
- Release the proximal portion of the semitendinosus and gracilis tendons and the surrounding fascia from the musculotendinous junction, using either blunt or sharp dissection or a tendon stripper. If a tendon stripper is used, release all the fascial attachments to allow smooth passage of the tendon stripper. Without this step, the stripper may transect the tendons prematurely, resulting in an excessively short graft.

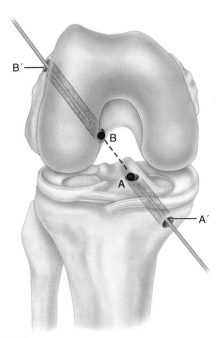

FIGURE 1.118   Anterior cruciate ligament (ACL) reconstruction with hamstrings. Lines AA′ and BB′ coincide with anatomic center of normal ACL. **SEE TECHNIQUE 1.23.**

- After release of the tendons, allow the muscle bellies to retract.
- Deliver both tendons through the distal portion of the medial parapatellar incision with their tibial insertions remaining intact.
- If a tendon remains attached distally, be sure to free the tendons completely from their bony insertion sites on the tibia. Otherwise, some creeping can occur at the tibial side after the tendons have been passed through the knee and tensioned.
- Free the tendons from any remaining muscle tissue and suture the tendons to each other under tension with a 2-0 absorbable suture.
- Weave a Bunnell stitch of no. 2 nonabsorbable material into the free tendon ends.
- Wrap the tendons deep to the remaining sartorius tendon to the anteromedial flare of the tibia 3.5 to 4.0 cm below the joint line.
- Insert a guide pin at this location and direct it proximally and medially to enter the joint area of the normal tibial attachment of the ACL (Fig. 1.118).
- Use a cannulated reamer to create a 5-mm tunnel in the tibial condyle over the guide pin.
- Bring the tendons of the semitendinosus and gracilis through the tunnel into the interior of the joint.
- If a free tendon graft is preferred, dissect the tendons at their tibial attachments with care. Between 1 and 2 cm of additional length can be harvested, including the periosteum of the tibial crest where the tendons insert.
- Weave a Bunnell stitch of no. 2 nonabsorbable material into the free tendon ends of all four strands.
- Place the tendons on a commercially available tensioning board so that all four strands can be placed under equal tension.
- Suture the strands together with a 2-0 absorbable suture.

- Measure the diameter of this construct. The tibial drill hole should be of the same diameter as that of the hamstring construct. Most constructs are between 7 and 8 mm in diameter when doubled on themselves. Research at our institution has indicated that the fixation of the tibial tunnel is improved if the tibial tunnel is reamed to 2 mm smaller than the diameter of the construct and then dilated to the appropriate size. Initially, ream the external tibial cortex to the appropriate diameter of the construct and then ream the medullary canal 2 mm smaller to facilitate passing the dilators through the external tibial cortex.
- The femoral fixation can be achieved either with a second lateral skin incision and rear-entry technique or with a transtibial femoral guide system and a single-incision technique.
- If the two-incision technique is chosen, make a lateral skin incision longitudinally in the region of the lateral femoral epicondyle.
- Split the fascia lata in line with the skin incision, reflecting the vastus lateralis anteriorly off the lateral intermuscular septum.
- Expose the lateral femoral epicondylar area.
- Direct a guide pin from without inward to emerge in the intercondylar notch near the normal femoral attachment of the ACL. Various commercial guides are available to aid in placement of this guide pin.
- Once satisfactory placement of the guide pin has been achieved, create a tunnel in the lateral femoral condyle with a cannulated reamer.
- Pull the hamstring tendons through the tunnel in the lateral femoral condyle. When the tendons are of sufficient length, secure them with multiple sutures or a staple in the lateral femoral epicondylar area.
- If the tendons are not long enough to reach the surface of the tunnel, drill a second hole obliquely into the tunnel and pass one end of the Bunnell suture through this hole with a suture passer and tie the two sutures over the bridge of bone in the lateral femoral epicondylar area.
- Alternatively, the ends of the Bunnell suture can be tied around the shank of a screw in the screw post technique or secured with a biodegradable screw using an interference technique.
- Close the fascia lata, the lateral skin incision, and the anteromedial arthrotomy.
- If the transtibial femoral tunnel is chosen, use of commercially available guides can assist in the placement of the guide pin in the roof of the intercondylar notch.
- Place the knee between 70 and 90 degrees of flexion and pass a Beath pin through the femur and then out through the anterolateral thigh.
- Ream with a cannulated acorn-type reamer, which minimizes injury to the PCL.
- The position of the femoral tunnel should leave 1.5 to 2.0 mm of posterior wall to prevent posterior blowout. The femoral tunnel should be at the 1 to 2 o'clock position on the left knee and the 10 or 11 o'clock position on the right knee. The depth of the tunnel should be at least 2 cm, and the diameter of the tunnel should correspond to the diameter of the graft. Because the bone of the distal femur is denser than the tibial metaphysis, dilating the femoral tunnel probably is unnecessary.
- Mark the hamstring construct with indelible ink 2 cm from the tip to confirm that adequate tissue has been passed into the femoral tunnel.

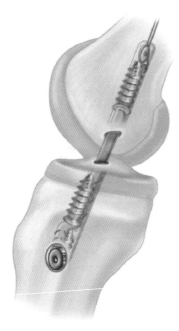

FIGURE 1.119 Two-screw fixation of hamstring graft in tibial tunnel. **SEE TECHNIQUE 1.23.**

- Secure the construct on the femoral side with either an interference screw or suspensory button on the lateral femoral cortex or transfixion pin.
- On the tibial side, choose an interference screw that is at least 1 mm larger than the diameter of the tunnel and graft. Research also has indicated that placement of the interference screw near the subchondral surface of the tibia minimizes pistoning of the graft as well as creep. However, maintaining contact between the interference screw and the external tibial cortex provides better initial fixation of the graft. Screws have been designed to achieve the desired length, and systems have been created that allow fixation both proximally and distally (Fig. 1.119).

See also Video 1.4.

POSTOPERATIVE CARE The knee is placed in a controlled motion brace locked in full extension. Protected range-of-motion exercises are begun immediately.

COMBINED ANTERIOR CRUCIATE LIGAMENT INSTABILITIES

Although a number of authors have recommended reconstruction of only the primary restraint (the ACL), ignoring the deficiencies in the secondary capsular restraints, we reconstruct only the ACL in patients with only mild or moderate (1+ to 2+) rotary instability under anesthesia. We have added capsular reefing (posterior oblique reconstruction) and extraarticular substitution techniques (e.g., iliotibial band tenodesis or ALL reconstruction) in patients with severe (3+ or 4+) rotary instability.

SYNTHETIC MATERIALS FOR LIGAMENT RECONSTRUCTION

Interest in the use of artificial ligaments for treatment of symptomatic knees with ACL deficiency remains despite disappointing early clinical results. Artificial ligaments offer a number of theoretical advantages compared with reconstruction by use of autogenous tissues—no autogenous tissues are sacrificed, and the increased morbidity associated with the harvest of autogenous tissues is avoided. If autogenous tissues have been used in a failed reconstruction or if they are unacceptable, the use of a readily available synthetic device is appealing. Artificial ligaments generally permit a simpler and easier reconstructive technique (frequently arthroscopic), and they allow a more rapid rehabilitation because they do not become weak during tissue revascularization and reorganization. Although there has been a rapid development of new materials and surgical techniques for artificial ligament implantation, the long-term effects of these devices are not yet known.

Artificial ligaments function in one of three ways: (1) as a prosthetic ligament, that is, the prosthesis is implanted as a permanent replacement for the normal ligament; (2) as a stent temporarily protecting or augmenting an autogenous graft; or (3) as a scaffold providing support for and stimulating the ingrowth of collagen tissue. Several materials have been found to be biocompatible and to have adequate strength to serve as permanent prosthetic ligaments. However, many have failed because they do not have the functional, physiologic, and biomechanical characteristics of the normal ACL. No long-term studies of the artificial ligaments currently used support their routine use. At present, it is prudent to use them cautiously and to reserve them for salvage procedures when autogenous grafting and reconstructive procedures have failed.

Scaffolds typically have an open-weave structure that promotes the ingrowth of fibrous tissue. Initially, they are biomechanically inferior to permanent prostheses, but their strength increases with the ingrowth of host collagenous tissue. Although these synthetic ligaments have not been used widely in the United States, one of them, the Leeds-Keio prosthesis, has become popular elsewhere. It is composed of polyester with an open-weave tube to promote fibrous ingrowth. There is conflicting evidence regarding the quality of host tissue ingrowth into the Leeds-Keio prosthesis. Most reports have indicated unsatisfactory results and suggested that the Leeds-Keio artificial ligament is not an effective device for reconstruction of the ACL.

ALLOGRAFT LIGAMENT REPLACEMENT

The ideal ligament replacement should be readily available; it should be of sufficient length and diameter; it should have biomechanical properties similar to the ligament it replaces; it should not disturb normal structures; and it should retain or develop a vascular supply. Although autogenous tissues currently are the most commonly used grafts for reconstruction of the cruciate ligament, these transfers sacrifice a normal musculotendinous structure in an already deficient knee, adding to the functional disturbance. Extensive surgical exposure, long tourniquet times, and prolonged rehabilitation are other disadvantages of these techniques.

Because collagen allografts appear capable of fulfilling many of the requirements for an ideal ligament substitute, free allografts for ligament reconstruction have received growing attention during the past 20 years. Researchers have focused on the basic science of allografts and on early clinical results. Autografts and allografts both go through four stages after transplantation: necrosis, revascularization, cellular proliferation, and remodeling. However, after incorporation, neither autograft nor allograft tendons have been demonstrated to return to their original strength. Most reports show 30% to 40% ultimate load strengths. Because of this consistent reduction in strength, most surgeons prefer to use grafts or combinations of grafts that begin with more than 100% of ACL strength, which should result in sufficient strength after incorporation.

Early speculation that grafts could be transplanted with viable cells, allowing better graft incorporation, has proved incorrect. Unfortunately, even preservation of a vascular pedicle does not appear to provide any clinical benefit over avascular grafts. Maintaining vascular supply to primate and human patellar tendon autografts has not been shown to result in any clinically significant improvement.

During remodeling, autograft and allograft tendons both undergo conversion from large-diameter fibers to smaller fibers. Studies have indicated varying time frames for this conversion process; some indicate a similar time period for both tissues, and others show a delay in allografts.

Reports on the immunogenic properties of collagen allografts have been contradictory. Minami et al. studied collagen allografts after various treatment regimens both in vivo and in vitro. They found no evidence of cytotoxicity, no histologic signs of rejection, and no activity with antisera from collagen allografts pretreated by freezing and thawing. They also showed that the immunoreactivity of the allograft depended solely on the cellular component of the graft; they concluded that the freezing and thawing treatment effectively neutralized the immunologic antigens by killing the tendon cells. Sterilization and preservation techniques have been shown to affect immunologic response. Freeze-drying reduces the response more than fresh freezing does, although cryopreservation techniques that preserve cellularity still evoke an immunologic response. This seems to support the hypothesis that immune response is directed toward the cellular components within allografts rather than to the antigens of the collagen scaffold.

Other investigators have demonstrated elevated antibody titers predominantly in the joint rather than systemically after ACL reconstruction with a fresh frozen patellar tendon allograft. This finding raises concern for the potential for graft-versus-host reactions, which may account for the relative delay in the incorporation of allografts compared with autografts.

The cited advantages of allografts over autografts—no donor site morbidity, shorter operative times, smaller incisions, and greater availability—have been somewhat overshadowed by the risk of disease transmission, with reports of serious infection associated with allografts heightening these concerns. According to a report from the American Association of Tissue Banks (AATB) using data from 2003 and 2004, 192 suspected allograft-related infections were reported, 42% of which involved soft-tissue grafts and 37% involving bone grafts. Orthopaedic sports medicine procedures were involved in 59% of these infections. A major concern in use of allograft transplantation for ligament reconstruction remains the possibility of transmission of hepatitis or acquired immunodeficiency syndrome. Lochemes et al. demonstrated active viral replication in cells infected with human immunodeficiency virus 1 after exposure to 2.5 Mrad of gamma irradiation, the maximal dosage that can be used without destroying the clinical usefulness of the allograft.

Even though the donor may not demonstrate detectable antibodies to these viruses, a certain "window of vulnerability" exists between the time the patient may have contracted the virus and the production of measurable antibodies, which may be as long as several months. Emerging pathogens, such as West Nile virus, severe acute respiratory syndrome (SARS), coronavirus, and prion disease, also have become a concern in the use of allografts.

However, the risks of disease transmission are small when the allograft is obtained with sterile technique and disinfection and secondary sterilization procedures are carried out. Using the Kaiser Permanente ACL Reconstruction Registry, Yu et al. reviewed 10,190 primary ACL allograft surgeries and searched for 90-day postoperative deep infections. They looked at both processed allografts (8425, 82.7%), which were treated either chemically and/or irradiated, and nonprocessed allografts (1765, 17.3%), which were not treated. The overall incidence of deep infection was very low (0.15%), suggesting that the methods currently used by tissue banks to minimize the risk of infection are effective. No difference in the likelihood of infection between processed and nonprocessed allografts could be identified. From the same registry, Tejwani et al. examined outcomes after primary allograft ACL reconstruction and found that graft irradiation of more than 1.8 Mrad, BioCleanse graft processing, younger age, male patients, and bone–patellar tendon–bone allografts were all associated with a higher risk of clinical failure and subsequent revision surgery.

The use of ethylene oxide for sterilization has been questioned because of the residual of ethylene glycol remaining in the sterilized tissues, which has been cited as a cause of some sterile effusions in late failures. Freeze-drying of the allograft does not appear to significantly alter the mechanical properties compared with deep-freezing, but clinical reports reveal frequent late failures of freeze-dried allograft tissues. Gamma irradiation of the allografts with up to 2 Mrad has been shown not to significantly affect the initial mechanical properties of the allograft tissue, but effects are significant after use of 3 Mrad. Conversely, in a meta-analysis of the effect of irradiation on the clinical effectiveness of allogenic tissue when used for primary ACL reconstruction, Park et al. concluded that primary ACL reconstruction with nonirradiated allografts may provide better clinical outcomes than reconstructions using low-dose (<2.5 Mrad) irradiated grafts. Electron-beam radiation has been used for sterilization of soft-tissue grafts because of its lower penetrability compared with gamma irradiation and higher processing speed—seconds, compared with hours for gamma irradiation. Elenes and Hunter used electron beam sterilizations on tibial tendon and bone–patellar tendon–bone allografts and found that the biomechanical properties of the grafts sterilized with an e-beam at a dose range of 17.1 to 21.0 kGy were not different from those of aseptic, nonsterilized controls or gamma irradiated allografts. Currently, the most commonly used method of sterilization probably is a combination of lower doses of irradiation (1 to 3.5 Mrad) and other processing techniques, such as antibiotic soaks (Table 1.3). Several companies have proprietary processes for sterilization that each claims provides a disease-free graft.

The superiority of autograft or allograft for ACL reconstruction remains a matter of controversy. A systematic review of the literature that included 31 studies found that

TABLE 1.3

Process of Allograft Procurement, Sterilization, and Storage

DONOR SCREENING	PRECLUDED BY HISTORY OF:
	■ Autoimmune disease ■ Ingestion or exposure to toxic substances ■ Rheumatoid arthritis ■ Systemic lupus erythematosus ■ Polyarteritis nodosa ■ Sarcoidosis ■ Clinically significant bone disease
	BLOOD TESTING MUST BE NEGATIVE FOR:
	■ Antibodies to HIV ■ Nucleic acid test (NAT) for HIV-1 ■ Hepatitis B surface antigen ■ Total antibody to hepatitis B core antigen ■ Antibodies to hepatitis C virus (HCV) ■ NAT for HCV ■ Antibodies to human T-lymphotropic virus ■ Syphilis
Tissue harvest	Within 24 h of death if body cooled Within 15 h of death if body not cooled Aseptic technique Tissue cultured before processing
Disinfection: removal of contaminants	Antibiotic soaks
Secondary sterilization: destruction of all life forms	Ethyl oxide, other chemical sterilants Gamma/electron-beam irradiation Proprietary protocols (i.e., Allowash, BioClense, Clearant)
Storage	Fresh allograft (use within 24 days) Fresh freezing (3–5 years) Cryopreservation (up to 10 years) Lyophilization (3–5 years at room temperature)

the percentage of patients receiving a final IKDC score of "A" (normal knee) was statistically higher for allografts (44%) than for autografts (28%); however, the graft failure rate was 8.2 per 100 reconstructions for allograft compared with 4.7 for autografts, with a slightly higher complication rate for allografts. The authors concluded that, from currently available data, the graft source has a minimal effect on the outcomes of ACL reconstruction. Although a number of reports have documented good results with allograft reconstructions, worse outcomes have been reported with the use of anterior tibial tendon allografts in young, active patients. Singhal et al. reported an overall reoperation rate of 38% after primary ACL reconstruction with anterior tibial tendon allografts in 125 young patients (≤25 years of age); the failure rate in patients younger than 25 years was 55% compared with 24% in those older than 25 years. The MOON study also demonstrated that failure of ACL reconstruction was more frequent in young athletes when allografts were used. In a randomized controlled trial of 99 patients (100 knees) comparing hamstring autografts

to posterior tibial allografts (aseptically processed and fresh frozen without terminal irradiation), Bottoni et al. reported that at a minimum 10-year follow-up there were four (8.3%) autograft and 13 (26.5%) allograft failures. Yet, in the remaining patients whose graft was intact, there was no difference in the mean Single Assessment Numeric Evaluation, Tegner, or IKDC scores. The efficacy of augmenting small diameter hamstring autografts with allografts also has been disappointing. Pennock et al. reviewed 50 adolescent patients who had quadrupled autografts (semitendinosus-gracilis) less than 7 mm in size. Patients were grouped based on the surgeon's preference to either augment these grafts with allograft (augmented group, $n = 26$) or to accept the smaller autograft (nonaugmented group, $n = 24$). The augmentation of these small grafts with allograft tissue did not reduce graft failure rates and may, in fact, have led to higher retear rates with earlier graft failure.

■ REHABILITATION AFTER ANTERIOR CRUCIATE LIGAMENT RECONSTRUCTION

The goal of rehabilitation after ACL surgery is to restore normal joint motion and strength while protecting the ligament graft. Appropriate rehabilitation is crucial to the success of ACL reconstruction. Some stress to the graft is desirable for healing and remodeling but should not be excessive and disruptive. Current evidence indicates that intensive rehabilitation can help prevent early arthrofibrosis and restore strength and function earlier. Perhaps the most important step is the early restoration of full extension. Knee immobilization in a fully extended brace is started immediately after surgery to prevent development of a flexion contracture. We emphasize active and passive knee extension with the heel elevated and the knee supported posteriorly. Cold therapy with ice bags is used liberally, although its efficacy in decreasing hospital stay and limb swelling and in increasing knee range of motion has not been demonstrated. Commercial cold therapy units rarely are used because of the expense. We aggressively pursue a full range of knee flexion, actively and passively. Continuous passive motion machines are not used routinely except in knees treated for arthrofibrosis. The literature does not support any added benefit with the use of these machines.

After surgery, the thigh muscles atrophy quickly. Studies revealed that maximal thigh atrophy was recorded 6 weeks after surgery. The contralateral thigh girth difference was a mean of 4.2 cm. A tourniquet applied intraoperatively for ACL reconstructions with autogenous bone–patellar tendon–bone grafts decreased the quadriceps strength recovery at 12 weeks after surgery. However, at 52 weeks there was no significant difference in thigh girth and quadriceps strength recovery compared with a control group in which a tourniquet was not used.

Some investigators have suggested that quadriceps strength recovery is less for patients with patellar tendon grafts compared with hamstring grafts because of insult to the extensor mechanism. However, Carter and Edinger compared the hamstring and quadriceps isokinetic results 6 months postoperatively in 106 patients randomly allocated to ACL reconstruction with either autogenous patellar tendon or hamstring tendons. They found no statistically significant differences in knee extension or flexion strength in evaluating the different tissue sources. In addition, most patients had not achieved adequate strength to participate safely in unlimited activities at 6 months postoperatively.

While the use of a femoral nerve block for postoperative pain control has demonstrated effective analgesia, it also has been found to delay recovery of quadriceps strength. The adductor canal block, which is a purely sensory block, has been shown to provide equivalent pain relief without the motor block. We have found a faster recovery of quadriceps strength with the adductor canal block and it is now our preferred technique.

Recently, the use of blood flow restriction (placing an air tourniquet on the proximal portion of the extremity) during physical therapy rehabilitation has become popular. The protocol combines low-intensity exercise with vascular occlusion, promoting muscular hypertrophy or attenuating atrophy. The underlying mechanisms are postulated to include (1) additional recruitment of fast-twitch fibers in a hypoxic condition, (2) moderate production of reactive oxygen species promoting tissue growth, and (3) stimulated secretion of catecholamines and growth hormone. All of these processes also are thought to be associated with conventional heavy exercise, because strong muscular contractions produce a large amount of metabolic products and cause a transient intramuscular ischemia. The occlusive stimulus may result in promoting muscular hypertrophy or attenuate atrophy.

Electrical muscle stimulation does not significantly decrease muscle atrophy in patients after ACL surgery, nor does it have any long-term strengthening effect. We use electrical stimulation sparingly for muscle reeducation if the patient has a poor quadriceps set. The early emphasis of strengthening is on the hamstrings, which function in concert with the ACL to prevent anterior translation of the tibia. Also, their strengthening does not stress the graft. Early quadriceps strengthening concentrates on quadriceps sets and straight-leg raises. Certain resisted quadriceps exercises are worrisome because they put some strain on the ACL, especially in the last few degrees of extension of the knee if the limb is not bearing weight, so-called open chain exercises. In an effort to protect the ACL graft during quadriceps exercises, it has been suggested that the patient stand instead. The knee joint is thus loaded axially during motion, and perhaps the contours of the joint help stabilize the knee and protect the graft, so-called closed chain exercises. In a prospective randomized study of open and closed kinetic chain exercises during accelerated rehabilitation after ACL reconstruction, the closed kinetic chain group had lower mean KT-1000 arthrometer side-to-side differences and less patellofemoral pain. Furthermore, patients generally were more satisfied with the end result and more often thought they returned to normal daily activities and sports sooner than expected. It is not known whether strains induced by rehabilitation exercises always have negative effects on grafts, causing them to stretch, or if some strain actually is necessary to stimulate remodeling of the graft.

After isolated ACL reconstruction, partial weight bearing with crutches is allowed immediately. A straight-leg brace is worn to support the weakened quadriceps. Certain types of concurrent meniscal repairs or articular cartilage procedures may dictate a different weight-bearing status. Crutches usually are discontinued by 3 to 4 weeks postoperatively.

Proprioceptive training also is instituted in the first 2 weeks. Risberg and Holm found that the outcomes of a 6-month neuromuscular exercise training program and a traditional strength exercise training program were not significantly different at 2 years after ACL reconstruction; however, knee function and pain reduction were better in those with neuromuscular training while hamstring muscle strength was significantly better in those with strength training, leading the authors to recommend a postoperative program that combines neuromuscular and strength training. Return to full activity requires 80% return of thigh strength and the ability to perform sport-specific agility duties. We also usually delay return to sports for at least 6 months after surgery to allow maturation of the graft. Animal studies suggest that the graft should be spared significant loads for 6 to 12 months. A functional knee brace after ACL surgery sometimes is used for collision sports, although no data support this practice. The rehabilitation protocol for ACL reconstruction is outlined in other chapter.

In the current economic climate, more frequent use of home-based rehabilitation programs has been suggested to minimize costs, and several studies have reported them to be equally effective. In a comparison of home-based (four physical therapy sessions) and physical therapy–supervised (17 physical therapy sessions) patients, Grant and Mohtadi reported that the home-based group had a significantly higher mean score on the anterior cruciate ligament quality of life (ACL QOL) questionnaire, with no significant differences in secondary outcomes measures such as range of motion and strength. However, all of these patients were recreational athletes, not high-level competitive athletes.

Criteria for return to full activity or sports are evolving. Although attempts have been made to develop criteria-based progression in the rehabilitation process, validation of subjective and objective criteria for return to play has been difficult. The criteria should determine the athlete's physical ability as well as safety. In a meta-analysis and systematic review, Ardern et al. reviewed nearly 6000 patients after ACL reconstruction. Only 44% of patients were able to return to competitive sport despite the fact that 90% had normal or nearly normal function using objective outcome scores and 85% of patients had normal or nearly normal function on the basis of activity measures, such as IKDC subjective knee evaluation form. One proposed objective measure is hop testing, a functional rehabilitation measure that may signal the capacity for successful return to play. The common hop tests include single-leg hop for distance, single-leg triple hop for distance, single-leg timed hop, single-leg crossover hop for distance, and vertical jump test. A score of 85% or higher compared to the normal limb is required for release, but these tests have yet to be adopted as consensus guidelines. With the knowledge that graft maturation continues beyond 6 months and perhaps as long as 18 months and that early return to high level sports is a significant risk factor for ACL reconstruction failure, consideration should perhaps be given to a longer rehabilitation protocol. Similarly, the use of functional bracing following ACL reconstruction is controversial. Some data suggest that functional bracing may have some benefit with regard to in vivo knee kinematics and may offer increased protection of the graft, but limited evidence supports routine brace use to decrease the rate of reinjury.

■ RESULTS OF ANTERIOR CRUCIATE LIGAMENT RECONSTRUCTION

The goals of ligament surgery are to restore normal joint motion, to return the patient to full function, and to prevent secondary injury and joint arthrosis. As with all treatment evaluations, the results of the treatment must be compared with the natural history of the disease process and with other treatment methods. Although the scientific quality of the studies reporting results of ACL reconstruction has improved, serious deficiencies remain. As previously discussed, the full natural history of an ACL–injured knee is still unknown. Furthermore, current studies are flawed by various forms of bias. Detection bias results from the use of different scoring systems to report results and from subjective definitions of success. Studies that include patients with different associated injuries and consequently different prognoses create a susceptibility bias. Studies that include different surgeons, different techniques, and different rehabilitation protocols introduce performance bias. Finally, transfer bias occurs when unknown subsets of patients are lost to follow-up, creating a false impression by focusing only on patients who are available. With these limitations in mind, most current studies report a 90% to 95% success rate in restoring stability as defined by a KT-1000 side-to-side difference of 3 mm or less. Unfortunately, current evidence estimates that radiographic knee osteoarthritis appears in over 50% of patients from 10 to 20 years after ACL reconstruction, and the current literature does not support the prophylactic benefit of ACL reconstruction in reducing the rate of osteoarthritis after ACL injury.

The results are equivalent for single-incision and two-incision ACL reconstructions with autogenous patellar tendon and with hamstring tendons. Furthermore, the results reported with use of patellar tendon and hamstring tendons are comparable. Comparisons of the outcomes of ACL reconstruction with quadruple-stranded autograft hamstring tendon and autograft central-third patellar tendon have found that ligament stability, range of motion, and general symptoms are basically the same in both groups, but the hamstring graft must be at least 8 mm. Using the Kaiser Permanente ACL Registry in a case-control study of patients with primary ACL reconstruction with hamstring autografts, Spragg et al. compared those patients requiring revision (cases) with those not requiring revision (controls). Between the groups, there was no significant differences in sex distribution, median age, median BMI, or femoral and tibial fixation. The mean graft diameter was 7.9 ± 0.75 mm in the cases and 8.1 ± 0.73 mm in the controls. The likelihood of a patient needing revision ACL reconstruction in the study cohort was 0.82 times lower for every 0.5 mm increase in the graft diameter from 7.0 to 9.0 mm.

Several meta-analyses comparing patellar tendon and hamstring tendon autograft ACL reconstruction showed that the frequency of instability is not significantly different between the two techniques. However, bone–patellar tendon–bone grafting was shown to be more likely to result in reconstructions with normal Lachman score, normal pivot shift, KT-1000 manual maximal side-to-side difference of less than 3 mm, and less flexion loss. In contrast, hamstring grafts had a reduced incidence of patellofemoral crepitance, kneeling pain, and extension loss. More recent studies have noted no significant differences in outcomes related to graft choice. Holm et al. and Lecoq et al. found that the choice of a hamstring or patellar tendon–bone autograft had minimal effect on the prevalence of osteoarthritis at 10 years after surgery. In a randomized trial comparing hamstring and patellar tendon autografts, objective, subjective, and functional outcomes were similar 2 years after surgery. Similarly, Webster et al. reviewed 47 patients at a mean of 15.3 years after ACL reconstruction with 22 patellar tendon grafts and 25 hamstring grafts. There were no statistically significant differences between the groups for anterior knee pain and kneeling pain, knee laxity, or the degree of osteoarthritis. Extension deficits noted in the patellar tendon group at 3 years had resolved by 15 years, and a higher proportion of patients in the patellar tendon group were participating in sport on a weekly basis. Sajovic et al. reported a randomized, controlled trial comparing patellar tendon to semitendinosus and gracilis tendon autografts in 48 patients. At 17-year follow-up, there were no statistically significant differences with respect to graft failure and functional outcomes, but more patients in the hamstring group had increased instrumented laxity (more than 3 mm) measured with KT-1000 arthrometer, and patients in the patellar tendon group had a higher grade of osteoarthritis according to the IKDC grading system. Shelbourne et al. reviewed 1428 knees with primary ACL reconstruction without existing osteoarthritis or other ligamentous laxity and no reruptures. The prevalence rate of developing moderate to severe osteoarthritis at more than 20 years of follow-up was 28.6%. Significant factors predictive of osteoarthritis in the long-term were older age at surgery, medial meniscectomy, and knee extension loss. Bjornsson et al. also identified more signs of radiographic osteoarthritis in patients reconstructed with patellar tendon, but Belk et al., in a systematic review of eight randomized, controlled trials, found that at a mean follow-up of 11.5 years, there were no significant differences in clinical outcomes (graft failure rate, radiographic signs of knee osteoarthritis, or patient-reported outcomes) between patients who had ACL reconstruction with bone–patellar tendon–bone autograft or hamstring autograft. Reports from the Norwegian and Danish ACL registries demonstrated higher risk of revision with hamstring grafts, with hazard ratios of 1.41 to 2.3, respectively, but overall, both grafts provided good results. The choice of graft should be individualized, and the graft type may not be the primary determinant for successful outcomes after ACL surgery.

Most of these studies are short-term reports and are not indicative of the natural history of ACL reconstruction. The ultimate goals of reconstruction are to allow the patient to return to an active lifestyle and to prevent reinjury and the development of arthritis. In a cohort of 6576 active-duty army personnel who had been hospitalized for an ACL injury, the rate of reoperation was significantly lower among the ACL reconstruction group at 9 years after surgery compared with those treated nonoperatively. Proportional hazard regression analyses adjusted for age, sex, race, marital status, education, and physical activity level confirmed that ACL reconstruction was protective against meniscal and cartilage reinjury.

In one of the earliest attempts to examine the natural history of ACL–reconstructed knees, Daniel et al. observed for 64 months 292 patients who had an acute traumatic hemarthrosis. The patients were divided into four groups: I, early stable, no reconstruction; II, early unstable, no reconstruction; III, early reconstruction; and IV, late reconstruction. All patients were evaluated for joint arthrosis by radiographs and bone scans. Patients with reconstructed ligaments had a higher level of arthrosis, and Daniel et al. speculated that although objective stability was achieved, the function of the ACL had not been completely restored. The patients were given a knee that was stable enough to resume sports activities but perhaps not normal enough to prevent slowly progressive deterioration. In essence, they had been given a "license to abuse the knee." Long-term follow-up (average 14 years) of 502 patients with ACL reconstruction found that the loss of 3 to 5 degrees of knee extension, including loss of hyperextension, adversely affected subjective and objective outcomes, especially in patients with meniscectomy or articular cartilage damage. Kessler et al. reported a 94-patient matched-pair study comparing the postoperative function and osteoarthritis development in patients with isolated ACL ruptures treated with reconstructive surgery (47) to those treated conservatively (47). No additional lesions, extraarticular or intraarticular, were included in the study. At a mean 11.4-year follow-up, clinical and radiographic evaluations and Tegner and IKDC scoring were done; the degree of osteoarthritis was classified by the Kellgren-Lawrence scale. Significantly higher postoperative IKDC scores were found in the reconstructed group, but 42% of patients in that group developed definite osteoarthritis (grade II or more) compared with 25% in the conservative treatment group. In a review of administrative databases, Leroux et al. found that the cumulative incidence of knee arthroplasty 15 years after ACL reconstruction was low (1.4%); however, it was seven times greater than the cumulative incidence of knee arthroplasty among matched control patients from the general population (0.2%). Older age, female sex, higher comorbidity, low surgeon annual volume for ACL reconstruction, and reconstructions performed in a university-affiliated hospital were factors that increased knee arthroplasty risk. A controlled laboratory study of seven knees with ACL reconstruction showed that although anterior laxity was restored during KT-1000 arthrometer testing, reconstruction did not restore normal knee kinematics under weight-bearing loading conditions.

After ACL reconstruction, female athletes are more likely to rupture the contralateral ACL than are male athletes, but males are more likely to rupture the reconstructed knee. Although self-reported outcomes in the first 2 years after reconstruction are worse for females than males, longer-term studies demonstrate no difference. In a systematic review and meta-analysis, Tan et al. examined the association between patient sex and the subjective and objective outcomes after ACL reconstruction. Females had inferior outcomes in instrumented laxity, revision rate, Lysholm score, Tegner activity level, and incidence of not returning to sports. Females and males were equally likely to develop anterior knee pain and osteoarthritis; the graft rupture and graft failure rates did not differ significantly. Using data from the MOON, Jones and Spindler identified female sex, higher BMI, smoking, less education, allograft, medial meniscectomy or repair, and chondral injury as factors associated with worse patient reported outcomes. Kim et al. followed 163 patients with unilateral ACL reconstruction and divided them into two groups based on generalized joint laxity, with a score of 4 points or more, based on the Beighton and Horan criteria, considered generalized joint laxity and a score of 2 of less were without generalized joint laxity. They found that generalized joint laxity had a significant adverse effect on stability and functional outcomes for patients followed for 2 to 8 years.

Young age at the time of reconstruction has been identified as a risk factor for failure of ACL reconstruction. The literature indicates that in patients younger than 30 years, the failure rate of approaches 25%. From an analysis of the Kaiser Permanente ACLR Registry, Maletis et al. found that the highest probability of 5-year revision was in patients younger than 21 years and lowest in those older than 40. Higher risk of revision was also found in male patients, hamstring autografts, BMI less 30 kg/m², Caucasian race, and use of allografts in patients younger than 40 years. The 5-year survival rate for index ACL reconstruction was 95.1% and for the contralateral ACL, 95.8%. Factors associated with higher risk of contralateral ACL injury were younger age, female sex, and lower BMI. In a systematic review and meta-analysis, Wiggins et al. found that age and activity level were risk factors for reinjury after ACL reconstruction. The data indicated that nearly one in four young athletic patients who sustain an ACL injury and return to high-risk sport will sustain another ACL injury at some point in their career, and they will likely sustain it early in the return-to-play period. The high rate of secondary injury in young athletes who return to sport after ACL reconstruction equates to a 30 to 40 times greater risk of an ACL injury compared with uninjured adolescents. These data indicate that activity modification, improved rehabilitation and return-to-play guidelines, and the use of integrative neuromuscular training may help athletes safely reintegrate into sport and reduce second injury in this at-risk population. In addition to younger patient age, Parkinson et al. found that significant predictors of graft failure also included medial or lateral meniscal deficiency and shallow nonanatomic femoral tunnel positioning.

■ COMPLICATIONS OF ANTERIOR CRUCIATE LIGAMENT SURGERY

Complications of ACL surgery can be caused by preoperative, intraoperative, and postoperative factors. Preoperative factors include appropriate timing of surgery, adequate preoperative conditioning and strengthening, and graft and fixation choices. Although each of these has been debated, current opinion generally holds that early reconstruction is preferable for early return to sporting activities, better clinical and laxity testing results, and decreased risk of late osteoarthritic changes. Preoperative criteria for successful ACL reconstruction include minimal or no swelling, leg control, and full range of motion, including full hyperextension. The type of graft chosen and the fixation used have not been shown to have a significant influence on the incidence of complications. The incidences of complications also have not been significantly different if either the single-incision or two-incision technique is chosen.

Intraoperative complications include patellar fracture, inadequate graft length, mismatch between the bone plug and tunnel sizes, graft fracture, suture laceration, violation of the posterior femoral cortex, and incorrect femoral or tibial tunnel placement (Fig. 1.120). These complications and their prevention are discussed in detail in other chapter.

The most common postoperative complications are motion (primarily extension) deficits and persistent anterior knee pain. The incidence of these complications is difficult to determine from the literature, with reported frequencies of motion loss ranging from 1% to 13% and of postoperative pain ranging from 0% to 34%.

Motion loss after ACL reconstruction can result from preoperative, intraoperative, or postoperative factors. Preoperative effusion, limited range of motion, and concomitant knee ligament injuries make poor postoperative motion

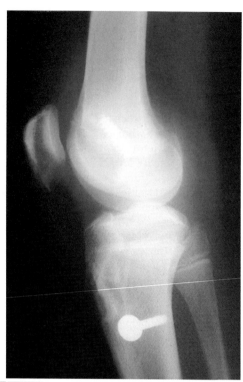

FIGURE 1.120 Frequent cause of failure of anterior cruciate ligament reconstruction is incorrect placement of tunnels for graft fixation. In this patient, tibial tunnel was placed too far anterior, resulting in graft stretching and knee laxity.

more likely. Intraoperative factors associated with motion deficits most often are incorrect tunnel position and inadequate notchplasty, which can result in overtightening or impingement of the graft, leading to loss of extension. Collateral ligament surgery and meniscal repair surgery have been reported to contribute to motion loss. Postoperative factors include prolonged immobilization and inadequate or inappropriate rehabilitation.

Anterior knee pain probably is the most common and most persistent complication after ACL reconstruction. Although its exact cause has not been determined, several studies have suggested a relationship between patellofemoral pain and persistent flexion contracture or quadriceps weakness.

In general, current postoperative protocols advocating limited or no immobilization and more aggressive rehabilitation have greatly decreased the frequency of both motion loss and anterior knee pain. Early concerns about possible stretching and failure of the graft have not been validated. Histologic analyses of patellar tendon autografts used for ACL reconstruction have shown that the grafts undergo "ligamentization" during a period of months to years, but a necrotic stage may not occur, and the grafts may be viable as early as 3 weeks after surgery.

Orthopaedic surgical procedures on the lower extremity are known to have a high risk of deep vein thrombosis (DVT) and pulmonary embolus (PE). Bokshan et al. queried the American College of Surgeons National Surgical Quality Improvement Program database for patients sustaining a postoperative DVT and or PE after ACLR. Of the 9146 patients identified who had ACL reconstructions, 46

(0.5%) developed DVT, eight (0.1%) developed PE, and five (0.05%) developed both. Risk factors for developing DVT in the 30-day postoperative period included age over 30 years, concomitant high tibial osteotomy, microfracture, hypertension requiring medication, and presence of wound infection. Cvetanovich et al. reviewed 4933 patients after ACL reconstruction and identified major complications in 27 patients (0.55%) and minor complications in 43 patients (0.87%). The most common complications were symptomatic DVT requiring treatment ($n = 27$; 0.55%), return to the operating room ($n = 18$; 0.36%), superficial infections ($n = 10$; 0.20%), deep infections ($n = 7$; 0.14%), and pulmonary embolism ($n = 6$; 0.12%).

While a postoperative deep infection is rare, it can be devastating; early recognition and aggressive treatment have proven successful. As with other orthopaedic procedures, diabetes has been identified to be a significant risk factor for infection following ACL reconstruction. Brophy et al., reviewing the MOON data, found that diabetics had an 18.8-times higher odds of postoperative infection than healthy patients. Schuster et al. reviewed 7096 consecutive arthroscopic ACL reconstructions (5907 primary and 1189 revision reconstructions) and found 36 cases (0.51%) of postoperative septic arthritis (0.41%, $n = 24$ primary; 1.01%, $n = 12$ revision). The first irrigation and debridement were performed a mean of 19.6 ± 10.6 days after the index procedure. Eradication was achieved in all patients after a mean of 2.25 ± 1.22 procedures, with graft retention in all but one patient (97.2%). The mean duration of antibiotic treatment was 5.4 ± 2.3 weeks. No recurrence of infection was seen. Coagulase-negative staphylococci (62.5%) and *Staphylococcus aureus* (21.9%) were the most common pathogens. Twenty-nine patients were available for follow-up at a mean of 4.7 ± 3.2 years. Two patients suffered recurrent nontraumatic ACL insufficiency (6.9%), and all the others (93.1%) had an intact graft. The mean KT-1000 arthrometer side-to-side difference was 1.4 ± 0.9 mm. The mean subjective IKDC score was 80.4 ± 11.2. No emergence or deterioration of osteoarthritis related to infections was seen.

REVISION ANTERIOR CRUCIATE LIGAMENT SURGERY

Recent reports suggest a range of 10% to 25% failures of ACL reconstruction. Also, the frequency of second ACL injuries in the first 12 months after reconstruction and return to sports in young, active patients has been reported to be 15 times greater than in previously uninjured patients. Paterno et al. found that the overall frequency of a second ACL injury within 24 months after reconstruction and return to sports was nearly six times greater than in healthy control participants. An accurate failure rate is difficult to determine because the meaning of "failure" of an ACL reconstruction is not well defined. One criterion, recurrent instability because of graft failure, is estimated to occur in 0.7% to 8% of reconstructions. Factors potentially involved in the failure of an ACL reconstruction include surgical technique, selection of graft material, problems with graft incorporation, integrity of the secondary restraints, condition of the articular and meniscal cartilage, postoperative rehabilitation, and motivation and expectations of the patient. Selection of patients and timing of surgery are crucial aspects of the preoperative plan. Early failure, usually within the first 6 months, most often is the result of technical errors, incorrect

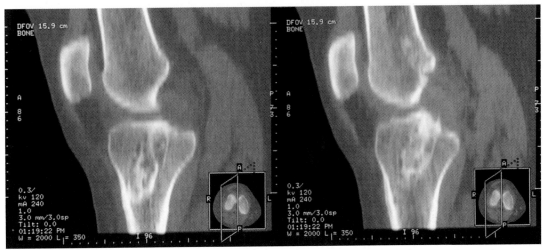

FIGURE 1.121 CT scan used to determine location and size of tunnels before anterior cruciate ligament revision.

or overly aggressive rehabilitation, premature return to sport, or failure of graft incorporation. Later failure, usually after 1 year, more typically is caused by recurrent injury.

The cause of ACL reconstruction failure may be difficult to determine, and more than one cause may be responsible. The most avoidable and most common cause is surgical technique. Errors in surgical technique can include improper tunnel placement, inadequate notchplasty, and errors in graft selection, size, physiometry, or tensioning. The most frequently cited reason for failure of the primary ACL reconstruction is inappropriate tunnel positioning, and the femoral tunnel is the most frequent culprit. These technique-related errors are discussed in detail in other chapter.

The main purpose for determining why an ACL reconstruction has failed is to prevent repetition of the cause if a revision is done. The causes of failure often cannot be determined. A detailed history, including events surrounding reinjury if present, is important. The patient's activity levels before and after primary ACL reconstruction should be noted. It is especially important to note if the patient was able to return to his or her previous level of activity after primary reconstruction and if instability and not pain is the primary complaint.

As with any knee examination, instability, meniscal signs, joint line tenderness, effusion, range of motion, quadriceps girth comparisons, and other parameters should be documented. A comparison with the opposite extremity, if it is uninjured, is helpful for objectively determining the baseline examination of the patient. Lower extremity alignment should be noted. The presence of combined instability patterns and the conditions of the secondary stabilizers also should be documented. Gait should be observed, including evaluation of varus or valgus thrust. Posterolateral instability is a commonly undiagnosed ligament instability pattern. Underlying ligamentous laxity of other joints also should be noted. Previous incisions should be documented with preoperative planning. Infection may need to be ruled out.

The patient's medical records, including operative reports and intraoperative photographs, can be helpful in determining why the graft initially failed. Numerous studies in the recent orthopaedic literature have investigated the impact of tobacco use on surgical results and complications. Cancienne et al., using a national insurance database, found that tobacco use led to a significantly higher risk of infection, venous thromboembolism, and subsequent ACL reconstruction. The surgeon should be prepared to correct any problems with graft fixation, implant removal, or bone deficiency, which might require a staged procedure.

Radiographic evaluation should include standard anteroposterior and lateral views, a 45-degree posteroanterior flexion weight-bearing view, and a patellofemoral view. Standing alignment radiographs of the lower extremity are helpful to determine the mechanical axis and if a concomitant osteotomy or staged osteotomy is necessary. The position of hardware, the position of tunnels, bony defects, osteolysis, and degenerative changes should be noted. CT, or preferably, MRI, is helpful in determining if the previous femoral and tibial tunnels are adequate for revision or if new tunnels are required, as well as in determining the extent of any tunnel widening (Fig. 1.121). MRI also provides information about the graft, the menisci, and the condition of the articular cartilage. Bone scanning may identify early degenerative changes.

GRAFT SELECTION

Reharvest of bone–patellar tendon–bone grafts typically is not recommended given the numerous other sources of autografts and allografts available for revision ACL reconstruction. Radiographic studies, including ultrasound and MRI, have shown that reharvest of the patellar tendon might be satisfactory because of suspected ligament regeneration and remodeling as demonstrated at progressive follow-up intervals up to 18 months. However, animal studies involving canine and goat models reported inferior biomechanical properties after tendon reharvest. A contralateral bone–patellar tendon–bone graft also may be a possibility but has the disadvantage of potential morbidity of the normal knee. We frequently have used the contralateral bone–patellar tendon–bone graft and found that rehabilitation of both knees has not been a problem. Shelbourne reported preferentially using the contralateral patellar tendon graft for initial reconstruction, citing improved rehabilitation and results in the ACL-reconstructed knee. Alternatively, we also have used the quadriceps–patellar bone plug graft with great success when patient or circumstances dictate avoidance of the contralateral bone–patellar tendon–bone graft.

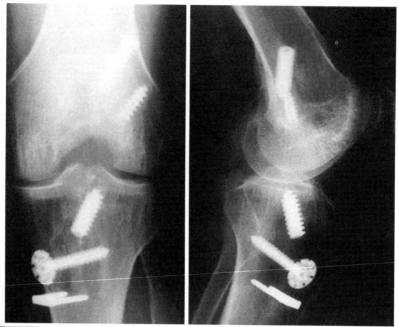

FIGURE 1.122   If possible, original fixation should be left in place during revision anterior cruciate ligament reconstruction.

Double, triple, or quadruple semitendinosus or quadruple-looped semitendinosus-gracilis grafts also are options for revision surgery. However, these grafts are smaller in diameter than the typical bone–patellar tendon–bone graft, possibly causing a graft-tunnel mismatch, which could result in problems with graft fixation and with "windshield wiper" effect of the graft.

The advantages of allografts include no donor site morbidity, smaller incisions, shorter tourniquet and operative times, and no size limitations. However, the cost is considerable. Their use also involves an acceptably low risk of disease transmission and a questionable potential for rejection, depending on graft preparation techniques. Sterilization techniques have been shown to have a significant impact on graft mechanical properties, immune response, and graft incorporation. Delayed graft incorporation has been demonstrated in a goat model study. The most common allografts for revision ACL surgery are bone–patellar tendon–bone grafts and Achilles tendon–bone grafts. Fascia lata and tibial tendon grafts also have been used. Although early reports found no significant functional or objective differences between revision ACL reconstruction with autografts and with allografts, this has been contradicted by more recent animal and clinical studies. It is helpful to have more than one graft option available at the time of revision; the surgeon should obtain preoperative consent from the patient if an allograft or autograft from the contralateral knee might be used.

■ TECHNICAL CONSIDERATIONS

Staged revision surgery should be considered if there is a problem with knee motion, specifically a lack of 5 degrees of extension or 20 degrees of flexion, when stability is not the problem. In addition, if large bony defects are present that cannot be adequately treated at the time of revision surgery, staged procedures should be considered. Harner et al. recommended a staged bone graft for a tunnel more than 15 mm

wide. Mitchell et al. compared the outcomes of one-stage revision versus two-stage. A bone–patellar tendon–bone allograft was considered for patients 50 years or older, for any patient with an insufficient ipsilateral or contralateral patellar tendon, or for those who chose not to have the contralateral patellar tendon graft harvested. Patients with malpositioned tunnels that would critically overlap with an anatomically placed tunnel or those with tunnels 14 mm or larger had bone grafting. In their study, objective outcomes and subjective patient scores and satisfaction were not significantly different between the two groups. Factors to be considered include the availability of autograft and whether the patient consents to the use of an allograft for the treatment of bony defects.

Previous incisions should be used or extended if possible. Skin bridges of less than 7 cm wide should be avoided to prevent problems with wound healing. Meniscal and articular cartilage disease should be treated at the time of revision surgery. The position of the original ACL graft should be noted and debrided.

Fixation should be removed only if necessary (Fig. 1.122). Unnecessary removal creates defects that require treatment. Typically, femoral fixation is the most difficult to remove, especially if the screw is buried. It is important to make sure the angle and seating of the screwdriver are accurate. If a screw has been in place for some time, the metal may have softened, and one turn of a screwdriver that is not properly seated may strip the screw head and make screw retrieval difficult. If the screw is cannulated, it is helpful to place a guide pin through the screw to avoid this problem. Removal of the tibial fixation usually is not as difficult, and intraoperative image intensification may help locate a screw that has been buried in or overgrown by bone. A bioabsorbable screw can still be present 2 years or more after surgery because the polylactic acid used to make the screws is not readily absorbable within this short period. Attempts to remove a bioabsorbable screw may cause fragmentation. It is best to leave it intact if

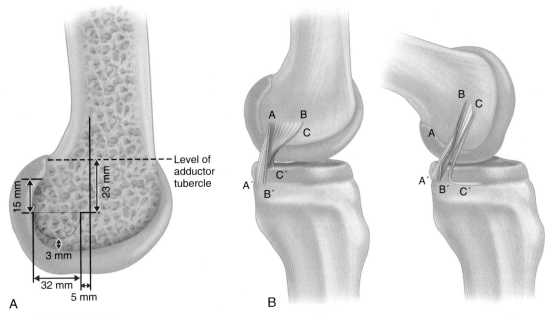

A

- Level of adductor tubercle
- 23 mm
- 15 mm
- 3 mm
- 32 mm
- 5 mm

B

FIGURE 1.123 Structure and attachments of posterior cruciate ligament. **A,** Lateral surface of medial condyle of femur showing average measurements and relationships of femoral attachment of posterior cruciate ligament *(shaded area).* **B,** Change in shape and tension of posterior cruciate ligament components in extension and flexion. With flexion, there is tightening of bulk of ligament (*BB′*) but less tension on small band (*AA′*). *CC′,* Ligament of Humphry attached to lateral meniscus.

possible or to ream through part or all of it if it is not readily removable. Prosthetic ligaments should be removed en bloc to avoid fragmentation of synthetic grafts.

Femoral or tibial fixation present from a previous two-incision technique and occasionally from an endoscopic technique can be left intact, depending on its location.

Screw and graft removal can cause large bony defects, which may require staged or simultaneous bone grafting. A cylinder-shaped graft can be taken from the tibia with a hand-held trephine harvester. In addition, the bony defects can be filled with oversized absorbable or metal interference screws, which can be stacked adjacent to one another to fill a defect. Harner et al. described the use of a large bone block allograft. For a posterior wall deficiency, it may be necessary to convert to an over-the-top technique or to use suspensory fixation. A generous revision notchplasty may be indicated. Adequacy of the notchplasty should be assessed after graft placement.

The clinical results of revision ACL reconstruction are not as good as those of primary reconstruction, and patients should be appropriately counseled about their expectations. The success rate for primary reconstructions is generally reported to be 90% to 95% compared with 65% to 75% for revisions. In a series of 63 patients with revision ACL reconstructions reported by Battaglia et al., approximately 60% were able to return to sports, most at lower levels than before revision. Significant progression of osteoarthritis, despite satisfactory stability and function, was reported by Diamantopoulos et al. at mid-term follow-up of 148 patients with revision ACL reconstructions. The MARS group determined that prior lateral meniscectomy and current grade 3 to 4 changes of the trochlea were associated with worse outcomes in terms of decreased sports participation, more pain, more stiffness, and more functional limitation at 2 years after revision, but no effect on activity level. Other factors contributing

to poorer clinical outcomes after revision ACL reconstruction included a higher BMI, female sex, and a shorter time since the patient's last ACL reconstruction. Better results were seen when a metal screw was used for interference femoral fixation and a notchplasty was not performed.

POSTERIOR CRUCIATE LIGAMENT
ANATOMY

The PCL is composed of two major parts, a large anterolateral bundle (ALB) that forms the bulk of the ligament and a smaller posteromedial bundle (PMB) that runs obliquely to the back of the tibia. It is an intrasynovial but extraarticular structure. The PCL attaches proximally to the lateral surface of the medial condyle (Fig. 1.123), and, like the anterior cruciate, it forms a segment of a circle. The tibial attachment is in a depression 1.0 to 1.5 cm behind and below the intraarticular portion of the tibia, with slips usually blending with the posterior horn of the lateral meniscus, the meniscofemoral ligaments of Humphrey and Wrisberg. Most investigators believe it is larger and stronger than the ACL. Harner et al. measured the cross-sectional shape and area of the ACL, PCL, and meniscofemoral ligaments in eight cadaver areas. The PCL increased in cross-sectional area from tibia to femur and was approximately 50% and 20% larger than the ACL at the femur and tibia, respectively. The meniscofemoral ligaments averaged approximately 22% of the entire cross-sectional area of the PCL. The insertion sites were 300% to 500% larger than the cross section of the midsubstance.

The attachment sites have been described according to arthroscopic and radiographic reference points. The center of the femoral insertion of the ALB is 7.4 mm from the trochlear point, 11.0 mm from the medial arch point, and 7.9 mm from the distal articular cartilage. The center of the tibial attachment site is 6.1 mm from the shiny white fibers of the posterior medial meniscus root, 4.9 mm from the bundle ridge, and 10.7 mm from the "champagne glass" drop-off. The bundle ridge is a horizontal bony prominence that separates the ALB from the PMB. The ALB is bordered medially and posteriorly by the PMB. At its femoral insertion, the PMB is bordered by the medial intercondylar ridge proximally, the ALB anteriorly, and the anterior meniscofemoral ligament, when present, distally. The center of its attachment was 11.1 mm from the medial arch point and 10.8 mm from the posterior point of the articular cartilage margin. The tibial attachment is more compact than the ALB. The PMB fans out in its attachment border along the posteromedial aspect of the ALB. It is described as having two "arms" and the thickest portion of the PMB, including the functional center of the bundle, is located posteromedial to the ALB. The functional center is 3.1 mm lateral from the medial groove of the medial tibial plateau articular surface and 4.4 mm anterior to the champagne glass drop-off.

BIOMECHANICS

Investigators evaluating the biomechanical properties of ligaments found that the anterolateral component of the PCL had a significantly greater linear stiffness and ultimate load than both the posteromedial component and meniscofemoral ligaments. Classically, the two bundles were thought to function independently, with the ALB primarily functioning in flexion and the PMB in extension; however, recent biomechanical studies suggest a more synergistic and co-dominant relationship between the two bundles.

The PCL is more vertically than obliquely oriented and is the axis around which rotation of the knee occurs. It appears to guide the "screw-home" mechanism on internal rotation of the femur during terminal extension of the knee. Selected cutting of the posterior cruciate shows that it is important in flexion; when it is lost, posterior drawer displacement is increased with no change in the anterior drawer sign. Most PCL fibers lengthen with progressive knee flexion. Rotational stability is unchanged in extension but altered in flexion after the posterior cruciate is cut. The PCL accounts for 89% of the resistance to posterior translation of the tibia on the femur and acts as a check of hyperextension only after the ACL has been ruptured. Secondarily, the PCL restrains external, internal, and varus-valgus rotation. The function of the meniscofemoral ligaments is debated, but biomechanical evidence suggests that they act as secondary restraints to posterior tibial translation.

PHYSICAL EXAMINATION

On physical examination, the posterior drawer test result is positive with a PCL tear; however, the true direction of translation of the tibia often is missed. The examiner frequently does not realize that the tibia is starting in a posteriorly subluxed position. Further posterior stress on the tibia does not produce any additional translation, suggesting a negative posterior drawer test result. An anterior drawer does result in anterior translation, and the diagnosis of an ACL injury is mistakenly made. The examiner does not realize that the tibia is simply moving from a posteriorly subluxed position to neutral instead of neutral to anteriorly subluxed. The confusion can be prevented by placing both knees in the drawer position (hips flexed 45 degrees and knees flexed 90 degrees), with

the examiner's thumbs being placed on the anteromedial joint line of each knee (see Fig. 1.43). Normally, there should be 5 to 10 mm of anterior offset of the tibia relative to the medial femoral condyle. With a PCL injury, this anterior offset is lost and the tibia appears flush with the femoral condyle.

Stress radiography assists in the diagnosis of the PCL injuries. Hewett et al. performed stress radiography on 21 patients with isolated unilateral PCL tears, 10 complete and 11 partial. An 89-N posterior load was applied to the proximal tibia and a lateral radiograph taken of each knee in 70 degrees of flexion. Stress radiographs were compared with KT-1000 arthrometer measurements and posterior drawer test results. Stress radiography was found to be superior to both. Increased posterior translation of 8 mm or more in stress radiographs is indicative of complete rupture. Alternatively, stress radiographs can be performed by having the patient kneel on an elevated firm bolster with the weight borne on the proximal tibia and the knee at 90 degrees. A true lateral radiograph of both knees taken individually allows comparison measurements of posterior displacement of the tibia relative to the femur using body weight as the posterior stress. MRI studies are more reliable for diagnosis of PCL tears than for ACL tears and are routinely obtained. Studies have shown that the sensitivity, specificity, and accuracy of MRI approach 100%. If an MRI study reveals associated meniscal disease (which is much less common than with ACL injuries) or other lesions, surgical treatment of these lesions is indicated and surgical treatment of the PCL is considered.

NATURAL HISTORY

The natural history of the disrupted PCL is still debated, with some investigators describing untreated patients with minimal symptoms many years later. Others reported significant osteoarthritic changes in knees with a PCL deficiency in an exceptionally high percentage (80%) of patients when repair or reconstruction was delayed beyond 4 years. The PCL has been reported to have an intrinsic healing ability after injury, although this healing may occur in a lax or attenuated position. The natural history of the isolated PCL–deficient knee varies considerably. Although trends toward moderate deterioration of the articular surfaces, mild decrease in knee function, and moderate increase in symptoms have been noted in patients with PCL-deficient knees, some patients have essentially normal knees and some have signs and symptoms of significant degeneration. Most reports on PCL insufficiency consider the problem of functional instability, and few emphasize the potential for early degenerative arthritis. However, functional instability may not be the major symptom of an isolated posterior cruciate insufficiency. Pain, aching during activity, and effusion may be the result of articular cartilage degeneration, which often begins several years before radiographic changes are evident. Long-term studies have found degenerative changes after PCL injury primarily in the medial and patellofemoral compartments.

As with the ACL, "isolated" tears of the PCL are relatively rare; as a rule, ruptures of this ligament are associated with medial or lateral compartment disruptions, especially the latter. Clinically, however, isolated tears of the PCL can be caused by a fall on the flexed knee with the foot plantarflexed. This foot position allows the knee to contact the ground at the tibial tuberosity, driving the proximal tibia posteriorly. If the foot is dorsiflexed, the knee contacts the ground through the patella. There is no posteriorly directed force endangering the PCL, but a patellar fracture is a risk. Perhaps the most common mechanism occurs in a motor vehicle accident when the knee is flexed and the proximal tibia strikes the dashboard. Such a mechanism (the upper tibia driven posteriorly with the knee flexed) may produce PCL disruption as the only clinically detectable instability (the clinician should also look for associated femoral shaft and neck fractures and posterior hip dislocations). These isolated PCL disruptions can be difficult to diagnose acutely unless a fragment of bone is avulsed from the posterior tibial insertion and is noted on radiographs.

Recently, as with the ACL, attention has focused on the association of a reduced posterior tibial slope and the increased risk of PCL injuries. The mean native tibial slope has been described as 7 to 10 degrees posteriorly and has been suggested to have a significant impact on in situ forces affecting the cruciate ligaments. Increased posterior tibial slope counteracts posterior tibial translation and reduces the stress placed on the native PCL. However, in PCL- reconstructed knees, a decreased posterior tibial slope is correlated with significantly higher residual posterior tibial translation and lower reduction in posterior tibial translation. Bernhardson et al. compared 104 patients with PCL tears with 104 matched controls. Of the PCL tear cohort, 91 patients (87.5%) sustained a contact mechanism of injury, while 13 (12.5%) reported a noncontact injury mechanism. The PCL injured patients had a significantly lower slope than the controls, 5.7 ± 2.1 degrees versus 8.6 ± 2.2 degrees, respectively. Furthermore, noncontact injuries had a significantly lower slope than the contact injured patients, 4.6 ± 1.8 degrees versus 6.2 ± 2.2 degrees, respectively. While decreased posterior tibial slope appears to be a risk factor for PCL injury, the impact on PCL reconstructions has not been determined. In another study of posterior knee laxity with double-bundle PCL reconstruction, Bernhardson et al., using linear regression analysis, found no significant correlation between preoperative posterior tibial slope and the amount of side-to-side difference in posterior tibial translation on postoperative stress radiographs.

TREATMENT

Treatment of a PCL injury is one of the most controversial current topics in knee surgery, primarily because the natural history of this injury is unknown. Most reports in the literature have relatively short follow-up and include a mix of acute and chronic injuries, as well as isolated and complex ligament injuries. Treatment of a PCL injury must be based on an understanding of the natural history of this injury, as well as on an accurate understanding of the long-term results of various treatment alternatives.

■ NONOPERATIVE TREATMENT

Traditionally, most authors have recommended nonoperative treatment of isolated PCL tears. Proven methods for reconstruction of this ligament are few; most surgeons have had limited experience with these procedures, and results often are unpredictable. Some patients remain free of symptoms despite the lack of a PCL, often with no direct correlation between the amount of ligamentous instability and the severity of any symptoms. The true incidence of injury to the PCL is not known but has been estimated to be between 3% and 20% of all knee ligament injuries. Complete PCL tears are defined as a measurement of 8 mm or more of increased anteroposterior laxity on stress radiographs. Many isolated injuries go undetected or become clinically silent. A review of the literature can be somewhat confusing, with studies reaching contradictory conclusions. Historically, most studies indicate that grade I or grade II injuries respond well to nonoperative treatment, at least at short term. Parolie and Bergfeld found high levels of satisfaction, return to sport, and performance in 25 elite athletes who were treated nonoperatively. Satisfaction and return to activity were not related to the amount of knee instability measured instrumentally but were related to quadriceps function on Cybex testing. Grade III injuries in patients with mild symptoms or low activity demands may be considered candidates for nonoperative treatment, but many clinicians question the existence of an isolated grade III injury, suggesting that a grade III injury occurs only in combination with associated ligamentous injuries.

MRI can be used to evaluate meniscal or chondral pathologic conditions and to determine if the injury is an interstitial or partial tear. These tear types have been reported to heal during 6 months, with a reduction in posterior laxity from a 2+ posterior drawer to a 1+ or even a trace. The commonly quoted criteria for nonoperative treatment include (1) a posterior drawer of less than 10 mm (grade II) with the tibia in neutral rotation (posterior drawer excursion decreases with internal rotation of the tibia on the femur), (2) less than 5 degrees of abnormal rotary laxity (specifically, abnormal external rotation of the tibia with the knee flexed 30 degrees, indicating posterolateral instability), and (3) no significant valgus-varus abnormal laxity (no associated significant ligamentous injury).

Reports have indicated that short-term functional instability is minimal and that function usually is not correlated with objective stability. Several studies have reported a return to sports activities in approximately 85% of patients with nonoperatively treated isolated PCL injuries, regardless of the grade of objective laxity. Nonoperative treatment focuses on restoring quadriceps strength. Despite these encouraging reports of nonoperative treatment, it is clear that not all knees with an isolated PCL tear do well. More recent longer-term studies have shown that knee function tends to deteriorate over time and that most patients eventually are affected by some degree of disability: pain with walking long distances, standing, climbing, and squatting; knee stiffness; and giving way. Dejour et al. suggested that the natural history of isolated rupture of the PCL could be described in three phases: (1) functional adaptation lasting 3 to 18 months, (2) functional tolerance continuing for 15 to 20 years, and (3) osteoarthritic deterioration that does not become disabling until after 25 years.

The worsening of symptoms and the development of osteoarthritis probably are caused by abnormal forces adversely affecting the articular surfaces of all compartments in the knee. In an in vivo biomechanical study, Castle et al. suggested that rupture of the PCL results in posterior subluxation of the tibia. During activities that require more knee flexion (e.g., ascending or descending stairs), the patella and patellar ligament are forced to assume a prominent role in the resistance of posterior tibial translation. However, the abnormal posterior tibial sag produces a shortened moment arm for the quadriceps muscle group, resulting in a decreased mechanical advantage. Cadaver sequential sectioning studies have found patellofemoral pressures and quadriceps loads greatly elevated and medial compartment pressures significantly increased after sectioning of the PCL and the posterior lateral complex. Logan et al. evaluated tibiofemoral motion by open-access MRI with the patient weight bearing in a squat, through the arc of flexion from 0 to 90 degrees, in six patients with isolated ruptures of the PCL in one knee and a normal contralateral knee. They found that PCL rupture led to an increase in passive sagittal laxity in the medial compartment of the knee. In the weight-bearing scans, PCL rupture altered the kinematics of the knee, with persistent posterior subluxation of the medial tibia so that the femoral condyle rode up the anterior slope of the medial tibial plateau. This fixed subluxation was observed throughout the extension-flexion arc and was statistically significant at all flexion angles. The kinematics of the lateral compartment was not altered by the ligament tear. These altered kinematics and contact forces result in the recognized degeneration of the medial and patellofemoral compartments.

Despite dividing their 38 patients into three groups on the basis of time from injury, Boynton and Tietjens could not identify prognosticating variables. They found subjects in all groups who had essentially normal knees and subjects who had signs and symptoms of significant degeneration, leading the authors to conclude that the prognosis varies for knees with an isolated rupture of the PCL.

In addition to the confusing "natural history" of the isolated rupture of the PCL, the results of current treatment options have been unpredictable, and the ability of any to prevent, slow, or arrest degenerative changes is unproved. Regardless, patients treated nonoperatively should be observed closely for symptoms of degenerative changes or functional deterioration.

After extensive experience with both operative and nonoperative treatment of PCL injuries, Shelbourne recommended nonoperative treatment of most acute grade II and all acute grade I isolated PCL tears. He found no correlation between knee laxity and subjective knee scores or radiographic changes. In a high-demand athlete with isolated posterior laxity of grade II or more, acute PCL reconstruction or repair may be indicated. In a chronic, isolated PCL tear with residual grade II or greater laxity that is symptomatic, other associated injuries, such as meniscal or chondral damage, are identified that may account for the symptoms. If the posterior laxity is believed to be contributing to or causing the symptoms, a PCL brace is worn to evaluate potential results from a stabilizing procedure. If the symptoms diminish or subside, PCL reconstruction is recommended. However, the success of surgical reconstruction in terms of stability has varied and is far from predictable. Long-term results after posterior cruciate reconstruction with an autogenous bone–patellar tendon–bone graft have shown decreased posterior laxity to an approximate grade 1.0 to 1.5, but posterior laxity has not been consistently or predictably eliminated in all patients. Clancy also recommended nonoperative treatment of acute isolated

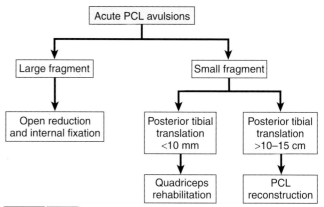

FIGURE 1.124 Treatment algorithm for posterior cruciate ligament *(PCL)* avulsion fracture. (From Veltri DM, Warren RF: Isolated and combined posterior cruciate ligament injuries, *J Am Acad Orthop Surg* 1:67, 1993.)

PCL tears because of the uncertainty of the natural history of this injury and the difficulty of consistently obtaining biomechanical stability. Furthermore, no studies have proved that PCL reconstruction prevents the development of articular cartilage degeneration. Gill et al. measured the patellofemoral joint contact pressures after PCL deficiency and after reconstruction in eight cadaver knees. Contact pressures were measured at 30, 60, 90, and 120 degrees of flexion under simulated muscle loads. PCL deficiency significantly increased the peak contact pressures measured in the patellofemoral joint relative to the intact knee under both an isolated quadriceps load of 400 N and a combined quadriceps-hamstrings load of 400 N-200 N. Reconstruction did not significantly reduce the increased contact pressures observed in the ligament-deficient knee.

■ OPERATIVE TREATMENT

We generally delay reconstruction for 1 to 2 weeks after injury to allow painful intraarticular reaction to subside and to allow the patient to regain full motion and some strength. "Clinically isolated" acute PCL disruptions are repaired if the ligament is avulsed with a fragment of bone (Fig. 1.124).

With knee dislocations, the PCL occasionally will be "peeled off" from its femoral attachment, and surgical repair produces good results. Repair of lesions at other sites is more controversial, with some authors concluding that suture alone cannot restore the PCL and is not strong enough to withstand the applied forces on the knee and that neither repair of the posterior cruciate alone nor semitendinosus augmentation of the proximal third or midthird substance tears provides adequate stabilization.

As with ACL repairs or reconstructions, we usually examine the knee arthroscopically before any open surgical procedure to better evaluate the intraarticular pathologic condition. Some PCL reconstruction techniques can be arthroscopically aided as to tunnel site placement and routing of the graft (see the section on arthroscopically aided ligament reconstruction in other chapter). Debate continues over the relative efficacy of single-bundle versus double-bundle PCL reconstructions and transtibial tunnel versus tibial inlay techniques. The following techniques are described as if only open techniques are used.

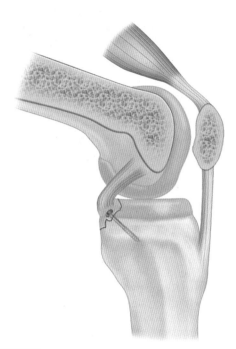

FIGURE 1.125 Screw reattachment of bone fragment avulsed with posterior cruciate ligament from posterior tibia. **SEE TECHNIQUE 1.24.**

REPAIR OF BONY AVULSION

TECHNIQUE 1.24

- If repair of an isolated posterior cruciate bony avulsion is the only anticipated procedure, begin a medial incision at a level 5 cm proximal to the superior pole of the patella and proceed distally across the medial epicondylar area paralleling the medial border of the patella and patellar tendon and ending at the level of the upper border of the pes anserinus.
- Reflect the skin and subcutaneous tissue anteriorly to the medial border of the patella and patellar tendon and posteriorly to the posteromedial corner.
- Make an anteromedial capsular incision and explore the joint.
- If the PCL is avulsed from the tibia and the repair is to be done through a medial approach, dissect the posterior skin and subcutaneous tissue as a single layer to the posteromedial corner and, with the knee flexed to 90 degrees, retract the medial head of the gastrocnemius and the popliteal structures posteriorly to adequately expose the tibial attachment of the ligament.
- In the absence of a major medial compartment disruption, a posteromedial capsular incision allows adequate exposure of the tibial attachment. The most medial portion of an intact posterior horn of the medial meniscus may make exposure and placement of the suture in the distal end of the ligament difficult, but excision of the intact medial meniscus is not necessary.
- Place nonabsorbable sutures through the avulsed tibial attachment of the ligament and drill parallel holes from the anteromedial aspect of the proximal tibia aimed posteriorly to exit near the normal tibial attachment of the PCL. These holes should exit the posterior aspect of the tibia approximately 5 mm below the posterior articular margin. As the drill penetrates the posterior tibial cortex, take care to protect

the popliteal vessels with a wide metallic retractor. Commercial drill guides can aid in placement of the drill holes.

- Pass the sutures previously placed in the avulsed fragment through the parallel drill holes with suture passers and tie them over the bridge of bone anteriorly to reattach the ligament to its normal insertion and to restore the tension within the ligament. If this is the only major repair required, use interrupted sutures to close both the anteromedial capsular incision used to explore the joint and the posteromedial capsular incision.
- If the isolated PCL disruption is characterized by avulsion of a large piece of bone from the posterior aspect of the tibia and a posterior approach is planned, the knee must be examined arthroscopically to rule out other orthopaedic disorders before making the approach. This approach does not permit exploration of the knee or correction of any other disorder.
- Fit the fragment of bone carefully into the crater and secure it with a cancellous screw if the fragment is large enough (Fig. 1.125) or with a nonabsorbable suture passed through parallel drill holes to the anterior aspect of the tibia.
- Repair the frequently found tear of the posterior capsule with interrupted sutures.

With the direct posterior approach for repair of bony avulsion of the PCL, detachment of the medial head of the gastrocnemius from the femoral condyle allows full exposure of the posterior capsule and the posterior intercondylar notch. Repair of avulsions at the tibial attachment, as well as repair of tears of the posterior capsule, is easily carried out with screws, suture anchors, or pull-through sutures.

Burks and Schaffer described an alternative approach to the posterior tibia for repair of an isolated tibial avulsion (see Technique 1.28).

Before closure of the capsular incision, some have advocated the insertion of a large Steinmann pin diagonally through the proximal tibia, entering the joint in the intercondylar area and then drilled into the intercondylar notch and the femoral condyle with the tibia held forward. Advocates of this technique believe that without this pin insertion there will be posterior sagging of the tibia and thereby stress on the PCL repair even if a long-leg cast is utilized. However, in an experimental study, Ogata et al. showed that no sagging of the tibia occurred at full extension in knees with "isolated" sectioning of the PCL. No sagging occurred when the posterior capsule also was sectioned if the knee remained fully extended. Sagging occurred in both instances as the knee was flexed. Only with sectioning of the MCL or LCL, or both, did posterior sagging and rotation occur in extension. This study suggests that after PCL injury immobilization in full extension is stable if the collateral ligaments are intact.

Müller and others advocated placing a 4.5-mm Steinmann pin through a predrilled hole in the patella and driving it into the tibia with the tibia and femur in appropriate alignment to prevent posterior sag of the tibia on the femur. Müller referred to this as "olecranization" of the patella. However, Weinstabl et al. investigated in vitro the influence of olecranization on PCL strain and showed that olecranization resulted in a strain five times greater than normal with the knee in extension below 20 degrees and in flexion above 40 degrees.

We do not use either of these techniques, preferring to place the knee in a controlled motion brace in full extension.

RECONSTRUCTION OF POSTERIOR CRUCIATE LIGAMENT

For PCL injuries in association with other significant ligament tears (including knee dislocation), reconstruction of the PCL is indicated. The lateral structures should be repaired or reconstructed as indicated; the medial structures can be repaired in knees with severe instability, or the knee can be braced in patients with mild-to-moderate laxity. Harner et al., in a biomechanical study, demonstrated that the PCL reconstruction is rendered ineffective and may be overloaded if the associated posterolateral structures are not repaired. Torg et al. found that the most significant predictive variable with regard to functional status is the presence of unidirectional rather than multidirectional instability at the time of injury. They established a direct correlation between combined multidirectional instability and the occurrence of associated problems of chondromalacia of the patella, meniscal derangement, quadriceps atrophy, and degenerative changes. The presence of a grade III posterior drawer (more than 10 mm of posterior laxity) is a relative indication for surgical reconstruction (Fig. 1.126).

Numerous techniques and tissues have been advocated to reconstruct the knee with a posterior cruciate deficiency. Since Hey-Groves reported reconstruction of the PCL with

the semitendinosus tendon, other authors have suggested extraarticular procedures, as well as intraarticular reconstruction with use of the lateral meniscus, the medial gastrocnemius, the semitendinosus and gracilis tendons, and bone–patellar tendon–bone autografts with arthroscopic or open techniques. We do not use the meniscus or the medial head of the gastrocnemius for reconstruction of the PCL and have had no experience with the use of the semitendinosus and gracilis tendons, but we doubt that they are long enough or strong enough to be used as a PCL replacement. We have found a free patellar tendon graft to produce the most predictable and satisfactory results for chronic PCL insufficiency.

In a systematic review of isolated PCL reconstructions of the ALB with at least 2 years of follow-up, Kim et al. found that Lysholm knee scores were significantly higher, 75% of patients had normal or nearly normal IKDC scores, and posterior knee laxity was significantly improved postoperatively. Mean postoperative posterior knee laxity varied in the reviewed articles from 2.0 to 5.9 mm, which was a considerable improvement over preoperative values ranging from 8.4 to 12.3 mm. However, it was concluded that normal knee stability was not achieved. Numerous other studies have shown similar results of improved clinical outcome scores but residual posterior laxity. In a study of 46 patients undergoing PCL reconstruction, Gwinner et al. measured posterior tibial translation with bilateral stress radiographs preoperatively and at 3, 6, 12, and 24 months postoperatively and at final follow-up. The mean side-to-side difference of posterior tibial translation improved from 10.9 ± 3.1 mm to 3.6 ± 3.8 mm at 3 months, but the translation significantly increased over time to 5.4 ± 3.4 mm at final follow-up. Flattening of the tibial slope resulted in a significantly higher posterior tibial translation compared to a high tibial slope.

If the patient will accept an allograft for PCL reconstruction, excellent results can be obtained with use of a deep-frozen bone–patellar tendon–bone graft (15 to 20 mm wide) or an Achilles tendon graft with bone on one end. These allografts are longer and stronger than grafts harvested from a patient's own tissues. In a systematic review and meta-analysis of five studies comparing allograft and autograft PCL reconstructions, Belk et al. reported no significant differences in subjective IKDC, Lysholm, and Tegner scores except in one study in which the Lysholm scores improved to a significantly greater extent in the autograft group. They did find average anteroposterior knee laxity was significantly higher in the allograft patients (3.8 mm) compared to autograft patients (3.1 mm), but the clinical significance of this small difference was unclear.

The controversy regarding management of PCL ruptures also extends to the technique for reconstruction. Most investigators agree that the anatomy of the PCLs should be re-created to provide the best opportunity for a stable knee, but the consensus ends there, and descriptions of the anatomy of this ligament vary among authors. Traditionally, the PCL has been described as consisting of two parts, the anterior, or anterolateral, band and the posterior, or posteromedial, band. Studies of the macroscopic and functional anatomy have added further complexity by characterizing the ligament as a continuum of fibers without truly separate bands or bundles. All studies agree that the anterior portion has the larger cross-sectional size, tightens with flexion of the knee, and relaxes with extension. The posterior fiber group has been estimated to constitute between 5% and 15% of the mass of the ligament, is lax with flexion, and tightens with extension. The amount of force

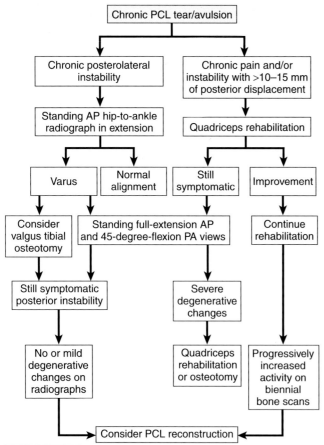

FIGURE 1.126 Treatment algorithm for chronic posterior cruciate ligament *(PCL)* injuries. *AP,* Anteroposterior; *PA,* posteroanterior. (From Veltri DM, Warren RF: Isolated and combined posterior cruciate ligament injuries, *J Am Acad Orthop Surg* 1:67, 1993.)

generated in the PCL during the posterior drawer test has been shown to depend on the angle of flexion at which the test is performed; when the angle is near 90 degrees of flexion, all the posterior force applied to the tibia is transmitted to the ligament.

The PCL attachment site on the medial femoral condyle is a broad semicircle with an average width of 32 mm. The tibial insertion site lies in a depression (fovea) 1 cm below the medial tibial articular surface. The ligament is oriented vertically in the frontal plane and angles forward 30 to 45 degrees in the sagittal plane, depending on the amount of knee flexion. Galloway et al. found that the restoration of knee stability in flexion depended greatly on the femoral attachment location. A femoral attachment that was nonisometric by intraoperative measurement but within the PCL anatomic footprint most closely reproduced the intact knee's posterior limits. Variations in the tibial attachment site produced only minor changes in the posterior motion limits. Grood et al. concluded that no absolutely isometric point exists within the femoral attachment zone.

Most surgeons have chosen to place the femoral tunnel in the anterior portion of the femoral footprint, replacing the ALB and tensioning the graft near 90 degrees of knee flexion (Fig. 1.127). Posterior placement creates a graft that is much more vertically oriented than the normal PCL. Investigators disagree as to whether it is better to place the PCL graft in a position where it will function isometrically or to replace the larger and stronger anterior bulk of the ligament, which is anatomic but nonisometric. Each option has its proponents, and there is conflicting evidence to support tensioning of the graft in full extension, 90 degrees of flexion, and points in between.

Robotic testing systems have delineated several important concepts concerning graft tensioning: PCL reconstruction with graft fixation at full extension with no load results in an overconstrained knee with significantly decreased total anteroposterior translation, whereas PCL reconstruction with graft fixation at 90 degrees of flexion results in kinematics similar to those of the intact knee, and graft fixation at full extension may overconstrain the knee and elevate in situ graft forces.

The controversy regarding PCL reconstruction continues to grow. Some authors have recommended reconstructing both portions of the ligament. Usually, an anatomic transtibial double-bundle PCL reconstruction involves the reaming of two femoral tunnels and one tibial tunnel. The insertions of the ALB and PMB are broader on the femoral side, which allows reaming of two separate tunnels, a larger tunnel for the ALB and a smaller one for the PMB. The tibial tunnel is more compact, and usually only a single tunnel can be reamed. To date, most of the studies have been biomechanical evaluations using cadaver models. These studies showed the double-bundle technique to restore posterior laxity levels and knee kinematics to more nearly normal than a single-bundle technique; however, a similar study found that the addition of a second posteromedial graft reduced laxity, but did so at the expense of higher than normal forces in the posteromedial graft. More recent cadaver and biomechanical studies have reached differing conclusions. In view of relatively high graft forces at full extension that could cause the graft to permanently elongate with time, Markolf et al. questioned the need for a posteromedial graft, whereas Whiddon et al. compared single-bundle and double-bundle techniques in a cadaver model and concluded that double-bundle reconstruction offers measurable benefits in terms of rotational stability and posterior translation in the presence of an untreated posterolateral corner injury. With the posterolateral corner intact, however, it provided more rotational constraint but did not further reduce posterior translation. There are few published clinical reports, and what is available is limited by short-term follow-up. Although the effectiveness of a double-bundle PCL reconstruction has yet to be proved, research suggests it offers the possibility of improving the results of reconstruction.

LaPrade et al. described 100 primary endoscopic double-bundle PCL reconstructions for isolated (31 patients) and

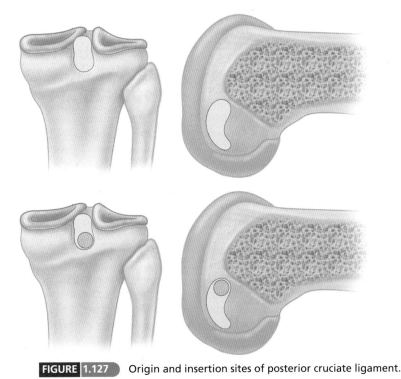

FIGURE **1.127** Origin and insertion sites of posterior cruciate ligament.

combined (69 patients) PCL injuries. At a mean follow-up of 2.9 years, functional and objective outcomes were significantly improved, regardless of concomitant ligamentous injury or timing to surgery (acute vs. chronic). The mean side-to-side difference in posterior tibial translation on kneeling stress radiographs improved from 11.0 ± 3.5 mm preoperatively to 1.6 ± 2.0 mm postoperatively ($P < .001$). Furthermore, comparable subjective and functional clinical outcomes were achieved compared with an isolated ACL reconstruction control cohort. Conversely, Houe and Jorgenson found no significant differences between single-bundle and double-bundle reconstructions with respect to instrumentally measured posterior tibial translation, activity level, Tegner and Lysholm knee scores, or patient satisfaction. In a randomized study using hamstring autograft reconstructions, Wang et al. did not identify any difference between reconstructions regarding functional assessment, posterior tibial translation, knee scores, or radiographic changes. Yoon et al. found similar outcome scores and range of motion between reconstruction types but identified a considerable decrease in posterior tibial translation of 1.4 mm in the double-bundle reconstruction group. They were uncertain of the clinical or functional relevance of this difference. Yoon et al. reviewed 64 patients (28 with single-bundle reconstruction and 36 with double-bundle techniques) at a minimum 10-year follow-up. There were no significant differences between groups in clinical, radiographic, and survivorship outcomes.

Concern has been expressed regarding the acuteness of the angle taken by the graft as it exits the tibial tunnel and proceeds anteriorly to its femoral attachment. This angle has been called the "killer turn" because of graft abrasion and graft thinning and fraying the can occur. Consequently, the tibial inlay technique was developed, which theoretically offered bony healing posteriorly in the trough, avoidance of graft abrasion, and use of larger graft sizes. The superiority of either technique has not been proven. Recently, attention has also focused on the angle of graft entry into the femoral tunnel. Investigators have compared the contact pressures on the graft using the outside-in and the inside-out techniques. Jang et al., using 3D-CT analysis, evaluated the graft bending angles at the femoral tunnel aperture in single-bundle PCL reconstructions using both inside-out and outside-in techniques. The graft bending angles were more acute in the sagittal and axial planes with the inside-out technique, but only by less than 10 degrees, and it was unclear if this difference would have any effect on graft survival. Using synthetic femurs, Narvy et al. established two groups with eight specimens in each group: an outside-in or inside-out femoral tunnel creation. Using an Achilles tendon allograft fixed with a suspensory device and a pressure sensor between the allograft and the femoral tunnel, they measured force, contact area, contact pressure, and peak pressure at the aperture. Outside-in creation of the femoral tunnel for the ALB reconstruction of the PCL resulted in decreased mean and peak contact pressures at the femoral aperture compared to inside-out tunnel creation.

Seon et al. compared 66 patients with either transtibial or open tibial inlay reconstruction and found no significant differences in knee scores, activity levels, or instrumentally measured posterior tibial translation. In a meta-analysis of biomechanical and clinical outcomes, Lee et al. determined that both techniques can restore normal knee kinematics and improve knee function, but they were unable to identify which produced better improvements in stability and functional recovery. Transtibial PCL reconstruction resulted in higher graft forces,

but the clinical significance was unclear. The tibial inlay technique tended to entail more perioperative complications. No differences in translation between a double-bundle graft and a single-bundle graft in tibial inlay PCL reconstructions were found in eight cadaver knees subjected to six cycles from a 40-N anterior reference point to a 100-N posterior translational force at 10, 30, 60, and 90 degrees of flexion, leading the authors to conclude that the use of a double-bundle graft may not offer any advantages over a single-bundle graft for tibial inlay posterior cruciate reconstructions. Apsingi et al. reached similar conclusions after comparing single- and double-bundle reconstruction in cadaver models of combined PCL and posterolateral corner injuries, noting that the added complexity of the double-bundle reconstruction does not seem to be justified by their results. Wiley et al. determined in a cadaver model that, because drilling two tunnels removes additional bone from the medial femoral condyle, the double-bundle technique increases the risk of medial femoral condyle fracture. Testing with a robotic testing system determined that an anterior position of the bone tunnels in double-bundle PCL reconstruction more nearly restored the normal knee kinematics than did a posterior position. Stannard et al. reported the results of reconstruction of the PCL by combined tibial inlay and two-femoral tunnel technique in 29 patients with 30 PCL ruptures. Twenty-three knees had no laxity, and seven had a 1+ laxity. The KT-2000 arthrometer data documented less than 0.5 mm of side-to-side difference for both posterior displacement and total anteroposterior displacement at both 30 and 70 degrees of knee flexion.

As with ACL repairs or reconstructions, we usually examine the knee arthroscopically before any open surgical procedure to better evaluate the intraarticular pathologic condition. Some PCL reconstruction techniques can be arthroscopically aided as to tunnel site placement and routing of the graft (see the section on arthroscopically aided ligament reconstruction in other chapter). The following techniques are described as if only open techniques are used.

RECONSTRUCTION OF POSTERIOR CRUCIATE LIGAMENT WITH PATELLAR TENDON GRAFT

The following technique for reconstruction of the PCL was described by Clancy in 1983. Any of the commercial drill guides or systems can be used to determine the tunnel locations. Interference screw fixation of the bone plugs in the femoral and tibial tunnels is preferred by most surgeons, although it may be more difficult than with ACL reconstructions. The length especially of the tibial tunnel for PCL reconstruction is greater than that for ACL reconstruction; therefore, the distal bone plug can be more difficult to see in the tunnel for interference screw fixation. A longer plug of bone from the tibial tuberosity is advised. However, a long fragment of bone on the proximal end of the graft can make its entrance into the femoral tunnel more difficult. An anterolateral rather than anteromedial tibial tunnel starting point has been recommended to avoid the "killer turn" as the graft emerges from the tibia. This position was found to be associated with improved objective outcomes, but clinical results were not significantly correlated to a specific graft position.

Proper tibial and femoral attachment sites are just as important in PCL reconstruction or augmentation as in ACL reconstruction. Similar to the ACL, the PCL tibial attachment site is not as crucial to isometry as the femoral site. This tibial attachment site often is difficult to expose for direct vision. Because the length pattern is relatively insensitive to either proximal-distal or medial-lateral location on the tibia, a widely exposed and visible tibial fossa is not as necessary as it is in choosing a femoral attachment site. Placing a gloved finger in the fovea and placing a guidewire by commercial guide or by touch may be good enough. Radiographs of the knee after guide pin insertion confirm that the guidewire exits in the fovea just inferior to the articular margin of the posterior tibia and just lateral to the midline. The femoral attachment site for the PCL substitute is crucial. Fortunately, this is visible through the intercondylar notch. When the ligament is augmented or reconstructed, any errors should be in the anteroposterior direction, not in the proximal-distal direction. In reconstructions of acute tears, the remaining PCL stump helps locate the proper femoral attachment site. Morgan et al. studied the femoral attachment site in 20 knees to define the location of the anatomic origin of both bands of the posterior cruciate ligament in reference to local anatomy to develop landmarks that can be used to reproducibly position two femoral tunnels. The central origin point for the anterolateral band was 13 ± 0.5 mm posterior to the medial articular cartilage–intercondylar wall interface and 13 ± 0.5 mm inferior to the articular cartilage–intercondylar roof interface. The posteromedial band centrally originated 8 ± 0.5 mm posterior to the medial articular cartilage–intercondylar wall interface and 20 ± 0.5 mm inferior to the articular cartilage–intercondylar roof interface. These distances were noted to be relatively constant despite varying knee morphologic features and size.

TECHNIQUE 1.25

(CLANCY)

- Prepare and drape the leg in the standard fashion and inflate the tourniquet.
- Make a standard medial parapatellar incision, curved posteriorly at the superior aspect in line with the medial femoral epicondyle but approximately two fingerbreadths proximal. Incise the subcutaneous tissue in a similar fashion.
- Make a medial arthrotomy close to the medial aspect of the patellar tendon. Inspect the knee joint and excise and repair any meniscal tears or excise the meniscus if necessary. If the tear of the PCL is acute, place sutures through the larger remnant.
- In isolated PCL injury, the ligament of Humphry usually is intact and can be mistaken for an intact PCL. However, careful dissection shows that its most anterior fibers follow a lateral course to the posterior horn of the lateral meniscus.
- The ligament of Wrisberg also may be present; it is composed of fibers attaching to the PCL and also travels in a lateral direction toward the posterior horn of the lateral meniscus.
- If either of these ligaments is intact, the tibia will move only slightly backward when it is held in marked internal rotation and a posterior drawer maneuver is done. These ligaments decrease the expected excessive internal rotation and posterior translation of the tibia and can lead to a mistaken diagnosis of pure posterolateral rotary instability. If neither ligament is intact, the tibia will have significant posterior and internal rotational excursions on the femur.
- Now direct attention to the posteromedial aspect of the knee.
- With the knee flexed to 90 degrees, sharply dissect the subcutaneous tissue and overlying skin to expose the anteromedial aspect of the medial gastrocnemius and semimembranosus tendons.
- Make a posterior incision in the capsule just anterior to the medial gastrocnemius tendon. Make the incision through the synovium and posterior capsule, keeping it posteromedially from the medial meniscus so that the meniscus can be preserved if it is intact.
- If necessary for exposure, release the medial third of the medial gastrocnemius tendon just distal to its insertion onto the femur.
- With the knee flexed to 90 degrees, use a curved retractor to retract the posterior capsule and synovium, exposing the old insertion of the PCL onto the tibia.
- Place a drill guide or a gloved finger posterolateral to the anatomic center of the PCL attachment on the tibia (Fig. 1.128A).
- Place the anterior part of the drill guide or a Kirschner wire distal and medial to the tibial insertion of the patellar tendon (Fig. 1.128B).
- Drill a tunnel from distal to proximal through the tibia at an angle of approximately 45 degrees (Fig. 1.128C).
- Place the Kirschner wire, with or without the drill guide, at the anterior site so that it will exit posterolaterally to the anatomic center of the PCL insertion (Fig. 1.128A). Then overdrill the Kirschner wire with a 10-mm drill bit.
- Use the drill guide to insert the Kirschner wire through the medial femoral condyle so that it exits anterosuperior to the anatomic center of the original PCL attachment, usually at the edge of the osteochondral junction (Figs. 1.128D,E and 1.129).
- Drill it to enter posterosuperior to the femoral epicondyle and then overdrill the wire with a 10-mm reamer.
- Undermine the vastus medialis inferiorly and retract it to expose the exit tunnel.
- Now harvest the graft. Free the medial third of the patellar tendon (leaving a 5-mm intact border) from the remaining patellar tendon.
- Use power instruments to remove a patellar bone block 10 mm wide, 4 mm deep, and 25 mm long; do not take any quadriceps tendon with the bone block.
- Drill three holes through the bone block with a 0.062-inch Kirschner wire and place a no. 5 nonabsorbable suture through each hole.
- Remove a bone block the same size as the patellar bone block from the tibial tuberosity insertion of the patellar tendon (Fig. 1.128F).
- Drill three holes through this block and place a no. 5 nonabsorbable suture through each hole (Fig. 1.128G).
- Place the patellar bone block in the femoral tunnel so that it lies entirely within the medial femoral condyle (Fig. 1.128H).

- Tie the femoral sutures loosely over a button placed over the exit of the femoral tunnel (Fig. 1.128I).
- Pass a suture passer into the posteromedial capsular incision and then into the intercondylar notch.
- Place the sutures into the tibial graft and pull them out through the posteromedial capsular incision, pulling the tibial graft gently through the intercondylar notch.
- Pass the suture passer into the tibial tunnel anteriorly and curve it out through the posteromedial capsular incision.
- Pass the tibial graft sutures through the suture passer and bring them out anteriorly. Tilt the tibial bone graft so that its inferior tip is angled anteriorly to allow easy passage into the tibial tunnel posteriorly.
- If the graft is difficult to place in the tunnel, soft tissue may be blocking the tunnel entrance, the tibial graft may be too long to be angled sufficiently to enter the tunnel, or the tunnel may be too low. If the tunnel is too low, enlarge it by reaming with gentle anterosuperior pressure on the reamer.
- Insert an AO malleolar screw and washer 5 mm longer than measured by the depth gauge at the inferior edge of the tibial tunnel.
- At the femoral tunnel, tie the patellar bone sutures over a button.
- Then, with the knee in 90 degrees of flexion, pull forward on the tibia and tie the tibial bone sutures over the AO screw and washer.
- Tighten one suture with the knee in 90 degrees of flexion; bring the knee to 30 degrees of flexion and retighten the suture while maintaining the anterior drawer.
- Secure the remaining ties and tighten the screw.
- Perform a posterior drawer test and examine the knee for the normal step-off of the medial and lateral femoral condyles. Place the knee through a full range of motion and perform a posterior drawer test.
- Close the capsular arthrotomies in the standard fashion and place a drain in the medial side.
- Close the subcutaneous tissue and skin in the standard fashion.

Both open and arthroscopic modifications of Clancy's technique have been described. If the central third autogenous patellar tendon is chosen as the graft source, a limited incision placed anteriorly over the patellar tendon, similar to that used for ACL reconstruction, can be made for graft harvest. The intraarticular portion of the procedure can be done arthroscopically, or the menisci and intercondylar notch can be exposed through the defect in the patellar tendon after graft harvest, as described by Sallay and McCarroll. The fat pad should be incised vertically in its midportion, and two curved knee retractors are used to retract the medial and lateral portions of the patellar tendon or fat pad. Typically, it is unnecessary to resect the fat pad; however, Sallay and McCarroll did not observe any complications in knees in which a portion of the fat pad was excised. Flexing the knee to 90 degrees provides the best exposure of the intercondylar notch so that the surgeon's line of sight is parallel to the intercondylar roof. Use of a headlight can improve visibility.

RECONSTRUCTION OF POSTERIOR CRUCIATE LIGAMENT WITH PATELLAR TENDON GRAFT

TECHNIQUE 1.26

(SALLAY AND MCCARROLL)

- Carefully identify the plane between the scarred PCL and the ACL to prevent damage to the ACL while excising remnants of the PCL. Preserve a minimal amount of tissue at the femoral attachment site to identify the anatomic footprint.
- Make a second incision to identify the tibial insertion of the PCL to safely drill the tibial tunnel and to facilitate graft passage. Many surgeons elect to make a small posteromedial incision, identical to the exposure for a medial meniscal repair, regardless of the basic technique chosen for PCL reconstruction (including arthroscopic), to protect the neurovascular structures and to facilitate graft passage. Sallay and McCarroll based the site of their incision on the need to treat associated medial or lateral injury. In the absence of injury to the lateral side, the standard approach has been a 4-cm posteromedial incision.
- Begin the proximal portion of the incision below and posterior to the medial femoral epicondyle, extending it vertically downward, parallel to the lines of skin cleavage (Fig. 1.130A).
- Incise the investing fascia (layer I) in line with the skin incision superior to the leading edge of the sartorius muscle. Protect the infrapatellar branch of the saphenous nerve in the inferior aspect of the wound.
- Retract the pes tendons posteriorly, exposing the MCL and the POL.
- Make a vertical arthrotomy between the POL and the medial head of the gastrocnemius tendon.
- Sharply dissect the capsule off its tibial attachment, leaving the meniscotibial ligament intact. In chronic tears, this plane may be obscured by scarring of the posterior capsule to the PCL. To prevent injury to the popliteal contents, carefully mobilize the scar tissue by blunt dissection to reflect the capsule off the tibial insertion of the PCL.
- Now identify the posterior tibial sulcus by palpation and observation.
- If there is an associated injury to the posterolateral corner, a lateral approach is preferred (Fig. 1.130B). Make a short, oblique incision, 6 cm long, just posterior to the LCL.
- Incise the iliotibial band (layer I) in line with its fibers.
- The LCL lies beneath a superficial lamina (layer II). Divide this layer posterior to the LCL, exposing the deep capsular lamina (layer III).
- Divide the capsule in line with the posterior aspect of the LCL, exposing the posterolateral joint space. Protect the popliteal tendon in the inferior aspect of the wound.
- Release the capsule and its attachment to the popliteus and meniscotibial ligament as described for the medial approach. In patients with acute injury of the PCL and the posterolateral corner, much of the exposure and dissection has been done by the disruption.

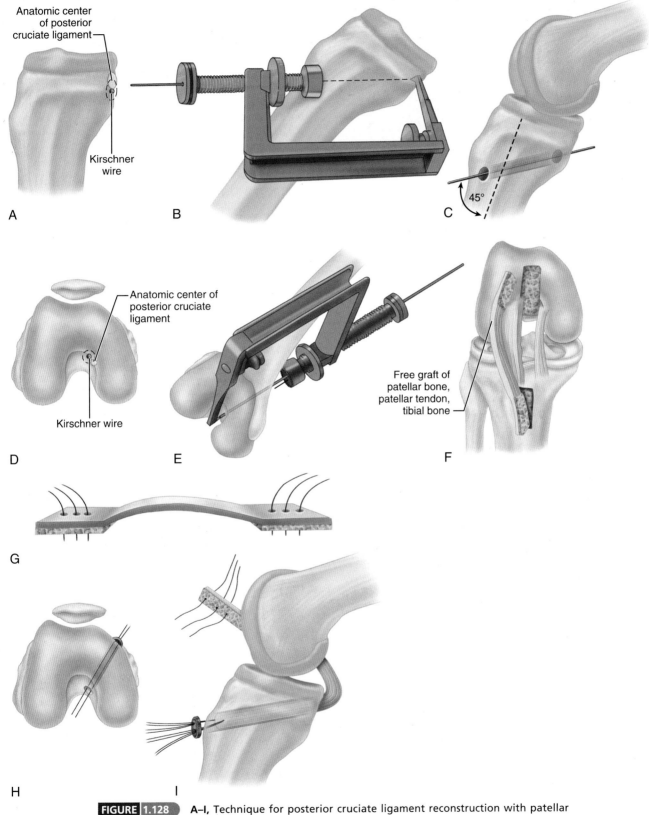

Anatomic center
of posterior
cruciate ligament

Kirschner
wire

A

B

45°

C

Anatomic center of
posterior cruciate
ligament

Kirschner wire

D

E

Free graft of
patellar bone,
patellar tendon,
tibial bone

F

G

H

I

FIGURE 1.128   A–I, Technique for posterior cruciate ligament reconstruction with patellar tendon graft. **SEE TECHNIQUE 1.25.**

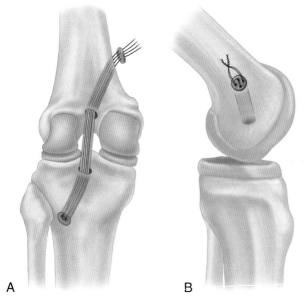

A   B

FIGURE 1.129   **A** and **B,** Technique for posterior cruciate ligament reconstruction with patellar tendon graft. **SEE TECHNIQUE 1.25.**

- To create the tibial tunnel, make an L-shaped periosteal flap 1 cm medial to the distal portion of the tibial tubercle just proximal to the pes tendon group insertion.
- With use of a commercially available drill guide, advance a guide pin from this site in a posterolateral and proximal direction, exiting at the inferior and lateral quadrant of the posterior tibial sulcus.
- Confirm and document the proper position of the guide pin with an intraoperative radiograph.
- Bone guides allow calculation of the distance of the tibial tunnel, and the guide pin can be "chucked down" to the proper length to prevent overpenetration; placing a finger through the posteromedial incision to palpate the tibial fovea also protects the neurovascular structures from overpenetration. Some surgeons prefer to perform this step under imaging guidance to ensure proper placement of the guidewire.

- Overream the pin with the 10-mm reamer, again using a finger to protect the neurovascular structures. Some surgeons remove the power source and complete the last portion of the reaming by hand because certain reamers pull tissue toward the reamer as they advance along a guidewire. Paulos et al. used an oscillating reamer and drill stop to prevent vascular complications. Sallay and McCarroll used a reamer with a conical profile because the standard square profile reamers have been shown to cut out the posterior tibial cortex as far as 2 cm inferior to the intended exit site.
- Be careful not to apply counterpressure at the level of the popliteal fossa because this could compress the popliteal structures against the posterior tibia during the reaming process.
- By use of an angled curet or sharp dissection over the tip of the reamer while it is still in the tunnel, debride the edge of the tunnel of residual soft tissue to avoid entrapment of the bone plug during later passage of the graft.
- Chamfer the edges of the tunnel with a rasp.
- The femoral tunnel can be prepared by one of two methods. The standard method begins with exposure of the anteromedial femoral cortex, using the superior portion of the medial incision.
- Elevate the vastus medialis proximally to allow access to the anteromedial aspect of the distal femur.
- Use a commercial drill guide to advance a guide pin from a point just proximal to the medial femoral epicondyle into the intercondylar notch. Pin entry should be at the junction of the anterior and middle thirds of the intercondylar notch (approximately 10 mm proximal to the articular surface) and at the 2 o'clock position for the right knee (10 o'clock position for the left knee), corresponding to the center of the anatomic insertion of the anterolateral fibers.
- Overream the pin with a 10-mm reamer and chamfer the tunnel edges with a rasp.
- The second technique for preparation of the femoral tunnel does not require dissection of the medial femoral cortex.
- Advance a long Beath pin through the capsule lateral to the patellar tendon to obtain the appropriate tunnel trajectory. The point of entry should correspond to the anatomic insertion of the anterior fibers.

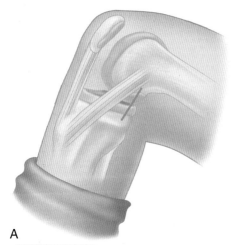
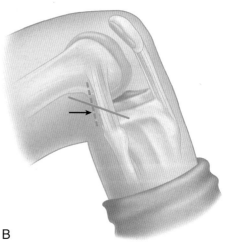

A   B

FIGURE 1.130   Posterior cruciate ligament reconstruction. **A,** Posteromedial incision over "soft spot" below and posterior to medial femoral epicondyle. **B,** Lateral incision is made in line with iliotibial band. **SEE TECHNIQUE 1.26.**

- Advance the pin through the vastus medialis muscle and skin.
- Ream over the guide pin from the intercondylar side with a 10-mm reamer, stopping short of the medial femoral cortex (Fig. 1.131).
- Withdraw the reamer, leaving the Beath pin in place. This creates a blind-end tunnel from inside to out.
- The graft can be passed in two ways, depending on the preference of the surgeon.
- The first technique begins by passing the smaller, bullet-shaped bone plug through the tibial tunnel from anterior to posterior.
- Use a suture passer to retrieve the traction sutures into the posteromedial (lateral) wound.
- With constant tension applied parallel to the direction of the tibia tunnel, deliver the bone plug into the posterior recess (Fig. 1.132). Avoid pulling at an angle oblique to the tunnel because this causes the bone plug to bend at the posterior tunnel opening.
- Use the suture passer to retrieve the bone plug into the intercondylar notch.
- Direct the graft into the femoral tunnel with the traction suture.
- The second technique uses the Beath pin to assist in passage of the femoral bone plug.
- Thread the traction sutures of the bone plug through the eyelet at the end of the guide pin.
- Withdraw the pin from the medial aspect of the knee, leaving the traction sutures in the tunnel exiting the medial soft tissues.
- Advance the bone plug into the tunnel with the tendon portion facing the articular surface until the end of the bone plug is flush with the wall of the intercondylar notch. Abrasion of the graft is minimized because the tendon does not rest against the edge of the femoral tunnel.

- Thread the sutures of the other bone plug through a DePuy graft passer (DePuy, Warsaw, IN). Advance the free end of the graft passer through the patellar tendon defect and the notch into the posterior recess. Apply gentle tension to the sutures to seat the end of the bone plug firmly in the mount of the graft passer.
- Thread the free end of the graft passer through the tibial tunnel from posterior to anterior, using an arthroscopic clamp.
- Place a heavy clamp on the end of the graft passer, preventing relative motion between the passer and the graft. Apply firm tension to the graft passer to deliver the graft through the notch and into the tibial tunnel. Maintaining an anterior drawer force on the tibia also aids graft passage into the tunnel.
- Fixation can be achieved by tying the sutures over ligament buttons, interference screws, or both.
- Fix the femoral bone plug first.
- Move the knee through a full range of motion to evaluate relative motion of the tibial bone plug with respect to the tibial tunnel. An appropriately placed graft should have no more than 2 mm of relative motion.
- Fix the tibial side with the knee flexed to 90 degrees with an anterior drawer force applied to re-create the normal femoral-tibial relationship. Secure the bone plug with a 9 × 20-mm cannulated interference screw. If the end of the graft is difficult to see, place the arthroscope into the tibial tunnel to allow more accurate screw fixation. As an alternative, tie the sutures over a ligament button.
- Perform a posterior drawer test to ensure adequate stability. Residual laxity should be grade I or less.
- Close in routine fashion over a drain.

POSTOPERATIVE CARE Restoring motion and reducing swelling take priority within the first week. Patients are encouraged to perform active range-of-motion exercises, quadriceps training, and full weight bearing in an extension brace in the immediate postoperative period.

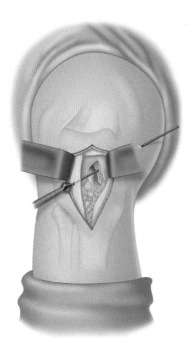

FIGURE 1.131 "Inside-out" method of drilling femoral tunnel uses lateral arthroscopic capsulotomy to advance Beath guide pin and to drill blind-end tunnel through intercondylar notch. **SEE TECHNIQUE 1.26.**

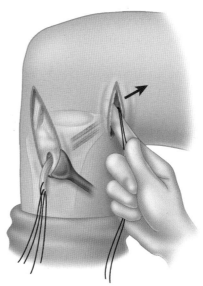

FIGURE 1.132 Graft is passed through tibial tunnel from anterior to posterior, pulling in line with direction of tunnel. **SEE TECHNIQUE 1.26.**

Immobilization is continued in extension for 3 weeks in patients in whom medial or lateral capsuloligamentous structures were repaired. Strengthening and functional activities are introduced in a stepwise program.

RECONSTRUCTION OF POSTERIOR CRUCIATE LIGAMENT WITH BONE–PATELLAR TENDON–BONE OR ACHILLES TENDON–BONE GRAFTS

Allografts, either bone–patellar tendon–bone or Achilles tendon–bone, also are popular graft sources for reconstruction of the PCL because of their large size. In addition, the Achilles tendon allograft has the advantages of extra length and only soft tissue at one end, which makes graft passage easier. Harner described an arthroscopic technique for Achilles tendon allograft. He emphasized that the tibial guide pin should course just anterior and parallel to the slope of the posterior tibial cortex, which is approximated by a line parallel to the slope of the proximal tibiofibular joint. The anterolateral

fibers are re-created by placing the femoral tunnel within the anterior portion of the PCL footprint. The guide pin enters 5 to 10 mm from the intraarticular cartilage of the medial femoral condyle. On the extraarticular side of the femoral condyle, the guide pin should exit 1.0 to 1.5 cm from the articular cartilage margin to avoid disruption of the subchondral bone. The bone plug should be advanced until its bone-tendon edge is flush with the cortex to minimize graft bending and abrasion. The bone plug is fixed in the femoral tunnel with an interference screw, and the soft-tissue end of the Achilles tendon allograft is secured outside the tibial tunnel with a screw and spiked washer or, in rare cases, a staple. After the graft has been fixed in the femoral tunnel, the knee is moved through a range of motion to check for isometricity and stability and to pretension the graft. The tibial side is secured with the knee in 70 to 80 degrees of flexion and 10 pounds of tension because the ALB is under maximal tension in this position, minimizing the risk of overtensioning the graft.

After surgery, the knee is placed in full extension in a commercially available knee brace with hinges locked in

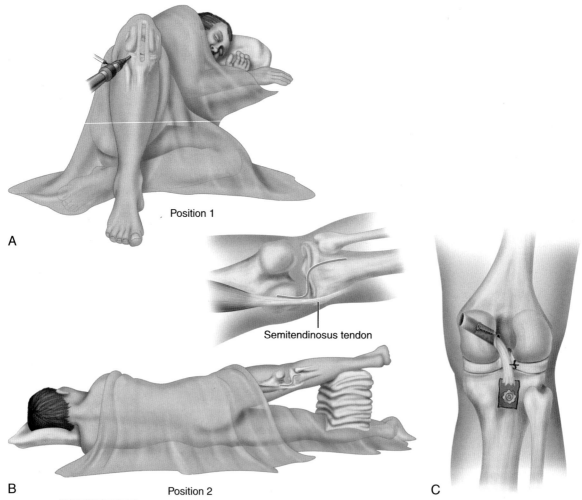

Position 1

A

Semitendinosus tendon

B

Position 2

C

FIGURE 1.133 **A,** Decubitus position with thigh abducted and knee and hip flexed allows access to anterior knee for arthroscopic and standard open technique. **B,** In second position, hip and knee are extended and table is tilted toward prone position to allow access to popliteal fossa, where vertical incision is made in line with semitendinosus tendon *(inset).* **C,** Patellar tendon bone block is inlaid within tibial window and secured to cancellous bone with screw and spiked washer. **SEE TECHNIQUE 1.27.**

extension. A range-of-motion exercise program of 0 to 90 degrees is initiated immediately. Limited weight bearing in the brace with crutches is allowed. Quadriceps exercises are started immediately with active knee extension from 90 to 0 degrees and straight-leg raises. Passive knee flexion exercises are used to gain knee flexion, but hamstring exercises are avoided because of the posterior translation stress they would place on the graft. Running begins at the fourth month, followed by sport-specific agility drills at 5 to 6 months. A full return to sports is allowed when adequate quadriceps and hamstring strength has been achieved and sport-specific agility and proprioceptive skills have been mastered.

All the previous techniques require the graft to turn at a right angle as it exits the tibial tunnel posteriorly and heads anteriorly toward the femoral tunnel. This acute bend creates the potential for graft abrasion and may make effective graft tensioning difficult. Posterior approaches to the tibial attachment of the PCL have been described with tibial inlay reconstruction to avoid this. Other methods to improve graft position include (1) placing the patient in the lateral decubitus position with the affected extremity up so that moving the leg and rotating the table allows access to both the anterior and posterior aspects of the knee, and (2) harvesting of the graft first and fixing the graft in the femoral tunnel with the patient supine, and then repreparing and redraping with the patient prone to make the posterior exposure and fixing the graft on the tibial side.

Both laboratory and cadaver studies have found no significant differences between the two techniques at any knee flexion angle, and a systematic review of the literature on clinical outcomes of transtibial and inlay reconstructions found satisfactory results for both techniques.

RECONSTRUCTION OF POSTERIOR CRUCIATE LIGAMENT WITH BONE–PATELLAR TENDON–BONE OR ACHILLES TENDON–BONE GRAFTS

TECHNIQUE 1.27

(BERG)
- Before beginning the operation, determine the size of the autogenous patellar tendon; if it is too long, the bony portion of the tendon graft will be recessed proximally within the femoral tunnel, which may subject the tendon to abrasive attenuation. Size the autogenous patellar tendon on a calibrated, 30-degree flexed, lateral knee radiograph with 3 mm or less of perfect posterior femoral condylar overlap. Use a high-intensity illuminator to discern the exact tibial tuberosity insertion site of the patellar tendon just anterior to the fat pad density. PCL strength is increased from the anterior margin of the intercondylar line to a point 1 cm below the posterior tibia. If the autogenous patellar tendon is longer than the measured PCL length by more than 1.5 cm, consider using an allograft of specified tendon length.
- Place the patient in the decubitus position with the operative leg up.

- Circumferentially prepare and drape the limb from the proximal thigh to midcalf.
- Abduct and externally rotate the hip 45 degrees and flex the knee 90 degrees; the anterior knee faces the surgeon (Fig. 1.133A).
- Harvest a 1-cm-wide central-third bone–patellar tendon–bone autograft.
- Drill and tap the tibial tubercle bone to accept a 6.5-cm cancellous screw and spiked washer.
- Use either standard anterior arthroscopic portals and an incision through the patellar tendon defect and fat pad or a medial parapatellar arthrotomy to examine intraarticular structures and perform meniscal surgery as needed.
- Place a femoral jig in the anterosuperior femoral origin of the PCL, 4 mm from the anterior articular margin of the medial femoral condyle.
- Make a 5-cm incision proximal to the medial femoral epicondyle.
- Divide the patellar retinaculum and expose the condyle subperiosteally.
- After guide pin placement, use a cannulated reamer to create a 1-cm-diameter interosseous tunnel in the medial femoral condyle. Chamfer the tunnel margins with a rasp.
- Pass an 18-gauge wire loop through the femoral tunnel, directed toward the posterior joint, and use it to pass the patellar tendon graft retrograde into the femoral tunnel later in the case.
- If a combined arthroscopic ACL and open PCL procedure is planned, perform the ACL reconstruction first because the popliteal arthrotomy will allow extravasation of the arthroscopic irrigant.
- Extend the knee, tilt the table toward the prone position, and abduct the thigh with stacked towels to allow access to the popliteal fossa (Fig. 1.133B).
- Make a vertical incision in line with the palpable semitendinosus tendon. Veer the incision laterally in the popliteal crease and extend it distally over the posterior calf (Fig. 1.133, inset).
- Expose the deep fascia overlying the gastrocnemius muscle and incise it vertically.
- Identify and protect the sural nerve between the two heads of the gastrocnemius muscle.
- Develop bluntly the plane between the medial head of the gastrocnemius and the semimembranosus tendon. Slightly flexing the knee improves exposure and allows relief of tension on the popliteal vessels.
- Incise the medial head of the gastrocnemius near its insertion and retract it laterally, protecting its tibial nerve motor branch.
- Identify and ligate the inferior medial geniculate artery and vein, which overlie the posterior joint capsule at the superior margin of the popliteus.
- Make a vertical incision through the OPL and posterior capsule.
- Identify the PCL and expose the posterior tibial plateau subperiosteally.
- Advance the tendon graft traction sutures with the wire loop retrograde into the medial femoral condyle tunnel.
- Use a 7- or 9-mm-diameter cannulated screw to secure interference fixation of the bone graft in the femoral tunnel. Optimally, the bone portion of the graft should not be recessed within the condylar tunnel but should lie

at the tunnel margin interface to prevent tendon–tunnel wall abrasion.

- Avoiding recurvatum, position the knee in full extension, which reduces posterior tibial subluxation through the geometric congruity of the femoral condyle and tibial plateau.
- Place the patellar tendon graft under slight manual tension to determine the site of posterior tibial fixation.
- Use an osteotome to create a unicortical window in the posterior tibia equal in size to the bony portion of the patellar tendon graft.
- Inlay the patellar tendon graft and secure it with a 6.5-mm titanium screw and spiked washer to the cancellous tibial bone (Fig. 1.133C).
- If the tendinous portion of the graft is too long, advance the tibial insertion site distally.
- If the meniscofemoral ligaments (Wrisberg and Humphry) are incompetent, suture the peripheral lateral meniscus to the PCL substitute.
- Repair the medial head of the gastrocnemius and perform a routine closure.

POSTOPERATIVE CARE After surgery, the knee is braced in full extension for 2 weeks and partial weight bearing on crutches is allowed. Full weight bearing is allowed at 2 weeks, and knee motion is permitted over a 0- to 90-degree arc of motion. Isometric quadriceps exercises are begun with the knee at 70 to 90 degrees of flexion. At 6 weeks, the patient is allowed to walk without crutches, and prone quadriceps and hamstring exercises over a full arc of motion are begun.

Burks and Schaffer described a posterior approach that does not require division of the medial head of the gastrocnemius. It does require repositioning, repreparing, and redraping of the patient after the graft has been harvested and secured in the femoral tunnel; however, the full prone position may be easier on the surgical team than the lateral decubitus or semi-prone position described by Berg.

RECONSTRUCTION OF POSTERIOR CRUCIATE LIGAMENT WITH BONE–PATELLAR TENDON–BONE OR ACHILLES TENDON–BONE GRAFTS

TECHNIQUE 1.28

(BURKS AND SCHAFFER)
- With the patient prone, make a gently curved incision, with a horizontal limb near the flexion crease of the knee and a vertical limb overlying the medial aspect of the gastrocnemius muscle.
- Carry the dissection to the deep fascial layer and incise it vertically over the medial head of the gastrocnemius.
- Protect the medial sural cutaneous nerve (posterior cutaneous nerve of the calf), which usually perforates the deep fascia distal to the horizontal limb of the incision.

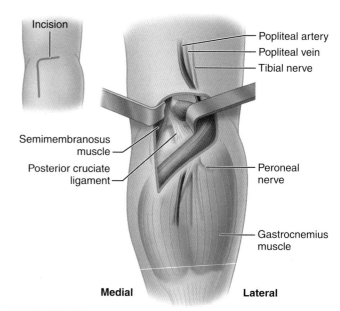

FIGURE 1.134 Posterior approach for reconstruction of posterior cruciate ligament. **SEE TECHNIQUE 1.28.**

- Identify the medial border of the medial gastrocnemius and bluntly develop the interval between it and the semimembranosus tendon, exposing the posterior joint capsule (Fig. 1.134). The middle geniculate artery may be encountered near the midposterior capsule and can be ligated if necessary. By lateral retraction on the medial head of the gastrocnemius, no tension is directly applied to the motor branch to the medial head of the gastrocnemius, the only motor branch from the tibial nerve in the popliteal fossa that traverses medially. The thick muscle belly protects the neurovascular structures as the capsule is exposed. Dissection on this protected medial side of the popliteal fossa is therefore relatively safe.
- Expose the posterior aspect of the proximal tibia and posterior margins of the femoral condyle.
- If further lateral exposure is necessary, release a portion of the tendinous origin of the medial head of the gastrocnemius from the distal femur and joint capsule. Slight knee flexion will aid exposure, and complete sectioning of the medial head of the gastrocnemius rarely is needed.
- Make a vertical incision through the posterior capsule to expose the contents of the posterior intercondylar notch and the tibial attachment of the PCL.
- Proceed as described by Berg (see Technique 1.27).
- Suture the capsular incision, allow the gastrocnemius to settle into position, approximate the subcutaneous layers, and close the skin in a routine fashion.

■ ARTHROSCOPICALLY AIDED POSTERIOR CRUCIATE LIGAMENT RECONSTRUCTION

As described in the section on ACL reconstruction, the PCL also can be replaced by arthroscopic surgical techniques. see other chapter for descriptions of these techniques.

■ COMPLICATIONS OF POSTERIOR CRUCIATE LIGAMENT RECONSTRUCTION

Aside from the usual postoperative complications, the most common problem associated with PCL reconstruction is residual posterior laxity, usually defined as more than 4 mm of increased posterior translation on PCL stress radiographs.

Loss of motion is the second most frequent complication. Flexion loss is more common than extension loss. Many studies report between a 10- and 20-degree loss of flexion, most likely caused by improper graft placement or inadequate rehabilitation. The position of the femoral tunnel is more critical than that of the tibial tunnel. Femoral attachments anterior and distal to the most isometric region result in increased graft tension, with flexion loss resulting from an increase in distance between the femoral and tibial attachment sites. Loss of extension or a flexion contracture most likely is caused by prolonged immobilization in flexion.

Poor graft selection has been implicated in the failure of reconstructions that use the iliotibial band, the medial head of the gastrocnemius, or the hamstring tendons. These tissues may have insufficient strength to prevent posterior sag and drawer. Improper tunnel placement can result in graft abrasion and subsequent failure. Femoral tunnel placement posterior and proximal to the most isometric region results in decreased graft tension in flexion secondary to a decrease in distance between femoral and tibial attachment sites. This results in graft laxity with an inability to prevent posterior sag and drawer.

Failure of the reconstruction may be the result of untreated associated ligamentous injuries, such as of the posterolateral corner, that allow excessive forces to be applied to the graft.

Neurologic injuries can result from excessive tourniquet time and manifest as neurapraxia. Direct injury to the tibial nerve can result from penetration by either the tibial guide pin or drill and can be avoided by ensuring direct exposure of the tip of the pin and drill during preparation of the tibial tunnel.

Vascular complications include laceration, thrombosis, and intimal injury to the popliteal artery. Viewing the tip of the guide pin and reamer at all times can prevent this injury.

Osteonecrosis of the medial femoral condyle has been reported. It may occur months to years after the surgery. The cause is thought to be local trauma to the blood supply of the subchondral bone from both soft-tissue dissection and drilling of the condyle. This complication has been treated successfully with curettage and autogenous bone grafting of the defect.

TRAUMATIC DISLOCATIONS

In comparison with other injuries of the knee, dislocations are relatively uncommon; however, some knee dislocations probably are never recognized because of spontaneous reduction before medical evaluation. In an acutely dislocated knee, the diagnosis usually is obvious because of deformity, pain, and swelling. The diagnosis may be more difficult in obese patients, in those with spontaneous reduction, and in patients with multiple trauma. McKee et al. noted that there is increasing evidence in the literature that morbid obesity is associated with low-energy knee dislocation and that this should be considered when assessing this group of patients with an acute

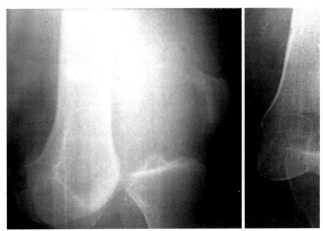

FIGURE 1.135 Ultralow-velocity knee dislocation in an obese patient.

knee injury. Failure to correctly diagnose a knee dislocation diminishes the likelihood of recognizing injury to the popliteal artery, which can result in devastating complications.

Knee dislocations have historically been described as high-velocity or low-velocity injuries. High-velocity dislocations most often occur in motor vehicle accidents, falls from a height, or severe crush injuries, whereas most low-velocity dislocations occur during sporting activities. Reports of low-velocity knee dislocations have focused primarily on dislocations occurring during sports. Although high-velocity injuries have historically been cited as having worse outcomes, we identified a subset of morbidly obese patients with what we termed ultralow-velocity knee dislocations that occurred during activities of daily living, such as stepping off a curb or stair or simply falling while walking (Fig. 1.135). The average age of the 17 patients (11 women and 6 men) was 28.6 years, and all 17 patients were clinically obese, with an average BMI of 48 (a BMI of 30 or more is considered clinical obesity). Popliteal artery injuries occurred in 7 of the 17 patients, and 7 had neurologic injuries. Two patients with vascular repairs required above-knee amputations because of tissue ischemia. We found a correlation between the BMI and the severity of injury: of patients with nerve injuries, the average BMI was 48.26; of those with vascular injuries, 56.28; and of those with both nerve and vascular injuries, 60.29. Only six patients did not have either vascular or nerve injury; their average BMI was 39.58. Regardless of BMI, patients with ligament reconstructions, especially posterolateral corner repair, had better subjective and objective outcomes than did those without ligament reconstructions. Since this study, others have reported similar findings.

In skeletally immature patients, stress radiographs should be obtained to rule out physeal injury.

CLASSIFICATION

Various classifications for knee dislocations have been proposed, including open or closed; high velocity, low velocity, or ultralow velocity; and reducible or irreducible. Dislocations also have been classified according to the position of the tibia relative to the femur (anterior, posterior, medial, lateral, or rotary). Anterior dislocations are most common, followed by posterior dislocations; medial, lateral, and rotatory combinations are less frequent. A classification of knee dislocations that focuses on identifying which structures are injured and the severity of injury to specific structures (Table 1.4) is more useful for preoperative planning. This classification aids with the timing of repair or reconstruction of specific ligaments. However, it is limited by the difficulty in obtaining an accurate examination. MRI and examination under anesthesia are useful to confirm the diagnosis and to identify injured structures. The ACL and PCL usually are both injured with a knee dislocation. In addition, either or both of the collateral ligaments and the posterolateral corner structures also may be injured. The most common pattern of injury is that of bicruciate ligament injuries with an associated MCL or LCL tear, depending on the direction of the deforming force (KD-III).

TABLE 1.4
Classification of Knee Dislocations (Schenck)

GRADE	DESCRIPTION
KD-I	PCL-intact knee dislocation, usually ACL and LCL torn; also includes ACL-intact knee dislocation with complete PCL tear
KD-II	ACL and PCL torn, collateral ligaments intact
KD-IIIM	ACL, PCL, and MCL—corner torn, lateral side intact
KD-IIIL	ACL, PCL, and LCL—corner torn, medial side intact
KD-IV	All four ligaments torn (ACL, PCL, MCL, LCL)

ACL, Anterior cruciate ligament; *KD*, knee dislocation; *LCL*, lateral collateral ligament; *MCL*, medial collateral ligament; *PCL*, posterior cruciate ligament.

EXAMINATION AND RADIOGRAPHIC EVALUATION

Completion and documentation of a thorough neurovascular examination are mandatory at the time of initial evaluation, before reduction, and after reduction. The extremity should be examined thoroughly for color, temperature, and capillary refill. Posterior tibial and dorsalis pedis pulses should be palpated and compared with the contralateral side. The ankle-brachial indices (ABIs) should be obtained in all patients with a knee dislocation. If necessary, arteriography should be carried out. Indications for arteriography are discussed in the section on vascular injuries.

Physical examination of patients with knee dislocations is not always reliable because of pain and guarding, spontaneous reduction, or ipsilateral fractures. However, once the neurovascular status is determined, the usual tests for ligamentous laxity should be carefully attempted. The extensor mechanism should be evaluated, and the limb should be examined for signs of compartment syndrome.

Initial radiographic evaluation focuses on determining the direction of dislocation and the presence of any concomitant bony injuries (Fig. 1.136). Anteroposterior, lateral, and oblique views should be obtained before and after reduction. MRI allows better evaluation of soft-tissue injuries, such as the actual site of cruciate and collateral ligament injury, meniscal disorders or injuries, and the status of the popliteal tendon when posterolateral corner injury is suggested (see earlier section on posterolateral instability). Most ACL injuries associated with knee dislocations are midsubstance tears (45%), followed by femoral avulsions (34%) and tibial avulsions (21%). The PCL injury is most often a femoral avulsion

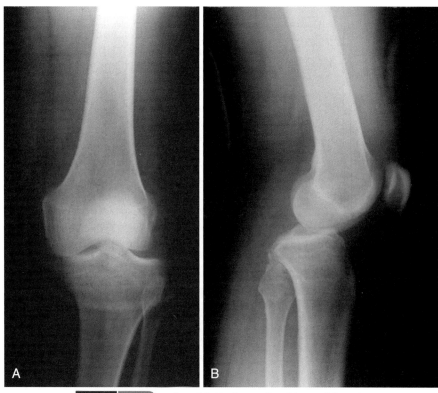

FIGURE 1.136   **A** and **B,** Radiographs of knee dislocation.

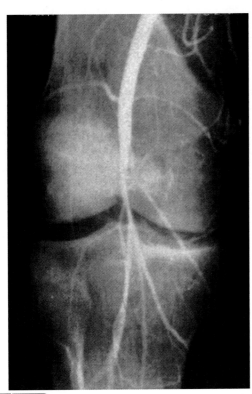

FIGURE 1.137 Arteriogram in patient with knee dislocation.

(76%), followed by midsubstance tear (17%) and tibial avulsion (7%). Occasionally, imaging by CT can be helpful in treatment planning if bone pathology is present. MRI has been found to be a sensitive measure of cruciate and collateral ligament injury (high sensitivity, lower specificity) in acute knee dislocations; however, it does not reliably diagnose injury to the posterolateral corner (low sensitivity, high specificity) or the menisci (low sensitivity, moderate specificity).

VASCULAR AND NERVE INJURIES
■ VASCULAR INJURIES

The first priority in the assessment and treatment of traumatic dislocations of the knee is not the ligaments but the vascular status of the extremity. Popliteal artery injury is common in dislocations of the knee, especially in anterior dislocations, because the relatively fixed popliteal artery is stretched, with intimal disruption and possible subsequent vascular occlusion. The incidence of popliteal artery injury has been reported in the literature to range from 5% to over 60%; however, some more recent studies cite a range of 7% to 25%, and a large database study involving 8050 knees found vascular injury in only 3.3%. This is in contrast to a systematic review that identified a frequency of 18% in 862 patients. Vascular injuries are more common with high-velocity injuries than with low-velocity injuries, and we have found them to be more common with ultralow-velocity injuries. Stewart et al. also found vascular injury more frequent with ultralow-velocity injuries (21%) than low-energy (17%) or high-energy (13%) injuries, and Johnson et al. found vascular injuries to be far more common in obese and morbidly obese patients than nonobese patients.

When the patient is first seen, if the peripheral circulation in the extremity is deficient, the dislocation should be reduced as quickly as possible and the circulatory status of the limb again carefully assessed. Several authors have suggested that even if pulses are present, the ABI should be calculated and rechecked several times. The ABI is the systolic pressure in the ankle divided by the systolic pressure in the arm. According to proponents of this method, if the ABI is more than 0.85 to 0.90, close observation is warranted; if the ABI is less than 0.85, arteriography is indicated. In a prospective study, the sensitivity, specificity, and positive predictive value of an ABI lower than 0.90 were 100% and the negative predictive value of an ABI that reached 0.90 or higher was 100%.

Femoral arteriography is indicated for any patient with questionable circulation or absent peripheral pulses either before or after reduction of a dislocated knee (Fig. 1.137).

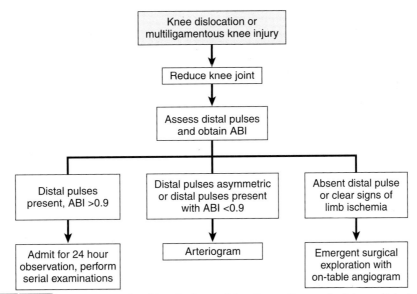

FIGURE 1.138 Treatment algorithm for knee dislocation with vascular injury. (Adapted from Nicandri GT, Chamberlain AM, Wahl CJ: Practical management of knee dislocations: a selective angiography protocol to detect limb-threatening vascular injuries, *Clin J Sport Med* 19:125, 2009.)

Femoral arteriography also is indicated in an extremity that originally has no pulses, even though satisfactory pulses are restored after reduction, because intimal tears may be present even though the patency of the popliteal artery is sufficient for satisfactory circulation. Sometime later, the tear may dissect free, resulting in thrombosis behind the intimal flap and occlusion of circulation. Although arteriography carries a 5% false-positive rate and an 8% complication rate, impaired or questionably impaired peripheral circulation at any time calls for arteriography to be done as soon as possible so that potential revascularization is not delayed. We avoid any potential delay by consulting with a vascular surgeon as soon as a vascular injury is suspected. Often, arteriography is done in the operating room at the time of emergency revascularization. We do not routinely obtain an arteriogram of extremities with knee dislocations when there is no sign of peripheral circulatory compromise before or after reduction. During the first 48 to 72 hours after injury, the extremity is monitored closely for an intimal tear that may progress and cause thrombosis even when the ABI is within normal limits.

CT angiography can be used more often as an alternative to femoral angiography; cited advantages include less invasive procedure, lower radiation dose, and high sensitivity and specificity. MR angiography also has been proposed as an alternative to define the vascular anatomy and diagnose asymptomatic vascular lesions; in one small series of knee dislocations, findings were comparable to those of standard angiography. Arterial duplex ultrasonography has been reported to be 100% sensitive and 97% specific for identifying arterial injuries, but this technique is highly operator dependent and is not always available for evaluation of acute injuries.

An evidence-based algorithm has been developed for diagnosis of vascular injury that provides a reasonable approach in line with current consensus and available evidence (Fig. 1.138).

■ NERVE DAMAGE

Nerve damage has been reported to occur in 10% to 40% of knee dislocations. Usually the peroneal nerve is injured, and nearly half of these nerve injuries result in permanent neurologic deficit. Although most common with posterolateral dislocations, peroneal or posterior tibial nerve injuries have been reported with all types of dislocations. In dislocations with disruption of the PCL and the posterolateral corner, the frequency of peroneal nerve injury has been reported to be as high as 45%. Transient or permanent peroneal nerve neurapraxias have been reported to occur in over half of patients with knee dislocations with arterial injuries. A systematic review of the literature determined that 87% of patients with partial peroneal nerve palsy achieved full motor recovery, whereas only 38% of patients with complete lesions had full recovery. Krych et al. also found that patients with partial nerve injury were more likely to regain antigravity strength; however, they found no difference between patients with peroneal nerve injury and those without on Lysholm or IKDC scores after multiligament reconstruction at 6-year follow-up. Posterior tibial tendon transfer has been recommended for treatment of foot drop that persists for at least 1 year after knee dislocation. Samson et al. developed an evidence-based algorithm for the management of common peroneal nerve

injury (Fig. 1.139) in which treatment depends on whether the palsy is complete or incomplete based on clinical examination and electromyography testing. Using these two criteria, Woodmass et al. found in a systematic literature review that 87% of patients with an incomplete palsy achieved full motor recovery, while fewer than 40% of those with complete palsy did so.

OTHER ASSOCIATED INJURIES

Traumatic knee dislocations that occur in isolation typically result in better outcomes than those that occur with associated injuries. The intercondylar eminences are frequently fractured, and other osteochondral fractures and meniscal tears have been reported. In addition, one study of 122 dislocated knees identified meniscal or chondral injuries in 76%. Fractures of the distal femur or proximal tibia are present in approximately 16% of knee dislocations. Darcy et al., in 88 patients with 90 knee dislocations, found that 57% had associated injuries (meniscal damage, tendon and/or ligament damage, fractures, dislocations of other joints, neurovascular compromise, organ damage). Those with isolated knee dislocations had better outcomes (45% good recovery) than those with multitrauma dislocations (25% good recovery). This finding was supported in the study by Woodmass et al., who found that comparison of knees with similar multiligament and neurovascular injury patterns showed that those with multitrauma have significantly lower functional scores after reconstruction. Although dislocation of the knee probably cannot occur without disruption of both cruciate ligaments, in straight anterior or posterior dislocations some stability may be retained because the femoral condyles are stripped cleanly out of the capsular and collateral ligament attachments and slip back inside them when the dislocation is reduced. On occasion, with avulsion fractures of the cruciate ligaments, the ligaments can be repaired rather than reconstructed. Midsubstance ACL tears occur in approximately 50% of knee dislocations, followed in frequency by injury to the femoral attachment and the tibial attachment. The PCL is torn from its femoral attachment in nearly 75% of knee dislocations, followed by midsubstance tears and tibial avulsions.

TREATMENT

Early ligament repair or reconstruction and aggressive rehabilitation is the optimal approach. Straight anterior or posterior dislocations—stable to varus and valgus stress after closed reduction—are most likely to have good results after closed reduction and brief immobilization. Other types of dislocations tend to be more unstable after reduction, and for these we generally prefer operative repair or reconstruction of all torn structures, especially in young patients.

Instability should be determined when the knee is reduced, and careful inspection of postreduction radiographs is necessary to determine that the reduction is anatomic. On occasion, the medial capsule and medial collateral ligamentous structures are trapped within the joint when a posterolateral dislocation is reduced. This is indicated by a slightly nonanatomic reduction on the radiographs and often a dimpling, puckering, or furrow along the medial joint line; immediate open reduction may be required. Other indications for immediate surgery include arterial injuries, open injuries, and compartment syndrome of the leg.

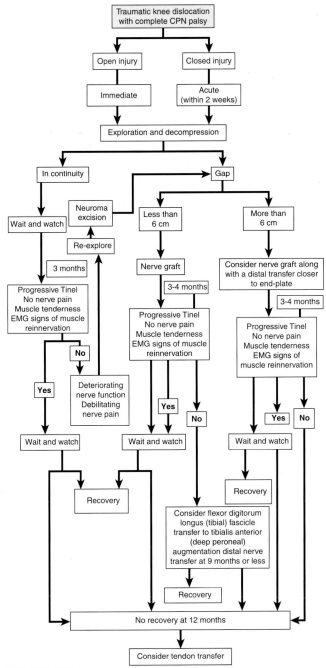

FIGURE 1.139 Evidence-based algorithm for management of common peroneal nerve injury associated with traumatic knee dislocation. (Adapted from Samson D, Ng CY, Power D: An evidence-based algorithm for the management of common peroneal nerve injury associated with traumatic knee dislocation, *EFORT Open Rev* 1:362, 2017.)

When anatomic closed reduction is achieved, the knee is immobilized in a splint or brace in its most stable position; 30 to 45 degrees of knee flexion is desirable if the knee is stable in this position because this approximates the posterior capsular and posteromedial and posterolateral corner structures and removes tension on the popliteal vessels. A circumferential cast should be avoided to allow careful monitoring of the neurocirculatory status. Spanning external fixation is recommended to maintain reduction if splinting is inadequate. Mercer et al., in a biomechanical study, determined that the

stiffest construct was achieved when pins were placed anterolateral on the femur and two connecting rods were used. A stiffer construct may provide a better clinical outcome. Transarticular pinning or olecranization of the patella should be avoided.

It has been well documented in the literature and we are convinced that the best results and the most stable knees can be obtained with repair or reconstruction of all disrupted ligaments when circumstances are optimal for surgery. A meta-analysis of studies of knee dislocations published over a decade ago (2001) concluded that, overall, reconstruction of the ligaments produced better results and a significantly lower risk of knee stiffness than did nonoperative treatment. Current literature continues to support this observation. This also was true in our group of patients with ultralow-velocity knee dislocations. Even though their mobility was limited before injury, those with surgical ligament reconstruction had better function than those treated nonoperatively. Vaidya et al. also found better outcomes with operative reconstruction in their 19 patients with ultralow velocity knee dislocations. Other factors to be considered include related injuries, other damage within the knee and surrounding tissues, the circulatory status, the age of the patient, and future demands on the knee. An elderly person with a sedentary lifestyle and few physical demands on the extremity may have a satisfactory result with closed conservative measures, but a young person who desires maximally stable function will benefit from early repair or reconstruction of the disrupted structures. In addition, the preexisting alignment of the lower extremities should be considered. A preexisting varus knee alignment should be treated surgically to prevent a subsequent lateral thrust gait. The same may hold true for a preexisting valgus knee alignment with a severe medial injury.

When circulation is impaired and abnormality is confirmed by angiography, immediate repair of the damaged popliteal vessel may save the limb. To delay with a nonsurgical approach or expectation that collateral circulation around the joint will provide sufficient peripheral circulation is to invite disaster. The amputation rate is approximately 6% when vascular repair is performed within 6 hours. This increases to 11% when repair is performed within 8 hours, to 86% when repair is delayed more than 8 hours, and to 90% when the vascular injury is untreated. When repair of the popliteal artery is required, we usually do not perform extensive ligamentous reconstruction at the same time. A few well-placed sutures in the capsular structures while the popliteal artery is exposed are justified, but extensive repair and reconstruction should be delayed. Repair of collateral and capsular structures and repair or reconstruction of cruciate ligaments can be carried out safely and effectively up to 3 weeks after vascular repair. The previous surgical incision should then be healed, the integrity of the popliteal artery established, and the ligamentous tissue quality still satisfactory for reconstruction or repair. The use of a tourniquet is left up to the discretion of the vascular surgeon. We usually await clearance from the vascular surgeon to use a tourniquet within the first 2 weeks of revascularization, and we have noted no recurrent vascular problems.

Current treatment recommendations focus on early reconstruction of the cruciate ligaments combined with repair or reconstruction of the collateral structures, followed by aggressive rehabilitation. This approach has been shown to improve knee stability and range of motion. In general, we prefer immediate repair or reconstruction (within 10 to 14 days) for the following injury patterns: ACL and PCL and posterolateral corner, PCL and posterolateral corner, ACL and PCLs and MCL (grade III injuries, distal tears), and PCL and MCL (grade III injuries, distal tears). Repair or reconstruction can be delayed for anterior and PCL injuries with intact collateral ligaments and for ACL, PCL, and MCL injuries (grade I or II) with an intact POL. Although tears of the medial patellofemoral ligament are frequent with multiligament knee injuries, they rarely cause patellar instability and, in most patients, do not require operative treatment.

The choice of graft for reconstruction of cruciate ligaments depends on the structures injured, the severity of the injury, the timing of the surgery, and the experience of the surgeon. We generally prefer allografts for reconstruction of multiple ligament–injured knees: bone–patellar tendon–bone graft for ACL reconstruction, Achilles tendon graft for PCL reconstruction, tibialis graft for reconstruction of the posterolateral corner, and tibialis or Achilles tendon graft for reconstruction of the medial or posteromedial corner. Autograft choices include bone–patellar tendon–bone, hamstring, and quadriceps tendon grafts. Artificial ligaments have

been studied, and their use has come under investigation for multiple-ligament reconstructions. A study of 71 patients with artificial ligament reconstructions found subjective and objective outcomes comparable with other graft choices at 54-month follow-up. Graft choices for knee ligament reconstruction are discussed in more detail in the earlier section on ACLs and in other chapter.

The operative treatment of a dislocated knee begins with a thorough examination with the patient under anesthesia to confirm the preoperative identification of injured structures. Maslaris et al. developed an updated "universal" treatment algorithm focusing on evaluation and treatment before ligament reconstruction (Fig. 1.140). Arthroscopy is especially helpful for evaluation of meniscal and chondral injuries, and some ligament repairs and reconstructions can be done arthroscopically or with arthroscopic assistance (see other chapter). However, arthroscopy of an acute injury should be limited because of the risk of fluid extravasation, which could precipitate a compartment syndrome in patients with acute injuries. In this situation, a dry arthroscopy may be helpful. Meniscal and articular cartilage injuries are treated before ligament injuries. The approach used depends on the structures injured (Fig. 1.141). A curved medial utility incision allows

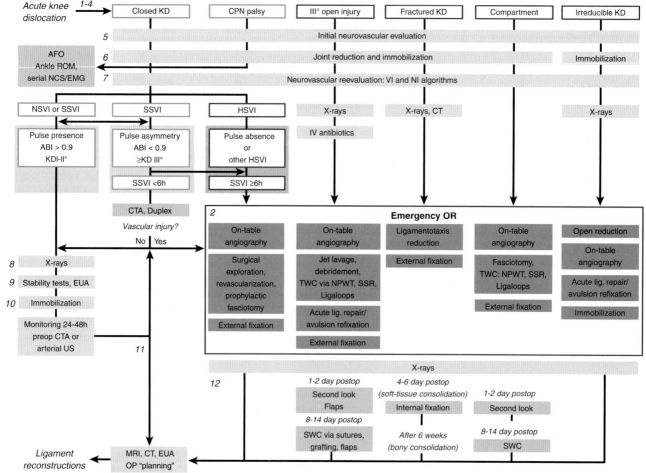

FIGURE 1.140 "Universal" treatment algorithm for evaluation and management of knee dislocation before ligament reconstruction. (From Maslaris A, Brinkmann O, Bungratz M, et al: Management of knee dislocation prior to ligament reconstruction: what is the current evidence? *Eur J Orthop Surg Traumatol* 28:1001, 2018.)

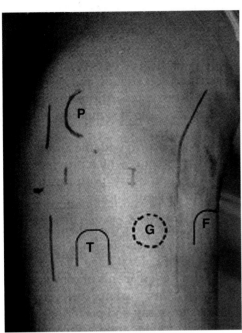

FIGURE 1.141   Skin incisions for open lateral or posterolateral reconstruction combined with arthroscopic reconstruction of anterior and posterior cruciate ligaments. *F*, Fibular head; *G*, Gerdy's tubercle; *P*, patella; *T*, tibial tubercle. (From L'Insalata JC, Dowdy PA, Harner CD: Multiple ligament reconstruction. In Harner CD, Vince KG, Fu FH, editors: *Techniques in knee surgery*, Philadelphia, 2000, Lippincott Williams & Wilkins.)

BOX 1.2

Sequence of Surgery for Traumatic Knee Dislocation

Examination under anesthesia
Arthroscopic examination
Treatment of meniscal and osteochondral injuries
   Reconstruction of cruciate ligaments:

PCL tibial tunnel		PCL tibial tunnel
PCL femoral tunnel	*or*	ACL tibial tunnel
ACL tibial tunnel		ACL femoral tunnel
ACL femoral tunnel		PCL femoral tunnel

Passage and fixation of PCL graft in femoral tunnel
Passage and fixation of ACL graft in femoral tunnel
Tensioning and fixation of PCL graft with knee flexed 90 degrees
Tensioning and fixation of ACL graft with knee in full extension
Repair, augmentation, and reconstruction of collateral ligaments
Range of motion and examination under anesthesia to ensure proper fixation
Radiographic confirmation of knee joint reduction

ACL, Anterior cruciate ligament; *PCL*, posterior cruciate ligament.

---

exposure of the cruciate ligaments, the MCL, and the posteromedial corner; a posterior L-shaped incision (Burks and Schaffer) allows exposure of the tibial insertion of the PCL for repair of an avulsion fracture or for tibial inlay reconstruction; and straight medial and lateral incisions allow exposure of the medial and posteromedial and the lateral and posterolateral structures, respectively. A straight midline incision allows exposure to all structures. Regardless of the approach used, full-thickness skin flaps should be developed and appropriate skin bridges (more than 7 cm) should be maintained. The suggested sequence of surgery is shown in Box 1.2.

Ferrari et al. described a technique for reconstruction in KDIII-M injuries that involves ACL reconstruction with a bone–patellar tendon–bone allograft, double-bundle PCL reconstruction with Achilles and anterior tibial tendon allografts, and augmentation of the superficial MCL with semitendinosus and gracilis autografts. The procedure begins with an open surgical approach to allow improved vision of the soft tissues and limit fluid extravasation into the operative site. Once the MCL reconstruction is completed (grafts are not fixed at this point), routine arthroscopic evaluation and reconstruction of the ACL and PCL are performed through standard anterolateral and anteromedial portals. After fixation of the ACL and PCL grafts, the semitendinosus and gracilis grafts are fixed.

An alternative early primary repair technique—one-stage anatomic repair and ligament bracing—was described by Heitmann et al. and was reported to have obtained good results in the treatment of KDIII or KDIV dislocations in 69 patients, with few complications and a low revision rate. The technique involves primary ACL and PCL transosseous sutures with additional suture augmentation. More data are needed to support the use of this technique.

Rehabilitation after surgery depends on the individual patient and the type and severity of injuries repaired or reconstructed. In general, protected weight bearing is continued for a minimum of 8 weeks, with the continued use of a functional brace for an additional 6 to 8 weeks. Full recovery may require 9 to 12 months. In their rehabilitation protocol after multiple ligament reconstruction (Fig. 1.142), Harner et al. delayed return to sports activities requiring changes in direction and pivoting for 9 to 12 months after surgery.

■ OUTCOME OF OPERATIVE TREATMENT OF KNEE DISLOCATIONS

Although a better understanding of knee dislocations and improved surgical techniques have resulted in better outcomes, the severe soft-tissue disruption associated with knee dislocations often precludes restoration of normal knee function. In three studies that included more than 100 patients, none of the knees was rated as normal according to the IKDC scores; 39% were nearly normal, 40% were abnormal, and 21% were severely abnormal. More recently, long-term follow-up (10 years) of 36 patients with traumatic knee dislocations found that 20 (56%) had "nearly normal" knee function. Current literature continues to indicate better outcomes with operative treatment. Vicenti et al., in a recent systematic review, found higher Lysholm scores, higher IKDC scores, and more frequent return to sport in those treated operatively. A high level of overall knee function after operative reconstruction in 36 patients was reported by Khakha et al.

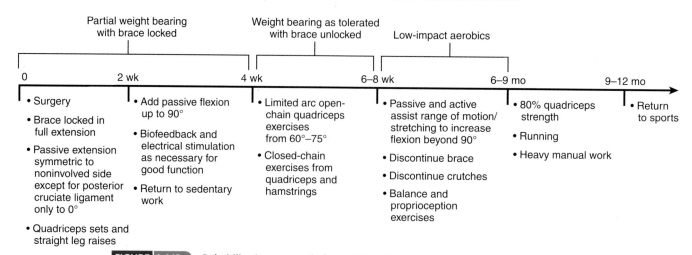

Rehabilitation Goal: Restore Range of Motion, Strength, and Function

Partial weight bearing with brace locked

Weight bearing as tolerated with brace unlocked

Low-impact aerobics

| 0 | 2 wk | 4 wk | 6–8 wk | 6–9 mo | 9–12 mo |

- Surgery
- Brace locked in full extension
- Passive extension symmetric to noninvolved side except for posterior cruciate ligament only to 0°
- Quadriceps sets and straight leg raises

- Add passive flexion up to 90°
- Biofeedback and electrical stimulation as necessary for good function
- Return to sedentary work

- Limited arc open-chain quadriceps exercises from 60°–75°
- Closed-chain exercises from quadriceps and hamstrings

- Passive and active assist range of motion/stretching to increase flexion beyond 90°
- Discontinue brace
- Discontinue crutches
- Balance and proprioception exercises

- 80% quadriceps strength
- Running
- Heavy manual work

- Return to sports

FIGURE 1.142 Rehabilitation protocol after multiple ligament reconstruction. (From Harner CD, Waltrip RL, Bennett CH, et al: Surgical management of knee dislocations, *J Bone Joint Surg* 86A:262, 2004.)

In a series of 119 patients with knee dislocations treated at a Level 1 trauma center, 32% had early complications and 9% required amputations; 47 patients (39%) required at least one unplanned secondary operation (total of 223 secondary operations) to treat instability or other complications. Limitations in knee motion were associated with high Injury Severity Score, infection, and heterotopic ossification. Despite these complications, in 31 patients (without amputation) who completed the Musculoskeletal Function Assessment (MFA) 31 scored excellent, 16 good, 16 fair, and three poor. Patients with popliteal artery injuries that require bypass grafting have significantly lower knee function scores than those with vascular injury.

Heterotopic ossification has been reported to occur in over 30% of patients with knee dislocations and may result in a stiff knee with loss of motion. In a study of 91 patients with knee dislocations, Whelan et al. cited PCL reconstruction as the only independent predictor of heterotopic ossification.

Studies of KDIV injuries have reported a poor prognosis compared to KDI, II, and III injuries. In a meta-analysis, patients with KDIV injuries had lower return-to-work and return-to-sport rates than those with KDIII injuries, and another study found that patients who had dislocations with multiple ligament injuries were more likely to require revision surgery for persistent instability. Patients with recurrent instability may have other concomitant pathologies, including limb malalignment, bone tunnel widening, retained implants, meniscal incompetence, and cartilage defects. Identification and treatment of these associated pathologies, often in a staged manner, can provide modest functional outcomes.

Patellar dislocations are discussed in other chapter.

SYNOVIAL PLICAE

During fetal development, the knee is separated into three compartments by synovial membranes. At 4 to 5 months of development, the partitions resolve to form a single cavity. Incomplete or partial resorption results in incomplete synovial shelves or plicae. The synovial plicae of the knee are commonly described as suprapatellar, mediopatellar, infrapatellar, and lateral (Fig. 1.143). Infrapatellar plicae usually are reported to be the most common.

Medial patellar plicae have been reported in 5% to 70% of individuals and suprapatellar plicae in approximately 17%.

Any condition that produces chronic irritation, trauma, or scarring may result in thickening of the plicae and the production of signs and symptoms suggesting internal derangement of the knee. Poorly placed medial arthrotomy incisions could damage the medial plica sufficiently to cause scarring and subsequent symptoms. Bumping the flexed knee on a hard object may traumatize a plica and inflame and thicken it sufficiently to cause symptoms. Careful examination should differentiate symptoms of a thickened plica that becomes inelastic from fibrosis or hyalinization from symptoms of a torn meniscus. A torn meniscus usually causes periodic episodes of giving way, buckling, locking, and pain localized along the joint line, and pain often is increased or reproduced by torsion of the tibia on the femur. A pathologic plica produces popping and catching in the knee by snapping across the patella or medial femoral condyle.

With the patient seated on the edge of the examining table and the leg dangling, palpation along the medial side of the patella as the patient flexes and extends the knee often localizes the abnormal plica as it flips over the medial femoral condyle and may produce a momentary "stuttering" of the patella. Kim et al. described a clinical test for medial patellar plica (MPP) that is reported to have a sensitivity of 90% and specificity of 89%, which was better than either ultrasound or MRI in a systematic literature review by Stubbings and Smith. The test is done with the patient supine and the knee extended. The examiner uses his or her thumb to apply manual force to

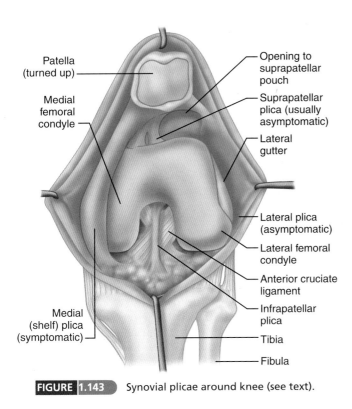

FIGURE 1.143   Synovial plicae around knee (see text).

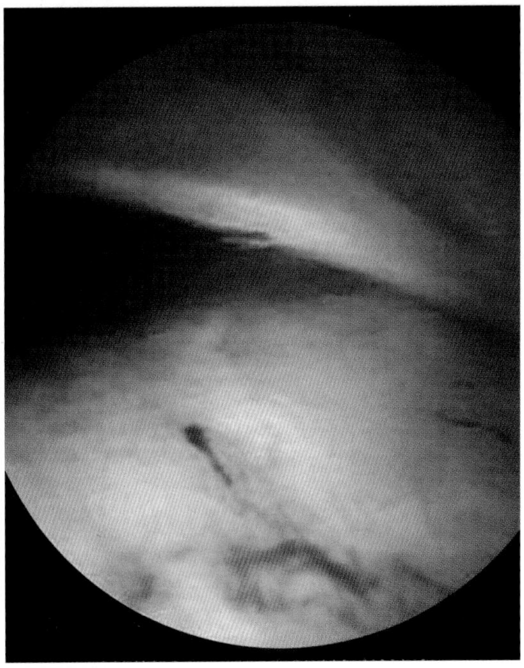

Labels on figure:
- Patella (turned up)
- Medial femoral condyle
- Opening to suprapatellar pouch
- Suprapatellar plica (usually asymptomatic)
- Lateral gutter
- Lateral plica (asymptomatic)
- Lateral femoral condyle
- Anterior cruciate ligament
- Infrapatellar plica
- Medial (shelf) plica (symptomatic)
- Tibia
- Fibula

FIGURE 1.144   Arthroscopic view of synovial plica.

the inferomedial portion of the patellofemoral joint to insert the medial pica between the medial femoral condyle and the patella. While this force is maintained, the knee is flexed 90 degrees. The MPP test is considered positive when pain is experienced with the knee in extension and is eliminated or markedly diminished with the knee in 90 degrees of flexion. Dynamic ultrasonography has been reported to have a diagnostic accuracy of 88%, sensitivity of 90%, and specificity of 83% in the evaluation of medial plica syndrome; however, this technique is highly operator dependent.

Abnormal plica is diagnosed best by arthroscopic examination of the knee. Careful assessment of the width and texture of the plica by viewing and probing is important. When it is sufficiently prominent (Fig. 1.144), a plica can present difficulties during arthroscopy as the arthroscope is introduced into the suprapatellar pouch.

Several authors have noted an association between the presence of plicae and the development of chondral lesions of the femoral condyle. These degenerative changes have been suggested to be caused by a pathologic medial plica that snaps or impinges against the underlying femoral condyle during knee motion. MRI or ultrasound may be helpful to confirm the diagnosis.

Treatment initially should be conservative. Restriction of activities, use of antiinflammatory agents, intraarticular corticosteroid injections with or without ultrasound guidance, and institution of an isometric exercise program for the quadriceps muscles often result in sufficient reduction of edema and synovitis so that the plica assumes a more normal resiliency and therefore does not produce symptoms. If a plica has become fibrotic and hyalinized and conservative measures fail to relieve a patient's symptoms, surgical excision should be curative. Excision usually is done by arthroscopic techniques, although a limited excision can be performed through a medial parapatellar incision. Simply incising or sectioning the plica is not recommended because of the possibility that the continuity of the plica will be restored by scar tissue.

ARTICULAR CARTILAGE INJURIES

Articular cartilage is a complex tissue that is able to withstand tremendous forces over many cycles but does not have the ability to heal even after a minor injury. More than 250 years ago, Hunter observed, "Ulcerated cartilage is a troublesome thing, once destroyed is not repaired." The health and function of a joint depend on the viability of the articular cartilage; without articular cartilage, arthritis develops. In young athletic individuals, articular cartilage changes usually are caused by trauma, whereas these changes are degenerative in older individuals. Knee arthroscopy studies have found articular cartilage lesions in 60% to 66% of patients.

Patients with articular cartilage injuries usually complain of pain, effusion, and mechanical symptoms. In patients with femoral lesions, pain generally is localized to the medial or lateral tibiofemoral compartment and is worse with weight bearing or high-impact activity. Patients with patellar lesions report pain with kneeling, stair climbing, and prolonged sitting.

Evaluation of a patient suspected of having a chondral or osteochondral lesion of the knee should include weight-bearing anteroposterior, 45-degree posteroanterior, lateral, and patellar (Merchant or sunrise) views of the involved extremity, as well as bilateral standing hip-knee-ankle anteroposterior views. Clinical suspicion of an articular cartilage lesion should prompt evaluation with cartilage-sensitive MRI to determine lesion location, size, and grade. Several classification systems have been developed to indicate the severity and type of articular cartilage injuries (Tables 1.5 and 1.6). Arthroscopic evaluation usually is necessary for definitive classification, but advances in cartilage-sensitive MRI techniques have made this method effective in providing valuable information about the size and grade of a lesion before surgery.

TABLE 1.5	
Classification of Articular Lesions by Configuration (Bauer and Jackson)	
TYPE	**CONFIGURATION**
I	Linear
II	Stellate
III	Flap
IV	Crater
V	Fibrillation
VI	Degrading

Articular cartilage lesions often are accompanied by significant hemarthrosis and occult subchondral trabecular microfractures (bone bruises, bone blisters). Occult subchondral bone bruises have been found in up to 80% of patients with complete ruptures of the ACL.

TREATMENT

Treatment recommendations for articular cartilage injuries and resulting arthritis include nonoperative and operative management. Nonoperative treatment involves decreasing the load on the joint. Having the patient lose weight, alter activities, and strengthen the muscles across the joint may help absorb some of the load. Orthoses or braces also are beneficial, as are analgesics and antiinflammatory medications.

Operative treatment generally is indicated if nonoperative methods fail to relieve pain and mechanical symptoms. Treatment options include debridement, marrow stimulation, transplantation to fill the defect, cell-based therapy, and the use of growth factors or pharmacologic agents (Table 1.7). The choice of procedure is based primarily on the size of the lesion (Table 1.8) and the activity demands of the patient.

■ ARTHROSCOPIC DEBRIDEMENT

For patients with minimal symptoms and small lesions (<2 cm^2) in areas of limited weight bearing, arthroscopic debridement to remove loose flaps or edges that impinge in the joint can provide short-term relief (see other chapter).

The goal of arthroscopic debridement and lavage is to reduce the inflammation and mechanical irritation within the joint. Debridement may include smoothing of the fibrillated articular surface (chondroplasty), meniscal trimming, shaving of osteophytes, and removal of inflamed synovium. Joint lavage is thought to reduce synovitis and pain by washing fragments of cartilage and calcium phosphate crystals from the knee. Scilla et al. reported that, at 6-year follow-up, 67% of National Football League players had been able to return to play after arthroscopic chondroplasty; those who had concomitant microfracture were less likely to return. Results after debridement are not as good in patients with significant knee arthritis.

■ ABRASION CHONDROPLASTY, MICROFRACTURE

Abrasion chondroplasty or microfracture techniques (Fig. 1.145) may stimulate a reparative process for small lesions (<2 cm^2) in low-demand patients. These procedures, which involve penetration of the avascular cartilage layer into the vascular subchondral bone to stimulate extrinsic repair, are the most commonly used procedures for cartilage restoration. According to the American Board of Orthopaedic Surgery (ABOS) Part II database (queried from 2002 to 2013), chondroplasty was the most common procedure (80%), followed by microfracture (21%) and osteochondral grafting (2%). Both patient age and frequency in chondroplasty had dramatic decreases since 2011. Improvement in symptoms has been reported in 60% to 70% of patients after abrasion or microfracture, but the fibrocartilaginous repair appears to deteriorate with time, beginning at about 18 months after surgery. In a review of the literature involving 3122 patients, functional outcomes were improved in 75% to 100% of patients at short-term follow-up after microfracture; however, at 2-year follow-up, 47% to 80% had a decline in function, and at long-term follow-up (6 to 7 years) functional decline was seen in 67% to 85% of patients. Results are significantly better in patients younger than 40 years than in patients older than 40 years. Advantages of microfracture are the simplicity of the procedure, the relatively low cost, and the low risk of patient morbidity. It also does not prevent the later use of other, more complex procedures.

TABLE 1.6			
Classification of Articular Cartilage Lesions by Severity			
GRADE	**OUTERBRIDGE**	**MODIFIED OUTERBRIDGE**	**ICRS**
0	Normal cartilage	Intact cartilage	Intact cartilage
I	Softening and swelling	Chondral softening or blistering with intact surface	Superficial (soft indentation or superficial fissures and cracks)
II	Fragmentation and fissures in area less than 0.5 inch in diameter	Superficial ulceration, fibrillation, or fissuring less than 50% of depth of cartilage	Lesion less than half the thickness of articular cartilage
III	Fragmentation and fissures in area larger than 0.5 inch in diameter	Deep ulceration, fibrillation, fissuring, or chondral flap more than 50% of cartilage without exposed bone	Lesion more than half the thickness of articular cartilage
IV	Exposed subchondral bone	Full-thickness wear with exposed subchondral bone	Lesion extending to subchondral bone

ICRS, International Cartilage Repair Society.

TABLE 1.7

Treatment Options for Articular Cartilage Lesions

PROCEDURE	INDICATIONS	OUTCOME
Arthroscopic debridement and lavage	Minimal symptoms	Palliative
Marrow stimulation	Smaller lesions, low-demand patient	Reparative
Osteochondral autograft	Smaller lesions, low- or high-demand patients	Restorative
Osteochondral allograft	Larger lesions with bone loss, low- or high-demand patients	Restorative
Autologous chondrocyte implantation	Small and large lesions with and without bone loss, high-demand patients	Restorative
Genetic engineering	Investigational	Restorative

From Garrick JG, editor: *Orthopaedic knowledge update: sports medicine*, ed 3, Rosemont, IL, 2004, American Academy of Orthopaedic Surgeons.

TABLE 1.8

Operative Treatment of Articular Cartilage Lesions

LESION SIZE	OPERATIVE TREATMENT
≤1.0 cm	Observation Abrasion chondroplasty Microfracture Osteochondral autograft transfer
1.0–2.0 cm	Abrasion chondroplasty Microfracture Osteochondral autograft transfer
2.0–3.5 cm	Fresh osteochondral allograft Autologous chondrocyte implantation
3.5–10 cm	Autologous chondrocyte implantation
Multiple (2 or 3)	Autologous chondrocyte implantation

Five factors have been identified as affecting the quality of the cartilaginous repair tissue after microfracture of a chondral defect: (1) during debridement, the calcified cartilage layer must be removed, but the abrasion of the subchondral bone must be avoided; (2) a 1- to 2-mm bridge of bone must be left between penetrations to allow connective tissue to fill the defect and adhere to the base of the defect; (3) joint function must be maintained after surgery by the use of early continuous passive motion; (4) protected weight bearing must be strictly enforced, depending on the location of the lesion; and (5) any significant abnormality in the mechanical axis must be corrected in conjunction with the microfracture procedure. This technique is described in other chapter. In an attempt to improve long-term results, principles of tissue engineering currently are being applied to microfracture techniques ("enhanced microfracture"). Autologous matrix-induced chondrogenesis (AMIC) combines microfracture with the use of an exogenous scaffold to stabilize the marrow clot and allow the ingrowth of mesenchymal stem cells. Several such matrices are commercially available, but most

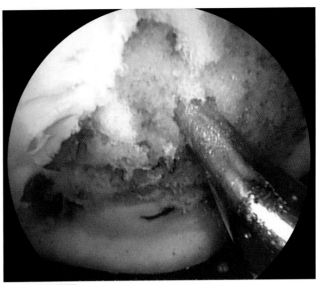

FIGURE 1.145 Microfracture of articular cartilage lesion. (From Canale ST, Azar FM: Osteochondritis dissecans. In Jackson DW, editor: *Master techniques in orthopaedic surgery: reconstructive knee surgery*, ed 3, Philadelphia, 2007, Lippincott Williams & Wilkins.)

are not approved by the U.S. Food and Drug Administration for use in the United States. Currently, there are few studies reporting the performance of these enhancements.

■ OSTEOCHONDRAL AUTOGRAFT TRANSPLANT, OSTEOCHONDRAL ALLOGRAFTING, AUTOLOGOUS CHONDROCYTE IMPLANTATION

For larger lesions or multiple lesions, especially in high-demand patients, restorative procedures such as osteochondral autograft transfer, osteochondral allografting, and autologous chondrocyte implantation (ACI) usually are indicated (Videos 1.5 and 1.6). Osteochondral autografts can be transplanted into damaged areas (up to 2 cm^2) from areas of less weight bearing on the femoral condyle as either a single large bone plug or multiple small plugs (mosaicplasty) (Fig. 1.146). For larger lesions (2 to 3.5 cm^2), allografts can be obtained from a fresh osteoarticular size-matched hemicondyle (Fig. 1.147). Chondrocyte viability of up to 80% has been reported at 4 weeks after implantation. Osteochondral allografts appear to be durable: short-term follow-up studies have indicated graft survival rates between 79% and 100%. In a long-term follow-up study of 129 knees with femoral condylar lesions treated with osteochondral allografts, survivorship was 82% at 10 years, 74% at 15 years, and 66% at 20 years. Graft failure was most likely in patients 30 years of age or older and in patients with two or more previous surgeries on the operative knee. Kyrch et al. reported a limited return to sport in 38 (88%) of 43 athletes at an average of 2.5 years after allograft transplantation, with full return to preinjury levels eventually achieved in 34 (79%). Risk factors for not returning to sports were age of 25 years or older and preoperative duration of symptoms of 12 months or more. A more recent study by Balazs et al. reported an 80% return to previous levels of competition in four professional and seven collegiate basketball players, and Nielsen et al. reported that 75% of patients had returned to sport or recreation 6 years after osteochondral allograft transplantation.

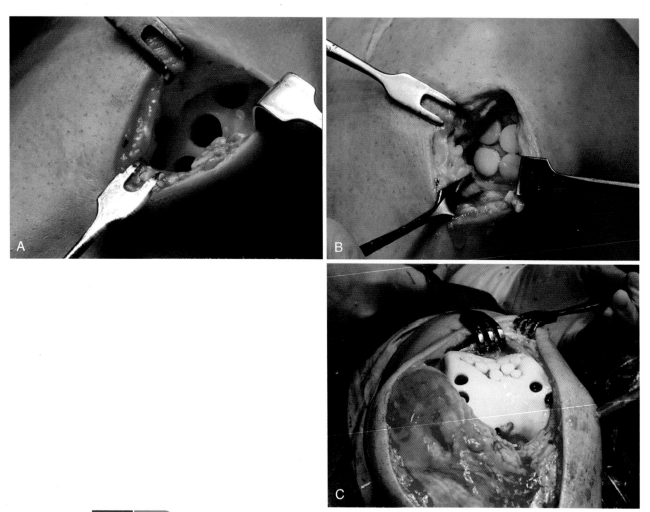

FIGURE 1.146 **A,** Miniarthrotomy mosaicplasty. Donor site area can be reached by extending knee. **B,** Recipient area is reached by flexing knee. **C,** Open mosaicplasty on femoral trochlea. (From Hangody L, Füles P: Autologous osteochondral mosaicplasty for the treatment of full-thickness defects of weight-bearing joints: ten years of experimental and clinical experience, *J Bone Joint Surg* 85A:25, 2003.)

Tirico et al. described osteochondral autograft transplantation (OAT) procedures in 371 patients (396 knees). At an average follow-up of 5.5 years, patient satisfaction rate was 88%, which was constant over time. OAT was used by Wang et al. in 43 revision surgeries after previous cartilage repair procedures. At a mean 3.5-year follow-up, significant improvements were noted in SF-36 Physical Function, SF-36 Pain, KOS-ADL, IKDC Subjective Knee Score, and Cincinnati Overall Symptom Assessment. Over 90% of grafts remained in place at latest follow-up. Using the National Surgical Quality Improvement Program Database, Gowd et al. analyzed 15,609 procedures and found linear increases in open and arthroscopic osteochondral autograft and allograft transplantation. The most frequent concomitant procedure was meniscectomy. Complication rates were low with all procedures (<1% to 2%), and no significant differences were found among procedures. A comparison of microfracture and mosaicplasty in 40 patients found that mosaicplasty resulted in better clinically relevant outcomes at short, medium, and long term (minimum 15 years) than microfracture.

Patients with irregular or ovoid lesion or multicompartmental focal lesions present challenging situations. Cotter et al. compared adjacent-plug OAT (snowman technique)

used for larger, high-grade chondral lesions to multicompartmental or bipolar OAT. Patients with unicondylar, multiplug OAT had inferior clinical outcomes, higher reoperation rates, and greater failure rates than those who had isolated single-graft transplantation, suggesting that multifocal OAT may be a better knee preservation technique for young, active patients with multifocal chondral lesions.

The biggest disadvantage to the use of fresh allografts is that the patients must be "on call" for immediate surgery when a suitable graft becomes available. To alleviate this problem, a preshaped, cylindrical sterilized and decellularized osteochondral allograft (SDOCA) has recently been developed as a treatment option. Farr et al. used these allografts in 32 patients with a mean age of 35 years and mean defect size of 2.9 cm^2. Twenty-three (72%) of these knees were considered failures, defined as structural damage of the graft or any reoperation resulting in removal of the graft; implant survival was only 20% at 2 years.

■ AUTOLOGOUS CHONDROCYTE IMPLANTATION

For lesions up to 10 cm or for multiple lesions, ACI can be an effective restorative procedure. This procedure is done in two

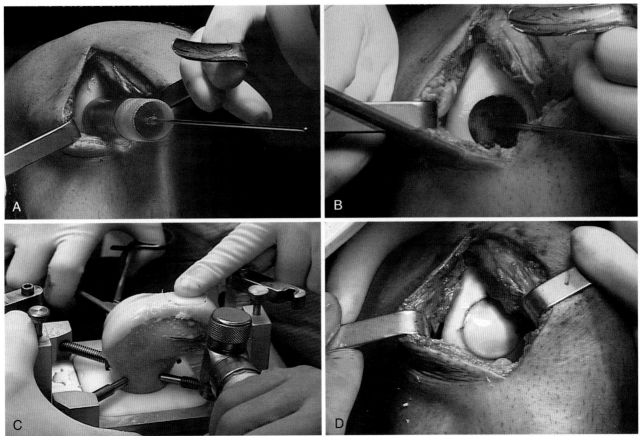

FIGURE 1.147 Allografting of osteochondral lesion. **A** and **B,** Preparation of recipient bed. **C,** Removal of graft from donor bone. **D,** Graft in place. (From Canale ST, Azar FM: Osteochondritis dissecans. In Jackson DW, editor: *Master techniques in orthopaedic surgery: reconstructive knee surgery,* ed 3, Philadelphia, 2007, Lippincott Williams & Wilkins.)

stages. First, a small amount of articular cartilage or chondral bone is removed arthroscopically for growing of the autologous chondrocytes. Then, usually 3 to 6 weeks later, an open procedure is done to implant the cells in the chondral defect. A periosteal graft is sutured over the defect, and the chondrocytes are injected under the graft into the defect (Fig. 1.148). The injection site is closed with one or two additional sutures and sealed with fibrin glue. Malalignment, ligament instability, and meniscal deficiencies must be corrected before or at the time of ACI. Good to excellent results have been reported in 80% to 89% of patients at 2 to 9 years after surgery. Some authors have reported better results in patients younger than 40 years of age at the time of surgery, whereas others have found no differences in the outcomes of ACI. Ogura et al. reported a 20-year survival rate of 63% in 23 patients with first-generation ACI; 79% of patients maintained their native knee for which they initially sought treatment and were satisfied with their outcomes. ACI also has been reported to be successful in treating large (average approximately 500 mm^2) chronic articular cartilage lesions. In 104 patients who had symptoms for nearly 8 years before treatment, 26% experienced graft failure at an average of 6 years after ACI; of the patients in whom the graft did not fail, 88% had excellent or good results. The most common complications are articular adhesions (2%) and detachment or delamination (<1%).

To avoid multiple operative procedures, an ACI "sandwich" technique (Fig. 1.149) was developed in which cancellous bone graft is used to fill the bone defect, periosteum is sutured above the bone graft at the level of the subchondral bone with the cambium layer facing the joint, more periosteal membrane is sutured to the rim of the chondral defect with the cambium layer facing the defect, fibrin glue is used to secure a watertight seal, and chondrocytes are injected between the membranes. One variation of this sandwich technique uses a porcine type I to type III membrane rather than periosteum, and another matrix-induced ACI technique uses a porcine collagen bilayer seeded with chondrocytes and secured directly to the base of a prepared chondral defect by fibrin glue.

Because of the frequency of periosteal hypertrophy and the difficulty of harvesting the periosteum and sewing it in place, bioabsorbable collagen covers were developed as an alternative (second-generation ACI). The implantation of cultured chondrocytes in suspension, as is done in both periosteal and collagen covers, raised concerns about uneven distribution of the chondrocytes in the defect and the possibility of cell leakage. To avoid these problems, chondrocytes have been seeded directly onto biodegradable scaffolds that are collagen based (e.g., MACI, Genzyme Biosurgery, Cambridge, MA) or hyaluronan based (e.g., Hyalograft-C, Anika Therapeutics, Bedford, MA; BioCart II, ProChon Biotech, Woburn, MA; Cartilix, polymer hydrogel, Biomet, Warsaw, IN; Cartipatch, agarose-alginate matrix, TBF Tissue Engineering, Mions, France). Because these membrane scaffolds are naturally "sticky," they can be placed into the defect arthroscopically

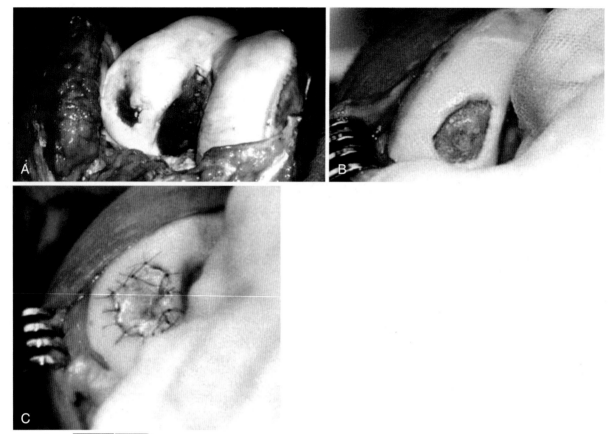

FIGURE 1.148 Autologous chondrocyte implantation. **A,** Femoral defect. **B,** After debridement. **C,** Cells held in place by periosteum sutured over defect.

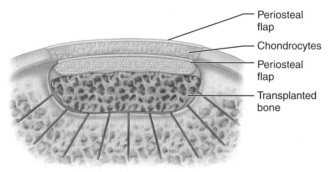

Periosteal flap
Chondrocytes
Periosteal flap
Transplanted bone

FIGURE 1.149 "Sandwich" technique of autogenous chondrocyte implantation uses layers of transplanted bone, periosteal flap, chondrocytes, and periosteal flap. (From Peterson L: International experience with autologous chondrocyte transplantation. In Scott WN, editor: *Insall & Scott surgery of the knee*, ed 4, Philadelphia, 2006, Churchill Livingstone Elsevier.)

without additional fixation or covering. Results comparable to those obtained with standard ACI have been reported in the European literature. Hoburg et al. reported a third-generation MACI technique using spheroids for treatment of 71 patients (29 adolescents, 42 young adults). All patients achieved high functional values, and there were no significant differences in rates of treatment failure between adolescents (3%) and young adults (5%). However, Zaffagnini et al., reported a low rate of return to pre-injury sport levels 10 years after MACI procedures in 31 competitive athletes. The best results were obtained

in young patients with traumatic dislocations without previous surgery. At even longer follow-up (12 years), Kreuz et al. reported significant improvement in the IKDC, the Lysholm, the KOOS, and the Noyes scores in 21 patients, with complete defect filling in 10 of 14 patients evaluated with MRI.

Other investigators (NeoCart, Histogenics, Northampton, MA) have cultured a scaffold seeded with autologous chondrocytes inside a bioreactor that continuously applies hydrostatic pressure to the scaffold; the company ceased Phase 3 clinical trials in 2018 and has suspended development of the implant. A Belgian company (ChondroCelect, Tigenix, Inc., Leuven, Belgium) identified and developed a mechanism to selectively culture more potent chondrocytes for implantation, but this was withdrawn from the market in November of 2016. To eliminate the need for a two-stage procedure, minced donor cartilage was placed on a bioabsorbable scaffold, which was then stapled into the chondral defect. Suggested advantages of this system (CAIS, DePuy-Mitek, Norwood, MA) are the avoidance of multiple surgeries for cartilage biopsy harvesting and chondrocyte implantation, simplification of the surgical technique by staple fixation rather than suturing of the periosteum, and reduction of the high costs associated with the mechanical and logistical complexities of current methods of ACI. However, slow trial enrollment and concerns about return on investment led to discontinuation of the trial. A more recent product is particulated juvenile cartilage allograft (DeNovo NT, Zimmer, Warsaw, IN), which consists of allograft articular cartilage from donors younger than 13 years old that has been cut into approximately 1-mm cubes. Juvenile chondrocytes have 100-fold increased ability to produce proteoglycans and have the potential to increase the ability of adult cartilage fragments to produce matrix. DeNovo NT has a shelf life similar to a fresh osteochondral allograft (40 to 45 days). Each package of DeNovo NT is intended to cover defects up to 2.5 cm², so multiple packets may be necessary for larger lesions. DeNovo NT is applied to cartilage lesions in a monolayer and held in place with a fibrin sealant (Fig. 1.150). Currently, there are few reports of clinical outcomes of this technique, most involving patellar or talar lesions. In a prospective study of 25 patients with 29 lesions of the femoral condyles or trochlea treated with DeNovo NT, Farr et al. reported significant improvements in pain and function as early as 3 months after surgery and maintained at 2-year follow-up. Although CARGEL (Smith & Nephew Inc., Memphis TN), a chitosan-based polymer scaffolding biomaterial, has been used since 2012 for treating articular cartilage lesions, limited data are available on patient outcomes. Most recently, Steinwachs et al. reviewed 91 patients (93 lesions) treated with

CARGEL and microfracture. Significant decreases were found in pain and swelling and significant increases were found in MOCART II scores. No patients required reoperation.

Regardless of the specific technique used, a disadvantage of ACI is the prolonged postoperative rehabilitation that requires strict compliance of the patient with weight-bearing and activity restrictions. However, one study found that activity levels in patients with characterized chondrocyte implantation were comparable to those of patients with microfracture at 2 years after surgery, and in both groups a lack of low-load activities after surgery adversely affected functional outcomes.

The popularity of the use of PRP in treating osteoarthritis of the knee has led to its use in the treatment of chondral defects of the knee, although clinical follow-up data are limited. A small comparative study of 20 patients found that functional recovery and resolution of pain were quicker with the addition of PRP to microfracture. Currently, there is no

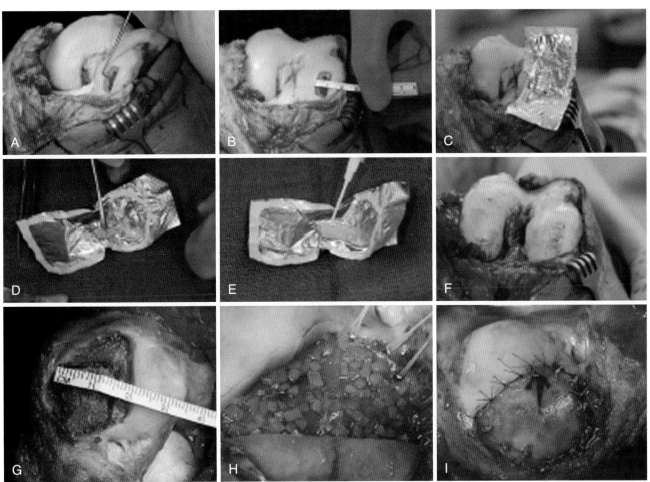

FIGURE 1.150 Use of particulated articular cartilage for chondral defects of the knee. **A,** Parapatellar arthrotomy and debridement of defect. **B,** Sizing of defect. **C,** Placement of thin sheet of sterile foil in defect to create negative mold. **D,** Placement of particulated cartilage fragments as single layer into mold. **E,** Filling of mold with fibrin glue. **F,** Application of layer of fibrin glue to base of defect, insertion of implant, and final layer of fibrin glue to secure graft. **G,** For large defects, particulated cartilage can be applied directly to bed of defects **(H)**, fixed with fibrin glue, then covered with collagen I/III membrane, which is sewn in place using standard techniques from autologous chondrocyte implantation **(I)**. (From Ribboh JF, Cole BJ, Farr J: Particulated articular cartilage for symptomatic chondral defects of the knee, *Curr Rev Musculoskelet Med* 8:429, 2015.)

conclusive, high-quality evidence to support the use of PRP for either traumatic or degenerative chondral lesions.

A recent prospective randomized study evaluated the use of hyaluronic acid after intraarticular knee fractures to decrease the frequency of posttraumatic arthritis and osteochondral damage. Patients with hyaluronic acid injections had significantly less pain, but no differences were found in other KOOS-related outcome measures, complications, functional outcome, or quality of life. Monckeberg et al. used intraarticular injections of peripheral blood stem cells in 20 patients to determine if they improved the regeneration of articular cartilage in patients with osteochondral knee injuries. They reported improvements in all outcome measures at 5-year follow-up and no infections, tumors, or synovitis.

One strategy currently being developed is the manipulation of the repair process at the cellular and molecular levels by the transfer of new genetic information to cells that contribute to the healing process ("gene therapy"). Research is focused on finding the most efficient vector for delivering this genetic information and the candidate genes most likely to improve cartilage repair and regeneration. Cell-based therapy also is being investigated using mesenchymal stem cells; the use of cell-based therapies allows the versatility of using scaffolds, growth factors, recombinant proteins, and gene therapy in various combinations.

With any of these procedures, malalignment, ligament instability, patellar instability, or any other coexisting patellofemoral pathologic process should be corrected to improve outcome. A systematic review of treatment methods that included microfracture, osteochondral autologous transplantation, ACI, and matrix-associated ACI found that all operative procedures produced comparable improvements in Lysholm scores, with no procedure proven superior. A prospective comparative study of microfracture, OAT, and ACI also found no differences in functional scores or MRI grades among the groups, with good results in 80% after microfracture, 82% after OAT, and 80% after ACI. Using a large US commercial database, Frank et al. compared reoperation rates after 47,207 cartilage restoration procedures in the knee (microfracture, ACI, OAT, and osteochondral allograft). Microfracture had the greatest risk of conversion to arthroplasty, and cell-based approaches had a significantly increased risk for reoperation.

■ EMERGING TECHNOLOGIES

Tissue engineering has the potential to provide a more sustainable and effective treatment of osteochondral defects by replacing the damaged tissue with a long-lasting bio-manufactured replacement tissue. Generally, the most common approach involves the use of a suitable biocompatible scaffold, stem cells, and a combination of bioactive molecules including growth factor proteins. The use of scaffolds for treatment of osteochondral defects is limited by the lack of availability; only a few scaffold designs have made it to clinical trials. The continued development of materials and techniques for tissue engineering, including 3D printing, holds promise for improved outcomes of osteochondral lesion treatment.

OSTEOCHONDRITIS DISSECANS

Osteochondritis dissecans (OCD) is the most common source of loose bodies in the knee joint. Other sources are (1) synovial chondromatosis, (2) osteophytes, (3) fractured articular surfaces, and (4) damaged menisci. In OCD, an area of subchondral bone becomes necrotic and degenerative changes usually occur in the cartilage overlying it. During the course of the disease, unless it is interrupted by surgery, other treatment, or spontaneous healing, the necrotic bone and the cartilage overlying it gradually separate from adjacent bone and cartilage and together become a loose body. It occurs most often in the knee joint, but it can occur in any joint, including the elbow, ankle, shoulder, and hip, and on any part of the articular surfaces (Fig. 1.151). OCD is most common in individuals aged 12 to 19 years.

In OCD of the knee (Fig. 1.152), the lesion usually is located on the lateral aspect of the medial femoral condyle near the attachment of the PCL (80%), but it can occur elsewhere on the articular surface of this condyle and occasionally on that of the posterolateral aspect of the femoral condyle (15%) or the inferomedial quadrant of the patella (5%). OCD is bilateral in 20% to 30% of patients.

OCD occurs in two groups of patients: (1) young patients, before physeal closure, in whom treatment can be expected to produce good results (Fig. 1.153); and (2) adults, in whom the cause may be a vascular phenomenon and the results less satisfactory. OCD of the knee joint is more common during adolescence.

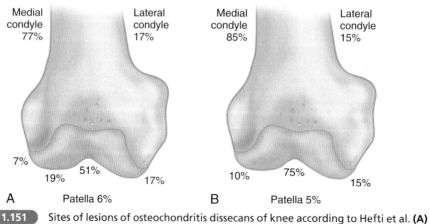

FIGURE 1.151 Sites of lesions of osteochondritis dissecans of knee according to Hefti et al. **(A)** and Aichroth **(B)**.

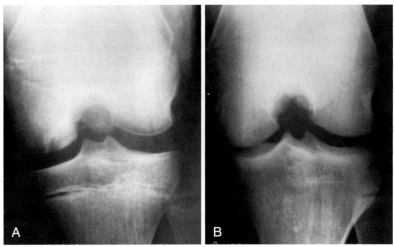

FIGURE 1.152   Osteochondritis dissecans of knee, nonoperative treatment. **A,** Lesion in adolescent treated nonoperatively in cast for 9 months. **B,** Several years later, complete healing is apparent and knee is asymptomatic.

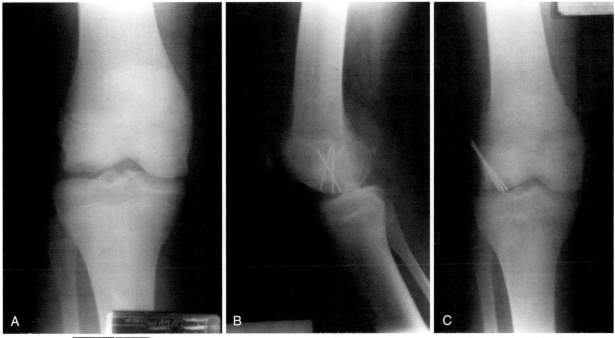

FIGURE 1.153   Osteochondritis dissecans. **A,** Osteochondritis dissecans involving weight-bearing portion of lateral femoral condyle in 15-year-old boy. **B** and **C,** Fragment internally fixed with multiple Kirschner wires.

ETIOLOGY

The etiology of OCD is controversial and remains unclear. Theories include ischemia, repetitive microtrauma, familial predisposition, endocrine imbalance, epiphyseal abnormalities, accessory centers of ossification, growth disorders, osteochondral fracture, repetitive microtrauma with subsequent interruption of interosseous blood supply to the subchondral area of the epiphysis, anatomic variations in the knee, and congenitally abnormal subchondral bone. Mechanical factors have been implicated in the development of OCD by the finding of an association between medial condylar lesions and a varus mechanical axis of the leg and between lateral condylar lesions and a valgus axis. A comparison of 35 skeletally immature patients with OCD of the medial femoral condyle to matched controls determined that femoral notch width measured on MRI was significantly smaller in those with OCD. The authors suggested that this anatomic factor may increase the likelihood of tibial eminence impingement and contribute to OCD lesion formation.

CLINICAL AND RADIOGRAPHIC FINDINGS

OCD of the knee occurs twice as often in males as in females. It is rare in patients younger than 10 years or older than 50 years. There are two distinctly different clinical pictures, one in a child or young adolescent 5 to 15 years of age with open physes and the other in an older adolescent or adult. The most common symptom is vague, aching discomfort in the knee, frequently of several months' duration. Approximately 80% of juvenile patients have symptoms for an average of 14 months before initial presentation. A history of trauma to the knee is given by 40% to 60% of patients. Examination also may reveal effusion, joint line tenderness or tenderness over the lesion, limitation of motion, presence of McMurray sign, and quadriceps atrophy. The patient may walk with an externally rotated gait to avoid contact of the medial femoral condyle with the medial tibial spine (Wilson sign). A thorough history and physical examination are necessary to rule out other causes of knee disease.

Catching and popping may be prominent symptoms once the lesion becomes separated or partially separated, and these may be due to a slight effusion. These symptoms can mimic those of meniscal derangement. Once complete separation has occurred, the patient experiences mechanical symptoms and may be able to palpate a loose body within the joint.

Radiographic examination is diagnostic. Because the lesion most commonly is on the inner aspect of the medial femoral condyle, the tunnel or intercondylar notch view may be the most revealing. Routine anteroposterior, lateral, and patellofemoral radiographs should be made in addition to the tunnel view. Comparison radiographs should be obtained in juvenile and adolescent patients because an OCD lesion may be confused with bilateral anomalous ossification centers, which may cause transient symptoms but usually resolve spontaneously within 6 to 12 months. OCD is bilateral in up to 30% of patients.

MRI is helpful in assessing fragment attachment and viability. Common MRI characteristics include a high-signal intensity line or cystic area beneath the lesion, a high-signal intensity line through the articular cartilage, and a focal articular cartilage defect on T2-weighted spin-echo and short tau inversion recovery images. Currently, a spoiled gradient-echo sequence using fat suppression and three-dimensional acquisition is considered the optimal technique for evaluating articular cartilage lesions. Fluid around the fragment and focal cystic areas beneath the fragment are the best indicators of instability; the absence of a zone of high signal intensity at the interface of the fragment and the bone is a reliable sign of lesion stability. MRI also is useful for identification of associated ligamentous and meniscal injuries.

Primary prognostic factors, in addition to the age of the patient, include progression, size, stability, amount of subchondral bone present, and location of the lesion, especially as it relates to weight bearing.

Technetium-99m bone scans may be helpful to follow the healing activity of lesions and to help predict the results of treatment. In addition, scan-negative ossific anomalies and scan-positive unhealed OCD lesions can be distinguished. Sequential single-photon emission CT (SPECT) scans obtained at 8-week intervals can be helpful. If CT is performed, it should be done in the coronal plane.

Several classification schemes for OCD have been proposed (Table 1.9). Dipaola et al. classified lesions according to their appearance on MRI and associated specific findings with the potential for fragment detachment and correlated these with arthroscopic and radiographic findings (Table 1.10).

TABLE 1.9

Classification of Osteochondritis Dissecans Based on Bone Scan

STAGE	FINDING
0	Normal radiographic and scintigraphic appearance
I	Lesion visible on plain radiographs, bone scan normal
II	Increased uptake in area of lesion on bone scan
III	Increased isotopic uptake in entire femoral condyle
IV	Uptake in tibial plateau opposite lesion

Based on data from Cahill BR: Osteochondritis dissecans of the knee: treatment of juvenile and adult forms, *J Am Acad Orthop Surg* 3:237, 1995.

TABLE 1.10

Staging Systems for Osteochondritis Dissecans

STAGE	ARTHROSCOPY	MAGNETIC RESONANCE IMAGING	RADIOGRAPHY
I	Irregularity and softening of articular cartilage; no definable fragment	Thickening of articular cartilage; low signal changes	Compression lesion; no visible fragment
II	Articular cartilage breached; definable fragment not displaceable	Articular cartilage breached; low signal rim behind fragment indicating fibrous attachment	Fragment attached
III	Articular cartilage breached; definable fragment, displaceable but attached by some overlying cartilage	Articular cartilage breached; high signal changes behind fragment indicating synovial fluid between fragment and underlying subchondral bone	Nondisplaced fragment without attachment
IV	Loose body	Loose body	Displaced fragment

From Dipaola JD, Nelson DW, Colville MR: Characterizing osteochondral lesions by magnetic resonance imaging, *Arthroscopy* 7:101, 1991.

TREATMENT

The treatment of OCD depends on the patient's age and the degree of involvement. The lesions often heal with conservative treatment in young patients with open physes. Although nonoperative treatment has a limited role in patients with symptomatic osteochondral lesions, multiple forms of nonoperative treatment have been described, including periods of immobilization, activity modification, and non–weight bearing. Prolonged immobilization should be avoided because joint motion affects articular cartilage attrition. Sanders et al. described nonoperative treatment of OCD in 86 patients, with a cumulative incidence of arthritis of 30% at 35 years after diagnosis. Diagnosis of OCD as an adult and a BMI at diagnosis of more than 25 kg/m were cited as predisposing factors for arthritis. Weiss et al. also noted a worse prognosis after nonoperative treatment in older patients with OCD, with progression to surgery strongly correlated with patient age at the time of diagnosis.

In older adolescents and adults, the prognosis is less satisfactory than in younger patients, regardless of treatment. In their systematic literature review, Sacolick et al. found that, although all patients had improvements in symptoms after ACI, better results occurred in younger, active male patients with smaller lesions, while Hevesi et al. found that persistent knee pain risk in skeletally immature patients was highest with patellar and unstable lesions and female sex. Other authors have found similar rates of healing in skeletally immature and mature patients.

Many forms of surgical treatment have been described in the literature, including drilling or excision of the fragment, debridement or microfracture of the crater, and different forms of fixation and grafting. There seems to be no argument that the object of treatment is to promote healing of the lesion before closure of the physis and concomitantly to prevent detachment of the lesion. Careful assessment of the patient and the lesion is mandatory, and correlation of the size and location of the lesion with the patient's age and symptoms is important.

Determination of the surface topography by MRI, CT, or arthroscopy is essential. Arthroscopy is useful not only because the diagnosis can be established but also because a lesion can be drilled, curetted, or pinned through the arthroscope and loose bodies can be removed with minimal morbidity. Suggested advantages of arthroscopy in treating OCD include immediate evaluation of the surface topography, decrease in total rehabilitation time, avoidance of open surgery and the risk of infection, decreased morbidity, avoidance of the physical and psychologic scars of knee surgery, and decreased length and cost of hospitalization. Indications for operative treatment include a symptomatic knee in a patient who is skeletally older than 12 years, a lesion larger than 1 cm in diameter, and involvement of the weight-bearing surface. Lesions with intact articular cartilage are simply drilled. Those with early separation are drilled and occasionally pinned in place. Because partial detachment leads to a break in the cartilaginous border and protrusion of fibrous tissue, removal of the fibrous tissue to bleeding bone is recommended followed by pinning of the fragment in place. Craters are trephined and drilled, and fresh loose bodies are replaced and pinned. Cancellous grafts are used in selected lesions to restore surface congruity. One must be extremely proficient in surgical arthroscopic techniques to pin and bone graft such lesions. Treatment of larger lesions is much the same as that discussed in the earlier section on osteochondral lesions and may include osteochondral autografting (see other chapter) or allografting and ACI techniques.

Although we use arthroscopic techniques to treat most patients with OCD lesions that require surgery, open arthrotomy techniques can be done through a mini-incision if arthroscopy does not allow for optimal fixation. Also, lesions involving areas inaccessible by arthroscopic techniques can be treated by open procedures.

The most commonly used open techniques are removal of loose bodies or loose fragments, curettage and drilling of the base of craters, and replacement and pinning of fragments. A well-done arthrotomy is preferable to a poorly done arthroscopic procedure. Arthrotomy also is indicated for lesions larger than 3 cm for which more than one graft is needed, when reshaping of a large loose body for replacement is required, and when multiple, salvageable loose fragments are present.

When arthroscopy is performed, injection of methylene blue may better define the lesion. The knee should be flexed fully to view the entire lesion or to locate posterior lesions. Fluoroscopy may be needed to locate a lesion that is intact with little or no articular change. Holes should be drilled to a depth of 1.0 to 1.5 cm to promote vascular healing. Retrograde drilling, pinning, or bone grafting should not cross the physis.

■ EXCISION OF LOOSE BODIES

The indications for removal of loose bodies include small fragments (<2 cm), multiple fragments, fragments with inadequate bone stock (usually purely cartilaginous), and fragments that cannot be secured with internal fixation. Most loose bodies currently are removed by arthroscopic techniques (see other chapter). In searching for and removing loose bodies, it is important to remember that some may be composed entirely of cartilage and therefore may not be visible on radiographs. If an arthrotomy is used for reduction and fixation of a detached fragment or for removal of loose bodies, it is important to remember that loose bodies often move freely from one compartment to another when the joint is moved or manipulated. Therefore, radiographs should be made in the operating room, after the tourniquet has been applied but before the incision is made. The loose body or bodies may have moved to another part of the joint since radiographs were made, and any plan for the surgical approach may have to be changed (Fig. 1.154).

Sanders et al. compared arthritis occurrence after fragment excision, fragment preservation, and chondral defect grafting, and found that patients treated with fragment excision had higher rates of osteoarthritis and knee arthroplasty at long-term follow-up.

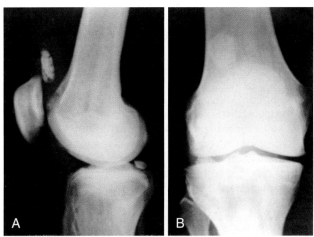

FIGURE 1.154 **A** and **B,** Large loose body in lateral portion of suprapatellar pouch; smaller body in posterolateral compartment. Small fragment of bone opposite posterior surface of lateral condyle of femur is sesamoid bone in lateral head of gastrocnemius muscle, not loose body.

FIXATION OF FRAGMENTS

Good results have been reported with the fixation of loose fragments with headless screws, cannulated screws, and biodegradable pins and screws. Biodegradable implants are currently the preferred method of fixation; however, one study of 21 knees fixed with bioabsorbable fixation found a low rate of clinical healing and a high rate of complications with this method. A more recent study by Adachi et al. of fixation with bioabsorbable pins in 30 juvenile patients (33 lesions) reported a healing rate of 97% with no complications. All patients regained normal range of motion, and 25 of 28 patients who had been involved in sports returned to their previous sports activity levels within 6 months. Fabricant et al. described fixation of chondral-only fragments with bioabsorbable implants in 15 patients. All 15 returned to sports a median of 26 weeks after surgery, and 12 of 14 patients who participated in team sports preoperatively returned to the same sport(s) postoperatively, competing at or above the preoperative level. Whatever implant is used, it needs to provide appropriate compression across the fixation point.

We have had no experience with the use of bone pegs for fixation or bone grafting of OCD defects. With this technique, small matchstick grafts are fashioned, the crater bed is curetted to cancellous bone, and the fragment is carefully replaced; with the appropriate-size drill, the fragment is perforated to receive two, three, or four matchstick grafts that are tapped through the holes and into the underlying cancellous bone. These grafts can be used alone for fixation or can be supplemented with Kirschner wires.

DRILLING OF THE LESION

Isolated drilling of an osteochondritic lesion currently is done arthroscopically and is most commonly indicated for stable lesions in immature patients in whom nonoperative treatment fails. Three drilling techniques are commonly used in the knee—transarticular, retroarticular, and notch—all three of which have demonstrated high rates of healing and good return to function. A comparison of transarticular and retroarticular techniques showed healing rates of 90% for both, with no reported complications. For descriptions of open loose body removal and open drilling and pinning, see earlier editions of this text.

OUTCOMES OF TREATMENT OF OSTEOCHONDRITIS DISSECANS OF THE KNEE

The prognosis after surgery varies with the size and location of the lesion and with the treatment. Reported results of operative treatment vary considerably among techniques and among authors, with good results reported in from 65% to 95% of patients. ACI was successful in 85% of patients with failed previous treatment, and 6-year follow-up of 34 knees with stage III or IV OCD found a statistically significant improvement in function after ACI. Osteochondral autologous grafting was reported to obtain significant increases in function in 64 patients. Follow-up evaluation of 48 knees surgically treated for OCD with a variety of methods (debridement, drilling, loose body removal, arthroscopic reduction and internal fixation, microfracture, osteochondral allograft, ACI) found significant improvement in all outcome measures, including function and symptom relief, at 4-year follow-up. A 6-year follow-up study found that, regardless of the type of cartilage repair, knee function improved over 5 to 8 years after surgery but remained significantly less than the contralateral knee.

COMPLICATIONS

Complications, in addition to typical postoperative knee complications such as infection and hemarthrosis, include iatrogenic cartilage damage, implant loosening, and abrasion of the articular cartilage by implants. Aggressive drilling of an intact lesion can cause fragmentation of the lesion. Metallic screws that are prominent or become prominent as surrounding articular cartilage wears down can damage adjacent articular cartilage; removal usually is recommended. Absorbable fixation devices have been reported to cause foreign body reactions on occasion. Damage to adjacent articular cartilage has been attributed to loosening and failure of bioabsorbable screws that backed out, and unabsorbed screw heads have been found as intraarticular loose bodies. Fibrocartilage hypertrophy has been reported at osteochondral autograft donor sites, causing knee pain and occasional locking that required arthroscopic trimming of the fibrocartilage. Delayed union or nonunion of an internally fixed lesion may require an additional procedure if it is symptomatic.

DISORDERS OF THE PATELLA

OSTEOCHONDRITIS DISSECANS OF THE PATELLA

OCD of the patella is less frequent than that of the femoral condyles and typically has a worse prognosis. It usually occurs in the second and third decades and is most often located in the lower half of the patella. Involvement is bilateral in up to one third of patients and should be distinguished from dorsal defects of the patella. OCD of the patella is best seen on a slightly overexposed lateral radiograph. An axial ("skyline") radiographic view determines whether the lesion is in the medial or lateral facet.

Treatment is essentially the same as described for OCD of the distal femur; however, in the patella, it usually is associated with chondromalacia that extends considerably beyond the peripheral margins of the avascular bone. Residual disability after treatment usually is proportional to the size of the chondromalacic area. Rarely is chondromalacia so extensive as to require patellectomy; the patella should almost always be preserved. (It can be excised later if too much disability persists.) Excision of the lesion followed by curettage and drilling of the lesion, arthroscopic screw (metallic and bioabsorbable) fixation, and ACI have been described for OCD of the patella.

DORSAL DEFECT OF THE PATELLA

Dorsal defect of the patella is a circular, well-circumscribed, radiolucent, benign lesion of approximately 1 cm that abuts the articular cartilage and invariably is in the superolateral aspect of the patella. In half the patients the lesion is asymptomatic. Differential diagnoses include OCD, Brodie abscess, eosinophilic granuloma, enchondroma, osteoid osteoma, and, in older individuals, metastatic disease.

Although the cause is unknown, most authors believe that dorsal defect of the patella is a variant of ossification. It has been attributed to a traction injury at the insertion of the vastus lateralis muscle during ossification of the patella; ossification anomalies, such as patellar cartilage depressions and perforations lend support to this hypothesis. Some have proposed that dorsal defect of the patella may be a fibrous cortical defect or nonossifying fibroma of the patella.

The lesion usually is self-limited and heals spontaneously. In patients with symptomatic defects, treatment should be conservative, with reduction of physical activity and follow-up evaluation. Operative treatment rarely is required, but curettage and bone grafting have been reported to hasten healing. The most important aspect of dorsal defects of the patella is differentiating them from OCD so that unnecessary surgery is not done in a self-limited condition.

BIPARTITE PATELLA

Bipartite patella is usually asymptomatic and is noted incidentally on an anteroposterior or tunnel tangential radiograph. When present, it occurs bilaterally in approximately 40% of patients. The most commonly used classification system identifies three types of bipartite patella. Type I, which accounts for 5%, occurs at the inferior pole and may be associated with Sinding-Larsen-Johansson syndrome. Type II, which accounts for 20%, occurs along the entire lateral border of the patella and may be associated with a nonunion of a patellar fracture. Type III, the most common type, occurs as an elliptical area in the superolateral portion of the patella and accounts for 75% of cases. A more recent classification scheme considers location (superolateral or lateral) and number of fragments (bipartite, tripartite, multipartite) (Fig. 1.155). In their study of 139 knees, the authors found that most (83%) were superolateral bipartite, 12% were lateral bipartite, 4% were superolateral and lateral tripartite, and 1% were superolateral tripartite.

Pain is unusual in bipartite patella; when present, it is caused by overuse. A diagnostic radiographic test to determine if pain is caused by a nonunion at the bipartite site uses a normal skyline view followed by a skyline view taken with the patient in a squatting weight-bearing position. The test result is considered positive if the separation is greater in the squatting weight-bearing position than on the normal skyline view. MRI usually is not necessary for diagnosis but has been shown to identify bone marrow edema within the bipartite fragment in about half of patients. Abnormally high scintigraphic uptake has been found to be frequent in both symptomatic and asymptomatic bipartite patella, and treatment decisions should not be based on bone scans.

If pain does occur with a bipartite patella, we have had success by limiting and restricting activity, correcting the activity that is causing an overuse syndrome, and prescribing nonsteroidal antiinflammatory agents and a short-arc exercise program. Immobilization for 3 weeks or more relieves the

symptoms of repetitive microtrauma of the synchondrosis. Operative treatment rarely is necessary.

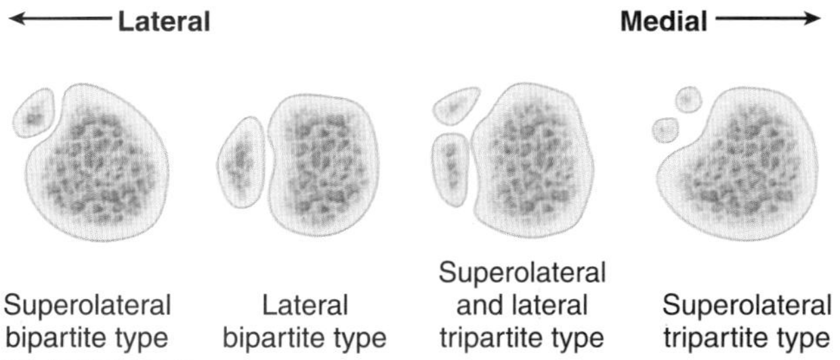

Fracture and traumatic separation of bipartite patellae have been described in the literature, but these are rare occurrences. We have had success with excision of the bipartite fragment, especially in the superolateral quadrant. One systematic review of the literature found that 86% of athletes made a full return to athletic activity after operative treatment of a painful bipartite patella; excision of the painful fragment produced the best results (91% return to sport). Arthroscopic excision of a painful bipartite patella fragment results in less morbidity than open excision. However, excision of large fragments with an articular surface may produce patellofemoral incongruity; internal fixation of separated fragments has been reported but has limited support in the literature. Lateral retinacular release and detachment of the vastus lateralis muscle insertion have been reported to produce good pain relief and union of the fragments by reducing the traction force of the vastus lateralis on the loose fragment.

Ogata described a subperiosteal release of the lateral quadriceps mechanism that inserts into the bipartite portion of the patella. The continuity of the tendon periosteal complex to the main portion of the patella is preserved. The fragment is thus relieved from muscle traction without causing a mediolateral imbalance that would affect patellofemoral tracking.

SUBPERIOSTEAL RELEASE OF THE LATERAL QUADRICEPS MECHANISM

TECHNIQUE 1.29

(OGATA)
- After arthroscopic examination of the knee, make a longitudinal skin incision over the distal portion of the vastus lateralis tendon, extending just distal to the midportion of the separated area of the patella (Fig. 1.156A).
- Split the tendon, which usually is thickened, along its middle fibers, and detach its insertion to the painful patellar fragment subperiosteally while preserving the continuity of its expansion to the main mass.
- Dissect the tendon-periosteum complex, consisting of the tendinous expansion and the periosteal tissues, and sharply denude the fragment completely (Fig. 1.156B,C).
- Observe the area of separation of the smaller portion of the patella after it has been exposed as bending stress is applied to the fragment by grasping it and attempting to move it with the thumb and finger. In general, a groove at the area of separation widens with such bending stress if the patellar fragment is unstable.
- Ogata recommended removal of the fragment if it is shown to be grossly mobile but leaving the fragment in situ if it shows little mobility with bending stress.
- Repair the longitudinal incision in the vastus lateralis with 0 absorbable sutures and close the skin incision.

FIGURE 1.155 Classification of bipartite patella according to location (superolateral or lateral) and number of fragments (bipartite, tripartite, multipartite). (Redrawn from Oohashi Y, Koshino T, Oohashi Y: Clinical features and classification of bipartite or tripartite patella, *Knee Surg Sports Traumatol Arthrosc* 18:1465, 2010.)

Lateral ← → Medial

Superolateral bipartite type | Lateral bipartite type | Superolateral and lateral tripartite type | Superolateral tripartite type

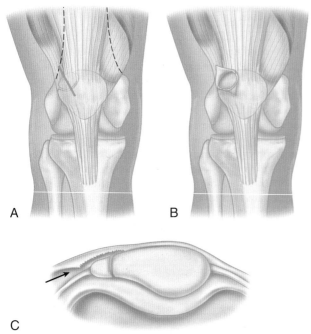

FIGURE 1.156 Ogata technique for bipartite patella. **A,** Oblique skin incision is made over distal portion of vastus lateralis tendon, extending just distal to midportion of separated area of patella. **B,** Vastus lateralis tendon is split along its middle fibers, and insertion to painful patellar fragment is detached subperiosteally. Continuity of tendon-periosteum complex to main portion of patella is preserved. **C,** Fragment is relieved from muscle traction without causing mediolateral imbalance that would affect patellofemoral tracking. Care should be taken not to injure synovial capsule to preserve some blood supply to fragment. **SEE TECHNIQUE 1.29.**

POSTOPERATIVE CARE Postoperative management is the same regardless of whether the patellar fragment was removed. The patient is immediately allowed to walk with full weight bearing and progress with range-of-motion exercises. Sports activity is gradually allowed by 2 to 4 weeks if the patient is asymptomatic.

CHONDROMALACIA OF THE PATELLA

The term *chondromalacia of the patella* was introduced in the literature in 1928 by Aleman, who described the degeneration of articular cartilage of the patella. Unfortunately, the term *chondromalacia* has become synonymous with patellofemoral pain. Numerous terms have been proposed to describe the syndrome, such as patellofemoral syndrome, patellofemoral arthralgia, extensor mechanism dysplasia, anterior knee pain syndrome, and others, but these do not accurately reflect the pathologic condition present in chondromalacia. Some patients with minimal changes in the articular surface have marked patellofemoral joint symptoms and, conversely, some patients with no patellofemoral joint pain have marked changes in the articular surface of the patella. Chondromalacia of the patella should describe a pathologic condition of the cartilage and not a clinical syndrome.

The basic pathologic lesion in chondromalacia of the patella is not the same as that in traumatic arthritis. In chondromalacia of the patella, the initial lesion is a change in the ground substance and collagen fibers at the deep levels of the cartilage. It is a disorder of the deep layers of the cartilage that involves the surface layer only late in its development. Such a change is tangible but not visible, and the surface is smooth and intact. In contrast, in osteoarthritis, the initial changes occur on the surface of the cartilage, with loss of continuity of the transverse fibers followed by fibrillation, which usually becomes grossly visible.

Chondromalacia is attributed to a decrease in sulfated mucopolysaccharides in the ground substance. This can be demonstrated by loss of basophilia on hematoxylin and eosin preparations. The changes occur most commonly at one of two sites in the deep layer of cartilage. The first is an area about 1 cm in diameter astride the ridge that separates the lateral facet from the medial facet; the second area straddles the inferior part of the central ridge that separates the medial and lateral facets. These areas are close together and sometimes are confluent (Fig. 1.157). If these noncontact areas were never subjected to the mechanical stresses of articulation, chondromalacia at these sites might be of little significance. However, when parts of these areas do articulate, usually at some extreme range of motion, the softened cartilage is mechanically inadequate to support the collagen framework. Its complex structure begins to break up, and the next phase of degeneration, fibrillation, occurs. These changes may deepen progressively until all the layers of cartilage are affected down to the subchondral bone. Pain has been suggested to result from the disorganization of the fibrous structure of the intermediate zone of collagen fibers, which subjects the subjacent bone plates to pressure variations from which they normally are protected by the energy-absorbing function of that zone of cartilage (Fig. 1.158), which may act as a pain stimulus on the nerve endings in the subchondral bone plate. Some authors have pointed out the tendency in other joints for articular cartilage that habitually is out of contact with other articular cartilage to undergo surface fibrillation. These changes are age-dependent, nonprogressive, surface changes; they do not progress to an advanced, full-thickness cartilage loss.

In most human knees, a ridge of varying height crosses the medial femoral condyle at its osteochondral junction, and

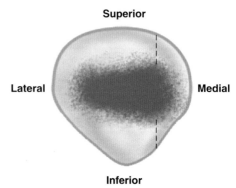

FIGURE 1.157 Dark areas represent most common areas of patellar chondromalacia from maps of 105 patellas. It was most severe in central zone but extended equally onto medial and lateral facets.

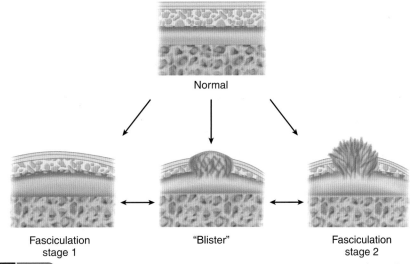

Normal

Fasciculation
stage 1

"Blister"

Fasciculation
stage 2

FIGURE 1.158 Stages of lesion of basal degeneration of articular cartilage of patella.

friction of the medial facet on the cartilage as the patella rides over this ridge during the normal movement of the knee has been proposed as a cause of chondromalacia of the patella.

CLASSIFICATION AND ETIOLOGY

Several authors have attempted to classify the macroscopic and microscopic pathologic changes. Some have based their classification on the cartilage changes; others, on the size of the lesion. In general, grade I changes include minimal articular cartilage changes. The cartilage may have localized softening with minimal or no break in the surface. A blunt instrument pressed on the surface may sink into the cartilage, and the cartilage may appear slightly discolored and soft. Grade II changes include an area of fibrillation or fissuring and an irregular surface. Grade III changes have definite fibrillation with fissuring extending down to the subchondral bone, which presents a classic arthroscopic picture frequently described as "crab meat appearance." Grade IV changes are those in which the articular cartilage has disappeared, allowing exposure and erosion of the subchondral bone. Etiologic factors can be divided into two main categories: biomechanical causes and biochemical causes (Box 1.3).

CLINICAL FINDINGS

The signs and symptoms of chondromalacia of the patella are nonspecific; there is no pathognomonic symptom. Most patients with chondromalacia describe a dull, aching discomfort that is well localized to the anterior part of the knee and that is most prominent after sitting in one position for a long time. This has been called the "movie sign" or "theater sign." Crepitation in the patellofemoral joint also varies. The patient may describe a catching or giving way sensation with activity; pain and giving way both tend to be much more prominent while descending stairs. Puffiness or swelling may be noted, depending on the degree of synovitis present.

Articular cartilage is devoid of nerve endings and therefore cannot be the direct source of pain. The synovium and subchondral bone probably are the two areas producing pain in chondromalacia of the patella. The articular cartilage debris that is shed into the joint with chondromalacia of the patella can produce a chemical irritation of the synovium, resulting

---

BOX 1.3

Etiologic Factors in Chondromalacia of Patella

Biomedical Causes
Acute
- Dislocation of the patella with a chondral or osteochondral fracture
- Direct trauma (e.g., a fall on or blow to the patella)
- Fracture of the patella, resulting in incongruous surfaces

Chronic
- Recurrent subluxation or dislocation of the patella (secondary to femoral dysplasia, small patella, patella alta, femoral anteversion, external tibial torsion, or even anterior cruciate ligament insufficiency)
- Increased quadriceps angle
- Quadriceps muscle imbalance, either weakness or abnormal attachment of the vastus medialis
- Patella alta
- Posttraumatic malalignment after femoral shaft fracture
- Excessive lateral pressure syndrome
- Meniscal injury with alteration of synchronous pattern of patellar movement and loss of stability
- Reflex sympathetic dystrophy
- Medial femoral condylar ridge

Biochemical Causes
Disease
- Rheumatoid arthritis
- Recurrent hemarthrosis
- Alkaptonuria
- Peripheral synovitis
- Sepsis and adhesions

Iatrogenic
- Repeated intraarticular corticosteroid injections
- Prolonged immobilization

Degenerative
- Primary osteoarthritis

in swelling and pain. Pain in the patellofemoral syndrome, with or without chondromalacia, has been suggested to originate from the subchondral bone. One hypothesis is that the biomechanical failure of articular cartilage in chondromalacia of the patella results in an alteration of load transfer to the subchondral bone; another is that extensor mechanism malalignment, rather than the articular changes themselves, is responsible for the pain.

Arthroscopic examination of 56 young adults with anterior knee pain confirmed chondromalacia patellae in 45% and synovial plica in 45%. No association was found between the severity of the chondromalacia patellae seen at arthroscopy and the clinical symptoms of anterior knee pain syndrome, suggesting that the symptoms of anterior knee pain syndrome should not be used as an indication for knee arthroscopy.

Proton density fat suppression (PDFS) and T2 mapping MRI have been found to be only moderately accurate in predicting patellar chondromalacia found at arthroscopy.

■ TREATMENT

Treatment of chondromalacia of the patella depends on the underlying cause of the articular surface changes and should be directed to the cause rather than to the results. Most often, this involves nonsurgical measures, such as antiinflammatory medications, quadriceps exercises and hamstring stretching, bracing, taping, and orthotics. In addition, activity modification is encouraged to avoid lunges, squats, and leg presses beyond 90 degrees; no training is allowed on uneven terrain.

Operative treatment is divided into two phases: (1) treatment directed at malalignment and other abnormalities of the extensor mechanism and patellofemoral joint, and (2) treatment of the diseased cartilage. Surgery may be indicated for chronic patellofemoral pain after all attempts at nonoperative management been exhausted. Again, surgery should be directed at the cause, and a specific diagnosis must be established.

Arthroscopy has proved extremely reliable in diagnosis of chondromalacia of the patella. The degree of fibrillation and fragmentation of the surface can be probed under direct vision, and areas of abnormal softness can be identified by careful probing.

Malalignment of the extensor mechanism is believed to be one of the most common causes of patellofemoral pain and chondromalacic changes in the patellofemoral joint. Malalignment frequently results in subluxation or dislocation of the patella. Surgical procedures for those conditions are described in other chapter. Malalignment problems related to bony abnormalities, such as excessive femoral anteversion, excessive external tibial torsion, and severe genu valgum, may require osteotomy for skeletal realignment.

Lateral retinacular release by open, subcutaneous, or arthroscopic technique has been recommended for patellofemoral pain syndromes. Release of the strong tethering lateral structures has proved effective if the preoperative diagnosis has been accurate. However, before retinacular release, incongruity, lateral tilting, and lateral orientation of the patella in the patellofemoral joint should be established on axial radiographs. Surgery for chondromalacia of the patella has been unpredictable in patients with normal axial radiographic studies. Lateral retinacular release in patients with chondromalacia of the patella caused by patella alta is rarely successful, and an open procedure that reestablishes a more

normal relationship between the length of the patellar tendon and the length of the patella by moving the patellar insertion distally may be more appropriate.

In any surgery directed at the chondromalacic patellar surface, the healing of articular cartilage must be considered. Cartilage is an avascular tissue with limited healing capacity. Defects that extend through the articular cartilage, breaching the subchondral bone and thus opening an access channel for blood vessels to the surface, heal with a poor-grade fibrocartilaginous tissue that is disorganized, fibrous, and apparently prone to deterioration. This limited ability of the cartilage to heal or to replace itself is a major consideration in the treatment of the articular surface irregularities in chondromalacia of the patella. Procedures involving the articular surface include (1) arthroscopic patellar shaving, (2) local excision of defects with drilling of the subchondral bone, (3) microfracture, (4) osteochondral allograft implantation, (5) facetectomy, (6) mechanical decompression of the patellofemoral joint by anterior elevation of the tibial tuberosity (Maquet procedure), and (7) patellectomy. Patellar resurfacing and patellofemoral arthroplasty have been used for unicompartmental patellofemoral arthritis and severe chondromalacia of the patella, and newer techniques and implants have resulted in a resurgence of interest in patellofemoral arthroplasty. This procedure is discussed in other chapter.

Most investigators believe that the only benefit from shaving of the patella is arthroscopic removal of the fibrillated cartilage, which decreases to some degree the breakdown products that may be shed into the joint and cause a painful synovitis.

Local excision of the defect coupled with drilling of the subchondral bone has been a popular method of managing severe advanced chondromalacia of the patella. In this procedure, the area of chondromalacia is debrided with an arthroscopic shaver and all diseased articular cartilage is removed down to subchondral bone. The subchondral bone is then perforated or microfractured with multiple drill holes, allowing access for vascularity onto the surface defect to produce a replacement fibrocartilaginous covering.

Removal of the medial or lateral patellar facet for chondromalacia of the patella has been recommended to limit the pathologic condition to a single facet. We have had no experience with this procedure.

Anterior advancement or elevation of the insertion of the patellar tendon on the tibial tuberosity was designed to reduce the articular pressures in the patellofemoral joint. This has been used more often for patellofemoral arthritis than for chondromalacia of the patella. Patellectomy should be used only in advanced chondromalacia and severe patellofemoral joint degeneration.

ADVANCEMENT OF THE TIBIAL TUBEROSITY

Maquet and Murray recommended anterior advancement of the patellar tendon at the tibial tuberosity to relieve the compressive effect of the patella on the femoral condyles. They advanced the tibial tuberosity anteriorly by elevating the tibial crest (Fig. 1.159). In a modification of the technique, the proximal part of the tibia is regularly wid-

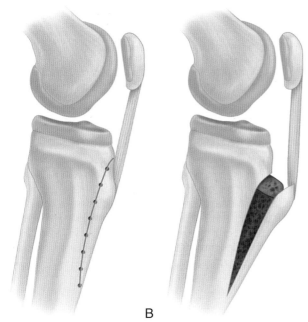

A   B

FIGURE 1.159   Maquet technique of advancement of tibial tuberosity by elevation of tibial crest. **A,** Drill holes and line of osteotomy. **B,** Osteotomy is sprung open and propped with iliac graft. **SEE TECHNIQUE 1.30.**

ened, without causing a cosmetically significant bulge at the level of the tibial tuberosity. A finite element study confirmed the effectiveness of this procedure in reducing patellofemoral contact forces, especially at smaller flexion angles; maximal contact stress was substantially decreased at full extension but increased at 90 degrees. Substantial effects of tuberosity elevation on tibial kinematics, cruciate ligament forces, tibiofemoral contact forces, and the extensor lever arm also were found. The authors cautioned that the effect of the procedure on the entire knee joint, not just the isolated compartment, should be considered.

TECHNIQUE 1.30

(MAQUET)
- Through a medial parapatellar incision carried distal to the tibial tuberosity on the anteromedial aspect of the tibia, outline the tuberosity.
- Dissect the patellar tendon along its posterior surface and loosen the infrapatellar fat pad sufficiently to permit the patella to ride free without tethering.
- Open the joint medially and correct intraarticular abnormalities as indicated.
- Carefully elevate a tongue of bone, composed of the tibial tuberosity and the attachment of the patellar tendon, that is 2.0 cm thick, 2.5 cm wide, and 11.5 cm long, and lever it anteriorly, leaving its distal attachment intact. This can be cut with an oscillating saw or by drilling multiple holes and connecting them with thin osteotomy cuts (Fig. 1.159A).
- Remove a block of bone 2.5 cm wide, 2.5 cm thick, and 5 cm long from the anterior iliac crest in the area of the iliac tubercle through another incision. We have found that bank bone is just as satisfactory.

- Elevate the tongue of bone and the tibial tuberosity carefully away from the tibia anteriorly and insert the block of iliac bone beneath it at its most proximal extent (Fig. 1.159B). Cut the block of bone to approximately 2.5 cm on all sides before its final insertion.
- We prefer to elevate the tibial tuberosity only 1.5 cm. The major decompression of the patellofemoral joint occurs with this amount of elevation, and complications are reduced. Usually the pressure of the tongue of tibial bone will hold this block in place securely, although Murray recommended a single stainless steel screw 5 cm long inserted as a lag screw for further stability. We prefer a 6.5-mm fully threaded unicortical cancellous screw.
- If the distal end of the tongue of bone fractures from the tibia, insert three screws along the tongue for fixation.
- Perform an anterior compartment fasciotomy.
- Undermine the subcutaneous tissues extensively, if necessary, to close the skin without tension. Insert a suction drain under the subcutaneous tissue and close the wound.

POSTOPERATIVE CARE The extremity is placed in a postoperative brace for 6 weeks. The patient is allowed immediate weight bearing to tolerance using crutches. Quadriceps exercises, leg-lifting exercises, and calf raises are begun on follow-up after surgery. Range-of-motion exercises with or without continuous passive motion are begun once the wound has healed, usually at 2 weeks.

PATELLECTOMY

Instead of patellaplasty, West and Soto-Hall and others recommended patellectomy. Today, patellectomy is used rarely and only as a salvage procedure because of the poor results and difficult rehabilitation after the procedure.

TECHNIQUE 1.31

(SOTO-HALL)
- Through a transverse incision at the level of the inferior third of the patella, incise the quadriceps expansion in line with the incision so that the suture line in the tendon will lie at the level of the fat pad rather than over the femoral condyles.
- By careful sharp dissection, excise the patella. Because this produces a relative lengthening of the quadriceps mechanism, proper tension can be restored by overlapping the cut edges about 1.5 cm and suturing them together. According to Soto-Hall, complete active extension will thus be regained more rapidly after surgery.
- When the quadriceps mechanism is in a valgus position and lateral instability of the patella has been demonstrated before surgery, extend the medial arm of the incision through the mechanism somewhat more proximally and remove or plicate a V-shaped section of capsule to restore balance between the medial and lateral muscles by effectively transferring part of the insertion of the vastus medialis distally.

POSTOPERATIVE CARE Quadriceps-setting exercises that have been practiced before surgery are resumed within the first week after surgery. Quadriceps-resistant exercises are started after 2 weeks, with particular attention given to the last 15 or 20 degrees of extension.

EXTRAARTICULAR ANKYLOSIS OF THE KNEE

Ankylosis of the knee, either intraarticular or extraarticular, may occur with the knee in complete extension, in flexion alone, or in flexion, external rotation, and valgus position. When the ankylosis is extraarticular, some motion can be preserved and radiographs even may reveal an apparently normal joint space.

When extraarticular ankylosis and contracture, in either flexion or extension, limit mobility, a soft-tissue release procedure, such as quadricepsplasty or capsulotomy, generally is indicated. The use of free tissue transfers has been recommended for soft-tissue augmentation in patients who have release procedures for posttraumatic knee joint stiffness to minimize wound problems, such as wound edge necrosis, wound dehiscence, and infection; to allow early initiation of postoperative physical therapy, which improves functional outcomes; and to obtain a more acceptable cosmetic result.

EXTRAARTICULAR ANKYLOSIS IN EXTENSION

After fractures of the femur or extensive soft-tissue wounds of the anterior aspect of the thigh, scarring or fibrosis of all or a part of the quadriceps mechanism can result in extraarticular ankylosis of the knee in extension. This deformity can be caused by one or more of the following: (1) fibrosis of the vastus intermedius muscle scarring down the rectus femoris to the femur in the suprapatellar pouch and proximally, (2) adhesions between the patella and the femoral condyles, (3) fibrosis and shortening of the lateral expansions of the vasti and their adherence to the femoral condyles, and (4) actual shortening of the rectus femoris muscle. Quadricepsplasty was devised to correct the deformity; its success depends on (1) whether the rectus femoris muscle has escaped injury, (2) how well this muscle can be isolated from the scarred parts of the quadriceps mechanism, and (3) how well the muscle can be developed by active use.

THOMPSON QUADRICEPSPLASTY

TECHNIQUE 1.32

(THOMPSON)
- Use an electrocoagulation unit throughout the operation.
- Make an anterior longitudinal incision through the skin and superficial fascia from the proximal third of the thigh to the distal pole of the patella, the exact location of the incision depending on the position of any scars.
- Divide the deep fascia along each side of the rectus femoris muscle from the proximal end of the skin incision to the patella and separate this muscle from the vastus medialis and lateralis.
- Then divide the anterior part of the knee capsule, including the lateral expansions of the vasti on both sides of the patella, far enough to overcome their contracture.
- Excise completely the vastus intermedius, which usually is a scarred band binding the posterior surfaces of the rectus femoris and patella to the femur, but leave a fibrous or periosteal covering on the anterior surface of the femur.
- If the tendon of the rectus has been destroyed by the injury, create a new one by making longitudinal incisions through the scar tissue in the distal third of the thigh.

- At this point, slowly flex the knee to 110 degrees to release the remaining intraarticular adhesions.
- If the vastus medialis and lateralis are badly scarred, interpose subcutaneous tissue and fat between them and the rectus. If these muscles are relatively normal, suture them to the rectus as far distally as the distal third of the thigh. If a tourniquet has been used, remove it and obtain complete hemostasis before closing the wound.

POSTOPERATIVE CARE The extremity is placed in a continuous passive motion machine, and range of motion is used until 90 degrees of passive flexion is achieved. Passive and active exercises for the quadriceps and hamstrings continue and are of critical importance to the success of this procedure. The knee is kept in full extension during the night and is exercised during the day with active and active-assisted exercises. If 90 degrees of flexion is not obtained after 3 months, gentle manipulation with the patient under anesthesia may be required. The patient should expect a very slow return of active quadriceps extension. Most patients can expect improvement in range of motion of the knee after quadricepsplasty but should expect severe quadriceps weakness for many months. If the patient is not skeletally mature, some of the improvement in flexion may be lost as growth occurs.

As an alternative to minimize damage to the quadriceps mechanism, a proximal-based, staged, sequential release of the intrinsic and extrinsic structures limiting knee flexion was developed, and several modifications to this technique have been developed. The three phases described by Judet were (1) release of the medial and lateral retinacula and release of the adhesions in the suprapatellar gutter and between the patella and femoral condyles through a longitudinal or medial (or both) parapatellar incision, (2) release of the vastus intermedius through a long posterolateral incision extending from the superior pole of the patella to the greater trochanter, and (3) detachment of the rectus femoris from its insertion at the anterior inferior iliac spine through a proximal anterolateral extension of the posterolateral incision. The final phase was used only if flexion was still limited after manipulation subsequent to the first two phases. Most reports of this procedure are small, with relatively short follow-up. Excellent or good results have been reported in approximately 81% of patients and fair results in 19%.

MINI-INVASIVE QUADRICEPSPLASTY

Endoscopically and arthroscopically assisted percutaneous techniques have been described for quadricepsplasty, but follow-up reports are few, and these techniques are not well established. Wang, Zhao, and He described an extraarticular "mini-invasive" quadricepsplasty followed by intraarticular arthroscopic lysis of adhesions. Their procedure is done in five stages; the range of flexion is measured after each stage of release, and the procedure is terminated when the desired degree of flexion (ideally 120 degrees) is obtained. Currently, the only report of results of this technique is that of the technique developers; they reported 16 excellent results, 5 good results, and 1 fair result in 22 patients with severely arthrofibrotic knees observed for an average of 44 months. Average maximal flexion

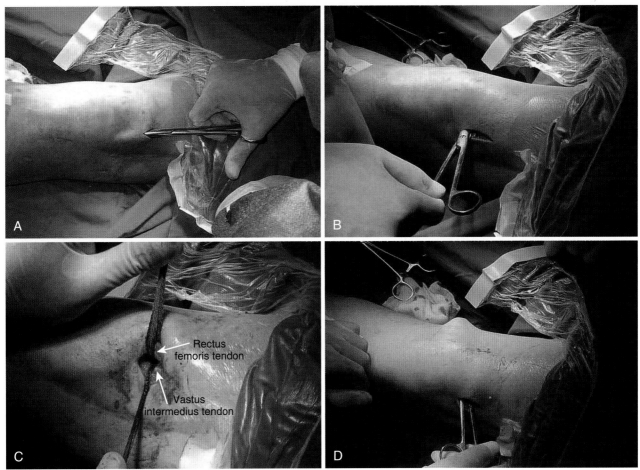

FIGURE 1.160 Mini-incision quadricepsplasty. **A,** Lateral patellar retinaculum is released. **B,** Adhesions in patellofemoral compartment are released. **C,** Tendinous tissue of vastus intermedius is separated from rectus femoris and anterior surface of femur. **D,** Medial patellar retinaculum is released.

increased from 15 degrees preoperatively to 115 degrees at most recent follow-up; only one patient had a persistent 15-degree extension lag. We have no experience with this technique, but it seems a reasonable alternative to open quadricepsplasty and certainly would produce a more pleasing cosmetic result.

TECHNIQUE 1.33

(WANG, ZHAO, HE)

STAGE 1

- With an inside-out technique, make a percutaneous parapatellar lateral arthrotomy by incising the lateral retinaculum from the patella along its lateral border, from the superolateral corner of the patella down to the lateral aspect of its lower pole (Fig. 1.160A).
- To restore the lateral recess, free the lateral retinaculum from the lateral femoral condyle and free the vastus lateralis tendon and the iliotibial band from the distal third of the femur.

STAGE 2

- Mobilize the suprapatellar pouch, the patellofemoral compartment, and the anterior interval by dividing the adhesions within these spaces (Fig. 1.160B). The anterior interval is the region of the knee posterior to the infrapatellar fat pad and anterior to the anterosuperior aspect of the tibial plateau.
- Separate the tendinous tissue of the vastus intermedius from that of the rectus femoris and the anterior surface of the femur (Fig. 1.160C).

STAGE 3

- With a percutaneous inside-out technique, release the medial patellar retinaculum through the suprapatellar pouch, patellofemoral compartment, and anterior interval that were reestablished in the second stage. Take care to delineate the medial arthrotomy margin, which starts from the medial epicondyle of the femur and slants laterally to the tibial tubercle, to avoid detachment of the vastus medialis from its insertion at the superomedial corner of the patella (Fig. 1.160D).
- Free the medial retinaculum from the medial femoral condyle, and free the vastus medialis from the distal third of the femur to restore the medial recess.

STAGE 4

- Transect the previously mobilized vastus intermedius at a level near its musculotendinous junction (Fig. 1.160E).

STAGE 5

- The fifth stage consists of lengthening the quadriceps tendon.

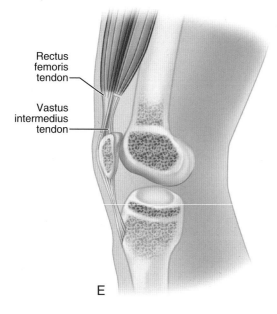

Rectus femoris tendon

Vastus intermedius tendon

E

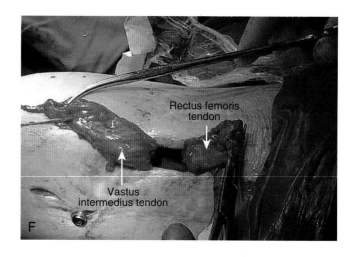

Rectus femoris tendon

Vastus intermedius tendon

F

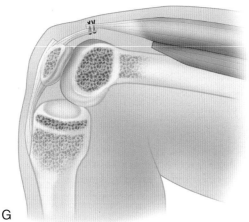

G

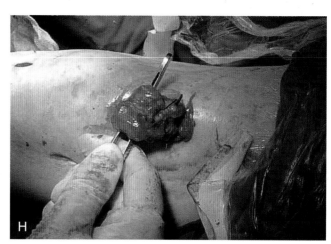

H

FIGURE 1.160 Cont'd **E** and **F,** Quadriceps is lengthened. **G** and **H,** Proximal portion of vastus intermedius tendon and distal portion of rectus femoris tendon are sutured together with knee in **90 degrees of flexion.** (From Wang JH, Zhao JZ, He YH: A new treatment strategy for severe arthrofibrosis of the knee: surgical technique, *J Bone Joint Surg* 89A[Suppl 2, pt 1]:93, 2007.) **SEE TECHNIQUE 1.33.**

- Transect the rectus femoris at a more distal level than the vastus intermedius, adjacent to its patellar insertion (Fig. 1.160E), and deliver the free tendinous ends of the vastus intermedius and rectus femoris through the wound (Fig. 1.160F).
- Gently manipulate the knee in flexion repeatedly until maximal flexion is achieved.
- Then overlap the proximal tendinous end of the vastus intermedius and the distal portion of the rectus femoris tendon and suture them with a no. 2 nonabsorbable Ethibond suture with the knee held in 90 degrees of flexion (Fig. 1.160G and H).
- Test the passive range of motion after repair of the quadriceps tendon to ensure that the lengthened tendon is under substantial tension but remains competent at 90 degrees of flexion.
- If the knee can be easily flexed beyond 90 degrees, increase the overlapping of the tendons by more proximal advancement of the vastus intermedius tendon to reduce the risk of creating an extension lag.

- If flexion is restricted, decrease the overlapping by more distal fixation of the vastus intermedius tendon.
- Throughout the procedure, manipulate the knee in flexion to release intraarticular adhesions, to assess the arc of knee flexion, and to determine if there are remaining intraarticular adhesions. Once flexion of more than 120 degrees has been achieved, the extraarticular portion of the procedure is terminated, closed suction drains are placed, and the skin is closed.

In knees of moderate arthrofibrosis, the first four stages often allow knee flexion of more than 120 degrees. With severe arthrofibrosis, the fifth stage (quadriceps lengthening) usually is necessary to gain more than 90 degrees of flexion. After the initial mini-invasive quadricepsplasty, the primary arc of knee flexion should reach 90 degrees and the suprapatellar pouch, patellofemoral compartment, anterior interval, lateral recess, and medial recess are reestablished. With these spaces restored, arthroscopic surgery can be safely done for lysis of any remaining adhesions.

POSTOPERATIVE CARE A compressive wrap with an elastic bandage is applied from the toe to the thigh to decrease swelling. Physical therapy is started on the day after surgery. When the quadriceps tendon is lengthened, the rehabilitation protocol is modified to protect its repair during the first 3 weeks. A continuous passive motion machine is used as tolerated; the range and speed of motion are increased gradually without exceeding 90 degrees of flexion during the first 3 weeks after surgery. Active-assisted flexion (with the same restriction of 90 degrees of flexion) and patellar mobility exercises are begun on the first postoperative day. Additional flexion and quadriceps-strengthening exercises, including active straight-leg raising, isometric quadriceps exercises, resistance exercises, and stationary bicycling, are deferred until 4 to 6 weeks after surgery. If the quadriceps tendon has not been lengthened, the rehabilitation program is more aggressive, without restriction of range of motion. Manipulation is necessary if less than 90 degrees of flexion is possible at 6 weeks after surgery.

EXTRAARTICULAR ANKYLOSIS IN FLEXION

Flexion contracture of the knee is much more common than extension contracture. It often is complicated by subluxation and external rotation of the tibia on the femur because the hamstring muscles pull the tibia posteriorly and the biceps femoris muscle and iliotibial band rotate the tibia externally. All of the soft tissues in the popliteal space are contracted.

Flexion contractures usually can be at least partially corrected conservatively; the amount of correction possible depends on the severity and duration of the deformity. Traction with balanced suspension, Buck extension, and static or dynamic splints, casts, or braces designed to extend the knee gradually are of value. These measures can be used before surgery to make the operation less extensive and after surgery to increase the correction. Regardless of how a contracture is corrected, it always must be remembered that the peroneal nerve is more susceptible to injury from stretching than is the popliteal artery and its branches, and extreme caution is indicated when signs of irritation develop along its course. Otherwise, prolonged or permanent paralysis can result after a flexion contracture has been corrected as little as 20 degrees.

Gradual distraction by either a circular external fixator or a monolateral external fixator has been reported to improve the function position of the arc of motion, although the total arc of motion remains essentially unchanged. Distal hamstring release with femorotibial external fixation also has been reported to allow complete extension or residual flexion contracture of less than 10 degrees.

POSTERIOR CAPSULOTOMY

Posterior capsulotomy is indicated for severe flexion contractures of the knee that cannot be corrected by more conservative means. The following operation is a modification of one described by Putti.

TECHNIQUE 1.34

(PUTTI, MODIFIED)
- Position the patient prone.
- Make a curvilinear incision 15 cm long through the skin and superficial fascia over the popliteal space.
- Expose the medial and lateral aspects of the posterior part of the joint capsule by separate approaches through the deep structures as follows.
- Dissect between the subcutaneous tissue and deep fascia to the lateral aspect of the popliteal space and incise the deep fascia longitudinally. Isolate and retract laterally the biceps femoris tendon and common peroneal nerve and expose the lateral head of the gastrocnemius; retract medially the popliteal vessels and nerves that lie in the midline.
- Under direct vision, divide the lateral head of the gastrocnemius, the lateral half of the posterior capsule, and the attachment of the PCL.
- Now dissect between the subcutaneous tissue and deep fascia to the medial aspect of the popliteal space. Incise the deep fascia to expose the lateral aspect of the semimembranosus and semitendinosus muscles, and retract these muscles medially; retract the popliteal vessels and nerves laterally.
- Divide the medial head of the gastrocnemius and medial half of the capsule.
- At this point, the knee may be completely extended by gentle manipulation if the hamstring tendons are not contracted. Avoid excessive force. During extension of the knee, fibrous adhesions may audibly rupture.
- This also can be accomplished through limited medial or lateral incisions, or both. This allows the patient to be in the supine position throughout the operation, in the event that additional procedures such as arthroscopic lysis of adhesions also are performed.
- On occasion, the biceps, semitendinosus, and semimembranosus tendons and the iliotibial band are severely contracted; in these instances, lengthen the tendons by Z-plasty and divide the iliotibial band and lateral intermuscular septum as described by Yount.

POSTERIOR CAPSULOTOMY

TECHNIQUE 1.35

(YOUNT)
- Expose the fascia lata through a lateral longitudinal incision just proximal to the femoral condyle.
- Divide the iliotibial band and fascia lata posteriorly to the biceps tendon and anteriorly to the midline of the thigh at a level 2.5 cm proximal to the patella.
- Now, at this level excise a segment of the iliotibial band and intermuscular septum 5 to 8 cm long.
- Before the wound is closed, determine by palpation that all tight bands have been divided. Suture only the subcutaneous tissue and skin.

POSTOPERATIVE CARE A brace locked in extension is fitted, and range-of-motion exercises are begun. Use of a continuous passive motion machine may be beneficial. The patient should be examined frequently to detect any recurrent flexion contracture, which may require serial casting for extension to be regained.

OPEN WOUNDS OF THE KNEE JOINT

Although the management of war-related open joint injuries has been reviewed extensively, much less information is available concerning the treatment of open joint wounds in the civilian population. As the incidence of civilian gunshot injuries has increased, gunshot injuries to the knee also have become more common. Of all open joint injuries, those of the knee are by far the most common (53% to 91%).

In one of the earliest articles on the "modern" management of open joint injuries, Patzakis et al. reviewed 140 patients with penetrating joint injuries treated during a 4-year period. They divided the injuries into three types: those associated with fractures, open joint injuries without fracture, and gunshot wounds. All patients were treated with antibiotics, surgical debridement, and irrigation, including the installation of polyethylene tubes into the joint for closed irrigation and suction. Their results were remarkably good, with infection developing in only three of the 140 patients (2.1%). A number of patients had positive cultures from the drainage tubes in the postoperative period. Because these same patients did not have positive cultures at the time of initial surgery, they concluded that the positive cultures from the tubes were secondary to the tubes themselves and that a closed irrigation and suction system must be considered a potential source of contamination. Therefore, they recommended that closed irrigation and suction not be used routinely for open joint injuries but only for those with initial severe contamination or when the soft-tissue injury was extensive and closure of the joint was desirable. We concur with these recommendations. They further concluded that open joint injuries should be treated with broad-spectrum antibiotic coverage before, during, and after arthrotomy, open surgical debridement, and irrigation and primary closure of the wound in most patients. More recently, Brubacher et al. developed an algorithm for diagnosis and treatment of traumatic arthrotomies based primarily on physical examination and CT scanning (Fig. 1.161). Konda et al. reported their experience in the treatment of 40 open knee joint wounds; 43% were gunshot wounds and 20% were sustained in motor vehicle accidents; no infections were reported, and only one patient had a vascular injury that ultimately required amputation. Twenty-one (53%) of these patients had an associated periarticular fracture, an association confirmed in other studies.

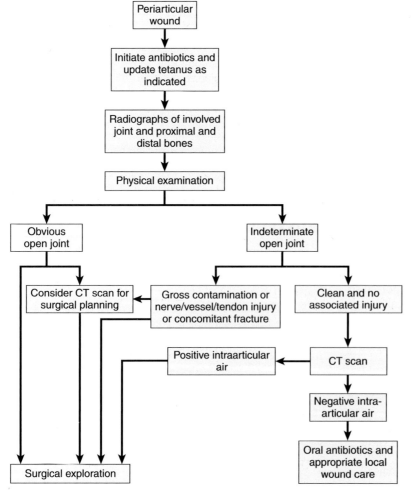

FIGURE 1.161 Treatment algorithm for traumatic arthrotomy. (From Brubacher JW, Grote CW, Tilley MB: Traumatic arthrotomy, *J Am Acad Orthop Surg* 28:102, 2020.)

In patients with gunshot wounds of the knee, evaluation of the neurovascular status is of primary importance (Fig. 1.162). Once neurovascular injuries have been identified and treated, if necessary, skeletal injuries can be evaluated. Anteroposterior and lateral radiographs are carefully scrutinized for fractures, air in the joint space, bullet fragments, and osteochondral fragments. CT also can provide valuable information about the extent and complexity of the fracture pattern. If intraarticular fractures are not evident, knee joint aspiration can help determine if the joint has been penetrated; a bloody aspirate indicates the need for joint irrigation. The treatment of open fractures caused by firearms is discussed in detail in other chapter.

If open fracture reduction is not required, irrigation and debridement can be done arthroscopically, resulting in a shorter postoperative hospital stay, less postoperative pain, and superior cosmetic results. It can also help identify intraarticular injuries. Fracture management depends on the stability of the fracture pattern and may include casting or bracing, open reduction and internal fixation, or external fixation. Large osteochondral fragments can be reattached and fixed with arthroscopic techniques (see other chapter). Soft-tissue coverage may require grafts or flaps (see other chapter). Damaged musculotendinous or ligamentous structures should be repaired or reconstructed as soon as possible to restore joint function.

A rare late complication of intraarticular gunshot injuries, including those of the knee, is lead poisoning, which has been reported from 2 days to 52 years after injury. Lead fragments in the soft tissues generally become encapsulated by fibrous tissue and are effectively inert; however, intraarticular bullet fragments in contact with synovial fluid can cause foreign-body reactions, mechanical articular cartilage damage, proliferative synovitis, and destructive arthritis. Lead can be absorbed into the systemic circulation through the inflamed synovial membrane. Bullet fragmentation and the surface area of lead exposed to synovial fluid correlate with increased levels of lead in the blood (Fig. 1.163). Adults with lead poisoning may be asymptomatic or may have nausea, diarrhea, abdominal pain, and weakness. Lead poisoning should be considered in a patient with a history of an intraarticular gunshot wound and microcytic anemia. Prompt therapy, including chelation and removal of the bullet fragments, is essential.

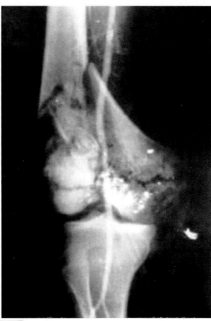

FIGURE 1.162 Anteroposterior view of right distal femur of 18-year-old woman with high-velocity rifle wound. Note "lead snowstorm" pattern and severe comminution. Arteriogram revealed no gross arterial damage. (From Bartlett CS, Helfet DL, Hausman MR, Strauss E: Ballistics and gunshot wounds: effects on musculoskeletal tissues, *J Am Acad Orthop Surg* 8:21, 2000.)

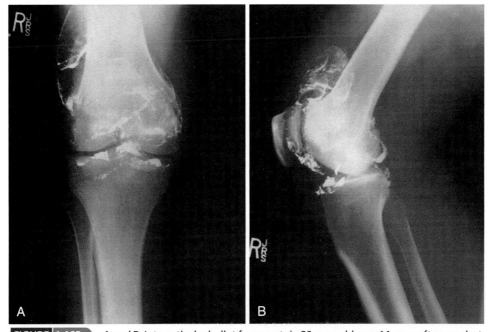

FIGURE 1.163 **A** and **B,** Intraarticular bullet fragments in 30-year-old man 14 years after gunshot injury. He was found to have microcytic anemia with high blood lead levels and was treated with chelation therapy and removal of the fragments. (From Rehani B, Wissman R: Lead poisoning from a gunshot wound, *South Med J* 104:57, 2011.)

REFERENCES

GENERAL

Guess TM, Razu S, Jahandar H: Evaluation of knee ligament mechanics using computational models, *J Knee Surg* 29:126, 2016.

Häfner SJ: The body's integrated repair kit: studying mesenchymal stem cells for better ligament repair, *Biomed J* 42:365, 2019.

Halewood C, Amis AA: Clinically relevant biomechanics of the knee capsule and ligament, *Knee Surg Sports Traumatol Arthrosc* 23:2789, 2015.

Hirschmann MT, Müller W: Complex function of the knee joint: the current understanding of the knee, *Knee Surg Sports Traumatol Arthrosc* 23:2780, 2015.

Hogan MV, Walker GN, Cui LR, et al.: The role of stem cells and tissue engineering in orthopaedic sports medicine: current evidence and future directions, *Arthroscopy* 31:1017, 2015.

Innocenti B, Salandra P, Pascale W, et al.: How accurate and reproducible are the indentification of cruciate and collateral ligament insertions using MRI? *Knee* 23:575, 2016.

Jung YB, Nam CH, Jung HJ, et al.: The influence of tibial positioning on the diagnostic accuracy of combined posterior cruciate ligament and posterolateral rotatory instability of the knee, *Clin Orthop Surg* 1:68, 2009.

La A, Nadarajah V, Jauregui JJ, et al.: Clinical characteristics associated with depression or anxiety among patients presenting for knee surgery, *J Clin Orthop Trauma* 11(Suppl 1):S164, 2020.

LaPrade RF, Heikes C, Bakker AJ, et al.: The reproducibility and repeatability of varus stress radiographs in the assessment of isolated fibular collateral ligament and grade-III posterolateral knee injuries: an in vitro biomechanical study, *J Bone Joint Surg* 90A:2069, 2008.

Levy BA, Stuart MJ, MacDonald PB, et al.: Comprehensive case-based review of knee ligament injuries, *Instr Course Lect* 68:513, 2019.

Musahl V, Zaffagnini S, LaPrade R, et al.: The challenge of treating complex knee instability, *Knee Surg Sports Traumatol Arthrosc* 23:2769, 2015.

Spang 3rd RC, Getgood A, Strickland SM, et al.: Optimizing anterior cruciate ligament (ACL) outcomes: what else needs fixing besides the ACL? *Instr Course Lect* 69:653, 2020.

Tsai WH, Chiang YP, Lew RJ: Sonographic examination of knee ligaments, *Am J Phys Med Rehabil* 94:e77, 2015.

Tsifountoudis I, Karantanas AH: Current concepts on MRI evaluation of postoperative knee ligaments, *Semin Musculoskelet Radiol* 20:74, 2016.

MENISCUS

Abram SGF, Judge A, Beard DJ, et al.: Long-term rates of knee arthroplasty in a cohort of 834, 393 patients with a history of arthroscopic partial meniscectomy, *Bone Joint Lett J* 101-B:1071, 2019.

Barber-Westin SD, Noyes FR: Clinical healing rates of meniscus repairs of tears in the central-third (red-white) zone, *Arthroscopy* 30:134, 2014.

Bedi A, Kelly N, Baad M, et al.: Dynamic contact mechanics of radial tears of the lateral meniscus: implications for treatment, *Arthroscopy* 28:372, 2012.

Bedi A, Kelly N, Baad M, et al.: Dynamic contact mechanics of the medial meniscus as a function of radial tear, repair, and partial meniscectomy, *J Bone Joint Surg* 92A:1398, 2010.

Bernthal NM, Seeger LL, Motamedi K, et al.: Can the repairability of meniscal tears be predicted with magnetic resonance imaging? *Am J Sports Med* 39:506, 2011.

Bhatia S, LaPrade CM, Ellman MB, LaPrade RF: Meniscal root tears: significance, diagnosis, and treatment, *Am J Sports Med* 42:3016, 2014.

Bin SI, Nha KW, Cheong JY, et al.: Midterm and long-term results of medial versus lateral meniscal allograft transplantation: a meta-analysis, *Am J Sports Med* 46:1243, 2018.

Brucker PU, von Cample A, Meyer DC, et al.: Clinical and radiological results 21 years following successful, isolated, open meniscal repair in stable knee joints, *Knee* 18:396, 2011.

Bumberger A, Killer U, Hofbauer M, et al.: Ramp lesions are frequently missed in ACL-deficient knees and should be repaired in case of instability, *Knee Surg Sports Traumatol Arthrosc*, 2019, [Epub ahead of print].

Choi NH, Kim TH, Son KM, Victoroff BN: Meniscal repair for radial tears of the midbody of the lateral meniscus, *Am J Sports Med* 38:2472, 2010.

Cox CL, Huston LJ, Dunn WR, et al.: Are articular cartilage lesions and meniscal tears predictive of IKDC, KOOS, and Marx activity level outcomes after anterior cruciate ligament reconstruction? A 6-year multicenter cohort study, *Am J Sports Med* 42:1058, 2014.

Cristiani R, Parling A, Forssblad M, et al.: Meniscus repair does not result in an inferior short-term outcome compared with meniscus resection: an analysis of 5,378 patients with primary anterior cruciate ligament reconstruction, *Arthroscopy*, 2019, [Epub ahead of print].

De Coninck T, Huyssse W, Verdonk R, et al.: Open versus arthroscopic meniscus allograft transplantation: magnetic resonance imaging study of meniscal radial displacement, *Arthroscopy* 29:514, 2013.

DePhillipo NN, Moatshe G, Chahla H, et al.: Quantitative and qualitative assessment of the posterior medial meniscus anatomy: defining meniscal ramp lesions, *Am J Sports Med* 47:372, 2019.

Dürselen L, Vögele S, Seitz AM, et al.: Anterior knee laxity increases gapping of posterior horn medial meniscus tears, *Am J Sports Med* 39:1749, 2011.

Edd SN, Netravali NA, Favre J, et al.: Alternations in knee kinematics after partial medial meniscectomy are activity dependent, *Am J Sports Med* 43:1399, 2015.

Griffin JW, Hadeed MM, Werner BC, et al.: Platelet-rich plasma in meniscal repair: does augmentation improve surgical outcomes? *Clin Orthop Relat Res* 473:1665, 2015.

Gülenc B, Kemah B, Yalcin S, et al.: Surgical treatment of meniscal RAMP lesion, *J Knee Surg*, 2019, [Epub ahead of print].

Hagmeijer MH, Kennedy NI, Tagliero AJ, et al.: Long-term results after repair of isolated meniscal tears among patients aged 18 years and younger: an 18-year follow-up study, *Am J Sports Med* 47:799, 2019.

Jauregui JJ, Wu AD, Meredith S, et al.: How should we secure our transplanted meniscus? A meta-analysis, *Am J Sports Med* 46:2285, 2018.

Karachalios T, Hantes M, Zintzaras E: Do physical diagnostic tests accurately detect meniscal tears? *Knee Surg Sports Traumatol Arthrosc* 19:1226, 2011.

Kim JG, Lee YS, Bae T, et al.: Tibiofemoral contact mechanics following posterior root of medial meniscus tear, repair, meniscectomy, and allograft transplantation, *Knee Surg Sports Traumatol Arthrosc* 21:2121, 2013.

Kim SJ, Lee SK, Kim SH, et al.: Does decreased meniscal thickness affect surgical outcomes after medial meniscectomy? *Am J Sports Med* 43:937, 2015.

Kocher MS, Logan CA, Kramer DE: Discoid lateral meniscus in children: diagnosis, management, and outcomes, *J Am Acad Orthop Surg* 25:736, 2017.

Krych AJ, Bernard CD, Kennedy NI, et al.: Medial vs. lateral meniscus root tears: is there a difference in injury presentation, treatment decisions, and surgical repair outcomes? *Arthroscopy*, 2020, [Epub ahead of print].

Krych AJ, Hevesi M, Leland DP, et al.: Meniscal root injuries, *J Am Acad Orthop Surg*, 2019, [Epub ahead of print].

LaPrade CM, James EW, Cram TR, et al.: Meniscal root tears: a classification system based on tear morphology, *Am J Sports Med* 43:363, 2015.

LaPrade CM, Jansson KS, Dornan G, et al.: Altered tibiofemoral contact mechanics due to lateral meniscus posterior horn root avulsions and radial tears can be restored with in situ pull-out suture repairs, *J Bone Joint Surg* 96A:471, 2014.

Lee BS, Bin SI, Kim JM, et al.: Partial meniscectomy for degenerative medial meniscal root tears shows favorable outcomes in well-aligned, nonarthritic knees, *Am J Sports Med* 47:606, 2019.

Lee SS, Ahn JH, Kim JH, et al.: Evaluation of healing after medial meniscal root repair using second-look arthroscopy, clinical, and radiological criteria, *Am J Sports Med* 46:2661, 2018.

Matsubara H, Okazaki K, Izawa T, et al.: New suture method for radial tears of the meniscus: biomechanical analysis of cross-suture and double horizontal suture techniques using cyclic load testing, *Am J Sports Med* 40:414, 2012.

Monk P, Garfield Roberts P, Palmer AJ, et al.: The urgent need for evidence in arthroscopic meniscal surgery, *Am J Sports Med* 45:965, 2017.

Nepple JJ, Dunn WR, Wright RW: Meniscal repair outcomes at greater than five years: a systematic literature review and meta-analysis, *J Bone Joint Surg* 94A:2222, 2012.

Noyes FR, Barber-Westin SD: Long-term survivorship and function of meniscus transplantation, *Am J Sports Med* 44:2330, 2016.

Ode GW, Van Thiel GS, McArthur SA, et al.: Effects of serial sectioning and repair of radial tears in the lateral meniscus, *Am J Sports Med* 40:1863, 2012.

Padfalecki JR, Jansson KS, Smith SD, et al.: Biomechanical consequences of a complete radial tear adjacent to the medial meniscus posterior root attachment site: in situ pull-out repair restores derangement of joint mechanics, *Am J Sports Med* 42:699, 2014.

Pujol N, Salle De Chou E, Boisrenoult P, Beaufils P: Platelet-rich plasma for open meniscal repair in young patients: any benefit? *Knee Surg Sports Traumatol Arthrosc* 23:51, 2015.

Salata MJ, Gibbs AE, Sekiya JK: A systematic review of clinical outcomes in patients undergoing meniscectomy, *Am J Sports Med* 38:1907, 2010.

Schillhammer CK, Werner FW, Scuderi MG, Cannizzaro JP: Repair of lateral meniscus posterior horn detachment lesions: a biomechanical evaluation, *Am J Sports Med* 40:2604, 2012.

Shelbourne KD, Dickens JF: Joint space narrowing after partial medial meniscectomy in the anterior cruciate ligament–intact knee, *J Am Acad Orthop Surg* 15:519, 2007.

Shrier I, Boudier-Revéret M, Fahmy K: Understanding the different physical examination tests for suspected meniscal tears, *Curr Sports Med Rep* 9:284, 2010.

Smith NA, Parkinson B, Hutchinson CE, et al.: Is meniscal allograft transplantation chondroprotective? A systematic review radiological outcomes, *Knee Surg Sports Traumatol Arthrosc* 24:2923, 2016.

Thaunat M, Fournier G, O'Loughlin P, et al.: Clinical outcome and failure analysis of medial meniscus bucket-handle tear repair: a series of 96 patients with a minimum 2 year follow-up, *Arch Orthop Trauma Surg*, 2020, [Epub ahead of print].

Trucker PU, von Campe A, Meyer DC, et al.: Clinical and radiological results 21 years following successful, isolated, open meniscal repair in stable knee joints, *Knee* 18:396, 2011.

van de Graaf VA, Wolterbeek N, Mutsaerts EL, et al.: Arthroscopic partial meniscectomy or conservative treatment for nonobstructive meniscal tears: a systematic review and meta-analysis of randomized controlled trials, *Arthroscopy* 32:1855, 2016.

Van Der Straeten C, Byttebier P, Eeckhoudt A, et al.: Meniscal allograft transplantation does not prevent or delay progression of knee osteoarthritis, *PLoS One* 11:e0156183, 2016.

Vangsness Jr CT, Farr 2nd J, Boyd J, et al.: Adult human mesenchymal stem cells delivered via intra-articular injection to the knee following partial medial meniscectomy: a randomized double-blind controlled study, *J Bone Joint Surg* 96A:90, 2014.

Verdonk PC, Demurie A, Almqvist KF, et al.: Transplantation of viable meniscal allograft: surgical technique, *J Bone Joint Surg* 88A(Suppl 1) Pt 1):109, 2006.

von Lewinski G, Kohn D, Wirth CJ, Lazovic D: The influence of nonanatomical insertion and incongruence of meniscal transplants on the articular cartilage in an ovine model, *Am J Sports Med* 36:841, 2008.

von Lewinski G, Pressel T, Hurschler C, et al.: The influence of intraoperative pretensioning on the chondroprotective effect of meniscal transplants, *Am J Sports Med* 34:397, 2006.

Xu C, Zhao J: A meta-analysis comparing meniscal repair with meniscectomy in the treatment of meniscal tears: the more meniscus, the better outcome? *Knee Surg Sports Traumatol Arthrosc* 23:164, 2015.

Yim JH, Seon JK, Song EK, et al.: A comparative study of meniscectomy and nonoperative treatment for degenerative horizontal tears of the medial meniscus, *Am J Sports Med* 41:1565, 2013.

Zaffagnini S, Marcheggiani Muccioli GM, Lopomo N, et al.: Prospective long-term outcomes of the medial collagen meniscus implant versus partial medial meniscectomy: a minimum 10-year follow-up study, *Am J Sports Med* 39:977, 2011.

KNEE LIGAMENTS

ANTEROLATERAL LIGAMENT

Ariel de Lima D, Helito CP, Lacerda de Lmia L, et al.: Anatomy of the anterolateral ligament of the knee: a systematic review, *Arthroscopy* 35:670, 2019.

Capogna BM, Kester BS, Shenoy K, et al.: The anterolateral ligament (ALL). The new ligament? *Bull Hosp Jt Dis* 77:64, 2013, 2019.

Cavaignac E, Ancelin D, Chiron P, et al.: Historical perspective on the "discovery of the anterolateral ligament of the knee, *Knee Surg Sports Traumatol Arthrosc* 25:991, 2017.

Coquart B, LeCorroller T, Laurent PE, et al.: Anterolateral ligament of the knee: myth or reality? *Surg Radiol Anat* 38:955, 2016.

Daggett M, Ockuly AC, CCullen M, et al.: Femoral origin of the anterolateral ligament: an anatomic analysis, *Arthroscopy* 32:835, 2016.

Hartigan DE, Carroll KW, Kosarek FJ, et al.: Visibility of anterolateral ligament tears in anterior cruciate ligament-deficient knees with standard 1.5-Tesla magnetic resonance imaging, *Arthroscopy* 32:2061, 2016.

Helito CP, Bonadio MB, Gobbi RG, et al.: Is it safe to reconstruct the knee anterolateral ligament with a femoral tunnel? Frequency of lateral collateral ligament and popliteus tendon injury, *Int Orthop* 40:821, 2016.

Helito CP, Demange MK, Bonadio MB, et al.: Radiographic landmarks for locating the femoral origin and tibial insertion of the knee anterolateral ligament, *Am J Sports Med* 42:2356, 2014.

Katakura M, Koga H, Nakamura K, et al.: Effects of different femoral tunnel positions on tension changes in anterolateral ligament reconstruction, *Knee Surg Sports Traumatol Arthrosc* 25:1272, 2017.

Kennedy MI, Claes S, Fuso FA, et al.: The anterolateral ligament: an anatomic, radiographic, and biomechanical analysis, *Am J Sports Med* 43:1606, 2015.

Kosy JD, Soni A, Venkatesh R, et al.: The anterolateral ligament of the knee: unwrapping the enigma. Anatomical study and comparison to previous reports, *J Orthop Traumatol* 17:303, 2016.

Kraeutler MJ, Welton KL, Chahla J, et al.: Current concepts of the anterolateral ligament of the knee: anatomy, biomechanics, and reconstruction, *Am J Sports Med* 46:1235, 2018.

Musahl V, Herbst E, Burnham JM, et al.: The anterolateral complex and anterolateral ligament of the knee, *J Am Acad Orthop Surg* 26:261, 2018.

Parsons EM, Gee AO, Spiekerman C, et al.: The biomechanical function of the anterolateral ligament of the knee, *Am J Sports Med* 43:669, 2015.

Pomajzi R, Maerz T, Shams C, et al.: A review of the anterolateral ligament of the knee: current knowledge regarding its incidence, anatomy, biomechanics, and surgical dissection, *Arthroscopy* 31:583, 2015.

Porrino Jr J, Maloney E, Richardson M, et al.: The anterolateral ligament of the knee: MRI appearance, association with the Segond frature, and historical perspective, *AJR Am J Roentgenol* 204:367, 2015.

Runer A, Birkmaier S, Pamminger M, et al.: The anterolateral ligament of the knee: a dissection study, *Knee* 23(8), 2016.

Saithna A, Daggett M, Helito CP, et al.: Clinical results of combined ACL and anterolateral reconstruction: a narrative review from the SANTI Study Group, *J Knee Surg*, 2020, [Epub ahead of print].

Schon JM, Moatshe G, Brady AW, et al.: Anatomic anterolateral ligament reconstruction of the knee leads to overconstraint at any fixation angle, *Am J Sports Med* 44:2546, 2016.

Sonnery-Cottet B, Vieira TD, Ouanezar H: Anterolateral ligament of the knee: diagnosis, indications, technique, outcomes, *Arthroscopy* 35:302, 2019.

Taneja AK, Miranda FC, Braga CA, et al.: MRI features of the anterolateral ligament of the knee, *Skeletal Radiol* 44:403, 2015.

Vincent JP, Magnussen RA, Gezmez F, et al.: The anterolateral ligament of the human knee: an anatomic and histologic study, *Knee Surg Sports Traumatol Arthrosc* 20:147, 2012.

COLLATERAL LIGAMENTS

Ahn JH, Wang JH, Lee SY, et al.: Arthroscopic-assisted anatomical reconstruction of the posterolateral corner of the knee joint, *Knee* 26:1136, 2019.

Bonadio MB, Helito CP, Foni NO, et al.: Combined reconstruction of the posterior cruciate ligament and medial collateral ligament using a single femoral tunnel, *Knee Surg Sports Traumatol Arthrosc* 25:3024, 2017.

Bushnell BD, Bitting SS, Crain JM, et al.: Treatment of magnetic resonance imaging-documented isolated grade iii lateral collateral ligament injuries in National Football League athletes, *Am J Sports Med* 38:86, 2010.

Chahla J, Murray IR, Robinson J, et al.: Posterolateral corner of the knee: an expert consensus statement on diagnosis, classification, treatment, and rehabilitation, *Knee Surg Sports Traumatol Arthrosc* 27:2520, 2019.

Coobs BR, Wijdicks CA, Armitage BM, et al.: An in vitro analysis of an anatomical medial knee reconstruction, *Am J Sports Med* 38:339, 2010.

Crawford MD, Kennedy MI, Bernolt DL, et al.: Combined posterior cruciate ligament and superficial medial collateral ligament reconstruction: avoiding tunnel convergence, *Arthrosc Tech* 8:e929, 2019.

Dean RS, LaPrade RF: ACL and posterolateral corner injuries, *Curr Rev Musculoskelet Med*, 2019, [Epub ahead of print].

DeLong JM, Waterman BR: Surgical techniques for the reconstruction of medial collateral ligament and posteromedial corner injuries of the knee: a systematic review, *Arthroscopy* 31:2258, 2015.

Devitt BM, Whelan DB: Physical examination and imaging of the lateral collateral ligament and posterolateral corner of the knee, *Sports Med Arthrosc* 23:10, 2015.

Dong JT, Chen BC, Men XQ, et al.: Application of triangular vector to functionally reconstruct the medial collateral ligament with double-bundle allograft technique, *Arthroscopy* 28:1445, 2012.

Elkin JL, Zamora E, Gallo RA: Combined anterior cruciate ligament and medial collateral ligament knee injuries: anatomy, diagnosis, management recommendatons, and return to sport, *Curr Rev Musculoskelet Med* 12:239, 2019.

Feeley BT, Muller MS, Sherman S, et al.: Comparison of posterolateral corner reconstructions using computer-assisted navigation, *Arthroscopy* 26:1088, 2010.

Gilmer BB, Crall T, DeLong J, et al.: Biomechanical analysis of internal bracing for treatment of medial knee injuries, *Orthopedics* 39:e532, 2016.

Grawe B, Schroeder AJ, Kakazu R, et al.: Lateral collateral ligament injury about the knee: anatomy, evaluation, and management, *J Am Acad Orthop Surg* 26:e120, 2018.

Hartshorn T, Otarodifard K, White EA, Hatch 3rd GF: Radiographic landmarks for locating the femoral origin of the superficial medial collateral ligament, *Am J Sports Med* 41:2527, 2013.

Hinckel BB, Demange MK, Gobbi RG, et al.: The effect of mechanical varus on anterior cruciate ligament and lateral collateral ligament stress: finite element analyses, *Orthopedics* 39:e729, 2016.

Innocenti B, Salandra P, Pascale W, et al.: How accurate and reproducible are the identification of cruciate and collateral ligament insertions using MRI? *Knee* 23:575, 2016.

Jakobsen BW, Lund B, Christiansen SE, et al.: Anatomic reconstruction of the posterolateral corner of the knee: a case series with isolated reconstructions in 27 patients, *Arthroscopy* 26:918, 2010.

James EW, LaPrade CM, LaPrade RF: Anatomy and biomechanics of the lateral side of the knee and surgical implications, *Sports Med Arthrosc* 23(2), 2015.

Kamath GV, Redfrm JC, Burks RT: Femoral radiographic landmarks for lateral collateral ligament reconstruction and repair: a new method of reference, *Am J Sports Med* 38:570, 2010.

Kennedy MI, Akamefula R, DePhillipo NN, et al.: Fibular collateral ligament reconstruction in adolescent patients, *Arthrosc Tech* 8:e141, 2019.

Kim MS, Koh IJ, In Y: Superficial and deep medial collateral ligament reconstruction for chronic medial instability of the knee, *Arthrosc Tech* 8:e549, 2019.

Kim SJ, Kim HS, Moon HK, et al.: A biomechanical comparison of 3 reconstruction techniques for posterolateral instability of the knee in a cadaveric model, *Arthroscopy* 26:335, 2010.

Kitamura N, Ogawa M, Kondo E, et al.: A novel medial collateral ligament reconstruction procedure using semitendinosus tendon autograft in patients with multiligamentous knee injuries: clinical outcomes, *Am J Sports Med* 41:1274, 2013.

Kramer DE, Miller PE, Berrhou IK, et al.: Collateral ligament knee injuries in pediatric and adolescent athletes, *J Pediatr Orthop* 40:71, 2020.

LaPrade MD, Kennedy MI, Wijdicks CA, LaPrade RF: Anatomy and biomechanics of the medial side of the knee and their surgical implications, *Sports Med Arthrosc* 23:63, 2015.

LaPrade RF, Spiridonov SI, Coobs BR, et al.: Fibular collateral ligament anatomical reconstructions: a prospective outcomes study, *Am J Sports Med* 38:2005, 2010.

LaPrade RF, Wijdicks CA: Surgical technique: development of an anatomic medial knee reconstruction, *Clin Orthop Relat Res* 470:806, 2012.

Levy BA, Dajani KA, Morgan JA, et al.: Repair versus reconstruction of the fibular collateral ligament and posterolateral corner in the multiligament-injured knee, *Am J Sports Med* 38:804, 2010.

Liu P, Wang J, Zhao F, et al.: Anatomic arthroscopically-assisted, mini-open fibular collateral ligament reconstruction: an in vitro biomechanical study, *Am J Sports Med* 42:373, 2014.

Malinowski K, Hermanowicz K, Góralczyk A, et al.: Medial collateral ligament reconstruction with anteromedial reinforcement for medial and anteromedial rotatory instability of the knee, *Arthrosc Tech* 8:e807, 2019.

Marchant Jr MH, Tibor LM, Sekiya JK, et al.: Management of medial-sided knee injuries, part 1: medial collateral ligament, *Am J Sports Med* 39:1102, 2011.

Marx RG, Hetsroni I: Surgical technique: medial collateral ligament reconstruction using Achilles allograft for combined knee ligament injury, *Clin Orthop Relat Res* 470:798, 2012.

Moulton SG, Geeslin AG, LaPrade RF: A systematic review of the outcomes of posterolateral corner knee injuries, part 2: surgical treatment of chronic injuries, *Am J Sports Med* 44:1616, 2016.

Moulton SG, Matheny LM, James EW, et al.: Outcomes following anatomic fibular (lateral) collateral ligament reconstruction, *Knee Surg Sports Traumatol Arthrosc* 23:2960, 2015.

Narvani A, Mahmud T, Lavelle J, et al.: Injury to the proximal deep medial collateral ligament: a problematical subgroup of injuries, *J Bone Joint Surg* 92B:949, 2010.

Niki Y, Matsumoto H, Otani T, et al.: A modified Larson's method of posterolateral corner reconstruction of the knee reproducing the physiological tensioning pattern of the lateral collateral and popliteofibular ligaments, *Sports Med Arthrosc Rehabil Ther Technol* 4:21, 2012.

Noyes FR, Barber-Westin SD: Long-term assessment of posterolateral ligament femoral-fibular reconstruction in chronic multiligament unstable knees, *Am J Sports Med* 39:497, 2011.

Pedersen RR: The medial and posteromedial ligamentous and capsular structures of the knee: review of anatomy and relevant imaging findings, *Semin Musculoskelet Radiol* 20:12, 2016.

Shea KG, Polousky JD, Jacobs Jr JC, Ganley TJ: Anatomical dissection and CT imaging of the posterior cruciate and lateral collateral ligaments in skeletally immature cadaver knees, *J Bone Joint Surg* 96A:753, 2014.

Stannard JP: Evaluation and treatment of medial instability of the knee, *Sports Med Arthrosc* 23:91, 2015.

Svantesson E, Hamrin Senorski E, Alentom-Geli E, et al.: Increased risk of ACL revision with non-surgical treatment of a concomitant medial collateral ligament injury: a study on 19,457 patients from the Swedish National Knee Ligament Registry, *Knee Surg Sports Traumatol Arthrosc* 27:2450, 2019.

Tibor LM, Marchant Jr MH, Taylor DC, et al.: Management of medial-sided knee injuries, part 2: posteromedial corner, *Am J Sports Med* 39:1332, 2011.

Westerman RW, Spindler KP, Huston LJ, et al.: Outcomes of grade III medial collateral ligament injuries treated concurrently with anterior cruciate ligament reconstruction: a multicenter study, *Arthroscopy* 35:1466, 2019.

Wijdicks CA, Ewart DT, Nuckley DJ, et al.: Structural properties of the primary medial knee ligaments, *Am J Sports Med* 38:1638, 2010.

Wijdicks CA, Michalski MP, Rasmussen MT, et al.: Superficial medial collateral ligament anatomic augmented repair versus anatomic reconstruction: an in vitro biomechanical analysis, *Am J Sports Med* 41:2858, 2013.

Wilson BF, Johnson DL: Posterior horn medial meniscal root repair with cruciate ligament/medial collateral ligament combined injuries, *Orthopedics* 4:986, 2011.

Yoon KH, Lee SH, Park SY, et al.: Comparison of anatomic posterolateral knee reconstruction using 2 different popliteofibular ligament techniques, *Am J Sports Med* 44:916, 2016.

Zaffagnini S, Bonanzinga T, Marcheggiarisonini Muccioli GM, et al.: Does chronic medial collateral ligament laxity influence the outcome of anterior cruciate ligament reconstruction?: a prospective evaluation with a minimum three-year follow-up, *J Bone Joint Surg* 83B:1060, 2011.

Zhang H, Bai X, Sun Y, Han X: Tibial inlay reconstruction of the medial collateral ligament using Achilles tendon allograft for the treatment of medial instability of the knee, *Knee Surg Sports Traumatol Arthrosc* 22:279, 2014.

Zhang H, Sun Y, Han X, et al.: Simultaneous reconstruction of the anterior cruciate ligament and medial collateral ligament in patients with chronic ACL-MCL lesions: a minimum 2-year follow-up study, *Am J Sports Med* 42:1675, 2014.

ANTERIOR CRUCIATE LIGAMENT

Abdel-Aziz A, Radwan YA, Rizk A: Multiple arthroscopic debridement and graft retention in septic knee arthritis after ACL reconstruction: a prospective case-control study, *Int Orthop* 38:73, 2014.

Achtnich A, Herbst E, Forkel P, et al.: Acute proximal anterior cruciate ligament tears: outcomes after arthroscopic suture anchor repair versus anatomic single-bundle reconstruction, *Arthroscopy* 32:2562, 2016.

Ahldén M, Sernert N, Karlsson J, Kaartus J: A prospective randomized study comparing double- and single-bundle techniques for anterior cruciate ligament reconstruction, *Am J Sports Med* 41:2484, 2013.

Ahlén M, Lidén M, Bovaller A, et al.: Bilateral magnetic resonance imaging and functional assessment of the semitendinosus and gracilis tendons a minimum of 6 years after ipsilateral harvest for anterior cruciate ligament reconstruction, *Am J Sports Med* 40:1735, 2012.

Åhlén M, Roshani L, Lidén M, et al.: Inflammatory cytokines and biomarkers of cartilage metabolism 8 years after anterior cruciate ligament reconstruction: results from operated and contralateral knees, *Am J Sports Med* 43:1460, 2015.

Ahmad SS, Hirschmann MT, Voumard B, et al.: Adjustable ACL suspension devices demonstrate less reliability in terms of reproducibility and irreversible displacement, *Knee Surg Sports Traumatol Arthrosc* 26:1392, 2018.

Ahn JH, Kim JG, Wang JH, et al.: Long-term results of anterior cruciate ligament reconstruction using bone–patellar tendon–bone: an analysis of the factors affecting the development of osteoarthritis, *Arthroscopy* 28:1114, 2012.

Ajuied A, Wong F, Smith C, et al.: Anterior cruciate ligament injury and radiologic progression of knee osteoarthritis: a systematic review and meta-analysis, *Am J Sports Med* 42:2242, 2014.

Andernord D, Desai N, Björnsson H, et al.: Patient predictors of early revision surgery after anterior cruciate ligament reconstruction: a cohort study of 16,930 patients with 2-year follow-up, *Am J Sports Med* 43:121, 2015.

Andernord D, Desai N, Björnsson H, et al.: Predictors of contralateral anterior cruciate ligament reconstruction: a cohort study of 9061 patients with 5-year follow-up, *Am J Sports Med* 43:295, 2015.

Anderson AF, Anderson CN: Correlation of meniscal and articular cartilage injuries in children and adolescents with timing of anterior cruciate ligament reconstruction, *Am J Sports Med* 43:275, 2015.

Ardern CL, Webster KE, Taylor NF, Feller JA: Hamstring strength recovery after hamstring tendon harvest for anterior cruciate ligament reconstruction: a comparison between graft types, *Arthroscopy* 26:462, 2010.

Andriolo L, Di Matteo B, Kon E, et al.: PRP augmentation for ACL reconstruction, *BioMed Res Int* 2015:373746, 2017.

Asai S, Maeyama A, Hoshino Y, et al.: A comparison of dynamic rotational knee instability between single-bundle and over-the-top anterior cruciate ligament reconstruction using triaxial accelerometry, *Knee Surg Sports Traumatol Arthrosc* 22:972, 2014.

Barenius B, Ponzer S, Shalabi A, et al.: Increased risk of osteoarthritis after anterior cruciate ligament reconstruction: a 14-year follow-up study of a randomized controlled trial, *Am J Sports Med* 42:1049, 2014.

Barker JU, Drakos M, Maak TG, et al.: Effect of graft selection on the incidence of postoperative infection in anterior cruciate ligament reconstruction, *Am J Sports Med* 38:281, 2010.

Barrera Oro F, Sikka RS, Wolters B, et al.: Autograft versus allograft: an economic cost comparison of anterior cruciate ligament reconstruction, *Arthroscopy* 27:1219, 2011.

Barrett AM, Craft JA, Replogle WH, et al.: Anterior cruciate ligament graft failure: a comparison of graft type based on age and Tegner activity level, *Am J Sports Med* 39:2194, 2011.

Battaglia 2nd MJ, Cordasco FA, Hannafin JA, et al.: Results of revision anterior cruciate ligament surgery, *Am J Sports Med* 35:2057, 2007.

Bedi A, Musahi V, O'Loughlin P, et al.: A comparison of the effect of central anatomical single-bundle anterior cruciate ligament reconstruction and double-bundle anterior cruciate ligament reconstruction on pivot-shift kinematics, *Am J Sports Med* 38:1788, 2010.

Benner RW, Shelbourne KD, Freeman H: Infections and patellar tendon ruptures after anterior cruciate ligament reconstruction: a comparison of ipsilateral and contralateral patellar tendon autografts, *Am J Sports Med* 39:519, 2011.

Benner RW, Shelbourne KD, Urch SE, Lazarus D: Tear patterns, surgical repair, and clinical outcomes of patellar tendon ruptures after anterior cruciate ligament reconstruction with a bone–patellar tendon–bone autograft, *Am J Sports Med* 40:1834, 2012.

Björnsson H, Desai N, Mushl V, et al.: Is double-bundle anterior cruciate ligament reconstruction superior to single-bundle? A comprehensive systematic review, *Knee Surg Sports Traumatol Arthrosc* 23:696, 2015.

Björnsson H, Samuelsson K, Sundemo D, et al.: A randomized controlled trial with mean 16-year follow-up comparing hamstring and patellar tendon autografts in anterior cruciate ligament reconstruction, *Am J Sports Med* 44:2304, 2016.

Bokshan SL, DeFroda SF, Panrello NM, et al.: Risk factors for deep vein thrombosis or pulmonary embolus following anterior cruciate ligament reconstruction, *Orthop J Sports Med* 6, 2018. 2325967118781328.

Born TR, Engasser WM, King AH, et al.: Low frequency of symptomatic venous thromboembolism after multiligamentous knee reconstruction with thromboprophylaxis, *Clin Orthop Relat Res* 472:2705, 2014.

Bottoni CR, Smith EL, Shaha J, et al.: Autograft versus allograft anterior cruciate ligament reconstruction: a prospective, randomized clinical study with a minimum 10-year follow-up, *Am J Sports Med* 43:2501, 2015.

Brambilla L, Pulici L, Carimati G, et al.: Prevalence of associated lesions in anterior cruciate ligament reconstruction: correlation with surgical timing and with patient age, sex, and body mass index, *Am J Sports Med* 43:2966, 2015.

Brophy RH, Wright RW, Huston LJ, et al.: Factors associated with infection following anterior cruciate ligament reconstruction, *J Bone Joint Surg* 97A:450, 2015.

Browning 3rd WM, Kluczynski MA, Curatolo C, et al.: Suspensory versus aperture fixation of a quadrupled hamstring tendon autograft in anterior cruciate ligament reconstruction: a meta-analysis, *Am J Sports Med* 45:2418, 2017.

Calvo R, Figueroa D, Anastasiadis Z, et al.: Septic arthritis in ACL reconstruction surgery with hamstring autografts. Eleven years of experience, *Knee* 21:717, 2014.

Canienne JM, Gwathmey FW, Miller MD, Werner BC: Tobacco use is associated with increased complications after anterior cruciate ligament reconstruction, *Am J Sports Med* 44:99, 2016.

Chalmers PN, Mall NA, Moric M, et al.: Does ACL reconstruction alter natural history? A systematic literature review of long-term outcomes, *J Bone Joint Surg* 96A:292, 2014.

Chisholm MF, Bang H, Maalouf DB, et al.: Postoperative analgesia with saphenous block appears equivalent to femoral block in ACL reconstruction, *HSS J* 10:245, 2014.

Cho Y, Jang SJ, Son JH: Transphyseal anterior cruciate ligament reconstruction in a skeletally immature knee using anterior tibialis allograft, *Orthopedics* 34:397, 2011.

Christensen JJ, Krych AJ, Engasser WM, et al.: Lateral tibial posterior slope is increased in patients with early graft failure after anterior cruciate ligament reconstruction, *Am J Sports Med* 43:2510, 2015.

Colombet P, Graveleau N, Jambou S: Incorporation of hamstring grafts within the tibial tunnel after anterior cruciate ligament reconstruction: magnetic resonance imaging of suspensory fixation versus interference screws, *Am J Sports Med* 44:2838, 2016.

Conte EJ, Hyatt AE, Gatt Jr CJ, Dhawan A: Hamstring autograft size can be predicted and is a potential risk factor for anterior cruciate ligament reconstruction failure, *Arthroscopy* 30:882, 2014.

Cox CL, Huston LJ, Dunn WR, et al.: Are articular cartilage lesions and meniscus tears predictive of IKDC, KOOS, and Marx activity levels after anterior cruciate ligament reconstruction? A 6-year multicenter cohort study, *Am J Sports Med* 42:1058, 2014.

Cox CL, Spindler KP, Leonard JP, et al.: Do newer-generation bioabsorbable screws become incorporated into bone at two years after ACL reconstruction with patellar tendon graft?: a cohort study, *J Bone Joint Surg* 96A:244, 2014.

Csintalan RP, Inacio MC, Funahashi TT, Maletis GB: Risk factors of subsequent operations after primary anterior cruciate ligament reconstruction, *Am J Sports Med* 42:619, 2014.

Cvetanovich GL, Chalmers PN, Verma NN, et al.: Risk factors for short-term complications of anterior cruciate ligament reconstruction in the United States, *Am J Sports Med* 44:618, 2016.

Delaloye JR, Murar J, Gonzalez M, et al.: Clinical outcomes after combined anterior cruciate ligament and anterolateral ligament reconstruction, *Tech Orthop* 33:225, 2018.

Demirag B, Aydemir F, Danis M, Ermutlu C: Incidence of meniscal and osteochondral lesions in patients undergoing delayed anterior cruciate ligament reconstruction, *Acta Orthop Traumatol Turc* 45:348, 2011.

Desai N, Björnsson H, Musahl V, et al.: Anatomic single- bersus double-bundle ACL reconstruction: a meta-analysis, *Knee Surg Sports Traumatol Arthrosc* 22:1009, 2014.

Desai N, Björnsson H, Samuelsson H, et al.: Outcomes after ACL reconstruction with focus on older patients: results from the Swedish National anterior cruciate ligament Register, *Knee Surg Sports Traumatol Arthrosc* 22:379, 2014.

Devitt BM, Bell SW, Ardern CL, et al.: The role of lateral extra-articular tenodesis in primary anterior cruciate ligament reconstruction: a systematic review with meta-analysis and best-evidence synthesis, *Orthop J Sports Med* 5:2325967117731767, 2017.

Dhawan A, Gallo RA, Lynch SA: Anatomic tunnel placement in anterior cruciate ligament reconstruction, *J Am Acad Orthop Surg* 24:443, 2016.

DiFelice GS, Villegas C, Taylor S: Anterior cruciate ligament preservation: early results of a novel arthroscopic technique for suture anchor primary anterior cruciate ligament repair, *Arthroscopy* 31:2162, 2015.

Duchman KR, Westermann RW, Spindler KP, et al.: The fate of meniscus tears left in situ at the time of anterior cruciate ligament reconstruction: a 6-year follow-up study from the MOON cohort, *Am J Sports Med* 43:2688, 2015.

Dunn WR, Spindler KP, Amendola A, et al.: Which preoperative factors, including bone bruise, are associated with knee pain/symptoms at index anterior cruciate ligament reconstruction (ACLR)? A Multicenter Orthopaedic Outcomes Network (MOON) ACLR cohort study, *Am J Sports Med* 38:1778, 2010.

Dunn WR, Spindler KP: MOON Consortium: predictors of activity level 2 years after anterior cruciate ligament reconstruction (ACLR): a Multicenter Orthopaedic Outcomes Network (MOON) ACLR cohort study, *Am J Sports Med* 38:2040, 2010.

Dunn WR, Wolf BR, Harrell Jr FE, et al.: Baseline predictors of health-related quality of life after anterior cruciate ligament reconstruction: a longitudinal analysis of a multicenter cohort at two and six years, *J Bone Joint Surg* 97A:551, 2015.

Edgar C, Kumar N, Ware JK, et al.: Incidence of posteromedial meniscocapsular separation and the biomechanical implications on the anterior cruciate ligament, *J Am Acad Orthop Surg* 27:e184, 2019.

Emond CE, Woelber EB, Kurd SK, et al.: A comparison of the results of anterior cruciate ligament reconstruction using bioabsorbable versus metal interference screws: a meta-analysis, *J Bone Joint Surg* 93A:572, 2011.

Engelman GH, Carry PM, Hitt KG, et al.: Comparison of allograft versus autograft anterior cruciate ligament reconstruction graft survival in an active adolescent cohort, *Am J Sports Med* 42:2311, 2014.

Erickson BJ, Cvetanovich G, Waliullah K, et al.: Two-stage revision anterior cruciate ligament reconstruction, *Orthopedics* 39:e456, 2016.

Eysturoy NH, Nissen KA, Nielsen T, et al.: The influence of graft fixation methods on revision rates after primary anterior cruciate ligament reconstruction, *Am J Sports Med* 46:524, 2018.

Figueroa D, Figueroa F, Calvo R, et al.: Platelet-rich plasma use in anterior cruciate ligament surgery: systematic review, *Arthroscopy* 31:981, 2015.

Foster TE, Wolfe BL, Ryan S, et al.: Does the graft source really matter in the outcome of patients undergoing anterior cruciate ligament reconstruction? An evaluation of autograft versus allograft reconstruction results: a systematic review, *Am J Sports Med* 38:189, 2010.

Frobell RB: Change in cartilage thickness, posttraumatic bone marrow lesions, and joint fluid volumes after acute ACL disruption: a two-year prospective MRI study of sixty-one subjects, *J Bone Joint Surg* 93A:1096, 2011.

Gagliardi AG, Carry PN, Parikh HB, et al.: ACL repair with suture ligament augmentation is associated with a high failure rate among adolescent patients, *Am J Sports Med* 47:560, 2019.

Gali JC, Bernardes AD, Dos Santos LC, et al.: Tunnel collision during simultaneous anterior cruciate ligament and posterolateral corner reconstruction, *Knee Surg Sports Traumatol Arthrosc* 24:195, 2016.

Gaskill T, Pullen M, Bryant B, et al.: The prevalence of symptomatic deep venous thrombosis and pulmonary embolism after anterior cruciate ligament reconstruction, *Am J Sports Med* 43:2714, 2015.

Ghodadra N, Mall NA, Karas V, et al.: Articular and meniscal pathology associated with primary anterior cruciate ligament reconstruction, *J Knee Surg* 26:185, 2013.

Ghodadra NS, Mall NA, Grumet R, et al.: Interval arthrometric comparison of anterior cruciate ligament reconstruction using bone–patellar tendon–bone autograft versus allograft: do grafts attenuate within the first year postoperatively? *Am J Sports Med* 40:1347, 2012.

Gifstad T, Foss OA, Engebretsen L, et al.: Lower risk of revision with patellar tendon autografts compared with hamstring autografts: a registry study based on 45,998 primary ACL reconstructions in Scandinavia, *Am J Sports Med* 42:2319, 2014.

Gobbi A, Mahajan V, Karnatikos G, Nakamura N: Single- versus double-bundle ACL reconstruction: is there any difference in stability and function at 3-year followup? *Clin Orthop Relat Res* 470:824, 2012.

Gagliardi AG, Carry PN, Parikh HB, et al.: ACL repair with suture ligament augmentation is associated with a high failure rate among adolescent patients, *Am J Sports Med* 47:560, 2019.

Granan LP, Inacio MC, Maletis GB, et al.: Sport-specific injury pattern recorded during anterior cruciate ligament reconstruction, *Am J Sports Med* 41:2814, 2013.

Grant JA, Mohtadi NG: Two- to 4-year follow-up to a comparison of home versus physical therapy-supervised rehabilitation programs after anterior cruciate ligament reconstruction, *Am J Sports Med* 38:1389, 2010.

Greenberg DD, Robertson M, Vallurupalli S, et al.: Allograft compared with autograft infection rates in primary anterior cruciate ligament reconstruction, *J Bone Joint Surg* 92A:2402, 2010.

Griffith TB, Allen BJ, Levy BA, et al.: Outcomes of repeat revision anterior cruciate ligament reconstruction, *Am J Sports Med* 41:1296, 2013.

Guillard C, Lintz F, Odri GA, et al.: Effects of graft retensioning in anterior cruciate ligament reconstruction, *Knee Surg Sports Traumatol Arthsc* 20:2208, 2012.

Guo L, Yang L, Duan XJ, et al.: Anterior cruciate ligament reconstruction with bone–patellar tendon–bone graft: comparison of autograft, fresh-frozen allograft, and (-irradiated allograft, *Arthroscopy* 28:211, 2012.

Häberli J, Jaberg L, Bieri K, et al.: Reinterventions after dynamic intraligamentary stabilization in primary anterior cruciate ligament repair, *Knee* 25:271, 2018.

Hampton DM, Lamb J, Klimkiewica JJ: Effect of donor age on patellar tendon allograft ACL reconstruction, *Orthopedics* 35:e1173, 2012.

Hart A, Sivakumaran T, Burman M, et al.: A prospective evaluation of femoral tunnel placement for anatomic anterior cruciate ligament reconstruction using 3-dimensional magnetic resonance imaging, *Am J Sports Med* 46:192, 2018.

Hashemi J, Chandrashekar N, Mansouri H, et al.: Shallow medial tibial plateau and steep medial and lateral tibial slopes: new risk factors for anterior cruciate ligament injuries, *Am J Sports Med* 38:54, 2010.

Herman DC, Barth JT: Drop-jump landing varies with baseline neurocognition: implications for anterior cruciate ligament injury risk and prevention, *Am J Sports Med* 44:2347, 2016.

Henle P, Bieri KS, Brand M, et al.: Patient and surgical characteristics that affect revision risk in dynamic intraligamentary stabilization of the anterior cruciate ligament, *Knee Surg Sports Traumatol Arthrosc* 26:1182, 2018.

Hewison CE, Tran MN, Kaniki N, et al.: Lateral extra-articular tenodesis reduces rotational laxity when combined with anterior cruciate ligament reconstruction: a systematic review of the literature, *Arthroscopy* 31:2022, 2015.

Hewett TE, Ford KR, Hoogenboom BJ, Myer GD: Understanding and preventing acl injuries: current biomechanical and epidemiologic considerations—update 2010, *N Am J Sports Phys Ther* 5:234, 2010.

Hexter AT, Thangarajah T, Blunn G, et al.: Biological augmentation of graft healing in anterior cruciate ligament reconstruction, *Bone Joint Lett J* 100-B:271, 2018.

Hoffelner T, Resch H, Moroder P, et al.: No increased occurrence of osteoarthritis after anterior cruciate ligament reconstruction after isolated anterior cruciate ligament injury in athletes, *Arthroscopy* 28:517, 2012.

Holm I, Oiestad BE, Risberg MA, Aune AK: No difference in knee function or prevalence of osteoarthritis after reconstruction of the anterior cruciate ligament with 4-strand hamstring autograft versus patellar tendon-bone autograft: a randomized study with 10-year follow-up, *Am J Sports Med* 38:448, 2010.

Hoogeslag RAG, Brouwer RW, Boer BC, et al.: Acute anterior cruciate ligament rupture: repair or reconstruct? Two-year results of a randomized controlled clinical trial, *Am J Sports Med* 47:567, 2019.

Hosseini A, Lodhia P, Van de Velde SK, et al.: Tunnel position and graft orientation in failed anterior cruciate ligament reconstruction: a clinical and imaging analysis, *Int Orthop* 36:845, 2012.

Hoogeslag RAG, Brouwer RW, Boer BC, et al.: Acute anterior cruciate ligament rupture: repair or reconstruct? Two-year results of a randomized controlled clinical trial, *Am J Sports Med* 47:567, 2019.

Hussein M, van Eck CF, Cretnik A, et al.: Prospective randomized clinical evaluation of conventional single-bundle, anatomic single-bundle, and anatomic double-bundle anterior cruciate ligament reconstruction: 281 cases with 3- to 5-year follow-up, *Am J Sports Med* 40:512, 2012.

Inacio MC, Paxton EW, Maletis GB, et al.: Patient and surgeon characteristics associated with primary anterior cruciate ligament reconstruction graft selection, *Am J Sports Med* 40:339, 2012.

Indelicato PA, Ciccotti MG, Boyd J, et al.: Aseptically processed and chemically sterilized BTB allografts for anterior cruciate ligament reconstruction: a prospective randomized study, *Knee Surg Sports Traumatol Arthrosc* 21:2107, 2013.

Janssen RP, van der Velden MJ, Pasmans HL, Sala HA: Regeneration of hamstring tendons after anterior cruciate ligament reconstruction, *Knee Surg Sports Traumatol Arthrosc* 21:898, 2013.

Janssen RP, van der Wijk J, Fielder A, et al.: Remodeling of human hamstring autografts after anterior cruciate ligament reconstruction, *Knee Surg Sports Traumatol Arthrosc* 19:1299, 2011.

Jones MH, Spindler KP: Risk factors for radiographic joint space narrowing and patient reported outcomes of post-traumatic osteoarthritis after ACL reconstruction: data from the MOON cohort, *J Orthop Res* 35:1366, 2017.

Jonkergouw A, van der List JP, DiFelice GS: Arthroscopioc primary of proximal anterior cruciate ligament tears: with or without additional suture augmentation? *Orthop J Sports Med* 6(7 (Suppl 4):2325967118S00063, 2018.

Kaeding CC, Aros B, Pedroza A, et al.: Allograft versus autograft anterior cruciate ligament reconstruction: predictors of failure from a MOON prospective longitudinal cohort, *Sports Health* 3:73, 2011.

Kamien PM, Hydrick JM, Replogle WH, et al.: Age, graft size, and Tegner activity level as predictors of failure in anterior cruciate ligament reconstruction with hamstring autograft, *Am J Sports Med* 41:1808, 2013.

Kato Y, Maeyama A, Lertwanich P, et al.: Biomechanical comparison of different graft positions for single-bundle anterior cruciate ligament reconstruction, *Knee Surg Sports Traumatol Arthrosc* 21:816, 2013.

Keays SL, Newcombe PA, Bullock-Saxton JE, et al.: Factors involved in the development of osteoarthritis after anterior cruciate ligament surgery, *Am J Sports Med* 38:455, 2010.

Khan M, Rothrauff BB, Merali F, et al.: Management of the contaminated anterior cruciate ligament graft, *Arthroscopy* 30:236, 2014.

Kim D, Asai S, Moon CW, et al.: Biomechanical evaluation of anatomic single- and double-bundle anterior cruciate ligament reconstruction techniques using the quadriceps tendon, *Knee Surg Sports Traumatol Arthrosc* 23:687, 2015.

Kim SJ, Lee SK, Kim SH, et al.: Does anterior laxity of the uninjured knee influence clinical outcomes of ACL reconstruction? *J Bone Joint Surg* 96A:543, 2014.

Kim SJ, Lee SK, Kim SH, et al.: Effect of cigarette smoking on the clinical outcomes of ACL reconstruction, *J Bone Joint Surg* 96A:1007, 2014.

Kim SJ, Moon HK, Chun YM, et al.: Is correctional osteotomy crucial in primary varus knees undergoing anterior cruciate ligament reconstruction? *Clin Orthop Relat Res* 469:1421, 2011.

Koch M, Matteo BD, Eichhorn J, et al.: Intra-ligamentary autologous conditioned plasma and healing response to treat partial ACL ruptures, *Arch Orthop Trauma Surg* 138:675, 2018.

Koga H, Muneta T, Yagishita K, et al.: Effect of notchplasty in anatomic double-bundle anterior cruciate ligament reconstruction, *Am J Sports Med* 42:1813, 2014.

Koga H, Muneta T, Yagishita K, et al.: Effect of posterolateral bundle graft fixation angles on clinical outcomes in double-bundle anterior cruciate ligament reconstruction: a randomized controlled trial, *Am J Sports Med* 43:1157, 2015.

Koga H, Nakame A, Shima Y, et al.: Mechanisms for noncontact anterior cruciate ligament injuries: knee joint kinematics in 10 injury situations from female team handball and basketball, *Am J Sports Med* 38:2218, 2010.

Kohl S, Evangelopoulos DS, Schar MO, et al.: Dynamic intraligamentary stabilisation: initial experience with treatment of acute ACL ruptures, *Bone Joint Lett J* 98-B:793, 2016.

Kraeutler MJ, Bravman JT, McCarty EC: Bone–patellar tendon–bone autograft versus allograft in outcomes of anterior cruciate ligament reconstruction: a meta-analysis of 5182 patients, *Am J Sports Med* 41:2439, 2013.

Krismer AM, Gousopoulos L, Kohl S, et al.: Factors influencing the success of anterior cruciate ligament repair with dynamic intraligamentary stabilisation, *Knee Surg Sports Traumatol Arthrosc* 25:3923, 2017.

Lamblin CJ, Waterman BR, Lubowitz JH: Anterior cruciate ligament reconstruction with autografts compared to non-irradiated, non-chemically treated allografts, *Arthroscopy* 29:1113, 2013.

LaPrade CM, Smith SD, Rasmussen MT, et al.: Consequences of tibial tunnel reaming on the meniscal roots during cruciate ligament reconstruction in a cadaveric model, Part 1: the anterior cruciate ligament, *Am J Sports Med* 43:200, 2015.

LaPrade RF, Johansen S, Agel J, et al.: Outcomes of an anatomic posterolateral knee reconstruction, *J Bone Joint Surg* 92A:16, 2010.

Larson AI, Bullock DP, Pevny T: Comparison of 4 femoral tunnel drilling techniques in anterior cruciate ligament reconstruction, *Arthroscopy* 28:972, 2012.

Leal-Blanquet J, Alentorn-Geli E, Tuneu J, et al.: Anterior cruciate ligament reconstruction: a multicenter prospective cohort study evaluating 3 different grafts using same bone drilling method, *Clin J Sport Med* 21:294, 2011.

Lecoq FA, Parienti JJ, Murison J: Graft choice and the incidence of osteoarthritis after anterior cruciate ligament reconstruction: a causal analysis from a cohort of 541 patients, *Am J Sports Med* 46:2842, 2018.

Lee JH, Bae DK, Song SJ, et al.: Comparison of clinical results and second-look arthroscopy findings after arthroscopic anterior cruciate ligament reconstruction using 3 different types of grafts, *Arthroscopy* 26:41, 2010.

Lee JK, Lee S, Seong SC, Lee MC: Anatomic single-bundle ACL reconstruction is possible with use of the modified transtibial technique: a comparison with the anteromedial transportal technique, *J Bone Joint Surg* 96A:664, 2014.

Leiter JR, Gourlay R, McRae S, et al.: Long-term follow-up of ACL reconstruction with hamstring autograft, *Knee Surg Sports Traumatol Arthrosc* 22:1061, 2014.

Leroux T, Ogilvie-Harris D, Dwyer T, et al.: The risk of knee arthroplasty following cruciate ligament reconstruction: a population-based matched cohort study, *J Bone Joint Surg* 96A:2, 2014.

Leys T, Salmon L, Waller A, et al.: Clinical results and risk factors for reinjury 15 years after anterior cruciate ligament reconstruction: a prospective study of hamstring and patellar tendon grafts, *Am J Sports Med* 40:595, 2012.

Li RT, Lorenz S, Xu Y, et al.: Predictors of radiographic knee osteoarthritis after anterior cruciate ligament reconstruction, *Am J Sports Med* 39:2595, 2011.

Li Y, Hong L, Feng H, et al.: Posterior tibial slope influences static anterior tibial translation in anterior cruciate ligament reconstruction: a minimum 2-year follow-up study, *Am J Sports Med* 42:927, 2014.

Li YL, Ning GZ, Wu Q, et al.: Single-bundle or double-bundle for anterior cruciate ligament reconstruction: a meta-analysis, *Knee* 21:28, 2014.

Lim HC, Yoon YC, Wang JH, Bae JH: Anatomical versus non-anatomical single bundle anterior cruciate ligament reconstruction: a cadaveric study of comparison of knee stability, *Clin Orthop Surg* 4:249, 2012.

Lind M, Menhert F, Pedersen AB: Incidence and outcome after revision anterior cruciate ligament reconstruction: results from the Danish registry for knee ligament reconstructions, *Am J Sports Med* 40:1551, 2012.

Liu X, Feng H, Zhang H, et al.: Arthroscopic prevalence of ramp lesion in 868 patients with anterior cruciate ligament injury, *Am J Sports Med* 39:832, 2011.

Lu W, Wang D, Zhu W, et al.: Placement of double tunnels in ACL reconstruction using bony landmarks versus existing footprint remnant: a prospective clinical study with 2-year follow-up, *Am J Sports Med* 43:1206, 2015.

Magnussen RA, Lawrence JT, West RL, et al.: Graft size and patient age are predictors of early revision after anterior cruciate ligament reconstruction with hamstring autograft, *Arthroscopy* 28:526, 2012.

Makhni EC, Steinhaus ME, Mehran N, et al.: Functional outcome and graft retention in patients with septic arthritis after anterior cruciate ligament reconstruction: a systematic review, *Arthroscopy* 31:1392, 2015.

Maletis GB, Chen J, Inacio MC, Funahashi TT: Age-related risk factors for revision anterior cruciate ligament reconstruction: a cohort study of 21,304 patients from the Kaiser Permanente Anterior Cruciate Ligament Registry, *Am J Sports Med* 44:331, 2016.

Maletis GB, Inacio MC, Desmond JL, Funahashi TT: Reconstruction of the anterior cruciate ligament: association of graft choice with increased risk of early revision, *J Bone Joint J* 95B:623, 2013.

Maletis GB, Inacio MC, Funahashi TT: Analysis of 16, 192 anterior cruciate ligament reconstructions from a community-based registry, *Am J Sports Med* 41:2090, 2013.

Maletis GB, Inacio MC, Reynolds S, et al.: Incidence of postoperative anterior cruciate ligament reconstruction infections: graft choice makes a difference, *Am J Sports Med* 41:1780, 2013.

Mall NA, Abrams GD, Azar FM, et al.: Trends in primary and revision anterior cruciate ligament reconstruction among National Basketball Association team physicians, *Am J Orthop (Belle Mead NJ)* 43:267, 2014.

Mall NA, Chalmers PN, Moric M, et al.: Incidence and trends of anterior cruciate ligament reconstruction in the United States, *Am J Sports Med* 42:2363, 2014.

Månsson O, Sernert N, Rostgard-Christensen L, Kartus J: Long-term clinical and radiographic results after delayed anterior cruciate ligament reconstruction in adolescents, *Am J Sports Med* 43:138, 2015.

Mariscalco MW, Flanigan DC, Mitchell J, et al.: The influence of hamstring autograft size on patient-reported outcomes and risk of revision after anterior cruciate ligament reconstruction: a Multicenter Orthopaedic Outcomes Network (MOON) cohort study, *Arthroscopy* 29:1948, 2013.

Mariscalco MW, Magnussen RA, Mehta D, et al.: Autograft versus nonirradiated allograft tissue for anterior cruciate ligament reconstruction: a systematic review, *Am J Sports Med* 42:492, 2014.

MARS Group: Effect of graft choice on the outcome of revision anterior cruciate ligament reconstruction in the Multicenter ACL Revision Study (MARS) cohort, *Am J Sports Med* 42:2301, 2014.

MARS Group, Allen CR, Anderson AF, et al.: Surgical predictors of clinical outcomes after revision anterior cruciate ligament reconstruction, *Am J Sports Med* 45:2586, 2017.

Mascarenhas R, Cvetanovich GL, Sayegh ET, et al.: Does double-bundle anterior cruciate ligament reconstruction improve postoperative knee stability compared with single-bundle techniques? A systematic review of overlapping meta-analyses, *Arthroscopy* 31:1185, 2015.

Mascarenhas R, Tranovich M, Karpie JC, et al.: Patellar tendon anterior cruciate ligament reconstruction in the high-demand patient: evaluation of autograft versus allograft reconstruction, *Arthroscopy* 26(Suppl 9):S58, 2010.

Matava MJ, Arciero RA, Baumgarten KM, et al.: Multirater agreement of the causes of anterior cruciate ligament reconstruction failure: a radiographic and video analysis of the MARS cohort, *Am J Sports Med* 43:310, 2015.

Mather 3rd RC, Hettrich CM, Dunn WR, et al.: Cost-effectiveness analysis of early reconstruction versus rehabilitation and delayed reconstruction for anterior cruciate ligament tears, *Am J Sports Med* 42:1583, 2014.

Matsubara H, Okazaki K, Osaki K, et al.: Optimal entry position on the lateral femoral surface for outside-in drilling technique to restore the anatomical footprint of anterior cruciate ligament, *Knee Surg Sports Traumatol Arthrosc* 24:2758, 2016.

McRae S, Leiter J, McCormack R, et al.: Ipsilateral versus contralateral hamstring grafts in anterior cruciate ligament reconstruction: a prospective randomized trial, *Am J Sports Med* 41:2492, 2013.

Mehta VM, Mandala C, Foster D, Petsche TS: Comparison of revision rates in bone-patella tendon-bone autograft and allograft anterior cruciate ligament reconstruction, *Orthopedics* 33:12, 2010.

Meister M, Koch J, Amsler F, et al.: ACL suturing using dynamic intraligamentary stabilization showing good clinical outcome but a high reoperation rate: a retrospective independent study, *Knee Surg Sports Traumatol Arthrosc* 26:655, 2018.

Melton JT, Murray JR, Karim A, et al.: Meniscal repair in anterior cruciate ligament reconstruction: a long-term outcome study, *Knee Surg Sports Traumatol Arthrosc* 19:1729, 2011.

Mihelic R, Jurdana H, Jotanovic Z, et al.: Long-term results of anterior cruciate ligament reconstruction: a comparison with non-operative treatment with a follow-up of 17-20 years, *Int Orthop* 35:1093, 2011.

Miura K, Woo SL, Brinkley R, et al.: Effects of knee flexion angles for graft fixation on force distribution in double-bundle anterior cruciate ligament grafts, *Am J Sports Med* 34:577, 2006.

Mohtadi N, Chan D, Barber R, Oddone Paolucci E: A randomized clinical trial comparing patellar tendon, hamstring tendon, and double-bundle ACL reconstructions: patient-reported and clinical outcomes at a minimal 2-year follow-up, *Clin J Sport Med* 25:321, 2015.

Monaco E, Maestri B, Labianca L, et al.: Clinical and radiological outcomes of postoperative septic arthritis after anterior cruciate ligament reconstruction, *J Orthop Sci* 15:198, 2010.

Mouton C, Theisen D, Meyer T, et al.: Noninjured knees of patients with noncontact ACL injuries display higher average anterior and internal rotational knee laxity compared with healthy knees of a noninjured population, *Am J Sports Med* 43:1918, 2015.

Muneta T, Hara K, Ju YJ, et al.: Revision anterior cruciate ligament reconstruction by double-bundle technique using multi-strand semitendinosus tendon, *Arthroscopy* 26:769, 2010.

Murawski CD, van Eck CF, Irrgang JJ, et al.: Operative treatment of primary anterior cruciate ligament rupture in adults, *J Bone Joint Surg* 96A:685, 2014.

Murray MM, Flutie BM, Kalish LA, et al.: The Bridge-Enhanced Anterior Cruciate Ligament Repair (BEAR) procedure: an early feasibility cohort study, *Orthop J Sports Med* 4:23259671166721767, 2016.

Murray JR, Lindh AM, Hogan NA, et al.: Does anterior cruciate ligament reconstruction lead to degenerative disease? Thirteen-year results after bone–patellar tendon–bone autograft, *Am J Sports Med* 40:404, 2012.

Musahl V, Voos JE, O'Loughlin PF, et al.: Comparing stability of single- and double-bundle anterior cruciate ligament reconstruction techniques: a cadaveric study using navigation, *Arthroscopy* 26(Suppl 9):S41, 2010.

Nakamae A, Adachi N, Deie M, et al.: Risk factors for progression of articular cartilage damage after anatomical anterior cruciate ligament reconstruction, *Bone Joint Lett J* 100-B:285, 2018.

Naraoka T, Kimura Y, Tsuda E, et al.: Is remnant preservation truly bene-fucial to anterior cruciate ligament reconstruction healing? Clinical and magnetic resonance imaging evaluations of remnant-preserved recon-struction, *Am J Sports Med* 45:1049, 2017.

Nazem K, Barzegar M, Hosseini A, Karimi M: Can we use peroneus longus in addition to hamstring tendons for anterior cruciate ligament reconstruc-tion? *Adv Biomed Res* 3:115, 2014.

Newman JT, Carry PM, Terhune EB, et al.: Factors predictive of concomitant injuries among children and adolescents undergoing anterior cruciate ligament surgery, *Am J Sports Med* 43:282, 2015. Orthop J Sports Med 3: 2325967115575719, 2015.

Ntoulia A, Paadopoulou F, Ristanis S, et al.: Revascularization process of the bone–patellar tendon–bone autograft evaluated by contrast-enhanced magnetic resonance imaging 6 and 12 months after anterior cruciate liga-ment reconstruction, *Am J Sports Med* 39:1478, 2011.

Nwachukwu BU, McFeely ED, Nasreddine A, et al.: Arthrofibrosis after anterior cruciate ligament reconstruction in children and adolescents, *J Pediatr Orthop* 38:811, 2011.

Oiestad BE, Holm I, Aune AK, et al.: Knee function and prevalence of knee osteoarthritis after anterior cruciate ligament reconstruction: a prospec-tive study with 10 to 15 years of follow-up, *Am J Sport Med* 38:2201, 2010.

Osti M, El Attal R, Doskar W, et al.: High complication rate following dynamic intraligamentary stabilization for primary repair of the anterior cruciate ligament, *Knee Surg Sports Traumatol Arthrosc* 27:29, 2019.

Packer JD, Bedi A, Fox AJ, et al.: Effect of immediate and delayed high-strain loading on tendon-to-bone healing after anterior cruciate ligament reconstruction, *J Bone Joint Surg* 96A:770, 2014.

Pallis M, Svoboda SJ, Cameron KL, Owens BD: Survival comparison of allograft and autograft anterior cruciate ligament reconstruction at the United States Military Academy, *Am J Sports Med* 40:1242, 2012.

Papalia R, Franeschi F, D'Adamio S, et al.: Hamstring tendon regeneration after harvest for anterior cruciate ligament reconstruction: a systematic review, *Arthroscopy* 31:1169, 2015.

Park SS, Dwyer T, Congiusta F, et al.: Analysis of irradiation on the clinical effectiveness of allogenic tissue when used for primary anterior cruciate ligament reconstruction, *Am J Sports Med* 43:226, 2014.

Parkinson B, Robb C, Thomas M, et al.: Factors that predict failure in ana-tomic single-bundle anterior cruciate ligament reconstruction, *Am J Sports Med* 45:1529, 2017.

Pascual-Garrido C, Carbo L, Makino A: Revision of anterior cruciate liga-ment reconstruction with allografts in patients younger than 40 years old: a 2- to 4-year results, *Knee Surg Sports Traumatol Arthrosc* 22:1106, 2014.

Paterno MV, Rauh MJ, Schmitt LC, et al.: Incidence of second ACL injuries 2 years after primary ACL reconstruction and return to sport, *Am J Sports Med* 42:1567, 2014.

Paterno MV, Schmitt LC, Ford KR, et al.: Biomechanical measures during landing and postural stability predict second anterior cruciate ligament injury after anterior cruciate ligament reconstruction and return to sport, *Am J Sports Med* 38:1968, 2010.

Paterno MV, Weed AM, Hewett TE: A between sex comparison of anterior-pos-terior knee laxity after anterior cruciate ligament reconstruction with patellar tendon or hamstrings autograft: a systematic review, *Sports Med* 42:135, 2012.

Pennock AT, o B, Parvanta K, et al.: Does allograft augmentation of small-diameter hamstring autograft ACL grafts reduce the incidence of graft retear? *Am J Sports Med* 45:334, 2016.

Pérez-Prieto D, Torres-Claramunt R, Gelber PE, et al.: Autograft soaking in vancomycin reduces the risk of infection after anterior cruciate ligament reconstruction, *Knee Surg Sports Traumatol Arthrosc* 24:2724, 2016.

Phegan M, Grayson JE, Vertullo CJ: No infections in 1300 anterior cruci-ate ligament reconstructions with vancomycin pre-soaking of hamstring grafts, *Knee Surg Sports Traumatol Arthrosc* 24:2729, 2016.

Piasecki DP, Bach Jr BR, Espinoza Orias AA, Verma NN: Anterior cruciate ligament reconstruction: can anatomic femoral placement be achieved with a transtibial technique? *Am J Sports Med* 39:1306, 2011.

Plante MJ, Li X, Scully G, et al.: Evaluation of sterilization methods following contamination of hamstring autograft during anterior cruciate ligament reconstruction, *Knee Surg Sports Traumatol Arthrosc* 21:696, 2013.

Porter MD, Shadbolt B: "Anatomic" single-bundle anterior cruciate ligament reconstruction reduces both anterior translation and internal rotation during the pivot-shift, *Am J Sports Med* 42:2948, 2014.

Quelard B, Sonnery-Cottet B, Zayni R, et al.: Preoperative factors correlating with prolonged range of motion deficit after anterior cruciate ligament reconstruction, *A J Sports Med* 38:2034, 2010.

Rahr-Wagner L, Thillemann TM, Pedersen AB, Lind M: Comparison of hamstring tendon and patellar tendon grafts in anterior cruciate liga-ment reconstruction in a nationwide population-based cohort study: results from the Danish registry of knee ligament reconstruction, *Am J Sports Med* 42:278, 2014.

Ralles S, Agel J, Obermeir M, Tompkins M: Incidence of secondary intra-articular injuries with time to anterior cruciate ligament reconstruction, *Am J Sports Med* 43:1373, 2015.

Reinhardt KR, Hetsroni I, Marx RG: Graft selection for anterior cruciate liga-ment reconstruction: a level 1 systematic review comparing failure rates and functional outcomes, *Orthop Clin North Am* 41:249, 2010.

Robb C, Kempshall P, Getgood A, et al.: Meniscal integrity predicts laxity of anterior cruciate ligament reconstruction, *Knee Surg Sports Traumatol Arthrosc* 23:3683, 2015.

Robin BN, Lubowitz JH: Disadvantages and advantages of transtibial tech-nique for creating the anterior cruciate ligament femoral socket, *J Knee Surg* 27:327, 2014.

Rodriguez-Merchan EC: Evidence-based ACL reconstruction, *Arch Bone Jt Surg* 3:9, 2015.

Rue JP, Ghodadra N, Lewis PB, Bach Jr BR: Femoral and tibial tunnel posi-tion using a transtibial drilled anterior cruciate ligament technique, *J Knee Surg* 21:246, 2008.

Ryan J, Magnussen RA, Cox CL, et al.: ACL reconstruction: do outcomes dif-fer by sex? A systematic review, *J Bone Joint Surg* 96A:507, 2014.

Sasaki N, Farraro KF, Kim KE, Woo SL: Biomechanical evaluation of the quadriceps tendon autograft for anterior cruciate ligament reconstruc-tion: a cadaveric study, *Am J Sports Med* 42:723, 2014.

Scannell BP, Loeffler BJ, Hoenig M, et al.: Biomechanical comparison of ham-string tendon fixation devices for anterior cruciate ligament reconstruc-tion: part 1. Five femoral devices, *Am J Orthop (Belle Mead NJ)* 44:32, 2015.

Schuster P, Schulz M, Immendoerfer M, et al.: Septic arthritis after arthroscopic anterior cruciate ligament reconstruction. Evaluation of an arthroscopic graft-retaining protocol, *Am J Sports Med* 43:3005, 2015.

Setiawati R, Utomo DN, Rantam FA, et al.: Early graft tunnel healing after anterior cruciate ligament reconstruction with intratunnel injection of bone marrow mesenchymal stem cells and vascular endothelial growth factor, *Orthop J Sports Med* 5:2325967117708548, 2017.

Shelbourne KD, Beck MB, Gray T: Anterior cruciate ligament reconstruction with contralateral autogenous patellar tendon graft: evaluation of donor site strength and subjective results, *Am J Sports Med* 43:648, 2015.

Shelbourne KD, Benner RW, Gray T: Return to sports and subsequent injury rates after revision anterior cruciate ligament reconstruction with patellar tendon autograft, *Am J Sports Med* 42:1395, 2014.

Shelbourne KD, Benner RW, Gary T: Results of anterior cruciate ligament reconstruction with patellar tendon autografts: objective factors associ-ated with the development of osteoarthritis at 20 to 33 years after surgery, *Am J Sports Med* 45:2730, 2017.

Shi D, Zhou J, Yapici C, et al.: Effect of graft fixation sequence on knee joint biomechanics in double-bundle anterior cruciate ligament reconstruc-tion, *Knee Surg Sports Traumatol Arthrosc* 23:655, 2015.

Siebold R, Branch TP, Freedberg HI, Jacobs CA: A matched pairs compar-ison of single- versus double-bundle anterior cruciate ligament recon-structions, clinical results and manual laxity testing, *Knee Surg Sports Traumatol Arthrosc* 19(Suppl 1):S4, 2011.

Smith TO, Postle K, Penny F, et al.: Is reconstruction the best management strategy for anterior cruciate ligament rupture? A systematic review and meta-analysis comprient anterior cruciate ligament reconstruction ver-sus non-operative treatment, *Knee* 21:462, 2014.

Snow M, Campbell G, Adlington J, Stanish WD: Two to five year results of primary ACL reconstruction using doubled tibialis anterior allograft, *Knee Surg Sports Traumatol Arthrosc* 18:1374, 2010.

Sohn OJ, Lee DC, Park KH, Ahn HS: Comparison of the modified transtibial technique, anteromedial portal technique and outside-in technique in ACL reconstruction, *Knee Surg Relat Res* 26:241, 2014.

Song EK, Seon JK, Kim JH, et al.: Progression of osteoarthritis after double- and single-bundle anterior cruciate ligament reconstruction, *Am J Sports Med* 41:2340, 2013.

Sonnery-Cottet B, Mogos S, Thaunat M, et al.: Proximal tibial anterior closing wedge osteotomy in repeat revision of anterior cruciate ligament reconstruction, *Am J Sports Med* 42:1873, 2014.

Sonnery-Cottet B, Thaunat M, Freychet B, et al.: Outcome of a combined anterior cruciate ligament and anterolateral ligament reconstruction technique with a minimum 2-year follow-up, *Am J Sports Med* 43:1598, 2015.

Spindler KP, Huston LJL, Wright RW, et al.: The prognosis and predictors of sports function and activity a minimum 6 years after anterior cruciate ligament reconstruction: a population cohort study, *Am J Sports Med* 39:348, 2011.

Stener S, Ejerhed L, Sernert N, et al.: A long-term, prospective, randomized study comparing biodegradable and metal interference screws in anterior cruciate ligament reconstruction surgery: radiographic results and clinical outcome, *Am J Sports Med* 38:1598, 2010.

Strauss EJ, Barker JU, McGill K, et al.: Can anatomic femoral tunnel placement be achieved using a transtibial technique for hamstring anterior cruciate ligament reconstruction? *Am J Sports Med* 39:1263, 2011.

Struewer J, Frangen TM, Ishaque B, et al.: Knee function and prevalence of osteoarthritis after isolated anterior cruciate ligament reconstruction using bone–patellar tendon–bone graft: long-term follow-up, *Int Orthop* 36:171, 2012.

Suijkerbuijk MA, Reijman M, Lodewijks SJ, et al.: Hamstring tendon regeneration after harvesting: a systematic review, *Am J Sports Med* 43:2591, 2015.

Sumalainen P, Moisala AS, Paaqkkala A, et al.: Double-bundle versus single-bundle anterior cruciate ligament reconstruction: randomized clinical and magnetic resonance imaging study with 2-year follow-up, *Am J Sports Med* 39:1615, 2011.

Sun K, Zhang J, Wang Y, et al.: A prospective randomized comparison of irradiated and non-irradiated hamstring tendon allograft for ACL reconstruction, *Knee Surg Sports Traumatol Arthrosc* 20:187, 2012.

Svanatesson E, Hamrin Senorski E, Alentorn-Geli E, et al.: Increased risk of ACL revision with non-surgical treatment of a concomitant medial collateral ligament injury: a study on 19,457 patients from the Swedish National Knee Ligament Registry, *Knee Surg Sports Traumatol Arthrosc* 27:2450, 2019.

Swank KR, Behn AW, Dragoo JL: The effect of donor age on structural and mechanical properties of allograft tendons, *Am J Sports Med* 43:453, 2015.

Swank KR, DiBartola AC, Everhart JS, et al.: The effect of femoral nerve block on quadriceps strength in anterior cruciate ligament reconstruction: a systematic review, *Arthroscopy* 33:1082, 2017.

Tan SH, Lau BP, Khin LW, Lingaraj K: The importance of patient sex in the outcomes of anterior cruciate ligament reconstructions: a systematic review and meta-analysis, *Am J Sports Med* 44:242, 2016.

Tashiro Y, Gale T, Sundaram V, et al.: The graft bending angle can affect early graft healing after anterior cruciate ligament reconstruction: in vivo analysis with two years' follow-up, *Am J Sports Med* 45:1829, 2017.

Tejwani SG, Chen J, Funahashi TT, et al.: Revision risk after allograft anterior cruciate ligament reconstruction: association with graft processing techniques, patients characteristics, and graft type, *Am J Sports Med* 43:2296, 2015.

Tejwani SG, Prentice HA, Wyatt RWB, et al.: Femoral tunnel drilling method: risk of reoperation and revision after anterior cruciate ligament reconstruction, *Am J Sports Med* 46:3378, 2018.

Tiamklang T, Sumanont S, Foocharoen T, Laopaiboon M: Double-bundle versus single-bundle reconstruction for anterior cruciate ligament rupture in adults, *Cochrane Database Syst Rev* (11):CD008413, 2012.

Todd MS, Lalliss S, Gracia E, et al.: The relationship between posterior tibial slope and anterior cruciate ligament injuries, *Am J Sports Med* 38:63, 2010.

Tohyama H, Kondo E, Hayashi R, et al.: Gender-based differences in outcome after anatomic double-bundle anterior cruciate ligament reconstruction with hamstring tendon autografts, *Am J Sports Med* 39:1849, 2011.

Trojani C, Elhor H, Carles M, Boileau P: Anterior cruciate ligament reconstruction combined with valgus high tibial osteotomy allows return to sports, *Orthop Traumatol Surg Res* 100:209, 2014.

Ulstein S, Årøen A, Engebretsen L, et al.: A controlled comparison of microfracture, debridement, and no treatment of concomitant full-thickness cartilage lesions in anterior cruciate ligament-reconstructed knees: a nationwide prospective cohort study from Norway and Sweden of 368 patients with 5-year follow-up, *Orthop J Sports Med* 6:2325967118787767, 2018.

Ulstein S, Årøen A, Engebretsen L, et al.: Effect of concomitant cartilage lesions on patient-reported outcomes after anterior cruciate ligament reconstruction: a nationwide cohort study from Norway and Sweden of 8470 patients with 5-year follow-up, *Orthop J Sports Med* 6:2325967118786219, 2018.

Ulstein S, Bredland K, Årøen A, et al.: No negative effect on patient-reported outcome of concomitant cartilage lesions 5-9 years after ACL reconstruction, *Knee Surg Sports Traumatol Arthrosc* 25:1482, 2017.

Usman MA, Kamei G, Adachi N, et al.: Revision single-bundle anterior cruciate ligament reconstruction with over-the-top route procedure, *Orthop Traumatol Surg Res* 101:71, 2015.

van Eck CF, Limpisvasti O, ElAttrache NS: Is there a role for internal bracing and repair of the anterior cruciate ligament? A systematic literature review, *Am J Sports Med* 46:2291, 2018.

van Eck CF, Schkrohowsky JG, Working ZM, et al.: Prospective analysis of failure rate and predictors of failure after anatomic anterior cruciate ligament reconstruction with allografts, *Am J Sports Med* 40:800, 2012.

van Yperen DT, Reijman M, van Es EM, et al.: Twenty-year follow-up study comparing operative versus nonoperative treatment of anterior cruciate ligament ruptures in high-level athletes, *Am J Sports Med* 46:1129, 2018.

Waltz RA, Solomon DJ, Provencher MT: Radiographic assessment of failed anterior cruciate ligament reconstruction: can magnetic resonance imaging predict graft integrity? *Am J Sports Med* 42:1652, 2014.

Wang C, Lee YH, Siebold R: Recommendations for the management of septic arthritis after ACL reconstruction, *Knee Surg Sports Traumatol Arthrosc* 22:216, 2014.

Wasserstein D, Khoshbin A, Dwyer T, et al.: Risk factors for recurrent anterior cruciate ligament reconstruction: a population study in Ontario, Canada, with 5-year follow-up, *Am H Sports Med* 41:2099, 2013.

Wiggins AJ, Grandhi RK, Schneider DK, et al.: Risk of secondary injury in younger athletes after anterior cruciate ligament reconstruction: a systematic review and meta-analysis, *Am J Sports Med* 44:1861, 2016.

Wright RW, Gill CS, Chen L, et al.: Outcome of revision anterior cruciate ligament reconstruction: a systematic review, *J Bone Joint Surg* 94A:531, 2012.

Wyatt RW, Inacio MC, Liddle KD, Maletis GB: Factors associated with meniscus repair in patients undergoing anterior cruciate ligament reconstruction, *Am J Sports Med* 41:2766, 2013.

Xie X, Liu X, Chen Z, et al.: A meta-analysis of bone–patellar tendon–bone autograft versus four-strand hamstring tendon autograft for anterior cruciate ligament reconstruction, *Knee* 22:100, 2015.

Xie X, Xiao Z, Li Q, et al.: Increased incidence of osteoarthritis of knee joint after ACL reconstruction with bone–patellar tendon–bone autografts than hamstring autografts a meta-analysis of 1,443 patients at a minimum of 5 years, *Eur J Orthop Surg Traumatol* 25:149, 2015.

Yu A, Prentice HA, Burfeind WE, et al.: Risk of infection after allograft anterior cruciate ligament reconstruction: are nonprocessed allografts more likely to get infected? A cohort study of over 10,000 allografts, *Am J Sports Med* 46:846, 2018.

Zhang H, Sun Y, Han X, et al.: Simultaneous reconstruction of the anterior cruciate ligament and medial collateral ligament in patients with chronic ACL-MCL lesions: a minimum 2-year follow-up study, *Am J Sports Med* 42:1675, 2014.

POSTERIOR CRUCIATE LIGAMENT

Ahn S, Lee YS, Song YD, et al.: Does surgical reconstruction produce better stability than conservative in the isolated PCL injuries? *Arch Orthop Trauma Surg* 136:811, 2016.

Anderson CJ, Ziegler CG, Wijdicks CA, et al.: Arthroscopically pertinent anatomy of the anterolateral and posteromedial bundles of the posterior cruciate ligament, *J Bone Joint Surg Am* 94:1936, 2012.

Araujo PH, Moloney G, Rincon G, et al.: Use of a fluoroscopic overlay to guide femoral tunnel placement during posterior cruciate ligament reconstruction, *Am J Sports Med* 42:2673, 2014.

Arøen A, Sivertsen EA, Owesen C, et al.: An isolated rupture of the posterior cruciate ligament results in reduced knee function in comparison with an anterior cruciate ligament injury, *Knee Surg Sports Traumatol Arthrosc* 21:1017, 2013.

Bedi A, Musahi V, Cowan JB: Management of posterior cruciate ligament injuries: an evidence-based review, *J Am Acad Orthop Surg* 24:277, 2016.

Belk JW, Kraeutler MJ, Purcell JM, et al.: Autograft versus allograft for posterior cruciate ligament reconstruction: an updated systematic review and meta-analysis, *Am J Sports Med* 46:1752, 2018.

Benedetto KP, Hoffelner T, Osti M: The biomechanical characteristics of arthroscopic tibial inlay techniques for posterior cruciate ligament reconstruction: in vitro comparison of tibial graft tunnel placement, *Int Orthop* 38:2363, 2014.

Bonadio MB, Helito CP, Foni NO, et al.: Combined reconstruction of the posterior cruciate ligament and medial collateral ligament using a single femoral tunnel, *Knee Surg Sports Traumatol Arthrosc* 25:3024, 2017.

Cooper JM, McAndrews PT, LaPrade RF: Posterolateral corner injuries of the knee: anatomy, diagnosis, and treatment, *Sports Med Arthrosc Rev* 14:213, 2006.

Dold A, Swensen S, Strauss E, et al.: The posteromedial corner of the knee: anatomy, pathology, and management strategies, *J Am Acad Orthop Surg* 25:752, 2017.

Geeslin AG, Moulton SG, LaPrade RF: A systematic review of the outcomes of posterolateral corner knee injuries, part 1: surgical treatment of acute injuries, *Am J Sports Med* 44:1336, 2015.

Gwinner C, Jung TM, Schatka I, et al.: Posterior laxity increases over time after PCL reconstruction, *Knee Surg Sports Traumatol Arthrosc* 27:389, 2019.

Gwinner C, Weiler A, Roider M, et al.: Tibial slope strongly influences knee stability after posterior cruciate ligament reconstruction: a prospective 5- to 15-year follow-up, *Am J Sports Med* 45:355, 2017.

Hudgens JL, Gillette BP, Krych AJ, et al.: Allograft versus autograft in posterior cruciate ligament reconstruction: an evidence-based systematic review, *J Knee Surg* 26:109, 2013.

Johannsen AM, Anderson CJ, Wijdicks CA, et al.: Radiographic landmarks for tunnel positioning in posterior cruciate ligament reconstructions, *Am J Sports Med* 41:35, 2013.

Kennedy NI, Wijdicks CA, Goldsmith MT, et al.: Kinematic analysis of the posterior cruciate ligament, part 1: the individual and collective function of the anterolateral and posteromedial bundles, *Am J Sports Med* 41:2828, 2013.

Kim SJ, Kim SH, Kim SG, Kung YP: Comparison of the clinical results of three posterior cruciate ligament reconstruction techniques: surgical technique, *J Bone Joint Surg* 92A(Suppl 1) Pt 2):145, 2010.

Kim SJ, Lee SK, Kim SH, et al.: Clinical outcomes for reconstruction of the posterolateral corner and posterior cruciate ligament in injuries with mild grade 2 or less posterior translation: comparison with isolated posterolateral corner reconstruction, *Am J Sports Med* 41:1613, 2013.

LaPrade CM, Civitarese DM, Rasmussen MT, et al.: Emerging updates on the posterior cruciate ligament: a review of the current literature, *Am J Sports Med* 43:3077, 2015.

LaPrade RF, Cinque ME, Dornan GJ, et al.: Double-bundle posterior cruciate ligament reconstruction in 100 patients at a mean 3 years' follow-up. Outcomes were comparable to anterior cruciate ligament reconstructions, *Am J Sports Med* 46:1809, 2018.

LaPrade CM, Smith SD, Rasmussen MT, et al.: Consequences of tibial tunnel reaming on the meniscal roots during cruciate ligament reconstruction in a cadaveric model, Part 2: the posterior cruciate ligament, *Am J Sports Med* 43:207, 2015.

Lee DW, Jang HW, Lee YS, et al.: Clinical, functional, and morphological evaluations of posterior cruciate ligament reconstruction with remnant preservation: minimum 2-year follow-up, *Am J Sports Med* 42:1822, 2014.

Li Y, Li J, Wang J, et al.: Comparison of single-bundle and double-bundle isolated posterior cruciate ligament reconstruction with allograft: a prospective, randomized study, *Arthroscopy* 30:695, 2014.

Markolf KL, Jackson SR, McAllister DR: Single- versus double-bundle posterior cruciate ligament reconstruction: effects of femoral tunnel separation, *Am J Sports Med* 38:1141, 2010.

May JH, Gillette BP, Morgan JA, et al.: Transtibial versus inlay posterior cruciate ligament reconstruction: an evidence-based systematic review, *J Knee Surg* 23:73, 2010.

Min BH, Lee YS, Lee YS, et al.: Evaluation of transtibial double-bundle posterior cruciate ligament reconstruction using a single-sling method with a tibialis anterior allograft, *Am J Sports Med* 39:374, 2011.

Moulton SG, Cram TR, James EW, et al.: The supine internal rotation test: a pilot study evaluating tibial internal rotation in grade III posterior cruciate ligament tears, *Orthop J Sports Med* 3:2325967115572135, 2015.

Moulton SG, Geeslin AG, LaPrade RF: A systematic review of the outcomes of posterolateral corner knee injuries, part 2, *Am J Sports Med* 44:1616, 2015.

Narvy SJ, Hatch 3rd GF, He I, et al.: Evaluating the femoral-side critical corner in posterior cruciate ligament reconstruction: the effect of outside-in versus inside- creation of femoral tunnels on graft contact pressure in a synthetic knee model, *Arthroscopy* 33:1370, 2017.

Nicodeme JD, Löcherbach C, Jolles BM: Tibial tunnel placement in posterior cruciate ligament reconstruction: a systematic review, *Knee Surg Sports Traumatol Arthrosc* 22:1536, 2014.

Ochiai S, Hagino T, Senga S, et al.: Prospective analysis using a patient-based health-related scale shows lower functional scores after posterior cruciate ligament reconstructions as compared with anterior cruciate ligament reconstructions of the knee, *Int Orthop* 40:1891, 2016.

Qi YS, Wang HJ, Wang SJ, et al.: A systematic review of double-bundle versus single-bundle posterior cruciate ligament reconstruction, *BMC Musculoskelet Disord* 17:45, 2016.

Rios CG, Leger RR, Cote MP, et al.: Posterolateral corner reconstruction of the knee: evaluation of a technique with clinical outcomes and stress radiography, *Am J Sports Med* 38:1564, 2010.

Sanders TL, Pareek A, Barrett IJ, et al.: Incidence and long-term follow-up of isolated posterior cruciate ligament tears, *Knee Surg Sports Traumatol Arthrosc* 25:3017, 2017.

Shelbourne KD, Clark M, Gray T: Minimum 10-year follow-up of patients after an acute, isolated posterior cruciate ligament injury treated nonoperatively, *Am J Sports Med* 41:1526, 2013.

Song EK, Park HW, Ahn YS, Seon JK: Transtibial versus tibial inlay techniques for posterior cruciate ligament reconstruction: long-term follow-up study, *Am J Sports Med* 42:2964, 2014.

Tompkins M, Keller TC, Milewski MD, et al.: Anatomic femoral tunnels in posterior cruciate ligament reconstruction: inside-out versus outside-in drilling, *Am J Sports Med* 41:43, 2013.

Westermann RW, Sybrowsky C, Ramme AJ, et al.: Three-dimensional characterization of the femoral footprint of the posterior cruciate ligament, *Arthroscopy* 29:1811, 2013.

Wijdicks CA, Kennedy NI, Goldsmith MT, et al.: Kinematic analysis of the posterior cruciate ligament, part 2: a comparison of anatomic single- versus double-bundle reconstruction, *Am J Sports Med* 41:2839, 2013.

Yang BS, Bae WH, Ha JK, et al.: Posterolateral corner reconstruction using the single fibular sling method for posterolateral rotatory instability of the knee, *Am J Sports Med* 41:1605, 2013.

Yi A, Kleiner MT, Lorenzana D, et al.: Optimal femoral tunnel positioning in posterior cruciate ligament reconstruction using outside-in drilling, *Arthroscopy* 31:850, 2015.

Yoon KH, Kim EJ, Kwon YB, et al.: Minimum 10-year results of single- versus double-bundle posterior cruciate ligament reconstruction: clinical, radiological, and survivorship outcomes, *Am J Sports Med* 47:822, 2019.

Yoon KH, Park SW, Lee SH, et al.: Does cast immobilization contribute to posterior stability after posterior cruciate ligament reconstruction? *Arthroscopy* 29:500, 2013.

Zhao JX, Zhang LH, Mao Z, et al.: Outcome of posterior cruciate ligament reconstruction using a single- versus double-bundle technique: a meta-analysis, *J Int Med Res* 43:149, 2015.

DISLOCATIONS OF THE KNEE JOINT

Angelini FJ, Helito CP, Bonadio MB, et al.: External fixation for treatment of the sub-acute and chronic multi-ligament-injured knee, *Knee Surg Sports Traumatol Arthrosc* 23:3012, 2015.

Arom GA, Yeranosian MG, Petrigliano FA, et al.: The changing demographics of knee dislocation: a retrospective database review, *Clin Orthop Relat Res* 472:2609, 2014.

Azar FM, Brandt JC, Miller 3rd RH, et al.: Ultra-low velocity knee dislocations, *Am J Sports Med* 39:2170, 2011.

Bonnevialle P, Dubrana F, Galau B, et al.: Common peroneal palsy complicating knee dislocation and bicruciate ligament tears, *Orthop Traumatol Surg Res* 96:64, 2010.

Boyce RH, Singh K, Obremskey WT: Acute management of traumatic knee dislocation for the generalist, *J Am Acad Orthop Surg* 23:761, 2015.

Darcy G, Edwards E, Hau R: Epidemiology and outcomes of traumatic knee dislocations: isolated vs multi-trauma injuries, *Injury* 49:1183, 2018.

Derby E, Imrecke J, Henckel J, et al.: How sensitive and specific is 1.5 Tesla MRI for diagnosing injuries in patients with knee dislocation? *Knee Surg Sports Traumatol Arthrosc* 25:517, 2017.

Eranki V, Begg C, Wallace B: Outcomes of operatively treated acute knee dislocations, *Open Orthop J* 4:22, 2010.

Fanelli GC: Timing of repair or reconstruction after knee dislocation, *J Knee Surg*, 2019 Nov 4, [Epub ahead or print].

Fanelli GC, Sousa PL, Edson CJ: Long-term followup of surgically treated knee dislocations: stability restored, but arthritis is common, *Clin Orthop Relat Res* 472:2712, 2014.

Fanelli GC, Stannard JP, Stuart MJ, et al.: Management of complex knee ligament injuries, *Instr Course Lect* 60:523, 2011.

Ferrari MB, Chahla J, Mitchell JJ, et al.: Multiligament reconstruction of the knee in the setting of knee dislocation with a medial-sided injury, *Arthroscopy Tech* 6:e341, 2017.

Gella S, Whelan DB, Stannard JP, et al.: Acute management and surgical timing of the multiligament-injured knee, *Instr Course Lect* 64:531, 2015.

Georgiadis AG, Mohammad FH, Mizerik KT, et al.: Changing presentation of knee dislocation and vascular injury from high-energy trauma to low-energy falls in the morbidly obese, *J Vasc Surg* 57:1196, 2013.

Gimbr LH, Scalcione LR, Rowan A, et al.: Multiligamentous injuries and knee dislocations, *Skeletal Radiol* 44:1559, 2015.

Gray JL, Cindric M: Management of arterial and venous injuries in the dislocated knee, *Sports Med Arthrosc* 19:131, 2011.

Halvorson JJ, Anz A, Langfitt M, et al.: Vascular injury associated with extremity trauma: initial diagnosis and management, *J Am Acad Orthop Surg* 19:495, 2011.

Heitmann M, Akoto R, Krause M, et al.: Management of acute knee dislocations: anatomic repair and ligament bracing as a new treatment option—results of a multicenter study, *Knee Surg Sports Traumatol Arthrosc* 27:2710, 2019.

Hirschmann MT, Meier MD, Amsler F, Friederich NF: Long-term outcome of patients treated surgically for traumatic knee dislocation: does the injury pattern matter? *Phys Sportsmed* 38:82, 2010.

Hirschmann MT, Zimmerman N, Rhychen T, et al.: Clinical and radiological outcomes after management of traumatic knee dislocation by open single stage complete reconstruction/repair, *BMC Musculoskelet Disord* 11:102, 2010.

Howells NR, Brunton LR, Robinson J, et al.: Acute knee dislocation: an evidence based approach to the management of the multiligament injured knee, *Injury* 42:1198, 2011.

Khakha RS, Day AC, Gibbs J, et al.: Acute surgical management of traumatic knee dislocations—average follow-up of 10 years, *Knee* 23:267, 2016.

Krych A, Sousa PL, King AH, et al.: Meniscal tears and articular cartilage damage in the dislocated knee, *Knee Surg Sports Traumatol Arthrosc* 23:3019, 2015.

Lachman JR, Rehman S, Pipitone PS: Traumatic knee dislocations: evaluation, management, and surgical treatment, *Orthop Clin North Am* 46:479, 2015.

LaPrade RF, Chahla J, DePhillipo NN, et al.: Single-stage multiple-ligament knee reconstructions for sports-related injuries: outcomes in 194 patients, *Am J Sports Med* 47:2563, 2019.

Levy BA, Boyd JL, Stuart MJ: Surgical treatment of acute and chronic anterior and posterior cruciate ligament and lateral side injuries of the knee, *Sports Med Arthrosc* 19:110, 2011.

Levy BA, Krych AJ, Shah JP, et al.: Staged protocol for initial management of the dislocated knee, *Knee Surg Sports Traumatol Arthrosc* 18:1630, 2010.

Maslaris A, Brinkmann O, Bungartz M, et al.: Management of knee dislocation prior to ligament reconstruction: what is the current evidence? Update of a universal treatment algorithm, *Eur J Orthop Surg Traumatol* 28:1001, 2018.

Matthewson G, Kwapisz A, Sasyniuk T, et al.: Vascular injury in the multiligament injured knee, *Clin Sports Med* 38:199, 2019.

McKee L, Ibrahim MS, Lawrence T, et al.: Current concepts in acute knee dislocation: the missed diagnosis? *Open Orthop J* 8:162, 2014.

Medina O, Arom GA, Yeranosian MG, et al.: Vascular and nerve injury after knee dislocation: a systematic review, *Clin Orthop Relat Res* 472:2621, 2014.

Mercer D, Firoozbakhsh K, Prevost M, et al.: Stiffness of knee-spanning external fixation systems for traumatic knee dislocations: a biomechanical study, *J Orthop Trauma* 24:693, 2010.

Merritt AL, Wahl C: Initial assessment of the acute and chronic multiple-ligament injured (dislocated) knee, *Sports Med Arthrosc* 19:93, 2011.

Moatshe G, Dornan GJ, Løken S, et al.: Demographics and injuries associated with knee dislocation: a prospective review of 303 patients, *Orthop J Sports Med* 5:2325967117706521, 2017.

Moatshe G, Dornan GJ, Ludvigsen T, et al.: High prevalence of knee osteoarthritis at a minimum 10-year follow-up after knee dislocation surgery, *Knee Surg Sports Traumatol Arthrosc* 25:3914, 2017.

Natsuhara KM, Yeranosian MG, Cohen JR, et al.: What is the frequency of vascular injury after knee dislocation? *Clin Orthop Relat Res* 472:2615, 2014.

Nicandri GT, Dunbar RP, Wahl CJ: Are evidence-based protocols which identify vascular injury associated with knee dislocation underutilized? *Knee Surg Sports Traumatol Arthrosc* 18:1005, 2010.

Nicandri GT, Slaney SL, Neradilek MB, et al.: Can magnetic resonance imaging predict posterior drawer laxity at the time of surgery in patients with knee dislocation or multiple-ligament knee injury? *Am J Sports Med* 39:1053, 2011.

Parker S, Handa A, Deakin M, Sideso E: Knee dislocation and vascular injury: 4-year experience at a UK Major Trauma Centre and vascular hub, *Injury* 47:752, 2016.

Peskun CJ, Levy BA, Fanelli GC, et al.: Diagnosis and management of knee dislocations, *Phys Sportsmed* 38:101, 2010.

Peskun CJ, Whelan DB: Outcomes of operative and nonoperative treatment of multiligament knee injuries: an evidence-based review, *Sports Med Arthrosc* 19:198, 2011.

Rajeswaran G, Williams A, Mitchell AW: Radiology and management of multiligament injuries of the knee, *Semin Musculoskelet Radiol* 15:42, 2011.

Ranger P, Renaud A, Phan P, et al.: Evaluation of reconstructive surgery using artificial ligaments in 71 acute knee dislocations, *Int Orthop* 35:1477, 2011.

Rhon DI, Perez KG, Eskridge SL: Risk of post-traumatic knee osteoarthritis after knee injury in military service members, *Muscoskel Care* 17:113, 2019.

Samson D, Ng CY, Power D: An evidence-based algorithm for the management of common peroneal nerve injury associated with traumatic knee dislocation, *EFFORT Open Rev* 1:362, 2017.

Sanders TL, Johnson NR, Levy NM, et al.: Effect of vascular injury on functional outcome in knees with multi-ligament injury: a matched-cohort analysis, *J Bone Joint Surg Am* 99:1565, 2017.

Sillanpää PJ, Kannus P, Niemi ST, et al.: Incidence of knee dislocation and concomitant vascular injury requiring surgery: a nationwide study, *J Trauma Acute Care Surg* 76:715, 2014.

Stannard JP, Nuelle CW, McGwin G, Volgas DA: Hinged external fixation in the treatment of knee dislocations: a prospective randomized study, *J Bone Joint Surg* 96A:184, 2014.

Stewart RJ, Landy DC, Khazai RS, et al.: Association of injury energy level and neurovascular injury following knee dislocation, *J Orthop Trauma* 32:579, 2018.

Tay AK, MacDonald PB: Complications associated with treatment of multiple ligament injured (dislocated) knee, *Sports Med Arthrosc* 19:153, 2011.

Tocci SL, Heard WM, Fadale PD, et al.: Magnetic resonance angiography for the evaluation of vascular injuries in knee dislocations, *J Knee Surg* 23:201, 2010.

Vaidya R, Roth M, Nanavati D, Prince M, Sethi A: Low-velocity knee dislocations in obese and morbidly obese patients, *Orthop J Sports Med* 3(4), 2015. 2325967115575719.

Vicenti G, Solarino G, Carrozzo M, et al.: Major concern in the multiligament-injured knee treatment: a systematic review, *Injury* 50(Suppl 2):S89, 2019.

Werner BC, Gwathmey Jr FW, Higgins ST, et al.: Ultra-low velocity knee dislocation: patient characteristics, complications, and outcomes, *Am J Sports Med* 42:358, 2014.

Woodmass JM, Johnson NR, Mohan R, et al.: Poly-traumatic multi-ligament knee injuries: is the knee the limiting factor? *Knee Surg Sports Traumatol Arthrosc* 26:2865, 2018.

Woodmass JM, O'Malley MP, Krych AJ, et al.: Revision multiligament knee reconstruction: clinical outcomes and proposed treatment algorithm, *Arthroscopy* 34:736, 2018.

Woodmass JM, Romatowski NP, Esposito JG, et al.: A systematic review of peroneal nerve palsy and recovery following traumatic knee dislocation, *Knee Surg Sports Traumatol Arthrosc* 23:2992, 2015.

Xu B, Xu H, Tu J, et al.: Initial assessment and implications for surgery: the missed diagnosis of irreducible knee dislocation, *J Knee Surg* 31:254, 2018.

SYNOVIAL PLICA

Benedetti M, Spinosa M, Mechelli F: Plica syndrome and bilateral osteochondritis dissecans, *J Orthop Sports Phys Ther* 49:762, 2019.

Guney A, Bilal O, Oner M, et al.: Short- and mid-term results of plica excision in patients with mediopatellar plica and associated cartilage degeneration, *Knee Surg Sports Traumatol Arthrosc* 18:1526, 2010.

Hayashi D, Xu L, Guermazi A, et al.: Prevalence of MRI-detected mediopatellar plica in subjects with knee pain and the association with MRI-detected patellofemoral cartilage damage and bone marrow lesions: data from the Joints on Glucosaine study, *BMC Musculoskelet Disord* 14:292, 2013.

Hufeland M, Treder L, Kubo HK, et al.: Symptomatic medial synovial plica of the knee joint: an underestimated pathology in young patients, *Arch Orthop Trauma Surg* 139:1625, 2019.

Kent M, Khanduja V: Synovial plicae around the knee, *Knee* 17:97, 2010.

Kosaka M, Nakase J, Kitaoka K, et al.: Arthroscopic treatment of symptomatic lateral synovial plica of the knee, *J Orthop Surg (Hong Kong)* 27: 2309499019834496, 2019.

Lee PYF, Nixion A, Chandratreya A, et al.: Synovial plica syndrome of the knee: a commonly overlooked cause of anterior knee pain, *Surg J* 3:e9, 2017.

Lee YH, Song HT, Kim S, et al.: Infrapatellar plica of the knee: revisited with MR arthrographies undertaken in the knee flexion position mimicking operative arthroscopic posture, *Eur J Radiol* 81:2783, 2012.

Ozcan M, Coporuglu C, Ciftdemir M, et al.: Does an abnormal infrapatellar plica increase the risk of chondral damage in the knee, *Knee Surg Sports Traumatol Arthrosc* 19:218, 2011.

Schindler OS: "The Sneaky Pica" revisited: morphology, pathophysiology and treatment of synovial plicae of the knee, *Knee Surg Sports Traumatol Arthrosc* 22:247, 2014.

Stubbings N, Smith T: Diagnostic test accuracy of clinical and radiological assessments for medial patella plica syndrome: a systematic review and meta-analysis, *Knee* 21:486, 2014.

Weckström M, Niva MH, Lamminen A, et al.: Arthroscopic resection of medial plica of the knee in young adults, *Knee* 17:103, 2010.

ARTICULAR CARTILAGE INJURIES

Ahmed TA, Hincke MT: Strategies for articular cartilage lesion repair and functional restoration, *Tissue Eng Part B Rev* 16:305, 2010.

Albrecht C, Reuter CA, Stelzeneder D, et al.: Matrix production affects MRI outcomes after matrix-associated autologous chondrocyte transplantation in the knee, *Am J Sports Med* 45:2238, 2017.

Anderson JA, Little D, Toth AP, et al.: Stem cell therapies for knee cartilage repair: the current status of preclinical and clinical studies, *Am J Sports Med* 42:2253, 2014.

Balazs GC, Wang D, Burge AJ, et al.: Return to play among elite basketball players after osteochondral allograft transplantation of full-thickness cartilage lesions, *Ortho J Sports Med* 6:2325967118786941, 2018.

Barakat AS, Ibrahim NM, Elghobashy O, et al.: Prevention of post-traumatic osteoarthritis after intra-articular knee fractures using hyaluronic acid: a randomized prospective pilot study, *Int Orthop* 43:2437, 2019.

Bedi A, Feeley BT, Williams 3rd RJ: Management of articular cartilage defects of the knee, *J Bone Joint Surg* 92A:994, 2010.

Behery O, Siston RA, Harris JD, Flanigan DC: Treatment of cartilage defects of the knee: expanding on the existing algorithm, *Clin J Sport Med* 24:21, 2014.

Benthien JP, Schwaninger M, Behrens P: We do not have evidence-based methods for the treatment of cartilage defects in the knee, *Knee Surg Sports Traumatol Arthrosc* 19:543, 2011.

Bentley G, Biant LC, Vijayan S, et al.: Minimum ten-year results of a prospective randomised study of autologous chondrocyte implantation versus mosiacplasty for symptomatic articular cartilage lesions of the knee, *J Bone Joint Surg* 94B:504, 2012.

Biant LC, Bentley G, Vigayan S, et al.: Long-term results of autologous chondrocyte implantation in the knee for chronic chondral and osteochondral defects, *Am J Sports Med* 42:2178, 2014.

Blackman AJ, Smith MV, Flanigan DC, et al.: Correlation between magnetic resonance imaging and clinical outcomes after cartilage repair surgery in the knee: a systematic review and meta-analysis, *Am J Sports Med* 41:1426, 2013.

Brittberg M: Cell carriers as the next generation of cell therapy for cartilage repair: a review of the matrix-induced autologous chondrocyte implantation procedure, *Am J Sports Med* 38:1259, 2010.

Chu CR, Williams AA, West RV, et al.: Quantitative magnetic resonance imaging UTE-T2* mapping of cartilage and meniscus healing after anatomic anterior cruciate ligament reconstruction, *Am J Sports Med* 42:1847, 2014.

Cole BJ, Farr J, Winalski CS, et al.: Outcomes after a single-stage procedure for cell-based cartilage repair: a prospective clinical safety trial with 2-year follow-up, *Am J Sports Med* 39:1170, 2011.

Cotter EJ, Hannon CP, Christian DR, et al.: Clinical outcomes of multifocal osteochondral allograft transplantation of the knee: an analysis of overlapping grafts and multifocal lesions, *Am J Sports Med* 46:2884, 2018.

Crawford ZT, Schumaier AP, Glogovac G, et al.: Return to sport and sports-specific outcomes after osteochondral allograft transplantation in the knee: a systematic review of studies with at least 2 years' mean follow-up, *Arthroscopy* 35:1880, 2019.

Devitt BM, Bell SW, Webster KE, et al.: Surgical treatment of cartilage defects of the knee: systematic review of randomised controlled trials, *Knee* 24:508, 2017.

Dhollander AA, Verdonk PC, Lambrecht S, et al.: Short-term outcome of the second generation characterized chondrocyte implantation for the treatment of cartilage lesions in the knee, *Knee Surg Sports Traumatol Arthrosc* 20:1773, 2012.

Dold AP, Zywiel MG, Taylor DW, et al.: Platelet-rich plasma in the management of articular cartilage pathology: a systematic review, *Clin J Sport Med* 24:31, 2014.

Ebert JR, Fallon M, Smith A, et al.: Prospective clinical and radiologic evaluation of patellofeoral matrix-induced autologous chondrocyte implantation, *Am J Sports Med* 43:1362, 2015.

Erdil M, Bilsel K, Taser OF, et al.: Osteochondral autologous graft transfer system in the knee: mid-term results, *Knee* 20:2, 2013.

Fabricant PPD, Yen YM, Kramer DE, et al.: Fixation of traumatic chondral-only fragments of the knee in pediatric and adolescent athletes: a retrospective multicenter report, *Orthop J Sports Med* 6:23259671177531, 2018.

Farr J, Tabet SK, Margerrison E, Cole BJ: Clinical, radiographic, and histological outcomes after cartilage repair with particulated juvenile articular cartilage: a 2-year prospective study, *Am J Sports Med* 42:1417, 2014.

Fazalare JA, Griesser MJ, Siston RA, Flanigan DC: The use of continuous passive motion following knee cartilage defect surgery: a systematic review, *Orthopedics* 33:878, 2010.

Filardo G, Kon E, Berruto M, et al.: Arthroscopic second general autologous chondrocytes implantation associated with bone grafting for the treatment of knee osteochondritis dissecans: results at 6 years, *Knee* 19:658, 2012.

Filardo G, Kon E, Di Martino A, et al.: Arthroscopic second-generation autologous chondrocyte implantation: a prospective 7-year follow-up study, *Am J Sports Med* 39:2153, 2011.

Filardo G, Di Matteo B, Di Martino A, et al.: Platelet-rich plasma intra-articular knee injections show no superiority versus viscosupplementation: a randomized controlled trial, *Am J Sports Med* 43:1575, 2015.

Frank RM, McCormick F, Rosas S, et al.: Reoperation rates after cartilage restoration procedures in the knee: analysis of a large US commercial database, *Am J Orthop (Belle Mead NJ)* 47(6):1, 2018.

Gigante A, Calcagno S, Cecconi S, et al.: Use of collagen scaffold and autologous bone marrow concentrate as a one-step cartilage repair in the knee: histological results of second-look biopsies at 1-year follow-up, *Int J Immunopathol Pharmacol* 24(1 Suppl 2):69, 2011.

Gobbi A, Karnatzikos G, Kumar A: Long-term results after microfracture treatment for full-thickness knee chondral lesions in athletes, *Knee Surg Sports Traumatol Arthrosc* 22, 1986, 2014.

Gomoli AH, Farr J, Gillogly SD, et al.: Surgical management of articular cartilage defects of the knee, *Instr Course Lect* 60:461, 2011.

Gou GH, Tseng FJ, Wang SH, et al.: Autologous chondrocyte implantation versus microfracture in the knee: a meta-analysis and systematic review, *Arthroscopy*, 2019 Nov 7, [Epub ahead of print].

Gowd AK, Cvetanovich GL, Liu JN, et al.: Management of chondral lesions of the knee: analysis of trends and short-term complications using the National Surgical Quality Improvement Program Database, *Arthroscopy* 35:138, 2019.

Hancock KJ, Westermann RR, Shamrock AG, et al.: Trends in knee articular cartilage treatments: an American Board of Orthopaedic Surgery database study, *J Knee Surg* 32:85, 2019.

Harris JD, Brophy RH, Siston RA, Flanigan DC: Treatment of chondral defects in the athlete's knee, *Arthroscopy* 26:841, 2010.

Harris JD, Hussey K, Wilson H, et al.: Biological knee reconstruction for combined malalignment, meniscal deficiency, and articular cartilage damage, *Arthroscopy* 31:275, 2015.

Harris JD, Siston RA, Pan X, Flanigan DC: Autologous chondrocyte implantation: a systematic review, *J Bone Joint Surg* 92A:2220, 2010.

Heyworth BE, Edmonds EW, Murnaghan ML, Kocher MS: Drilling techniques for osteochondritis dissecans, *Clin Sports Med* 33:305, 2014.

Hoburg A, Löer I, Körsmeier K, et al.: Matrix-associated autologous chondrocyte implantation is an effective treatment at midterm follow-up in adolescents and young adults, *Orthop J Sports Med* 7:2325967119841077, 2019.

Kanneganti P, Harris JD, Brophy RH, et al.: The effect of smoking on ligament and cartilage surgery in the knee: a systematic review, *Am J Sports Med* 40:2872, 2012.

Keng A, Sayre EC, Guermazi A, et al.: Association of body mass index with knee cartilage damage in an asymptomatic population-based study, *BMC Musculoskelet Disord* 18:517, 2017.

Khan WS, Johnson DS, Hardingham TE: The potential of stem cells in the treatment of knee cartilage defects, *Knee* 17:369, 2010.

Kon E, Filardo G, Berruto M, et al.: Articular cartilage treatment in high-level male soccer players: a prospective comparative study of arthroscopic second-generation autologous chondrocyte implantation versus microfracture, *Am J Sports Med* 39:2549, 2011.

Kon E, Filardo G, Condello V, et al.: Second-generation autologous chondrocyte implantation: results in patients older than 40 years, *Am J Sports Med* 39:1668, 2011.

Kreuz PC, Kalkreuth RH, Niemeyer P, et al.: Long-term clinical and MRI results of matrix-assisted autologous chondrocyte implantation for articular cartilage defects of the knee, *Cartilage* 10:305, 2019.

Kreuz PC, Müller S, von Keudell A, et al.: Influence of sex on the outcome of autologous chondrocyte implantation in chondral defects of the knee, *Am J Sports Med* 41:1541, 2013.

Krych AJ, Robertson CM, Williams 3rd RJ: Cartilage Study Group: return to athletic activity after osteochondral allograft transplantation in the knee, *Am J Sports Med* 40:1053, 2012.

Landsdown DA, Wang K, Cotter E, et al.: Relationship between quantitative MRI biomarkers and patient-reported outcome measures after cartilage repair surgery: a systematic review, *Orthop J Sports Med* 6:2325967118765448, 2018.

Lee S, Frank RM, Christian DR, et al.: Analysis of defect size and ratio to condylar size with respect to outcomes after isolated osteochondral allograft transplantation, *Am J Sports Med* 47:1601, 2019.

Levy YD, Görtz S, Pulido PA, et al.: Do fresh osteochondral allografts successfully treat femoral condyle lesions? *Clin Orthop Relat Res* 471:231, 2013.

Lim HC, Bae JH, Park YE, et al.: Long-term results of arthroscopic excision of unstable osteochondral lesions of the lateral femoral condyle, *J Bone Joint Surg* 94B:185, 2012.

Løken S, Heir S, Holme I, et al.: 6-year follow-up of 84 patients with cartilage defects in the knee: knee scores improved but recovery was incomplete, *Acta Orthop* 81:611, 2010.

Longley R, Ferreira AM, Gentile P: Recent approaches to the manufacturing of biomimetic multi-phasic scaffolds for osteochondral regeneration, *Int J Mol Sci* 19:1755, 2018.

Mall NA, Harris JD, Cole BJ: Clinical evaluation and preoperative planning of articular cartilage lesions of the knee, *J Am Acad Orthop Surg* 23:633, 2015.

McIlwraith CW, Frisbie DD, Rodkey WG, et al.: Evaluation of intra-articular mesenchymal stem cells to augment healing of microfractured chondral defects, *Arthroscopy* 27:1552, 2011.

Monckeberg JE, Rafols C, Apablaza F, et al.: Intra-articular administration of peripheral blood stem cells with platelet-rich plasma regenerated articular and improved clinical outcomes for knee chondral lesions, *Knee* 26:824, 2019.

Montgomery SR, Foster BD, Ngo SS, et al.: Trends in the surgical treatment of articular cartilage defects of the knee in the United States, *Knee Surg Sports Traumatol Arthrosc* 22, 2014, 2070.

Moran CJ, Pascual-Garrido C, Chubinskaya S, et al.: Restoration of articular cartilage, *J Bone Joint Surg* 96A:336, 2014.

Neilsen ES, McCauley JC, Pulida PA, et al.: Return to sport and recreational activity after osteochondral allograft transplantation in the knee, *Am J Sports Med* 45:1608, 2017.

Nepple JJ, Wright RW, Matava MJ, Brophy RH: Full-thickness knee articular cartilage defects in National Football League combine athletes undergoing magnetic resonance imaging: prevalence, location, and association with previous surgery, *Arthroscopy* 28:798, 2012.

Niemeyer P, Köstler W, Salzmann GM, et al.: Autologous chondrocyte implantation for treatment of focal cartilage defects in patients age 40 years and older: a matched-pair analysis with 2-year follow-up, *Am J Sports Med* 38:2410, 2010.

Niemeyer P, Porichis S, Steinwachs M, et al.: Long-term outcomes after first-generation autologous chondrocyte implantation for cartilage defects of the knee, *Am J Sports Med* 42:150, 2014.

Nishizawa Y, Matsumoto T, Araki D, et al.: Matching articular surfaces of selected donor and recipient sites for cylindrical osteochondral grafts of the femur: quantitative evaluation using a 3-dimensional laser scanner, *Am J Sports Med* 42:658, 2014.

Noyes FR, Fleckenstein CM, Barber-Westin SD: The development of postoperative knee chondrolysis after intra-articular pain pump infusion of an anesthetic medication: a series of twenty-one cases, *J Bone Joint Surg* 94A:1448, 2012.

Ogura T, Mosier BA, Bryant T, et al.: A 20-year follow-up after first-generation autologous chondrocyte implantation, *Am J Sports Med* 45:2751, 2017.

Oussedik S, Tsitskaris K, Parker D: Treatment of articular cartilage lesions of the knee by microfracture or autologous chondrocyte implantation: a systematic review, *Arthroscopy* 31:732, 2015.

Pareek A, Reardon PJ, Macalena JA, et al: Osteochondral autograft transfer versus microfracture in the knee: a meta-analysis of prospective comparative studies at midterm, *Arthroscopy* 32:2118, 2916.

Pereira H, Cengiz IF, Vilela C, et al.: Emerging concepts in treating cartilage, osteochondral defects, and osteoarthritis of the knee and ankle, *Adv Exp Med Biol* 1059:25, 2018.

Pisanu G, Cottino U, Rosso F, et al.: Large osteochondral allografts of the knee: surgical technique and indications, *Joints* 6:42, 2018.

Quatman CE, Quatman-Yates CC, Scmitt LC, Paterno MV: The clinical utility and diagnostic performance of MRI for identification and classification of knee osteochondritis dissecans, *J Bone Joint Surg* 94A:1036, 2012.

Redondo ML, Beer AJ, Yanke AB: Cartilage restoration: microfracture and osteochondral autograft transplantation, *J Knee Surg* 31:231, 2018.

Reed ME, Villacis DC, Hatch 3rd FJ, et al.: 3.0-Tesla MRI and arthroscopy for assessment of knee cartilage lesions, *Orthopedics* 36:e1060, 2013.

Richter DL, Schenck Jr RC, Wascher DC, et al.: Knee articular cartilage repair and restoration techniques: a review of the literature, *Sports Health* 8:153, 2016.

Rodriguez-Merchan EC, Valentino LA: The role of gene therapy in cartilage repair, *Arch Bone Jt Surg* 7:79, 2019.

Safran MR, Seiber K: The evidence for surgical repair of articular cartilage in the knee, *J Am Acad Orthop Surg* 18:259, 2010.

Schneider U, Rackwitz L, Andereya S, et al.: A prospective multicenter study on the outcome of type I collagen hydrogel-based autologous chondrocyte implantation (CaReS) for the repair of articular cartilage defects in the knee, *Am J Sports Med* 39:2558, 2011.

Scilla AJ, Aune KT, Andrachuk JS, et al.: Return to play after chondroplasty of the knee in National Football League athletes, *Am J Sports Med* 43:663, 2015.

Sgaglione NA, Chen E, Bert JM, et al.: Current strategies for nonsurgical, arthroscopic, and minimally invasive surgical treatment of knee cartilage pathology, *Instr Course Lect* 59:157, 2010.

Solheim E, Hegna J, Strand T, et al.: Randomized study of long-term (15-17 years) outcome after microfracture versus mosaicplasty in knee articular cartilage defects, *Am J Sports Med* 46:826, 2018.

Steinwachs M, Caqvalcanti N, Mauuva Venkatesh Reddy S, et al.: Arthroscopic and open treatment of cartilage lesions with BST-CARGEL scaffold and microfracture: a cohort study of consecutive patients, *Knee* 26:174, 2019.

Tírico LEP, McCauley JC, Pulido PA, et al.: Is patient satisfaction associated with clinical outcomes after osteochondral allograft transplantation in the knee? *Am J Sports Med* 47:82, 2019.

Van Assche D, Staes F, Van Caspel D, et al.: Autologous chondrocyte implantation versus microfracture for knee cartilage injury: a prospective randomized trial, with 2-year follow-up, *Knee Surg Sports Traumatol Arthrosc* 18:486, 2010.

Vanlauwe J, Saris DB, Victor J, et al.: Five-year outcome of characterized chondrocyte implantation versus microfracture for symptomatic cartilage defects of the knee: early treatment matters, *Am J Sports Med* 39:2566, 2011.

Vascellari A, Rebuzzi E, Schiavetti S, Coletti N: Implantation of matrix-induced autologous chondrocyte (MACI) grafts using carbon dioxide insufflation arthroscopy, *Knee Surg Sports Traumatol Arthrosc* 22:219, 2014.

Verdonk P, Dhollander A, Almqvist KF, et al.: Treatment of osteochondral lesions in the knee using a cell-free scaffold, *Bone Joint Lett J* 97:318, 2015.

Vijayan S, Bartlett W, Bentley G, et al.: Autologous chondrocyte implantation for osteochondral lesions in the knee using a bilayer collagen membrane and bone graft: a two- to eight-year follow-up study, *J Bone Joint Surg* 94B:488, 2012.

Wang D, Chang B, Coxe FR, et al.: Clinically meaningful improvement after treatment of cartilage defects of the knee with osteochondral grafts, *Am J Sports Med* 47:71, 2019.

Wang T, Wang DX, Burge AJ, et al.: Clinical and MRI outcomes of fresh osteochondral allograft transplantation after failed cartilage repair surgery in the knee, *J Bone Joint Surg Am* 100:2018, 1949.

Weber AE, Locker PH, Mayer EN, et al.: Clinical outcomes after microfracture of the knee: midterm follow-up, *Orthop J Sports Med* 6:2325967117753572, 2018.

Wyatt RW, Inacio MC, Liddle KD, Maletis GB: Prevalence and incide3nce of cartilage injuries and meniscus tears in patients who underwent both primary and revision anterior cruciate ligament reconstructions, *Am J Sports Med* 42:1841, 2014.

Wylie JD, Hartley MK, Kapron AL, et al.: What is the effect of matrices on cartilage repair? A systematic review, *Clin Orthop Relat Res* 473:1673, 2015.

Zaffagnini S, Vannini F, Di Martino A, et al.: Low rate of return to pre-injury sport level in athletes after cartilage surgery: a 10-year follow-up study, *Knee Surg Sports Traumatol Arthrosc* 27:2502, 2019.

OSTEOCHONDRITIS DISSECANS

Adachi N, Deie M, Nakamae A, et al.: Functional and radiographic outcomes of unstable juvenile osteochondritis dissecans of the knee treatment with lesion fixation using bioabsorbable pins, *J Pediat Orthop* 35:82, 2015.

Andriolo L, Crawford DC, Reale D, et al.: Osteochondritis dissecans of the knee: etiology and pathogenic mechanisms: a systematic review, *Cartilage*, 2018 Jul 1, [Epub ahead of print].

Bauer KL: Osteochondral injuries of the knee in pediatric patients, *J Knee Surg* 31:382, 2018.

Carey JL, Grimm NL: Treatment algorithm for osteochondritis dissecans of the knee, *Clin Sports Med* 33:375, 2014.

Chambers HG, Shea KG, Anderson AF, et al.: American Academy of Orthopaedic Surgeons clinical practice guideline on: the diagnosis and treatment of osteochondritis dissecans, *J Bone Joint Surg* 94A:1322, 2012.

Chambers HG, Shea KG, Anderson AF, et al.: Diagnosis and treatment of osteochondritis dissecans, *J Am Acad Orthop Surg* 19:297, 2011.

Chambers HG, Shea KG, Carey JL: AAOS Clinical Practice Guideline: diagnosis and treatment of osteochondritis dissecans, *J Am Acad Orthop Surg* 19:307, 2011.

Chow RM, Guzman MS, Dao Q: Intercondylar notch width as a risk factor for medial femoral condyle osteochondritis dissecans in skeletally immature patients, *J Pediat Orthop* 36:640, 2016.

Cole BJ, DeBerardino T, Brewster R, et al.: Outcomes of autologous chondrocyte implantation in study of the treatment of articular repair (STAR) patients with osteochondritis dissecans, *Am J Sports Med* 40, 2015, 2012.

Delcogliano M, Menghi A, Piacella G, et al.: Treatment of osteochondritis dissecans of the knee with a biomimetic scaffold. A prospective multicenter study, *Joints* 2:102, 2014.

Grimm NL, Ewing CK, Ganley TJ: The knee: internal fixation techniques for osteochondritis dissecans, *Clin Sports Med* 33:313, 2014.

Grimm NL, Weiss JM, Kessler JI, Aoki SK: Osteochondritis dissecans of the knee: pathoanatomy, epidemiology, and diagnosis, *Clin Sports Med* 33:181, 2014.

Hevesi M, Sanders TL, Pareek A, et al.: Osteochondritis dissecans of the knee of skeletally immature patients: rates of persistent pain, osteoarthritis, and arthroplast at mean 14 years' follow-up, *Cartilage*, 2018 Jul 1, [Epub ahead of print].

Jacobi M, Wahl P, Bouaicha S, et al.: Association between mechanical axis of the leg and osteochondritis dissecans of the knee: radiographic study on 103 knees, *Am J Sports Med* 38:1425, 2010.

Jacobs Jr JC, Archibald-Seiffer N, Grimm NL, et al.: A review of arthroscopic classification systems for osteochondritis dissecans of the knee, *Orthop Clin North Am* 46:133, 2015.

Jones MH, Williams AM: Osteochondritis dissecans of the knee: a practical guide for surgeons, *Bone Joint Lett J* 98B:723, 2016.

Kessler JI, Jacobs Jr JC, Cannamela PC, et al.: Childhood obesity is associated with osteochondritis dissecans of the knee, ankle, and elbow in children and adolescents, *J Pediatr Orthop* 38:e296, 2018.

Kessler JI, Nikizad H, Shea KG, et al.: The demographic and epidemiology of osteochondritis dissecans of the knee in children and adolescents, *Am J Sports Med* 42:320, 2014.

Kramer DE, Yen YM, Simoni MK, et al.: Surgical management of osteochondritis dissecans lesions of the patella and trochlea in the pediatric and adolescent population, *Am J Sports Med* 43:654, 2015.

Masquijo J, Kothari A: Juvenile osteochondritis dissecans (JOCD) of the knee: current concepts review, *EFFORT Open Rev* 4:2901, 2019.

Millington KL, Shah JP, Dahm DL, et al.: Bioabsorbable fixation of unstable osteochondritis dissecans lesions, *Am J Sports Med* 38:2065, 2010.

Ochs BG, Müller-Horvat C, Albrecht D, et al.: Remodeling of articular cartilage and subchondral bone after bone grafting and matrix-associated autologous chondrocyte implantation for osteochondritis dissecans of the knee, *Am J Sports Med* 39:764, 2011.

Sacolick DA, Kirven JC, Abouljoud MM, et al.: The treatment of adult osteochondritis dissecans with autologous cartilage implantation: a systematic review, *J Knee Surg* 32:1102, 2019.

Sanders TL, Pareek A, Johnson NR, et al.: Nonoperative management of osteochondritis dissecans of the knee: progression to osteoarthritis and arthroplasty at mean 13-year follow-up, *Orthop J Sports Med* 5: 2325967117704644, 2017.

Sanders TL, Pareek A, Obey MR, et al.: High rate of osteoarthritis after osteochondritis dissecans fragment excision compared with surgical restoration at a mean 16-year follow-up, *Am J Sports Med* 45:1799, 2017.

Sekiya JK: Bone grafting and matrix-associated autologous chondrocyte implantation for osteochondritis dissecans of the knee, *J Bone Joint Surg* 93A:1, 2011.

Smolders JM, Kock NB, Koëter S, Van Susante JL: Osteochondral autograft transplantation for osteochondritis dissecans of the knee: preliminary results of a prospective case series, *Acta Orthop Belg* 76:208, 2010.

Steinhagen J, Bruns J, Deuretzbacher G, et al.: Treatment of osteochondritis dissecans of the femoral condyle with autologous bone grafts and matrix-supported autologous chondrocytes, *Int Orthop* 34:819, 2010.

Stone KR, Pelsis JR, Crues 3rd JV, et al.: Osteochondral grafting for failed knee osteochondritis dissecans repairs, *Knee* 21:1145, 2014.

Weiss J, Nikizad H, Shea KG, et al.: The incidence of surgery in osteochondritis dissecans in children and adolescents, *Orthop J Sports Med* 4: 2325967116635515, 2016.

Wu IT, Custers RJH, Desai VS, et al.: Internal fixation of unstable osteochondritis dissecans: do open growth plates improve healing rate? *Am J Sports Med* 46:2394, 2018.

DISORDERS OF THE PATELLA

Brophy RH, Wojahn RD, Lamplot JD: Cartilage restoration techniques for the patellofemoral joint, *J Am Acad Orthop Surg* 25:321, 2017.

Ferrari MB, Sanchez A, Sanchez G, et al.: Arthroscopic bony resection for treatment of symptomatic bipartite patella, *Arthrosc Tech* 6:e1003, 2017.

Fonseca F, Oliveira JP, Marques P: Maquet III procedure: what remains after initial complications—long-term results, *J Orthop Surg Res* 8:11, 2013.

Kusnezov N, Watts N, Belmont Jr PJ, et al.: Incidence and risk factors for chronic anterior knee pain, *J Knee Surg* 29:248, 2016.

Kwee TC, Sonneveld H, Nix M: Successful conservative management of symptomatic bilateral dorsal patellar defects presenting with cartilage involvement and bone marrow edema: MRI findings, *Skeletal Radiol* 45:723, 2016.

Macmull S, Jaiswal PK, Bentley G, et al.: The role of autologous chondrocyte implantation in the treatment of symptomatic chondromalacia patellae, *Int Orthop* 36:1371, 2012.

Matic GT, Flanigan DC: Efficacy of surgical interventions for bipartite patella, *Orthopedics* 37:623, 2014.

Matic GT, Flanigan DC: Return to activity among athletes with a symptomatic bipartite patella: a systematic review, *Knee* 22:280, 2015.

McMahon SE, LeRoux JA, Smith TO, et al.: The management of the painful bipartite patella: a systematic review, *Knee Surg Sports Traumatol Arthrosc* 24:2798, 2016.

Oohashi Y, Koshino T, Oohashi Y: Clinical features and classification of bipartite or tripartite patella, *Knee Surg Sports Traumatol Arthrosc* 18:1465, 2010.

Pak J, Lee JH, Lee SH: A novel biological approach to treat chondromalacia patellae, *PloS One* 8:e64569, 2013.

Pihlajamäki HK, Kuikka PI, Leppänen VV, et al.: Reliability of clinical findings and magnetic resonance imaging for the diagnosis of chondromalacia patellae, *J Bone Joint Surg* 92A:927, 2010.

Radha S, Shenouda M, Konan S, et al.: Successful treatment of painful synchondrosis of bipartite patella after direct trauma by operative fixaton: a series of six cases, *Open Orthop J* 11:390, 2017.

Tuna BK, Semiz-Oysu A, Pekar B, et al.: The association of patellofemoral joint morphology with chondromalacia patella: a quantitative MRI analysis, *Clin Imaging* 38:495, 2014.

van Eck CF, Kingston RS, Crues JV, et al.: Magnetic resonance imaging for patellofemoral chondromalacia: is there a role for T2 mapping? *Orthop J Sports Med* 5: 2325967117740554, 2017.

Vieira TD, Thaunat M, Saithna A, et al.: Surgical technique for arthroscopic resection of painful bipartite patella, *Arthrosc Tech* 6:e751, 2017.

EXTRAARTICULAR ANKYLOSIS OF THE KNEE

Hahn SB, Choi YR, Kang HJ, Lee SH: Prognostic factors and long-term outcomes following a modified Thompson's quadricepsplasty for severely stiff knees, *J Bone Joint Surg* 92B:217, 2010.

OPEN WOUNDS OF THE KNEE JOINT

Brubacher JW, Grote CW, Tilley MB: Traumatic arthrotomy, *J Am Acad Orthop Surg*, 2019 Aug 13, [Epub ahead of print].

Konda SR, Howard D, Davidovitch RI, Egol KA: The role of computed tomography in the assessment of open periarticular fractures associated with deep knee wounds, *J Orthop Trauma* 27:509, 2013.

Lee SY, Miikura T, Miwa M, et al.: Negative pressure wound therapy for the treatment of infected wounds with exposed knee joint after patellar fracture, *Orthopedics* 34:211, 2011.

Prokuski L, Clyburn TA, Evans RP, Moucha CS: Prophylactic antibiotics in orthopaedic surgery, *Instr Course Lect* 60:545, 2011.

Rehani B, Wissman R: Lead poisoning from a gunshot wound, *South Med J* 104:57, 2011.

The complete list of references is available online at ExpertConsult.com.

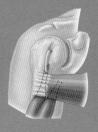

CHAPTER 2

SHOULDER AND ELBOW INJURIES
Robert H. Miller III, Frederick M. Azar, Thomas W. Throckmorton

SHOULDER INJURIES
ANATOMY AND BIOMECHANICS

The shoulder joint is composed of four articulations: the sternoclavicular, acromioclavicular, glenohumeral, and scapulothoracic that work together to allow smooth shoulder function. Together, they allow the shoulder joint to have the greatest range of motion of any joint in the body, and the relationship between these articulations must be considered when treating shoulder dysfunction. Normal function of the shoulder is a balance between mobility and stability. In addition to the four articulations, mobility is allowed by the "large ball–small socket" bony arrangement and the voluminous glenohumeral joint capsule, which does not restrict movement until the extremes of motion. The bony anatomy contributes little to stability and has been compared with a golf ball on a tee. The glenoid is encircled by the labrum, composed of dense fibrocartilaginous tissue, which increases the depth of the socket by 50% around the humeral head and increases stability. The glenoid articular surface and the labrum combine to create a socket that is approximately 9 mm deep in the superoinferior direction and 5 mm deep in the anteroposterior direction. Adding the glenoid labrum increases the glenoid surface to 75% of the humeral head vertically and 57% horizontally. Biomechanical testing of cadaver shoulder specimens showed that the labrum affects the distribution of contact stresses when a compressive load is applied to the shoulder at 90 degrees of abduction. Because there is very little bony constraint to the shoulder, most of the stability is provided by the surrounding muscles and ligaments.

The ligamentous constraints are the primary stabilizers at extremes of motion. The superior glenohumeral ligament is the primary restraint to inferior humeral subluxation in 0 degrees of abduction and is the primary stabilizer to anterior and posterior stress in the same position. Tightening of the rotator interval (which includes the superior glenohumeral ligament) decreases posterior and inferior translation. The middle glenohumeral ligament limits external rotation when the arm is in the lower and middle ranges of abduction but has little effect when the arm is in 90 degrees of abduction. The inferior glenohumeral ligament is composed of an anterior band that is quite thick, a posterior band that is less thick and distinct, and a thinner intervening axillary pouch, creating a hammock-type sling. With external rotation, the hammock slides anteriorly and superiorly, the anterior band tightens, and the posterior band fans out. With internal rotation, the opposite occurs. The anteroinferior glenohumeral ligament complex is the main stabilizer to anterior and posterior stresses when the shoulder is abducted 45 degrees or more.

The muscles of the shoulder joint can be divided into intrinsic and extrinsic groups. The extrinsic muscles primarily control movement of the scapula and include the rhomboids, levator scapulae, trapezius, and serratus anterior. The intrinsic muscles control the glenohumeral joint and include the rotator cuff muscles (subscapularis, supraspinatus, infraspinatus, and teres minor), the deltoid, the pectoralis major, the teres major, the latissimus dorsi, and the biceps brachii. The muscular constraints work in several ways to provide stability. First, they dynamically position the scapula to place the glenoid opposite the humeral head as the shoulder moves. Rowe compared the relationship to a "ball on a seal's nose." As the ball (humerus) moves, the seal (scapula and glenoid) moves to maintain the balanced relationship. Second, whereas ligaments work in a static fashion to limit translation and rotation, their stiffness and torsional rigidity are increased with concomitant muscle activity. Rotator cuff activity and biceps activity have been shown to stiffen the capsule and decrease glenohumeral translation. Third, intrinsic and extrinsic muscle groups serve as fine tuners of motion and power movers by working in "force couples." The force couples control and direct the force through the joint, contributing to stability. The most important such force couple involves the subscapularis and posterior rotator cuff. Together, these muscles provide a compressive force that centers the humeral head in the glenoid cavity and explains why some patients with massive superior rotator cuff tears can have remarkably well-preserved overhead activity. In particular, the teres minor has often been viewed as a minor contributor to rotator cuff function; however, there has been heightened attention to its contribution, particularly when the other cuff tendons fail.

The tendinous insertions of the rotator cuff muscles, the articular capsule, the coracohumeral ligament, and the glenohumeral ligament complex blend into a confluent sheet before insertion into the humeral tuberosities. The tendons of the infraspinatus and supraspinatus muscles join approximately 15 mm proximal to their insertion and cannot be readily separated by blunt dissection. The infraspinatus and teres minor fuse near their musculotendinous junctions. The supraspinatus and subscapularis tendons join as a sheath that surrounds the biceps tendon at the entrance of the bicipital groove. The roof of this sheath consists of a portion of the supraspinatus tendon, and a sheet of the subscapularis tendon forms the floor. This relationship is relevant to the frequent coexistence of subscapularis tendon tears with lesions and/or instability of the long head of the biceps. The coracohumeral ligament is a thick band of fibrous tissue extending from the coracoid process along the surface of the capsule to the tuberosities between the supraspinatus and subscapularis tendons. The ligament is deep to the tendinous insertion of the cuff and blends with the capsule and supraspinatus tendon to form part of the roof of the biceps sheath. A 1-cm wide thickening of fibrous tissue extends posteriorly from the coracohumeral ligament origin on the coracoid to the posterior margin of the infraspinatus. This band is an extension of the coracohumeral ligament and travels between the capsule and the cuff tendons. A sheet of fibrous tissue from the coracohumeral ligament origin also extends posterolaterally to form a sheet over the superficial supraspinatus and infraspinatus tendon insertions.

Histologic studies of the supraspinatus and infraspinatus tendons identified five distinct layers. The most superficial layer (layer one) contains large arterioles and comprises fibers from the coracohumeral ligament. This layer is 1 mm thick and contains fibers that are oriented obliquely to the long axis of the muscle bellies. Layer two is 3 to 5 mm thick and represents the direct tendinous insertion into the tuberosities. Large bundles (1 to 2 mm in diameter) of densely packed parallel tendon fibers compose layer two. The subscapularis tendinous insertion exhibits a similar structure, with collagen fiber bundles that parallel the long axis of the muscle and splay before insertion. A group of bundles from the subscapularis joins with fibers of the supraspinatus to serve as the floor of the biceps sheath, and the roof of the biceps sheath is formed by fibers from layer two of the supraspinatus. Layer three is approximately 3 mm thick and comprises smaller bundles of collagen with a less uniform orientation than in layer two. Fibers within this layer travel at 45-degree

angles to one another to form an interdigitating meshwork that contributes to the fusion of the cuff tendon insertion. Layer four comprises loose connective tissue and thick collagen bands that merge with the coracohumeral ligament at the most anterior border of the supraspinatus. Layer five (2 mm thick) represents the shoulder capsule and includes a sheet of interwoven collagen extending from the glenoid labrum to the humerus.

The insertion site of the rotator cuff tendon at the greater tuberosity often is referred to as the "footprint." Dugas et al. examined 20 normal cadaver rotator cuff specimens and mapped the footprint using a three-space digitizer. The mean medial-to-lateral insertion widths of the supraspinatus, infraspinatus, teres minor, and subscapularis tendons were 12.7 mm, 13.4 mm, 11.4 mm, and 17.9 mm, respectively. The mean minimal medial-to-lateral insertion width of the entire rotator cuff insertion occurred at the midportion of the supraspinatus and was 14.7 mm. The articular surface-to-tendon insertion distance was less than 1 mm along the anterior 2.1 cm of the supraspinatus-infraspinatus insertion. This distance progressively increased to a mean distance of 13.9 mm at the most inferior aspect of the teres minor insertion. The mean anteroposterior distances of the supraspinatus, infraspinatus, teres minor, and subscapularis insertions were noted to be 1.63 cm, 1.64 cm, 2.07 cm, and 2.43 cm, respectively.

An additional important concept relative to the rotator cuff is the rotator cable and rotator crescent. Viewed best from the articular side, the rotator cable is a thick bundle that acts as a suspensory support mechanism to bear forces applied to the rotator cuff (Fig. 2.1). In turn, it offloads and protects the rotator crescent. Rotator cuff tears involving the cable are believed to correlate more with pain than others.

The rotator interval is defined as the triangular area in the anterior and superior shoulder where no rotator cuff tendons are present. As such, the interval is bounded by the supraspinatus superiorly, the subscapularis inferiorly, and the coracoid medially. The apex of the triangle is marked laterally

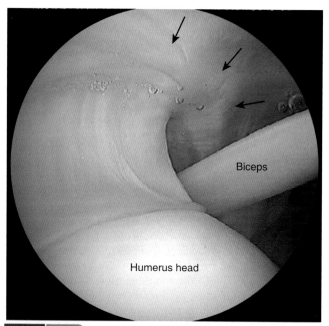

FIGURE 2.1 Arthroscopic view of the rotator cable *(arrows)*. (Courtesy Nickolas Garbis.)

by the transverse humeral ligament. The coracohumeral ligament, biceps tendon, and superior glenohumeral ligament are found in the rotator interval. The rotator interval is altered in pathologic states and has been found to be contracted in patients with adhesive capsulitis and expanded in those with shoulder instability.

The coracoacromial arch lies superior to the glenohumeral joint and is composed of the coracoid and the anterior acromion, which are spanned by the coracoacromial ligament. The distal clavicle usually is considered to be part of the arch as well. The rotator cuff tendons, the subacromial bursa, the biceps tendon, and the proximal humerus all pass beneath this arch. Any acquired or congenital process that narrows the space available for these structures can cause mechanical impingement. The coracoacromial arch also serves as a restraint to superior proximal humeral migration, and its disruption is considered the final step in the cascade of events culminating in anterosuperior escape in advanced degenerative shoulder disorders associated with massive rotator cuff tears. In escape, the humeral head dislocates anteriorly and superiorly with attempted forward elevation of the shoulder. As a result, the humeral head comes to rest in a palpable and visible position in the subcutaneous tissues.

CLINICAL PRESENTATION AND PHYSICAL EXAMINATION

Evaluation of a painful shoulder is challenging for several reasons. Different clinical conditions, such as the various impingement syndromes, rotator cuff tears (partial and complete), calcific tendinitis, adhesive capsulitis, and nerve entrapment syndromes, have similar histories, pain patterns, and findings on physical examination. All of these conditions can cause pain, weakness, and loss of motion of the affected extremity. The pain, usually exacerbated by overhead activities, is worse with active rather than passive motion and may awaken the patient from sleep. Pain may be referred to the area of the deltoid insertion. On physical examination, it often is impossible to reliably establish which structure in the shoulder is causing the pain because of the close anatomic proximity of these structures. Many tests are sensitive for detecting shoulder pathology but are not specific. Many conditions are painful with the same provocative maneuvers. Palpation is of limited benefit, especially in muscular or heavy patients. It is impossible to palpate the labrum or capsule, and although some authors have claimed to be able to palpate rotator cuff tears, we have not had that experience other than in very thin patients. Clicks and crepitus in the shoulder are not specific for any one pathologic condition, and often the reverberating quality of these clicks makes them unreliable for localization.

Although the physical examination often is inconclusive, it is an essential component of the evaluation of a patient with a painful shoulder and helps eliminate other potential causes of referred pain to the shoulder, such as disorders of the cervical spine (herniated disc, spondylosis, brachial plexopathy), chest cavity (Pancoast tumor, upper lobe pneumonia), breasts, axillary area, and abdomen (diaphragmatic irritation, gallbladder dysfunction).

The physical examination begins with inspection. The patient should be undressed above the waist. Women may cover up in a fashion similar to a strapless dress. This exposure allows observation of the anterior and the posterior aspects of the shoulder. Comparison of the shoulders may

reveal subtle atrophy, swelling, or deformity. Ecchymosis may suggest contusions or ruptures of structures such as the rotator cuff or the long head of the biceps tendon. Palpation of the superficial bony structures may identify a painful acromioclavicular joint, sternoclavicular joint, clavicle, or acromion. Palpation elsewhere around the shoulder may suggest potential sources of pain, but as previously mentioned this is not often specific. The joints above and below the area of pain should be examined; for the shoulder, the joint above is the cervical spine. Indeed, 5% of patients presenting with the chief complaint of shoulder pain will be found to have an isolated cervical spine disorder. Therefore, a neurovascular examination of both upper extremities should be included along with an assessment of motor strength. Range of motion is determined actively and passively, noting painful arcs and tendencies to substitute muscle function.

More than 100 tests have been described for detecting shoulder instability, tendinitis, and tears of the rotator cuff, with varying degrees of accuracy. In an exhaustive review of the literature, Hegedus et al. determined that no single physical examination test can be used to make an unequivocal diagnosis; combinations of tests provide only marginally better accuracy. The following tests are ones that we frequently use and are designed either to reproduce symptoms or to produce pain suggesting impingement of the rotator cuff or tendinitis.

■ NEER IMPINGEMENT SIGN AND IMPINGEMENT TEST

Neer first described the impingement test in 1972 (Fig. 2.2A). With the patient seated, the examiner raises the affected arm in forced forward elevation while stabilizing the scapula, causing the greater tuberosity to impinge against the acromion. This maneuver produces pain with impingement lesions of all stages. It also produces pain in many other shoulder conditions, such as adhesive capsulitis, osteoarthritis, calcific tendinitis, and bone lesions. Neer also described the impingement test with the use of a subacromial injection of 10 mL of 1% lidocaine (Xylocaine). Pain caused by impingement usually is significantly reduced or eliminated, but pain caused by other conditions (with the exception perhaps of calcific tendinitis) is not relieved. One study revealed sensitivity for the impingement sign of 75% for bursitis and 88% for cuff abnormalities, with specificities of 48% and 51%. The positive predictive values were 36% and 40%, and the negative predictive values were 83% and 89%. The test was positive, however, in 25% of patients with Bankart lesions, 46% of patients with superior labral anterior and posterior lesions, and 69% of patients with acromioclavicular arthritis.

■ HAWKINS-KENNEDY TEST

Hawkins and Kennedy described their test in 1980 as an alternative to the Neer test, but they did not believe that it was as reliable (Fig. 2.2B). The test is performed by forward flexing the humerus to 90 degrees and forcibly internally rotating the shoulder. This maneuver drives the greater tuberosity farther under the coracoacromial ligament, reproducing the impingement pain. Sensitivities of 92% for bursitis and 88% for cuff abnormalities were found in 85 consecutive patients, with specificities of 44% and 43%. The positive predictive values were 39% and 37%, and the negative predictive values were 93.1% and 90%. The test was positive, however, in 31%

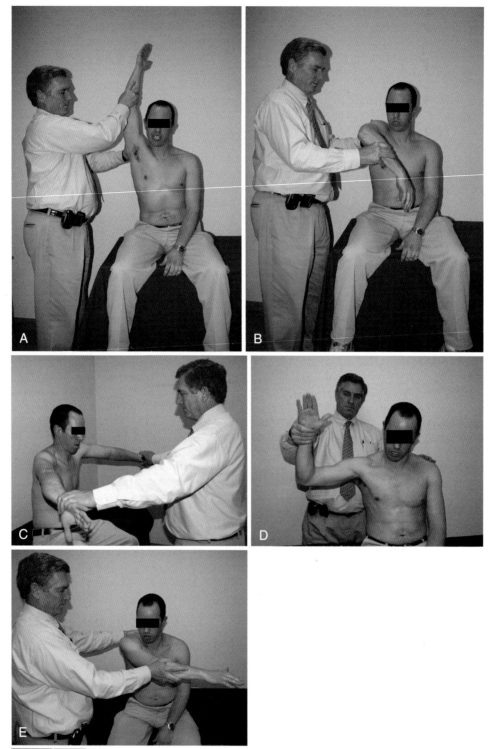

FIGURE 2.2   Impingement tests to reproduce symptoms or produce pain (see text). **A,** Neer impingement sign and impingement test. **B,** Hawkins-Kennedy test. **C,** Jobe supraspinatus test. **D,** Internal rotation resistance stress test. **E,** Gerber subcoracoid impingement test.

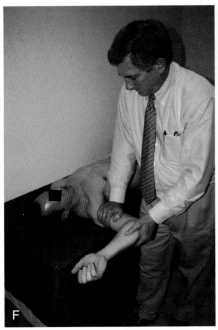 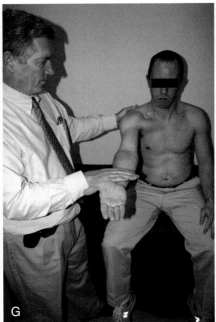 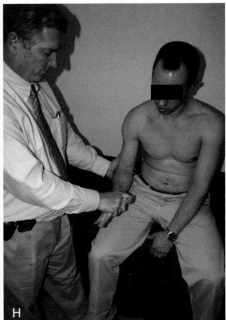

FIGURE 2.2 , Cont'd F, Jobe apprehension-relocation test. **G,** Speed test. **H,** Yergason "supination" sign.

of patients with Bankart lesions, 69% of patients with superior labral anterior and posterior lesions, and 94% of patients with acromioclavicular joint arthritis.

JOBE TEST

Jobe described the "supraspinatus test" in 1983 (Fig. 2.2C). The test is performed by placing the shoulder in 90 degrees of abduction and 30 degrees of forward flexion and internally rotated so that the thumb is pointing toward the floor. Muscle testing against resistance shows weakness or insufficiency of the supraspinatus owing to a tear or pain associated with rotator cuff impingement.

INTERNAL ROTATION RESISTANCE STRESS TEST

Zaslav described a test to differentiate between internal and classic outlet impingement (Fig. 2.2D). The test is performed with the patient seated and the examiner standing behind the patient. The patient's arm is positioned in 90 degrees of abduction in the coronal plane and approximately 80 degrees of external rotation. A manual isometric muscle test is performed for external rotation and compared with one for internal rotation in the same position. If a patient with a positive impingement sign has good strength in external rotation and weakness in internal rotation, the test is positive. A positive internal rotation resistance stress test suggests internal impingement, and a negative test (more weakness in external rotation) suggests classic outlet impingement. Zaslav reported a sensitivity of 88%, specificity of 96%, positive predictive value of 88%, and negative predictive value of 94%. All of the patients tested had been selected, however, because they had a previous positive Neer impingement test, resulting in a population of "impingers" rather than a population with unconfirmed shoulder abnormalities.

ACTIVE COMPRESSION TEST

This test, described by O'Brien for diagnosis of labral tears and acromioclavicular joint abnormalities, is performed with the physician standing behind the patient and asking the patient to forward flex the affected arm 90 degrees with the elbow in full extension. The arm is then adducted 10 to 15 degrees medial to the sagittal plane of the body and is internally rotated so that the thumb points downward. The examiner then applies a uniform downward force to the arm. With the arm in the same position, the palm is then fully supinated and the maneuver is repeated. The test is considered positive if pain is elicited with the first maneuver and is reduced or eliminated with the second maneuver. Pain localized to the acromioclavicular joint or on top of the shoulder is diagnostic of acromioclavicular abnormality. Pain or painful clicking described as inside the glenohumeral joint itself is indicative of labral abnormality. O'Brien et al. compared the physical examination findings to those identified on MRI or at surgery in 318 patients. The active compression test for labral abnormality revealed a sensitivity of 100%, a specificity of 98.5%, a positive predictive value of 100%, and a negative predictive value of 100%. For the acromioclavicular joint, the data revealed a sensitivity of 100%, a specificity of 95.2%, a positive predictive value of 91.5%, and a negative predictive value of 100%.

DYNAMIC LABRAL SHEAR TEST

O'Driscoll described the dynamic labral shear test to reproduce the shearing mechanism that can cause a superior labrum tear anterior and posterior (SLAP); it is reported to yield reliable results that isolate a SLAP lesion's causal role in symptoms and impaired function. The test is performed with the patient supine with the affected arm relaxed off the side of the examining table; the scapula is supported by the table, but the humerus is free. To test the right shoulder, the examiner flexes the right elbow 90 degrees and grasps the olecranon and distal humerus. The shoulder is passively rotated externally to its natural limit with the force of gravity alone pulling down on the forearm (approximately 90 degrees); the elbow is then dropped back into its natural limit of horizontal abduction (toward the floor), and the shoulder is passively elevated and depressed while horizontal abduction and external rotation are maintained. During elevation of the shoulder, the magnitude of horizontal abduction will vary and must be permitted to do so without constraint. The degree of external rotation also will vary throughout the arc of elevation and must be unconstrained. While the shoulder is being elevated, the examiner's right hand is kept on the acromion to stabilize the scapula and to detect any palpable click transmitted through the bony structures (Fig. 2.3). Usually the click will be felt by the left hand on the olecranon, as well as the distal humerus. After full overhead elevation, the entire motion is reversed and the arm is brought down to the side while the natural limits of shoulder external rotation and horizontal abduction are maintained. The test is considered positive if the patient's deep pain at the posterior glenohumeral joint is reproduced by the test through an arc from approximately 90 degrees to 120 degrees; it is considered negative if it is not painful in this range or it does not reproduce the patient's pain. The test can also be performed with the patient sitting or standing, and we have found this to be reliable in the clinical setting. Cheung and O'Driscoll reported sensitivity for diagnosis of a type II SLAP lesion of 86%, which was as good as MRI with gadolinium and better than MRI without gadolinium contrast dye. Kibler et al. found a sensitivity of 72%, specificity of 98%, accuracy of 97%, positive predictive value of 97%, and negative predictive value of 77% for detecting labral disease with this test.

KIM TEST FOR POSTEROINFERIOR LABRAL TEAR

This test is performed with the patient sitting with the arm in 90 degrees of abduction. The examiner holds the elbow and lateral aspect of the proximal arm, and applies a strong axial loading force (Fig. 2.4A). While the arm is elevated 45 degrees diagonally upward, downward and backward force is applied to the proximal arm (Fig. 2.4B). A sudden onset of posterior shoulder pain indicates a positive test result, regardless of accompanying posterior clunk of the humeral head. Because it is important to apply a firm axial compression force to the

glenoid surface by the humeral head, having the patient sit against the back of a chair rather than on a stool provides a good countersupport of the axial loading in the involved arm.

In both a study by Kim et al. and a systematic review, the Kim test was found to have a sensitivity of 80% and specificity of 94%. When the jerk test was used in combination with the Kim test, sensitivity increased to 97%.

JERK TEST FOR POSTERIOR LABRAL LESIONS

The jerk test is highly sensitive and specific for a posterior labral tear. It is performed with the patient sitting. While the examiner holds the scapula with one hand, the patient's arm is abducted 90 degrees and internally rotated 90 degrees. An axial force is applied with the examiner's other hand holding the patient's elbow (Fig. 2.5A), and a simultaneous horizontal adduction force is applied (Fig. 2.5B). A sharp pain, with or without posterior clunk or click, suggests a positive test result.

BICEPS LOAD II TEST FOR ISOLATED SLAP LESIONS

With the patient supine, the examiner places the patient's shoulder in 120 degrees of abduction, the elbow in 90 degrees of flexion, and the forearm in supination, and then externally rotates the shoulder (Fig. 2.6). The patient then flexes his or her elbow, and any pain while the examiner resists elbow flexion is a positive test. Reported sensitivity of the biceps load II test is 90%, specificity 97%, positive-predictive value 92%, and negative-predictive value 95%.

GERBER SUBCORACOID IMPINGEMENT TEST

The Gerber test is designed to identify impingement between the rotator cuff and the coracoid process (Fig. 2.2E). It is performed in a manner similar to the Hawkins-Kennedy impingement test. The arm is forward flexed 90 degrees and adducted 10 to 20 degrees across the body to bring the lesser tuberosity into contact with the coracoid. Pain with the maneuver indicates coracoid impingement.

JOBE APPREHENSION-RELOCATION TEST

Jobe described a combination test in 1989 to distinguish between primary impingement and secondary impingement owing to subtle anterior instability (Fig. 2.2F). With the patient supine, the arm is abducted 90 degrees and externally rotated, which produces pain from impingement. Application of a posteriorly directed force to the humeral head, relocating

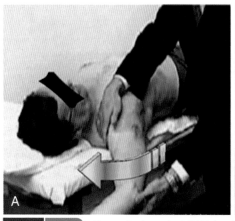
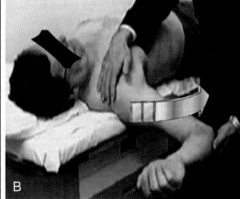

FIGURE **2.3**   Dynamic shear test (O'Driscoll).

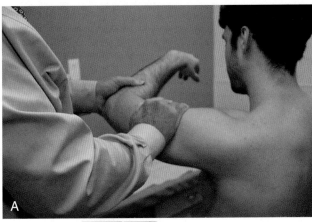
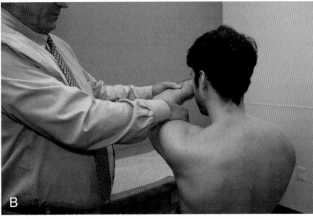

FIGURE 2.4 Kim test for posteroinferior labral tear. **A,** Examiner holds elbow and lateral aspect of proximal arm and applies a strong axial loading force. **B,** With arm elevated 45 degrees diagonally upward, examiner applies downward and backward force to the proximal arm. Sudden onset of posterior should pain indicates a positive test result.

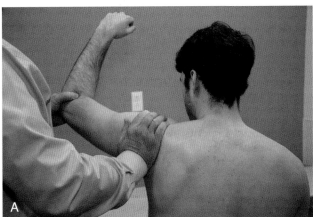
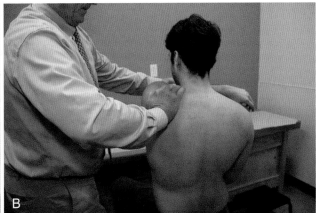

FIGURE 2.5 Jerk test for posterior labral lesions. **A,** Examiner holds scapula with one hand, patient's arm is abducted 90 degrees and internally rotated 90 degrees. **B,** Axial force is applied with examiner's other hand holding patient's elbow and simultaneous horizontal adduction force is applied. Sharp pain suggests positive test result.

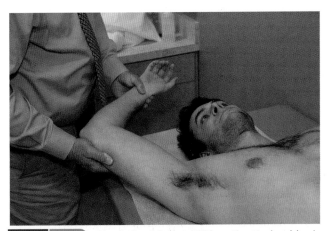

FIGURE 2.6 Biceps load II test. With patient's shoulder in 120 degrees of abduction, elbow in 90 degrees of flexion, and forearm supinated, examiner externally rotates shoulder. Patient then flexes his or her elbow, and any pain while examiner resists elbow flexion is positive result.

it in the glenoid, does not change the pain in patients with primary impingement but relieves the pain in patients with instability (subluxation) and secondary impingement, who tolerate maximal external rotation with the humeral head maintained in a reduced position. Evaluation of this test concluded that pain in the position of 90 degrees of abduction and 90 degrees of external rotation could be caused by a variety of disorders and would be diminished by a posteriorly directed force.

■ SPEED TEST

In 1966, Crenshaw and Kilgore described a test they attributed to Speed (Fig. 2.2G). The Speed test is performed by having the patient forward flex the shoulder to 90 degrees with the elbow extended and the forearm supinated. Resistance is applied to the forearm, and a positive result produces pain localized to the bicipital groove. In an arthroscopic analysis that included biceps tendinitis and superior labral anterior and posterior lesions as positive findings, Bennett found that the Speed test had a sensitivity of 90% and a specificity of 14%. The positive predictive value was 23%, and the negative

TABLE 2.1

Clinical Tests for Subacromial Impingement (Regardless of Severity of Rotator Cuff Disease)

TEST	SENSITIVITY (%)	SPECIFICITY (%)	POSITIVE PREDICTIVE VALUE (%)	NEGATIVE PREDICTIVE VALUE (%)	OVERALL ACCURACY (%)
Neer sign	68	68.7	80.4	53.2	68.3
Hawkins-Kennedy sign	71.5	66.3	79.7	55.7	69.7
Painful arc sign	73.5	81.1	88.2	61.5	76.1
Supraspinatus (Jobe) muscle test	44.1	89.5	88.4	46.8	60.2
Speed test	38.3	83.3	80.5	42.9	54.4
Cross-body adduction test	38.3	83.3	80.5	42.9	54.4
Drop-arm test	26.9	88.4	81	39.7	48.6
Infraspinatus muscle test	41.6	90.1	90.6	45.8	58.7

From Park HB, Yokota A, Gill HS, et al: Diagnostic accuracy of clinical tests for the different degrees of subacromial impingement syndrome, *J Bone Joint Surg* 87A:1446–1455, 2005.

predictive value was 83%. A study in 2005 showed the following values: sensitivity 38%, specificity 83%, positive predictive value 81%, and negative predictive value 43%.

■ YERGASON SIGN

Yergason described the "supination sign" in 1931 (Fig. 2.2H). The elbow is flexed to 90 degrees, and the forearm is pronated. The patient attempts to supinate the forearm actively against resistance applied by the examiner at the patient's wrist. Pain localized to the bicipital groove indicates inflammation of the long head of the biceps. Yergason noted that this test may be negative with partial or complete rupture of the supraspinatus tendon.

Park et al. evaluated eight impingement tests (Table 2.1) in 552 patients and determined that if the Hawkins-Kennedy sign, the painful arc sign, and the infraspinatus muscle (Jobe) test all were positive, the likelihood of a patient having an impingement syndrome of some degree was greater than 95%; if these three tests all were negative, the likelihood of impingement syndrome was less than 24%.

The tests described next (Fig. 2.7) are designed to assess rotator cuff integrity and fall into two types: tests that determine whether a movement can be undertaken actively and tests that determine whether a passive position can be maintained (the lag signs). The main finding on physical examination of patients with full-thickness tears depends on which tendons are torn, what percentage of the tendon width is torn, and the duration for which the tendons have been torn. During an examination of a patient with pain, it may be difficult to determine if weakness is caused by the pain or to a torn tendon. Weakness with pain should be interpreted with caution and not be assumed to indicate a full-thickness tear.

■ LIFT-OFF TEST

In 1991, Gerber and Krushell described the lift-off test for detection of an isolated rupture of the subscapularis tendon (Fig. 2.7A). With the patient seated or standing, the arm is internally rotated, and the dorsum of the hand is placed against the lower back. If the patient is unable to lift the dorsum of the

hand off the back, the test is positive. Electromyography has confirmed that the subscapularis muscle is maximally active with the hand in the midlumbar position and with resistance applied.

■ BELLY PRESS TEST

Gerber et al. described the belly press test for patients who have decreased internal rotation (Fig. 2.7B). In this test, the patient presses the abdomen with the flat of the hand and attempts to keep the arm in maximal internal rotation. If active internal rotation is strong, the elbow does not drop backward, meaning it remains in front of the trunk. If the strength of the subscapularis is impaired, maximal internal rotation cannot be maintained, the patient feels weakness, and the elbow drops back behind the trunk. The patient exerts pressure on the abdomen by extending the shoulder, rather than by internally rotating it. Other investigators have noted that when the subscapularis tendon is torn, patients tend to flex the wrist to press against the abdomen and are unable to hold the elbow forward.

▌ BEAR-HUG TEST FOR SUBSCAPULARIS TEAR

The bear-hug test is performed with the patient's palm of the involved side placed on the opposite shoulder with fingers extended (Fig. 2.8A) and the elbow positioned anterior to the body. The patient is asked to hold that position (resisted internal rotation), and the examiner tries to pull the patient's hand from the shoulder with an external rotation force applied perpendicular to the forearm (Fig. 2.8B). The test is considered positive if the patient is unable to hold the hand against the shoulder or if he or she shows weakness of resisted internal rotation of more than 20% compared with the opposite side. If strength is comparable to that of the opposite side, without any pain, the test is considered negative. A painful bear-hug test without weakness is considered negative.

■ EXTERNAL ROTATION STRESS TEST

The external rotation stress test is intended to test the integrity of the external rotators of the shoulder, specifically the

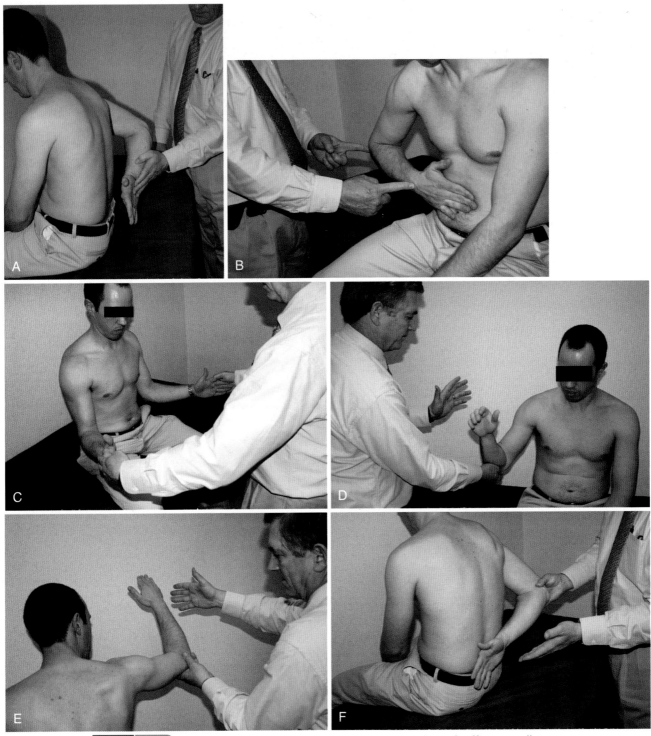

FIGURE 2.7   Tests for evaluating rotator cuff integrity (see text). **A**, Lift-off test. **B**, Belly press test. **C**, External rotation stress test. **D**, External rotation lag sign. **E**, Drop sign. **F**, Internal rotation lag sign.

infraspinatus and the teres minor (Fig. 2.7C). With the patient's arms by his or her side in neutral flexion and abduction, the shoulders are externally rotated 45 to 60 degrees. The examiner applies force against the dorsum of the hands, attempting to rotate the shoulders internally back to neutral while the patient is asked to resist. Pain and weakness suggest inflammation or tearing of the infraspinatus or the teres minor or both.

■ EXTERNAL ROTATION LAG SIGN

The external rotation lag sign test is designed to test the integrity of the supraspinatus and infraspinatus tendons (Fig. 2.7D). The patient is seated with his or her back to the examiner. The elbow is passively flexed to 90 degrees, and the shoulder is held at 20 degrees of elevation and near maximal external rotation (maximal external rotation −5 degrees to avoid elastic recoil in the shoulder) by the examiner. The

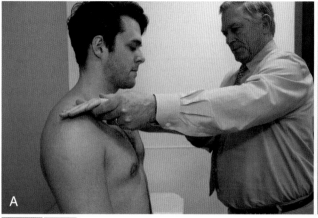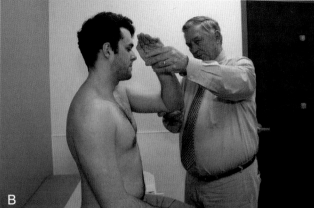

FIGURE 2.8   Bear-hug test for subscapularis tear.

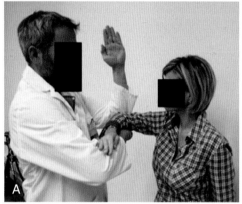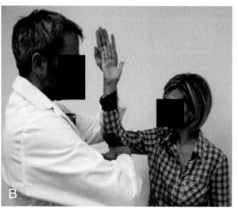

FIGURE 2.9   Patte test to determine strength of teres minor.

patient is asked to maintain the position of external rotation actively as the examiner releases the wrist, while maintaining support of the arm at the elbow. The sign is positive when a lag, or angular drop, occurs. As with all tests, performance and interpretation are complicated by pathologic changes in the passive range of motion. The external rotation lag sign of more than 40 degrees has been shown to have a sensitivity of 100% and a specificity of 92%.

■ PATTE (HORNBLOWER) SIGN

The Patte sign is used to determine the strength of the teres minor. With the patient standing, the examiner elevates the patient's arm to 90 degrees in the scapular plane and flexes the elbow to 90 degrees (Fig. 2.9). The patient is then asked to laterally rotate the shoulder. Weakness and/or pain constitutes a positive test. This sign was reported to have a sensitivity of 93% to 100% and a specificity of 72% to 93%.

■ DROP SIGN

The drop sign is intended to test the integrity of the infraspinatus (Fig. 2.7E). The patient is seated with his or her back to the examiner. The affected arm is held at 90 degrees of elevation in the scapular plane and at almost full external rotation with the elbow flexed at 90 degrees. The patient is asked to maintain this position actively as the examiner releases the wrist while supporting the elbow, which is mainly a function of the infraspinatus. The sign is positive if a lag or "drop"

occurs. The drop sign has a reported sensitivity of 87% and specificity of 88%.

■ INTERNAL ROTATION LAG SIGN

The internal rotation lag sign test is designed to test the integrity of the subscapularis tendon (Fig. 2.7F). The patient is seated with his or her back to the examiner. The affected arm is held by the examiner in almost maximal internal rotation. The elbow is flexed to 90 degrees, and the shoulder is held at 20 degrees of elevation and 20 degrees of extension. The dorsum of the hand is passively lifted away from the lumbar region until almost full internal rotation is reached. The patient is asked to maintain this position actively as the examiner releases the wrist while maintaining support at the elbow. The sign is positive when a lag occurs.

IMAGING

Plain radiographs should be obtained for initial evaluation of a patient with shoulder pain. The radiographs should be made in two planes, preferably at right angles to each other, and should include an anteroposterior view, axillary lateral view, and supraspinatus outlet view. Anteroposterior radiographs can be made with the shoulder in neutral, internal rotation, or external rotation with advantages to each view. The internal rotation view is useful for detecting Hill-Sachs lesions, and the external rotation view provides a good view of the greater tuberosity and proximal humeral physis in skeletally immature patients. A true anteroposterior radiograph of the glenohumeral joint (also known as the Grashey view) provides the best evaluation of the articular cartilage of the glenoid and the humeral head. The axillary lateral view has the advantage of showing the anatomy of the glenoid rim, the acromion, the coracoid, and the proximal humerus. An outlet view assists in the evaluation of patients with rotator cuff disease. This view is a lateral view of the scapula with the tube angled 10 degrees caudad. On this radiograph, the acromion can be classified into one of three types (flat, curved, or hooked). An association between a hooked acromion and rotator cuff disease has been shown, but the causal relationship between the two has not been established. This classification of the acromion also is subject to poor agreement between observers, and slight changes in how the radiographs are made may alter the classification of the acromial shape. Radiographs may reveal exostoses, greater tuberosity cysts or sclerosis, and subacromial sclerosis (sourcil sign), which indicate chronic cuff tears. Calcific deposits to the rotator cuff are consistent with calcific tendinitis. In addition, superior migration of the humeral head with narrowing of the acromiohumeral space to less than 7 mm suggests a rotator cuff tear, and a space less than 5 mm suggests a massive tear. A Stryker notch view is helpful to evaluate for Hill-Sachs lesions, and a West Point view is used to evaluate bony Bankart lesions.

Further imaging can assist with the diagnosis. Traditionally, an arthrogram has been used to document full-thickness rotator cuff tears. Leakage of contrast material into the subacromial and subdeltoid spaces after injection into the glenohumeral joint indicates a full-thickness tear. Tendinopathy or even partial-thickness tears are difficult, however, if not impossible, to diagnose with an arthrogram. The arthrogram does not provide any additional information, such as the size of the tear or the condition of the rotator cuff muscles. Arthrography is still useful for patients in whom MRI is contraindicated, such as patients with a pacemaker, cerebral aneurysm clip, intraocular metal, or recent cardiac stents. Arthrography can be combined with MRI to improve the diagnostic accuracy when evaluating rotator cuff repairs for failure or retears in which it is difficult to differentiate scar tissue from tendon, as well as for evaluation of entities such as labral tears, Bankart and reverse-Bankart lesions, and SLAP lesions, when additional information is needed for treatment decision-making.

MRI is currently the most commonly used test for evaluation of a rotator cuff pathologic process. It is highly accurate and shows detailed anatomic information, including the size of rotator cuff tears and the status of the rotator cuff muscles. In addition, partial tears and tendinopathy are well visualized by MRI. A patient with symptoms of subacromial impingement may show increased signal in the infraspinatus tendon on T2-weighted MRI consistent with tendinopathy; increased fluid in the subacromial bursa also is a sign of subacromial impingement. MR images typically are made in several orientations, including coronal oblique, sagittal oblique, and axial. Coronal oblique MR images assist in evaluating the supraspinatus tendon and muscle, delineating the extent of retraction and the size and quality of the supraspinatus muscle. Fatty replacement of the supraspinatus muscle and the supraspinatus fossa indicates chronic pathology. The size of the supraspinatus tear in the anterior and posterior direction can be determined by noting the tear on sequential images. The sagittal oblique images show the anterior and posterior extent of supraspinatus tearing and the quality of all of the rotator cuff muscles. Axial images are used to show the condition of the biceps tendon and of the subscapularis and infraspinatus tendons and muscles. One potential disadvantage of MRI is the significant potential for false-positive findings. Consequently, MRI findings should always be correlated with clinical findings. Another potential problem with MRI is overuse; specific indications rarely have been discussed. Patients with an insidious onset of shoulder pain and dysfunction do not require MRI evaluation until appropriate nonoperative treatment has failed. Patients for whom surgery is not a consideration do not need MRI unless there are concerns about another pathologic entity, such as an infection or neoplasm.

Ultrasound scanning has been reported to have a sensitivity of 58% to 100%, a specificity of 85% to 100%, and an overall accuracy of 80% to 94% in the detection of rotator cuff tears. In a comparison of MRI and ultrasound assessment of rotator cuff healing in 61 patients, ultrasound had 80% sensitivity and 98% specificity using MRI as the reference. A Cochrane Database Review concluded that MRI, MR arthrography, and ultrasound all have good diagnostic accuracy, and any could be used equally for detection of full-thickness tears in patients with shoulder pain for whom surgery is being considered, especially those with full-thickness tears; however, both MRI and ultrasound appear to have poor sensitivity for detecting partial-thickness tears. Advantages of ultrasonography over other imaging methods are that it is rapid, noninvasive, and inexpensive; a disadvantage is that the accuracy of ultrasound evaluation is highly dependent on the experience of the ultrasonographer and on the quality of the equipment used. Dynamic ultrasound also can be useful in confirming shoulder impingement syndrome, assessing glenohumeral laxity, and identifying biceps tendon pathology.

IMPINGEMENT SYNDROME

Current understanding of impingement syndrome has evolved considerably since Jarjavay's first description of subacromial bursitis in 1867. Codman, in 1931, was the first to note that many patients with inability to abduct the arm had incomplete or complete ruptures of the supraspinatus tendon, rather than primary bursal problems. In 1972, Neer described impingement syndrome characterized by a ridge of proliferative spurs and excrescences on the undersurface of the anterior process of the acromion, apparently caused by repeated impingement of the rotator cuff and the humeral head with traction of the coracoacromial ligament. Neer also noted that the anterior third of the acromion and its anterior lip seemed to be the offending structure in most cases. He introduced the concept of a continuum of impingement syndrome (Box 2.1). The supraspinatus insertion into the greater tuberosity that passes beneath the coracoacromial arch during forward flexion of the shoulder is susceptible to impingement (Fig. 2.10). Neer also described the temporary relief of pain with subacromial injection of lidocaine as a diagnostic test, now known as the *impingement test*, which is helpful in differentiating purely impingement-type symptoms from other pathologic processes.

The natural history of impingement syndrome remains unclear. In a group of 63 patients with subacromial impingement without rotator cuff tears who were evaluated 8 years after diagnosis, 44% had a relapsing course with asymptomatic periods between recurrences, 25% had no recurrences,

Developmental Stages of Impingement Syndrome

Stage 1: Edema and Hemorrhage
Typical age of patient: <25 years old
Differential diagnosis: subluxation, acromioclavicular joint arthritis
Clinical course: reversible
Treatment: conservative

Stage 2: Fibrosis and Tendinitis
Typical age of patient: 25-40 years old
Differential diagnosis: frozen shoulder, calcium deposits
Clinical course: recurrent pain with activity
Treatment: consider bursectomy or division of coracoacromial ligament

Stage 3: Bone Spurs and Tendon Rupture
Typical age of patient: >40 years old
Differential diagnosis: cervical radiculitis, neoplasm
Clinical course: progressive disability
Treatment: anterior acromioplasty, rotator cuff repair

Modified from Neer CS II: Impingement lesions, *Clin Orthop Relat Res* 173:70–77, 1983.

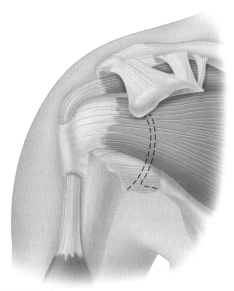

FIGURE 2.10 Impingement syndrome. Supraspinatus tendon is seen passing beneath coracoacromial arch.

and 30% had a chronic course. Of those with a chronic course, 37% eventually required surgery. Younger age, lower body mass index (BMI), more functional capacity, shorter symptomatic period, reversible changes on MRI, and higher Constant and American Shoulder and Elbow Surgeons (ASES) Standardized Shoulder Assessment scores at the first evaluation were good prognostic factors.

Since Neer's original description, the concept of impingement syndrome has evolved to encompass four types of impingement: (1) primary impingement, (2) secondary impingement, (3) subcoracoid impingement, and (4) internal impingement. Primary impingement is subcategorized further into intrinsic and extrinsic types. Primary impingement is the classic version and occurs without any other contributing pathology. Secondary impingement occurs when there is instability of the glenohumeral joint allowing translation of the humeral head, typically anteriorly, resulting in contact of the rotator cuff against the coracoacromial arch. When the structures passing beneath the coracoacromial arch become enlarged resulting in abutment against the arch, the cause of the impingement is considered to be intrinsic. Examples of this condition include thickening of the rotator cuff, calcium deposits within the rotator cuff, and thickening of the subacromial bursa. Extrinsic impingement occurs when the space available for the rotator cuff is diminished; examples include subacromial spurring, acromial fracture or pathologic os acromiale, osteophytes off the undersurface of the acromioclavicular joint, and exostoses at the greater tuberosity.

Acromial morphology has been implicated as contributing to impingement. Bigliani, Morrison, and April described three types of acromion morphology (Fig. 2.11) and noted an increase in rotator cuff tears with type III, or hooked, acromions. In a cadaver study of 140 shoulders, one third had full-thickness tears of the rotator cuff, 73% of which were in shoulders with type III acromions. A more recent comparison of patients with full-thickness supraspinatus tendon tears or subacromial impingement to a control group found that a low lateral acromial angle and a large lateral extension of the acromion were associated with a higher occurrence of impingement and rotator cuff tears. An extremely hooked anterior acromion with a slope of more than 43 degrees and a lateral acromial angle of less than 70 degrees occurred only in patients with rotator cuff tears. Patients with less slope to their acromion have been reported to have a propensity toward impingement because of subacromial stenosis. A cadaver study showed significantly lower angles in shoulders with rotator cuff tears than in shoulders with intact cuffs. A study investigating the association between kyphosis, subacromial impingement syndrome, and a reduction in shoulder elevation found a significant association between impingement and reduced shoulder elevation. The authors suggested that kyphosis might influence the development of impingement indirectly by reducing shoulder elevation because of restriction of thoracic spine extension and scapular dyskinesis. Based on these observations, the recommended treatment for impingement syndrome has been anterior acromioplasty to remove the offending structure.

Recently, numerous calculations of distances, angles, and slopes about the shoulder have been described that are based on measurements on radiographs and MRIs. These are attempts to provide objective support for the clinical diagnosis of impingement syndrome and to predict the presence or risk of development of a rotator cuff tear. Most measurements require precise shoulder positioning to be accurate and clinically helpful. The efficacy of these measurements has not been proven. Sasiponganan et al. correlated radiographic measurements of acromial index, lateral acromion angle, subacromial space on AP and Y-views, acromial anterior and lateral downsloping, and MRI findings of rotator cuff pathology. Studying 140 MRIs in 137 women, they concluded that subacromial impingement anatomy characteristics have no significant associations with supraspinatus

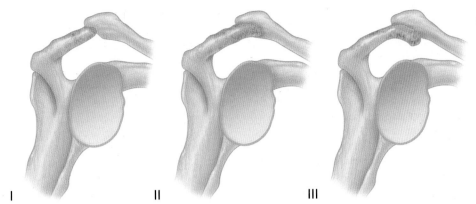

FIGURE 2.11 Three types of acromion morphology defined by Morrison and Bigliani. Type I had least compromise of supraspinatus outlet, and type III had highest rate of rotator cuff pathology.

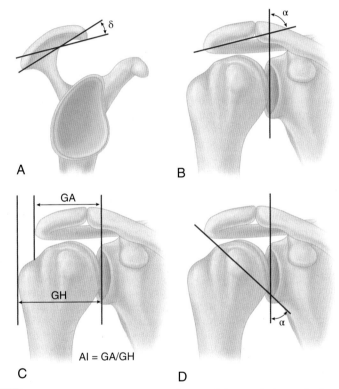

FIGURE 2.12 Radiographic parameters of acromial morphology. **A**, Acromial slope (σ). **B**, Lateral acromial angle (α). **C**, Acromion index (AI). **D**, Critical shoulder angle (α). (Redrawn from Balke M, Liem D, Greshake O, et al: Differences in acromial morphology of shoulders in patients with degenerative and traumatic supraspinatus tendon tears, *Knee Surg Sports Traumatol Arthrosc* 24[7]:2200–2205, 2016.)

or infraspinatus tears in symptomatic women. Balke et al. studied 136 patients with arthroscopic rotator cuff repair to determine if acromial morphology in degenerative supraspinatus tendon tears differs from that with traumatic tears. On preoperative radiographs, they evaluated Bigliani type, acromial slope, acromiohumeral distance, lateral acromial angle, acromion index, and critical shoulder angle (Fig. 2.12). They found that shoulders with degenerative tears had a narrower subacromial space, a larger lateral extension, and a steeper angulation of the acromion than traumatic tears.

Gumina et al. presented an intriguing study attempting to determine the relative role of genetics or external forces in determining the subacromial space width. They studied 29 pairs of twins, both monozygotic and dizygotic, and measured the acromiohumeral space on MRI scans. The intraclass correlation coefficient was substantially higher for monozygotic than for dizygotic twins, indicating a high degree of concordance of the acromiohumeral distance in pairs of individuals who shared 100% of their genes. There were no differences among subjects in different job categories. They concluded that the acromiohumeral distance is mainly genetically determined and only marginally influenced by external factors.

Other investigators have suggested that the shape of the acromion and the coracoacromial ligament are not the primary problems, but rather that intrinsic rotator cuff degeneration is the primary cause with subacromial changes occurring secondarily. Senescence of the tendon fibroblasts with resulting disruption of the tendon architecture is a common finding in the rotator cuff with aging. Age-related degenerative changes, including decreased cellularity, fascicular thinning and disruption, accumulation of granulation tissue, and dystrophic calcification, all have been noted and are likely irreversible. A zone of relative hypovascularity also is present on the articular surface of the rotator cuff. Differential shear stress within the tendon layers also has been cited as a cause of the disruption of the tendon fibers. Others have suggested that the rotator cuff tendons may fail in tension as a result of throwing a baseball or other overhead sports. Intrinsic degeneration leads to loss of the force couples, causing superior humeral head translation and impingement. As support for their theory of impingement as a secondary phenomenon, these authors cited the improvement of symptoms after rehabilitation (capsular stretching and rotator cuff strengthening). They recommended minimal or no acromioplasty at the time of surgery for rotator cuff repair and repair of the coracoacromial ligament rather than excision. Several systematic reviews and meta-analyses have failed to find differences in pain, function, and time to recovery between patients treated nonoperatively and those treated with acromioplasty. In addition, excision of the ligament is losing favor because of the potential for anterior and superior subluxation of the humeral head from underneath the acromion (anterior-superior escape) when the rotator cuff tear is irreparable or the repair fails and the ligament restraint is gone. A study of practice patterns in rotator cuff repair identified a trend toward increased arthroscopic rotator cuff repair without subacromial decompression and a decrease in isolated subacromial decompression.

In their study to identify shoulder motions that cause subacromial impingement, Park et al. measured the vertical displacement and peak strain of the coracoacromial ligament. They found that forward flexion, horizontal abduction, and internal rotation with the arm at 90 degrees of abduction showed higher vertical displacement and peak strain of the coracoacromial ligament, causing subacromial impingement. They recommended that patients with impingement syndrome or a repaired rotator cuff avoid these shoulder motions.

■ SUBCORACOID IMPINGEMENT

In 1909, Goldthwait first described pain in the shoulder caused by contact between the rotator cuff and the coracoid process. Gerber et al. suggested that this painful contact might be caused by a prominent coracoid, for which there may be numerous reasons, including idiopathic and iatrogenic conditions. The iatrogenic form was most common in their series, and it was found in patients who had undergone a Trillat osteotomy of the coracoid for the treatment of anterior instability. In their series of 475 patients with rotator cuff tears, Park et al. identified subcoracoid impingement in 13%; of 110 with subscapularis tears, 56% had subcoracoid impingement. Among patients with subacromial impingement but no rotator cuff tears, 41% had subcoracoid impingement. This entity has not been studied extensively, and it remains a diagnosis of exclusion.

Physical findings attributed to this condition include tenderness over the coracoid and a positive coracoid impingement test (see Fig. 2.2E). An injection of lidocaine into the subcoracoid region similar to the Neer impingement test (see Fig. 2.2A) has been used to evaluate patients for coracoid impingement. Relief of pain suggests the diagnosis, but the proximity of multiple structures in the subcoracoid region, including the glenohumeral joint itself, makes the accuracy of these injections questionable. CT has been used in the diagnosis of coracoid impingement; a suggested distance of 6.8 mm between the coracoid tip and the closest portion of the proximal humerus indicates impingement. For suspected impingement, open or arthroscopic coracoplasty has been recommended. A comparison of outcomes between patients with arthroscopic coracoplasty and those without found a significant increase in internal rotation in the treated group, especially in those with large to massive rotator cuff tears. We have no experience with this procedure.

■ INTERNAL IMPINGEMENT

In this condition, internal contact of the rotator cuff occurs with the posterosuperior aspect of the glenoid when the arm is abducted, extended, and externally rotated as in the cocked position of the throwing motion. This contact probably is a normal phenomenon but becomes pathologic in certain patients. It often occurs in throwers who have lost internal rotation of the shoulder. This loss causes the center of rotation of the humeral head to move upward so that the contact between the rotator cuff and the biceps tendon attachments increases. Several cadaver studies have attempted to identify factors related to the development of internal impingement. One such study determined that increased capsular laxity significantly increased horizontal abduction and contact pressure in the glenohumeral joint, resulting in impingement of the supraspinatus and infraspinatus tendons and posterosuperior labrum between the greater tuberosity and glenoid. In contrast, another cadaver study found that excessive posteroinferior capsular tightness caused forceful internal impingement of the shoulder at maximal external rotation, whereas another identified increased internal scapular rotation and decreased upward scapular rotation as significantly increasing glenohumeral contact pressure and the area of impingement of the rotator cuff. Arthroscopic findings include partial rotator cuff tears, posterior and superior labral tears, and anterior shoulder laxity. Early in the course of the condition, aggressive physical therapy with attention to regaining internal rotation and rotator cuff strengthening is often successful. Arthroscopic management of this problem is discussed in other chapter.

■ PRIMARY (EXTERNAL) IMPINGEMENT

The initial treatment of a patient with tendinopathy caused by classic primary extrinsic impingement is a well-planned and well-executed nonoperative regimen, including anti-inflammatory medications and one or at most two subacromial cortisone injections. Hyaluronic acid injections have been suggested to improve results, but a comparison of hyaluronic acid injections (51 patients) with corticosteroid (53 patients) or placebo injections (55 patients) found no benefit from hyaluronic acid injections; corticosteroid injections produced a significant reduction in pain in the short term (3 to 12 weeks), but in the long term the placebo injection produced the best results. Platelet-rich plasma (PRP) has been offered as a treatment for subacromial impingement, but a single-blinded randomized controlled trial comparing PRP to exercise therapy found that both were effective in reducing pain and disability. Medical treatment is followed by a physical therapy program focusing on stretching for full shoulder motion and strengthening the rotator cuff. A scapular motor control retraining protocol was reported to be successful in relieving symptoms in young patients. If the patient fails to respond after 3 to 4 months of conservative therapy, operative intervention may be indicated and should be directed to the specific lesion. Significantly greater improvements in Constant scores have been reported for patients with a positive Hawkins-Kennedy sign in the neutral position, and positive Neer and Jobe tests compared with those with negative signs. Patients with four positive tests out of the five studied (Neer, Hawkins-Kennedy in neutral and in abduction, Jobe empty can, and painful arc) had greater improvement than those with three or fewer positive test results.

Arthroscopic or open acromioplasty when indicated is the surgical treatment of choice for external impingement syndrome. The reported results of open anterior acromioplasty vary widely. In more than 20 large series of open acromioplasties, the overall success rate was approximately 85%. Failures were related to incorrect diagnosis, technical inadequacy, and other complications. For acromioplasty to be successful, impingement must be the cause of the pain and a thorough history and physical examination are necessary. Acromioclavicular arthritis, glenohumeral arthritis, subtle shoulder instability in throwing athletes, early adhesive capsulitis, and fibromyalgia all can present diagnostic dilemmas. Cervical spondylosis with nerve root irritation and suprascapular nerve injury also can mimic the symptoms associated with an impingement syndrome.

Recently, studies have questioned the superiority of acromioplasty over physical rehabilitation. Ketola et al. randomized 140 patients into a structured exercise program or an arthroscopic acromioplasty group that also did the therapy postoperatively. At follow-up, there were no statistically significant differences in either the amount of perforating ruptures of the supraspinatus tendon or in the changes in muscle volume at 5 years. Kolk et al. in a double-blind randomized clinical trial compared arthroscopic bursectomy alone with bursectomy combined with acromioplasty. Forty-three patients were examined at a median of 12 years postoperatively. Based on Constant score, Simple Shoulder test score, visual analog scale (VAS) pain score, and VAS shoulder function score, there were no relevant additional effects of arthroscopic acromioplasty on bursectomy alone with respect to clinical outcomes or rotator cuff integrity at 12 years follow-up. Paavola et al. compared arthroscopic acromioplasty, diagnostic arthroscopy, and physical therapy. There were no differences between acromioplasty and diagnostic arthroscopy at 2 years, and the differences between acromioplasty and therapy did not reach a minimum clinically important difference.

Technical inadequacy has been implicated as a cause of failed acromioplasties. Adequate bone must be removed to alleviate outlet stenosis. Inadequate bone removal seems to occur more often in arthroscopic than open acromioplasties. In addition to the anterior lip, the portion of the acromion anterior to the anterior clavicular border must be removed to obtain optimal results. Original technical descriptions called for resecting and removing a portion of the coracoacromial ligament to prevent the cut edge from scarring back to the acromion. Our current practice is to release the ligament. We believe that the ligament can be part of the pathologic process and anticipate that it would heal back to the acromion, restoring the coracoacromial arch and preventing anterosuperior subluxation of the humeral head.

We use arthroscopic and occasionally open techniques. We believe that either open or arthroscopic acromioplasty is satisfactory if the main principles of the original procedure as described by Neer are kept in mind, as follows:

- Release (but not resection) of the coracoacromial ligament
- Removal of the anterior lip and lateral edge of the acromion
- Removal of part of the acromion anterior to the anterior border of the clavicle
- Removal of the distal 1 to 1.5 cm of clavicle if significant degenerative changes are found

OPEN ANTERIOR ACROMIOPLASTY
TECHNIQUE 2.1

- Place the patient in a semi-upright position with the head elevated 30 to 35 degrees (beach chair position). Place a towel or an intravenous bag medial to the scapula to stabilize it. This degree of head elevation usually places the superior acromial surface perpendicular to the floor, allowing the acromial osteotomy to be made perpendicular to the floor. Drape the arm free to permit shoulder rotation.
- Outline the bony contour of the shoulder, including the lateral acromial border, coracoid, and acromioclavicular joint.
- Outline the proposed skin incision along the Langer line 4 to 6 cm long and infiltrate it with 10 mL of 1:500,000 epinephrine to minimize bleeding.
- Make the incision from lateral to the anterior acromion toward the coracoid and just lateral to it (Fig. 2.13).
- After mobilization of the subcutaneous tissue, identify the raphe between the anterior and middle deltoid and split it from a point 5 cm or less distal to the acromial border (to avoid axillary nerve injury) toward the anterolateral acromion (Fig. 2.14A).
- The deltoid can be left attached or can be detached from the corner of the acromion, depending on the surgeon's preference. We prefer to leave the deltoid attached initially, detaching it later if the procedure warrants.
- To use this approach, elevate a flap of deltoid with its periosteal attachment and the periosteal attachment of the trapezius approximately 2 cm onto the superior acromial surface (Fig. 2.14B).
- Carry this medially as far as the acromioclavicular joint (the anterior capsule of which usually is included in the flap) and 1 cm along the lateral acromion. Occasionally, these periosteal attachments are tenuous after elevation, and the deltoid must be detached, to be secured later to the acromion through drill holes. We have found that using electrocautery with a Bovie needle for elevation usually ensures thicker flaps.

- The importance of correct deltoid detachment cannot be overemphasized. A secure cuff of tissue must be maintained for later defect closure or reattachment to the acromion. Without secure deltoid attachment, the results of the acromioplasty would be compromised by lack of deltoid function.
- After completing the anterior limb of the elevation, resect the coracoacromial ligament. We use the electrocautery for this as well because the acromial branch of the coracoacromial artery is contained within the ligament, and electrocautery allows exposure of the entire subacromial space.
- With the subacromial space exposed, resect the bursa along with all adhesions and soft-tissue coverage from the acromial undersurface. The bursa can be quite thick and easily mistaken for the rotator cuff tendon. The bursa

can be identified by its continuity with the acromial undersurface and its unilaminar appearance, as opposed to the multilaminar appearance of the rotator cuff. Clark and Harryman showed five distinct layers with multiple interdigitations in the cuff tendons.

- After bursal resection, use an oscillating saw or rongeur to remove the portion of the acromion that projects anterior to the anterior border of the clavicle (Fig. 2.14C). This removes a portion of the offending acromial hook and squares off the surface, allowing easier completion of the acromioplasty with an oscillating saw or an osteotome. We prefer an oscillating saw for this portion of the procedure because it affords more control than an osteotome, which may propagate a fracture line into the posterior acromion.
- Begin the osteotomy at the anterosuperior aspect of the acromion and continue it through the junction of the anterior and middle thirds of the acromion, including the entire anterior acromion from medial to lateral.
- Use a curved, blunt Hohmann or malleable retractor to depress the humeral head and protect the cuff during this portion of the procedure.
- Smooth out any rough surfaces with a rasp.
- Palpate the acromioclavicular joint undersurface and remove any bony spurs.
- If severe degenerative changes are present, resect the distal 1.0 to 1.5 cm of the lateral clavicle. Preoperative radiographs and symptoms should indicate the necessity of this additional procedure, and it should not be done routinely.
- If the clavicle is resected, leave the superior acromioclavicular capsule intact to make deltoid repair in this area easier. Do not extend the clavicular cut beyond 1.5 cm to avoid violating the coracoclavicular ligaments and making the distal clavicle unstable.
- Carefully inspect the entire rotator cuff for tears before closure. The area just proximal to the supraspinatus insertion is the most common site for tears. Palpate this area for thinning, which may indicate a partial-thickness tear on the articular side.

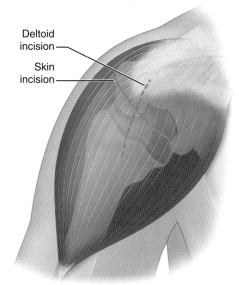

FIGURE **2.13** Anterior acromioplasty. Skin incision is made in skin lines across anterior corner of acromion. Acromion is exposed by incision in tendon between anterior and lateral deltoid. **SEE TECHNIQUE 2.1.**

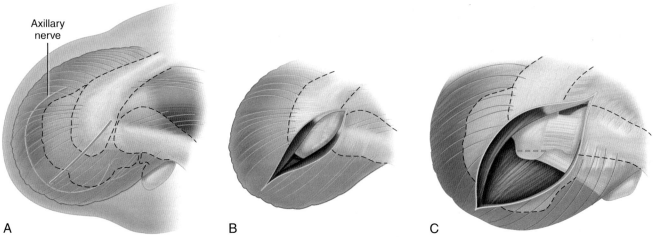

FIGURE **2.14** **A,** Incision centered on anterolateral corner of acromion, avoiding axillary nerve, and carried medially on superior surface of acromion. **B,** Deltoid origin elevated from acromion in continuity with acromial periosteum and trapezius insertion. **C,** Anterior extent of acromion to be removed. **SEE TECHNIQUE 2.1.**

- If preoperative studies show extreme degeneration without fresh tearing, resection of the diseased tendon and direct repair or suturing to a trough in bone should be considered (see Technique 2.2).
- Internally and externally rotate the shoulder to allow inspection of the entire bursal surface of the cuff.
- Copiously irrigate the area to remove all debris from the subacromial space.
- Suture the deltoid periosteum from side to side or, if necessary, through drill holes into the acromion with nonabsorbable sutures, ensuring that the reattachment is secure. The repair of the deltoid to the acromion through drill holes has become our preferred method of repair.
- Close the wound in layers in routine fashion.

POSTOPERATIVE CARE The arm is supported by a sling. Pendulum exercises are started the day after surgery. Passive abduction and internal and external rotation exercises are started at the end of 1 week. At 3 weeks, active exercises are begun. The sling is discarded as soon as the patient feels comfortable.

■ COMPLICATIONS

Complications after acromioplasty include, but are not limited to, infection, seroma formation, hematoma, synovial fistula, biceps rupture, pulmonary embolus, acromial fracture, and complex regional pain syndrome. Poor patient motivation, poor rehabilitation compliance, or a poorly designed rehabilitation program also can lead to failure because of continued pain and stiffness. Bouchard et al. cited co-planing and workers' compensation claims as poor prognostic indicators.

Without question, the worst common complication is loss of anterior deltoid function, which is caused by either axillary nerve injury or detachment of the deltoid from the acromion. Loss of anterior deltoid function produces a poor outcome despite technically adequate bone work and ligament resection. Very little can be done to restore function to a detached, retracted deltoid. Because deltoid detachment, retraction, and scarring are much more common after the "deltoid on" approach, we recommend suturing to the acromion with heavy sutures whenever tissue is unavailable for direct side-to-side repair.

ROTATOR CUFF TEAR

Although some patients present with a sudden onset of symptoms following an acute shoulder injury, most patients with a pathologic condition of the rotator cuff have insidious onset of progressive pain and weakness, with concomitant loss of active motion. Pain usually is present at night and may be referred to the area of the deltoid insertion. Passive motion initially remains full until pain limits active motion enough to cause development of adhesive capsulitis. Most patients cannot recall a specific traumatic incident referable to the onset of problems. Treatment recommendations are based on the patient's age, symptoms, and activity demands, and the natural history of rotator cuff tears.

The natural history of rotator cuff tears is not always predictable. On the one hand, many patients with full-thickness rotator cuff tears are asymptomatic or respond well to nonoperative treatment. On the other hand, studies indicate that some previously asymptomatic tears become symptomatic and some tears progress in size and become irreparable. Rotator cuff pathology is a common problem, and cadaver anatomic studies have reported rotator cuff tears in 30% to 50% of specimens, suggesting that they may be part of the normal aging process.

Full-thickness rotator cuff tears are compatible with normal function. In 1962, McLaughlin advanced five reasons to avoid early repair of the average rupture: (1) at least 25% of cadaver shoulders had a torn or degenerated cuff; (2) 50% of patients recovered spontaneously; (3) immediate repair had no advantages because rupture always occurred in diseased tendon; (4) results of early and late repair were the same; and (5) early diagnosis was difficult. Resolution of symptoms has been reported in 33% to 90% of patients treated nonoperatively, and we recommend nonoperative treatment initially for elderly patients or patients with low activity with suspected rotator cuff tears. Patients without pain or limitation of activities of daily living also should be treated nonoperatively. When the decision to treat nonoperatively is made, treatment should be instituted promptly and aggressively. The duration of symptoms seems to correlate inversely with the long-term success of nonoperative management because patients with symptoms for longer than 6 months had poorer outcomes.

The natural history of rotator cuff tears is not always predictable. When counseling a patient with a rotator cuff tear, the surgeon must remember that some asymptomatic tears become symptomatic and some tears do progress in size. A study of patients with bilateral rotator cuff tears found that, although all patients were asymptomatic on one side at presentation, at follow-up more than half had developed symptoms in the previously asymptomatic side. Medium-size tears have been shown to be at high risk of progression, whereas partial tears or small full-thickness tears appear to have little risk of early development of irreparable damage. The presence of rotator cuff disease has been shown to correlate with age; after the age of 66 years, there is a 50% likelihood of bilateral tears. Duration of symptoms also has been correlated with severity of rotator cuff disease: the longer the symptoms, the more extensive the fatty degeneration of the torn rotator cuff muscle. A retrospective review of 1688 patients with rotator cuff tears determined that moderate supraspinatus fatty infiltration appeared an average of 3 years after the onset of symptoms and that severe fatty infiltration appeared at an average of 5 years after the onset of symptoms. In an ultrasound study of 105 rotator cuff repairs, patients with intact repairs of large tears had outcomes that were equal to those in patients with small tears. As the size of the recurrent defect increased, the strength, motion, and function decreased. A more recent study confirmed these results in a group of patients aged 65 years or older: those with healed tears after surgery had function comparable to patients of a similar age without tears and better than that of patients with untreated tears. These findings indicate that early operative intervention, when most tears are small and less degeneration of the muscle has occurred, improves outcomes.

Loss of continuity of the rotator cuff can be described in several ways, including *acute* and *chronic*, *partial* or *full thickness*, and *traumatic* or *degenerative*. It is important to differentiate between the different types to plan appropriate treatment. Full-thickness rotator cuff tears also are classified based on their size (Box 2.2). The most common size classification (Cofield) is based on the largest dimension of the tear. Tears also can be classified according to the number of tendons involved. In addition, the extent of tendon retraction and tissue quality are important features not generally accounted for by classification schemes. Chronic tears can be classified based on the percentage of fatty infiltration of the muscle belly as seen on MRI or CT. Goutallier et al. proposed five stages of fatty degeneration. The presence and degree of fatty infiltration and atrophy of the muscle affect the success of the repair. Partial-thickness tears have been described by location, grade, and tear area (in mm^2). We have found it easier to classify partial tendon tears as involving less or more than 50% of the depth of the tendon and base treatment on this distinction.

PARTIAL-THICKNESS AND FULL-THICKNESS TEARS

Partial-thickness tears may be articular-sided, bursal-sided, or intratendinous. The true incidence of partial-thickness tears is unknown. Most of the information is from cadaver studies, which reflect an older population; the true incidence in young overhead-throwing athletes is unknown. Among partial-thickness tears, cadaver studies indicate that intratendinous tears are more common than articular-sided or bursal-sided tears, whereas a clinical study found that articular-sided tears constituted 91% of all partial-thickness tears in a population of young athletes. This discrepancy between cadaver and clinical studies may result because intratendinous tears are more difficult to diagnose with arthroscopy, MRI, or ultrasound than are bursal-sided or articular-sided tears. The true prevalence of partial-thickness tears is likely to be greater than that currently documented in the literature. In a systematic review of the literature, Lazarides et al. determined that among young patients with rotator cuff tears, most had full-thickness traumatic tears, but in a subgroup of elite throwers, most tears were partial-thickness tears resulting from chronic overuse.

The natural history of partial-thickness tears is not fully known. Imaging and clinical studies have suggested that partial-thickness tears progress in as many as 80% of patients.

For partial-thickness rotator cuff tears, a nonoperative program that includes activity modification, stretching and strengthening exercises, and antiinflammatory medication is appropriate as initial treatment. Operative management is indicated if conservative management fails. Arthroscopic evaluation is required to determine the extent of the lesion, and subacromial decompression is indicated when outlet impingement is present. The causes of the tear should be treated at the time of surgery. Debridement or repair of partial-thickness rotator cuff tears depends on the degree of the tear and the activity level and age of the patient. We currently perform arthroscopic debridement of partial-thickness tears when they are found on inspection during arthroscopic acromioplasty. If a lesion involves less than 50% of cuff thickness, acromioplasty and debridement are sufficient treatment. If a tear is longer or thicker, elliptical excision of the diseased tendon and repair are indicated. Good results have been reported with arthroscopic repair of bursal-side partial-thickness tears.

The results of nonoperative treatment of partial-thickness tears are unknown because no long-term follow-up studies using a standardized treatment protocol on a well-defined uniform patient population exist in the literature. Excellent and good results after arthroscopic debridement have been reported in from 80% to 90% of patients, with improvements in pain, function, active forward flexion, and strength. Studies also have shown no significant difference in outcome between patients with full-thickness and patients with partial-thickness tears or between patients with partial-thickness tears less than 50% of tendon thickness and patients without any tears.

The primary goal of operative management of rotator cuff tears is pain relief, and this is accomplished with predictable results. Improvement of function is a secondary but important consideration. Functional improvement is not as predictable as pain relief and depends on the age of the patient, the age and size of the tear (which suggests the quality of the tissue and the condition of the muscle), and the postoperative rehabilitation program. In elderly patients or patients with low activity, we attempt a course of conservative treatment (8 to 12 weeks). If there is a positive response, the nonoperative approach may be continued, but if there is no improvement, we proceed to surgery to minimize the atrophy of the rotator cuff musculature. Surgery is appropriate for an acute rotator cuff injury in a young patient or in an older patient (60 to 70 years old) with a defined injury who suddenly is unable to rotate the arm externally against resistance. In our experience, these patients usually have an excellent return of strength and function. Surgery is contraindicated in patients with rotator cuff tears and concomitant stiffness (secondary to adhesive capsulitis). Any significant preoperative stiffness must be corrected before rotator cuff repair to avoid severe postoperative stiffness. It is imperative that nearly full motion be regained before surgical intervention to prevent severe postoperative stiffness.

The clinical results of rotator cuff repair in symptomatic patients who have been followed for 10 years are good to excellent in a high percentage of cases, even though rerupture of the cuff occurs in 20% to 65%. In four large series (Hawkins et al., Neer et al., Ellman et al., and Cofield et al.) that included 476 patients, success rates ranged from 78% to 86%, with excellent or good results reported in 383 (80%) of the 476 patients. In a review of several series of rotator cuff repairs, overall pain relief was obtained in 87% of patients, with a 77% patient satisfaction rate. Most repair failures have been found to occur within the first 2 years after surgery; if the repair survives this initial period, its 10-year survival is likely. Our results with rotator cuff repair are similar, achieving pain control and return of function in approximately 80% of patients. Outcomes of repair generally are better in patients younger than 60 years of age, although clinical results often are good despite poor imaging results. Factors consistently found to be associated with failed repair include age of 65 years or older, large and massive tears (>3 cm), moderate to severe muscle atrophy, more than 50% fatty infiltration of the involved cuff, tear retraction of more than 2.5 cm, and diabetes. Some newer studies, however, have challenged these traditional risk factors. In a comparison of 40 patients older than 70 years and 40 patients younger than 50 years, Moraiti et al. found that functional gain was similar, even though healing was more frequent in younger patients. Although increasing age may predict a diminished healing environment, many studies have demonstrated excellent outcomes in older patients. Chung et al. reported that tendinosis severity assessed by preoperative MRI was the only factor associated with failure to heal in their 55 patients (mean age, 58 years), and Inderhaug et al. identified preoperative use of NSAIDs, long-standing symptoms before surgery, and nonacute onset of symptoms as predictors of inferior long-term outcomes in 147 patients. Other studies have noted that preoperative range of motion, obesity, fatty infiltration, or cuff retraction were not supported as prognostic factors for quality of life after arthroscopic rotator cuff repair. These conflicting reports emphasize the importance of careful preoperative evaluation and specific treatment plans tailored for the individual patient.

Several investigators have compared the results of decompression alone with repair and found much better results with repair. Satisfactory outcomes after decompression have ranged from 8% to 59%, and results have been reported to deteriorate over time. Most rotator cuff tears are now approached arthroscopically. The tear and size can be confirmed, and other intraarticular pathology can be treated. A decision can be made to treat the tear arthroscopically, or arthroscopically assisted (mini-open), or to convert to an open procedure. We currently believe that arthroscopic-assisted or arthroscopic repair is appropriate for partial-thickness and small to medium and some large full-thickness rotator cuff tears. Proposed advantages of arthroscopic repair include access for glenohumeral inspection and treatment of intraarticular lesions, no deltoid detachment, less soft-tissue dissection, and smaller incisions. Arthroscopic techniques can reliably assess rotator cuff tear size, tendon quality, tendon mobility, and suture anchor placement. A recent meta-analysis of randomized controlled trials comparing arthroscopic to mini-open repairs found no differences in surgery time, functional outcome scores, VAS pain scores, or functional outcomes. For the arthroscopic repair technique, see other chapter.

An arthroscopic-plus-open technique has been described for combined tears of the subscapularis, supraspinatus, and infraspinatus tendons. Repair of the posterosuperior rotator cuff is done arthroscopically, followed by open repair of the subscapularis tendon. Cited advantages of this method include an ability to treat concomitant pathology, relative ease of repair, and creation of a strong, reliable construct.

Open rotator cuff repairs also can be done through a miniarthrotomy deltoid-splitting approach.

OPEN REPAIR OF ROTATOR CUFF TEARS

TECHNIQUE 2.2

- Perform an anterior acromioplasty as described in Technique 2.1. This is an important part of rotator cuff surgery, and the results of repair without decompression are not as good as the results using the combined procedure.
- After standard acromioplasty, evaluate the rotator cuff tear carefully.
- Perform a subacromial bursectomy. Protect the biceps tendon unless biceps pathology is present; if so, a proximal biceps tendon release or tenodesis is indicated.
- Tears usually begin at the supraspinatus insertion, and the end retracts into its fossa under the acromioclavicular joint. Most tears not only are transverse but also have a longitudinal component, making them oval or triangular. All but the smallest tears need to be advanced anteriorly and laterally, not just laterally, to restore anatomic position and correct muscle-tendon unit length. In tears of more than 2 to 3 cm, the infraspinatus tendon is involved as well.
- When the defect has been identified and its size approximated, attention is turned to the repair itself. Typically some degree of mobilization is necessary.
- Begin mobilization posteriorly with the infraspinatus, using a blunt probe or a finger to release adhesions inside and outside the joint (Fig. 2.15A and B). Do not dissect below the level of the teres minor to avoid injury to the axillary nerve in the quadrangular space or the suprascapular nerve in the area of the spinoglenoid notch near the inferior border of the supraspinatus fossa.
- Continue mobilization anteriorly to the supraspinatus. If necessary, more exposure can be gained by resecting the distal 1.0 to 1.5 cm of the clavicle at the acromioclavicular joint, but this should not be done unless concomitant acromioclavicular arthrosis exists. Release of the coracohumeral ligament in this area allows further mobilization of the supraspinatus laterally.
- If the supraspinatus and infraspinatus tendons are retracted so far that adequate length cannot be obtained with tendon mobilization, incise the capsule at its insertion into the glenoid labrum (Fig. 2.15C and D). If necessary, carry this incision from the 8-o'clock position posterior to the 4-o'clock position posterior.
- The use of a second posterior incision over the scapular spine to increase mobilization has been described, but we have no experience with this technique.
- Debride the end of the mobilized tendon to obtain a raw edge, taking care not to confuse the tendon with the overlying bursa. The goals of mobilization are to obtain tissue of adequate strength, to position it anatomically for repair without damage to innervation and without compromise of deltoid function, and to decompress the subacromial space to prevent further mechanical impingement on repaired cuff tissue. When these goals are accomplished, the actual repair can be performed. We believe that the

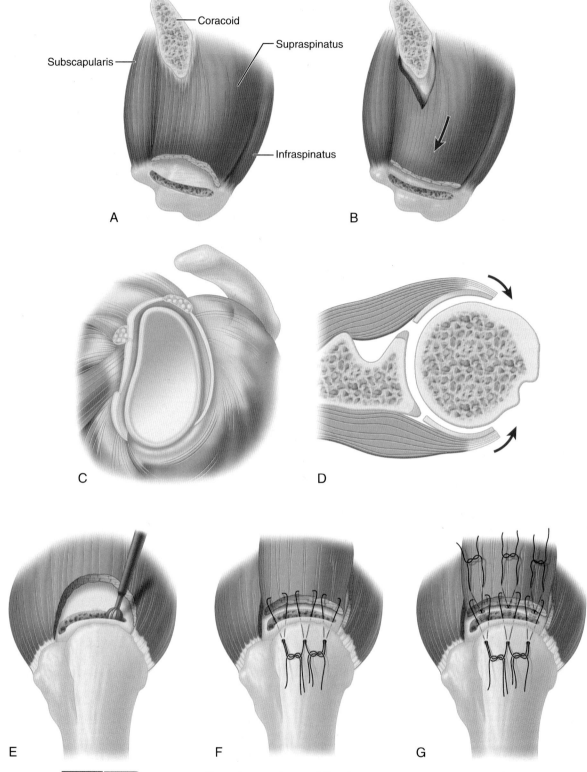

FIGURE **2.15** Rotator cuff repair. **A** and **B,** Mobilization. Supraspinatus and subscapularis muscles have fascial attachments to coracoid base via coracohumeral ligament. Lateral mobilization of retracted cuff is facilitated by release of these attachments. **C** and **D,** Substantial lateral advancement of cuff can be achieved by freeing capsule from glenoid by sharply incising capsule at its insertion into glenoid labrum. **E,** Osteotome is used to create trough. **F,** Holes for sutures are drilled 2 to 3 cm distal to trough. **G,** Suture anchors are inserted proximal to trough margin, passing proximal to proximal-most aspect of trough sutures. **SEE TECHNIQUE 2.2.**

best results are obtained with the double-row technique, suturing the tendon to bone in a cancellous trough in combination with suture anchor fixation. This reduces tension on the primary trough repair. Using transosseous tunnels through the greater tuberosity increases the surface area of tendon-to-bone healing, which more closely restores the anatomic footprint.

- With No. 2 nonabsorbable suture, use a double loop technique, superior to inferior and inferior to superior in a horizontal mattress manner. Place the sutures 5 to 10 mm from the free edge of the tear. This helps push the tendon down into the trough.

- Use a rongeur or burr to create a 3 mm wide shallow trough running the length of the exposed bone of the greater tuberosity (Fig. 2.15E) to accommodate the thickness of the supraspinatus and infraspinatus tendons.

- Place two or three rotator cuff suture anchors immediately medial to the trough at a 45-degree angle and pass the suture through the rotator cuff tendon 5 mm medial to the sutures in the free end of the tendon.

- Drill holes for sutures 2 to 3 cm distal to the trough, and connect them to the trough using a No. 5 Mayo needle, a towel clip, or a specialized instrument (Concept, Largo, FL; Fig. 2.15F). Take care not to fracture the thin cortical bone in this area, which may be osteoporotic. Space the holes at least 1 to 2 cm apart on the cortical humeral surface to give an adequate surface over which to tie the knots.

- Tie the suture of the anchor down on top of the tendon with four or five knots to prevent impingement of the suture material. The use of strong sutures rather than Kocher clamps or hemostats to pull on the tendon while suturing avoids crush injury to the tendon. We occasionally make longitudinal incisions along the extremes of the free tendon edge to allow placement of the tendon in the trough; these can be sutured before closure.

- Next secure the sutures from the suture anchors over the tendon, completing the double-row repair (Fig. 2.15G).

- Most repairs are done with the shoulder in 0 degrees of abduction.

- If the lateral humeral cortex is fractured during tying down of the suture or construction of the suture tunnel, the anchors can be used as a salvage procedure. The anchors reportedly have adequate holding power in cancellous bone and are reasonable alternatives in problematic situations. Use these sutures for additional leverage when tying down the trough sutures and tie them on top of the tendon with four knots to prevent impingement of the suture material.

- If the anterior deltoid has been detached, reattach it through 2-mm drill holes in the acromion and/or by periosteal repair.

- Close the wounds in the same manner as for open acromioplasty.

POSTOPERATIVE CARE Postoperative protocols are based on the size of the tear, condition of the tissue, and stability of the repair. The evidence supporting early motion protocols over immobilization is contradictory. After standard repair, a low-profile pillow sling is worn for 6 weeks. It is removed for assisted exercises in flexion and external rotation to avoid adhesions, disuse atrophy, and disruption of the repairs. The repair is weakest at 3 weeks, and tendon strength is less than at the time of surgery for the first 3 months after surgery. Empirically, we advance to isometric exercises of external rotation at 6 weeks, and at 12 weeks active motion is permitted. Patients are cautioned that over-aggressive use of the extremity can lead to disruption of the repair for 6 to 12 months, depending on the size of the repair and the quality of the tissue and repair.

■ MASSIVE AND IRREPARABLE TEARS

Cordasco and Bigliani identified five factors that improved results of operative treatment of large and massive rotator cuff tears:

1. Adequate subacromial decompression
2. Maintaining the integrity of the deltoid origin
3. Mobilizing torn tendons and performing an interval slide when indicated
4. Repairing tendons to bone
5. Carefully supervising and staging postoperative rehabilitation

In the ideal repair, the arm can be brought down to the patient's side without tension on the repair. Occasionally, despite the most diligent efforts to mobilize the tendons, tension remains on the repaired tendons. For these difficult problems, there are few options. If the tendon can be brought to the bony trough with the arm in abduction, the repair is completed and the shoulder is immobilized in an abduction orthosis for 6 weeks to permit tendon-to-bone healing. There are many problems with this technique, but we still believe it to be an option for certain patients.

Excessive tension at the repair that results in suture cutting through the tendon is believed to be the most common mechanism of failure of rotator cuff repair. The choice of suture type and technique can improve repair strength, as can decreasing the postoperative activity level. The latter option, however, has a significant problem with patient compliance. It is difficult to enforce the use of an abduction splint for 6 weeks because of problems with hygiene, comfort, and driving. Without early movement, adhesive capsulitis is likely and may produce a poorer result than the original tear and loss of collagen strength caused by immobilization. Overall results are consistent with improved pain relief and function; however, a decrease in range of motion and muscle strength may remain.

In an effort to decrease tension and increase strength and thus improve the rate and quality of biologic healing of rotator cuff repairs, a number of augmentation methods have been developed, including autografts (biceps, subscapularis, teres minor, latissimus dorsi, coracoacromial ligament), allografts (tendon, ligament, freeze-dried rotator cuff graft), xenografts, and synthetic grafts. The most frequently used augmentation methods involve scaffold devices, which have been developed from polylactic acid, poly(lactide-*co*-glycolide), and polytetrafluoroethylene; extracellular matrix (ECM) from human, porcine, bovine, and equine sources (Table 2.2); chitin; and chitosan-hyaluronan. Most of the published studies describe animal or biomechanical research involving ECM, with only a limited number of follow-up studies in human patients; these studies have reported mixed results in surgical outcomes and complication rates. Several studies, including one prospective comparative study, have reported improvements in outcomes after repairs of massive and recurrent rotator cuff tears with ECM augmentation, whereas others have

TABLE 2.2

Extracellular Matrix Scaffold Devices Currently Approved by the United States Food and Drug Administration for Rotator Cuff Repair

PRODUCT	TYPE	SOURCE	MANUFACTURER
Restore	SIS	Porcine	DePuy Orthopaedics (Warsaw, IN)
CuffPatch	SIS (crosslinked)	Porcine	Organogenesis (Canton, MA)
GraftJacket	Dermis	Human	Wright Medical Technology (Arlington, TN)
Conexa	Dermis	Porcine	Tornier (Edina, MN)
TissueMend	Dermis (fetal)	Bovine	Stryker Orthopaedics (Mahwah, NJ)
Zimmer Collagen Repair	Dermis (crosslinked)	Porcine	Zimmer (Warsaw, IN)
Bio-Blanket	Dermis (crosslinked)	Bovine	Kensey Nash (Exton, PA)
OrthADPAT Bioimplant	Pericardium (crosslinked)	Equine	Pegasus Biologics (Irvine, CA)
SYNTHETIC SCAFFOLD DEVICES			
SoftMesh Soft Tissue Reinforcement	Poly(urethane urea)		Biomet Sports Medicine (Warsaw, IN)
X-Repair	Poly-L-lactide		Synthasome (San Diego, CA)

SIS, Small intestinal submucosa.
From Derwin KA, Badylak SF, Steinmann SP, Iannotti JP: Extracellular matrix scaffold devices for rotator cuff repair, *J Shoulder Elbow Surg* 19:467–476, 2010.

found no significant improvement in outcomes. Other series have shown better results with synthetic patch augmentation than with biologic patch augmentation (retear rates of 17% and 51%, respectively). Studies of the use of a porcine xenograft scaffold have found not only worse outcomes with the scaffold but also severe postoperative inflammatory reactions requiring open debridement.

A number of factors influence the extent to which a scaffold device can augment the mechanical properties of a tendon repair, including the mechanical and suture retention properties and the surgical methods of scaffold application (e.g., the number, type, and location of fixation sutures; pretensioning of the scaffold at the time of repair). A study using an analytical model for rotator cuff repairs determined that 70% to 80% of the load is distributed to the tendon after repair, with 20% to 30% of the load carried by the augmentation device. The host response and remodeling of biologic scaffolds also are affected by the species and tissue of origin and the processing and sterilization methods used in preparing the scaffold. Because of the scarcity of clinical data on which to base indications for the use of biologic scaffolds, Derwin et al. developed a grading system that correlates tear size, geometry, and ability to be repaired to the appropriate use of ECM scaffolds (Table 2.3). We have limited experience with the use of ECM augmentation.

Molecular and cellular studies have targeted the tendon-bone interfaces, researching the use of growth factors and cell-coated scaffolds to improve healing. The delivery of transforming growth factor-β3 with an injectable calcium-phosphate matrix was reported to improve healing in a rat model, whereas other studies in a rat model found that application of mesenchymal stem cells genetically modified to overexpress bone morphogenetic protein-13 (BMP-13) did not improve healing, but that stem cells modified to overexpress the developmental gene *MT1-MMP* produced more fibrocartilage at the interface and improved biomechanical strength. Heringou et al. compared outcomes in rotator cuff tears with and without the use of mesenchymal stem cells and found significant improvements in healing time and substantial improvement in tendon integrity at 10 years after surgery.

In the late 1990s and early 2000s, platelet-rich plasma (PRP), which had been used successfully for many years in other medical specialties, became a popular treatment modality for a variety of orthopaedic conditions, including acute soft-tissue injuries and chronic tendinopathy. PRP is defined as a "volume of plasma that has a platelet count above the baseline of whole blood"; however, PRP preparations can vary markedly according to the amount of blood used and the efficacy of platelet recovery, the presence or absence of white or red blood cells, the activation of platelets with thrombin, and the level of fibrin production. The effect of PRP on healing also differs with different musculoskeletal structures, adding to the difficulty of determining its efficacy. Most studies of the efficacy of PRP in rotator cuff healing have found no benefit regarding retear rates or clinical outcomes. Five meta-analyses and two randomized controlled trials all reached the same conclusion: PRP does not improve early tendon-bone healing or functional recovery. Two comparative studies of leukocyte-plate-rich plasma (L-PRP) found no improvement in the quality of tendon healing or clinical outcomes with the use of L-PRP. A randomized comparison, however, found that PRP significantly decreased the rate of retears and increased the cross-sectional area of the supraspinatus in repair of large to massive rotator cuff repairs; there was no significant difference in clinical outcomes at 1 year.

Occasionally, despite the surgeon's best efforts and the use of all techniques of mobilization, some tears are so large or retracted, or both, that an anatomic repair is impossible. In this situation, several options are available, none of which is ideal. The two repair options are nonanatomic repair or partial repair. Muscle transfers or slides are another option. The final option is simple debridement.

TABLE 2.3

Grades of Rotator Cuff Pathology With Indications for Use of Extracellular Matrix in Repair

GRADE	TEAR CHARACTERISTICS	CURRENT TREATMENT(S)	OUTCOMES	INDICATION
VI	Massive, retracted irreparable tear with intraarticular pathology	Open reverse total shoulder replacement (aggressive)	Adequate, but limited function	Not indicated
V	Large, massive tear (3-5 cm, 2-3 tendons); not repairable (unable to reappose to tuberosity with low tension)	Open or arthroscopic attempt at repair, muscle transfer, debridement, and/or partial repair	High failure rate (≥50% retear and/or low outcome scores)	Interpositional in selected patients
IV	Large, massive tear (3-5 cm, 2-3 tendons); repairable	Open or arthroscopic repair	Moderate failure rate (≥30% retear rate, 85% pain free but function reduced)	Augmentation
III	Small to medium tear (<3 cm, 1 tendon)	Arthroscopic repair	Moderate failure rate (5%-10% retear rate; 85% pain free but >50% with reduced function)	Augmentation
II	Partial-thickness tear (>50% of articular or bursal surface)	Arthroscopic decompression/debridement or repair with acromioplasty	40% failure within 5 years with debridement only; 95% heal when repaired	Not indicated
I	Partial-thickness tear (<50% of articular or bursal surface)	Arthroscopic decompression/debridement or repair with acromioplasty	95% heal when repaired	Not indicated

From Derwin KA, Badylak SF, Steinmann SP, Iannotti JP: Extracellular matrix scaffold devices for rotator cuff repair, *J Shoulder Elbow Surg* 19:467–476, 2010.

McLaughlin described suturing the tendon to a trough in bone at whatever point it could be advanced onto the humeral head (Fig. 2.16). This may be more proximal (approximately 2 cm) through the anterior neck area. Although this repair allows a watertight closure, the mechanical advantage of the muscle-tendon unit is lost with this much proximal advancement. Partial repair of massive rotator cuff tears has been proposed to assist in closing large defects and as an alternative to debridement only or tendon transfers. The initial step is a side-to-side tendon repair that results in "marginal convergence" toward the greater tuberosity, which decreases the strain at the free margin of the rotator cuff tear, enhancing the mechanics of the construct. A combination of the tendon-to-tendon repair with tendon-to-bone repair can result in a functional rotator cuff. Partial repair has been shown to be superior to debridement, tendon transfers, and tendon augmentation procedures for the treatment of massive irreparable rotator cuff tears.

Tendon transfers for the treatment of irreparable rotator cuff tears may involve transfer of rotator cuff tendons or other muscle-tendon units. Cofield described subscapularis tendon transposition to fill large gaps in the supraspinatus insertion (Fig. 2.17). The flap is created by separating the outer portion of the subscapularis from the inner capsular portion. It is detached from the lesser tuberosity and mobilized superiorly to cover the humeral head. Other surgeons prefer to use the upper half of the subscapularis tendon by separating it from the anterior capsule and transferring it superiorly. This repair results in great tension in abduction and external rotation and disrupts the subscapularis force couple, which could prove detrimental to shoulder function.

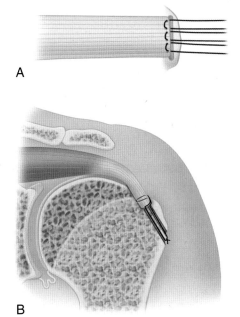

FIGURE 2.16 McLaughlin technique. **A** and **B,** Sutures are passed through appropriately placed bony holes, and cuff edge is drawn deep into trough.

For anterosuperior tears involving the subscapularis and the supraspinatus, transfer of the pectoralis major has been described. The coracoacromial arch should be intact. The technique involves sharply releasing the sternocostal portion of the pectoralis major from its common insertion site on the humerus and bluntly dissecting it from the more superficial clavicular head. Care should be taken not to injure its nerve supply. The sternocostal head is passed deep to the clavicular head and underneath the conjoined tendon to the lesser tuberosity. The musculocutaneous nerve should be identified and protected; the tendon is passed superficial to the nerve. Passing the tendon beneath the conjoined tendon improves the posterior and inferior vectors of the transferred tendon. This transfer also is indicated for treatment of anterior soft-tissue deficiencies and instability after shoulder arthroplasty.

For posterosuperior tears involving the infraspinatus and supraspinatus, the latissimus dorsi has been transferred. Clinically small but statistically significant gains can be expected in motion and strength. Factors reported to be associated with better clinical results include better preoperative function in active forward flexion and external rotation and synchronous in-phase contraction of the transferred latissimus dorsi by electromyography; poor shoulder function and generalized muscle weakness before surgery have been correlated with a poor clinical result. Patients with unsatisfactory results after this procedure may be clinically worse than they were preoperatively.

Transfer of the subcoracoid pectoralis major has been reported for patients with anterosuperior subluxation associated with massive rotator cuff tears, with approximately 80% satisfactory results. Other muscles used for transfer include the teres minor, deltoid, and trapezius, but these are used infrequently and are associated with compromised function. We have no experience with this technique.

Others have used free grafts (autologous or autogenous), such as the intrinsic portion of the biceps, the coracoacromial ligament, and fascia lata, or synthetics to augment or replace deficient rotator cuff tendon. There are few published reports of results, and most are not encouraging; however, successful closure of 14 massive cuff defects was reported with the use of a "tendon patch" fashioned from the long head of the biceps tendon. The disadvantages of the synthetic material are the potential for foreign body reaction to synthetics and tissue rejection. Such materials do not replace the atrophic and weakened rotator cuff musculature present with chronic massive tears.

LATISSIMUS DORSI TRANSFER

TECHNIQUE 2.3

(GERBER ET AL.)
- With the patient in the lateral decubitus position, make an 8-cm superolateral skin incision in the Langer lines immediately lateral to the acromioclavicular joint.
- With sharp dissection, detach the lateral deltoid from the acromion without leaving bone attached to the elevated tendinous origin; alternatively, use an osteotome to elevate the lateral deltoid with a thin layer of acromion attached to the deltoid origin.
- Leave the anterior deltoid untouched.
- After extensive mobilization of the retracted musculotendinous units, expose the rotator cuff and attempt to repair it directly to an osseous trough at the anatomic footprint.

- If mobilization of the supraspinatus, infraspinatus, and teres minor (including coracohumeral ligament release and capsulotomy) does not allow direct repair of the supraspinatus and infraspinatus tendons, proceed to latissimus dorsi transfer.
- Make a 12- to 15-cm posterior skin incision that follows the lateral border of the latissimus dorsi (Fig. 2.18A).
- Identify the muscle and release it from the humeral shaft (Fig. 2.18B), carefully protecting the axillary nerve, which lies immediately adjacent to the proximal end of the tendon, and the radial nerve, which curves around the humerus immediately distal to the tendon.
- Identify the neurovascular bundle and mobilize the latissimus dorsi distally.
- Pass two No. 3 braided polyester sutures through the tendon at its medial and lateral borders, and use a clamp to pull the tendon through the plane between the infraspinatus-teres minor and the deltoid muscles (Fig. 2.18C).
- Anchor the transferred tendon to a bony trough in the superolateral humeral head, pulling the heavy nonabsorbable sutures out through bone and tying the knots over the greater or lesser tuberosity (Fig. 2.18D).
- If possible, suture the remaining cuff to the transferred tendon. If this cannot be done, debride the remaining cuff and reattach the deltoid with transosseous sutures to the acromion. Close the deltopectoral fascia.

POSTOPERATIVE CARE The arm is splinted in 45 degrees of abduction and 30 to 45 degrees of external rotation; the splint is worn full time for 6 weeks. Passive range-of-motion exercises out of the splint are started the first postoperative day. After 6 weeks, the abduction splint is discontinued and active abduction and external rotation exercises are begun. Strengthening exercises are begun at 3 months and are continued for 6 to 9 months.

Another option that we recommend for many patients with massive tears without possibility for repair, even in abduction, is debridement and limited decompression. We attempt to leave the biceps in place as a humeral head depressor. The method is simple, does not disturb force couples, and is not overly restrictive postoperatively for the patient. We think it is a good choice, especially in elderly patients when pain control is the goal of surgery. Many short-term and midterm studies have shown satisfactory results with debridement and decompression of massive rotator cuff tears; however, long-term studies have shown that these results deteriorate over time.

We also have had success with subscapularis transposition (see Fig. 2.17); however, morbidity is higher with this procedure than with debridement and decompression, and the results are similar. Decompression and debridement should not be considered an alternative to direct repair or repair to a bone trough when such is possible.

We perform decompression and debridement of massive tears arthroscopically. The open technique is described here as an option, however. We have modified the technique by preserving and repairing the coracoacromial ligament to prevent anterosuperior subluxation of the humeral head postoperatively.

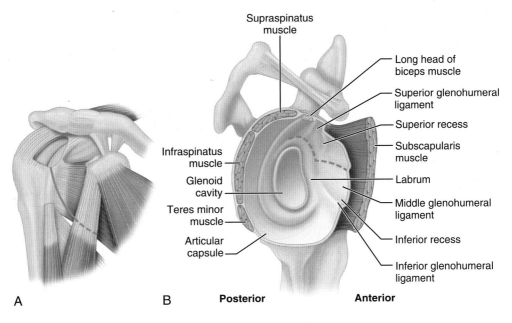

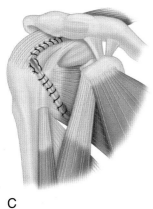

FIGURE 2.17 Cofield subscapularis transposition. **A,** Incision necessary for superior transposition of subscapularis tendon. **B,** Line of shoulder capsule incision. Inferior-middle glenohumeral ligament and subscapularis tendon and muscle are separated from capsule. **C,** Tendon-to-bone and tendon-to-tendon repair of transposed subscapularis. (**A** and **C** from Cofield RH: Subscapular muscle transposition for repair of chronic rotator cuff tears, *Surg Gynecol Obstet* 154[5]:667–672, 1982; **B** from Cofield RH: Subscapularis tendon transposition for large rotator cuff tears, *Tech Orthop* 3:58–64, 1989.)

DECOMPRESSION AND DEBRIDEMENT OF MASSIVE ROTATOR CUFF TEARS

TECHNIQUE 2.4

(ROCKWOOD ET AL.)
- Place the patient in a semi-seated position.
- Make an incision along the lateral border of the acromion along the lines of Langer.
- Open the interval between the anterior and lateral parts of the deltoid and resect the anterior part of the deltoid carefully from the anterior edge of the acromion.
- Remove 1 to 2 cm of the lateral part of the deltoid from the lateral edge of the acromion.
- With an osteotome, remove the portion of the acromion that extends beyond the anterior border of the clavicle vertically; excise the coracoacromial ligament along with this acromial fragment (as noted, we prefer to preserve the ligament).
- Remove the anteroinferior border of the acromion with an osteotome and smooth the surface on the remaining portion of the acromion with a rasp. We generally modify this portion by sharply detaching the coracoacromial ligament, performing an acromioplasty with an oscillating saw and reattaching the coracoacromial ligament to preserve coracoacromial arch stability.
- Debride the avascular tissue and try to mobilize, if possible, the vascularized tendons of the rotator cuff to repair the greater tuberosity of the humerus or the sulcus between the greater tuberosity and the articular surface of the humeral head without tension with the arm at the patient's side. This may be impossible if massive defects of 5 cm or more involving the supraspinatus and infraspinatus tendons are present. During mobilization, avoid injuring the suprascapular nerve.

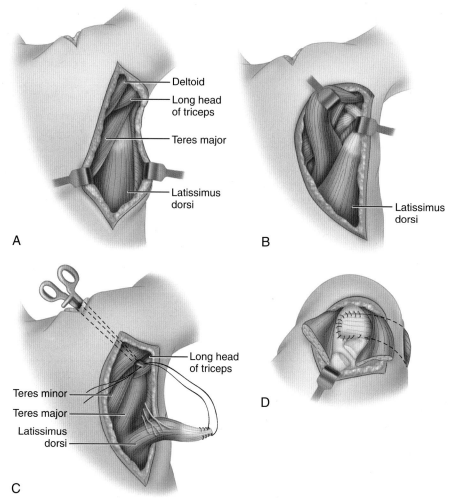

FIGURE 2.18 Latissimus dorsi transfer. **A,** Posterior skin incision. **B,** Release of muscle from humeral shaft. **C,** Braided sutures passed through end of tendon. **D,** Transferred tendon fixed to bony trough in humeral head. **SEE TECHNIQUE 2.3.**

- If adequate mobilization is impossible, sufficiently debride the cuff so that there are no residual components of the supraspinatus or infraspinatus tendons that can be caught, ground, or impinged between the head of the humerus and the acromion during flexion and rotation of the upper extremity. Greater tuberosity prominences must be excised to prevent impingement during passive flexion of the upper extremity.
- Apply bone wax to the base of the site of the excised exostosis to stop bleeding and prevent regrowth of the exostosis.
- Reattach the deltoid and the coracoacromial ligaments securely to the acromion with nonabsorbable No. 2 sutures.
- Close the incision in the usual manner.

POSTOPERATIVE CARE The upper extremity of the patient is supported in a commercially available shoulder-sling immobilizer. A single-shot or 3-day interscalene block can be placed preoperatively for pain control, and a cold therapy device can be used as desired. The initial objective is to obtain and maintain the maximal range of passive glenohumeral flexion and rotation while the deltoid muscle heals to the acromion. When the glenohumeral motion has been obtained, strengthening of the deltoid (especially the anterior portion), the remaining muscles of the rotator cuff, and the scapular stabilizers is the focus of therapy. Return to full activity usually requires 4 to 6 months.

■ COMPLICATIONS

Complications of rotator cuff repair occur with tears of all sizes, but especially with large and massive tears. Large amounts of retracted friable tissue are difficult to repair, and repair can be tenuous. Nonabsorbable suture material should be used for deltoid and rotator cuff tendon repair. Suture anchors alone seem to have sufficient endurance and pull-out strength compared with sutures pulled through bone tunnels. Although newer generations of suture anchors seem to have more favorable characteristics, we usually do not use them alone but rather combine them with sutures pulled through bone tunnels.

Because the suprascapular nerve lies only 1.8 cm from the posterosuperior glenoid rim, cuff mobilization should not exceed this. If more mobilization is necessary, capsular stripping can be done.

Transposition of the upper portion of the subscapularis tendon can result in anterior instability and weakness of internal rotation. Teres minor and infraspinatus transposition can result in external rotator weakness. Free grafts have been used with very little success and are not recommended.

Despite an excellent technical result, some patients do not return to previous activity levels. Some patients develop postoperative stiffness from immobilization, and some have persistent night pain. Although careful patient selection can decrease the frequency of these problems, only about 80% of patients have complete pain relief and return to nearly normal function. A special subset of patients comprises patients with workers' compensation claims in whom only a 40% to 50% success rate can be anticipated.

An unsolved complication of rotator cuff surgery involves coracoacromial arch deficiency with anterosuperior cuff tears resulting in subluxation of the humeral head, for which there is no effective treatment. Preservation of the coracoacromial arch is the best method to prevent this complication.

Outcomes after revision rotator cuff repair are not as good as after primary repair. Although short-term clinical results are similar, by 2 years, patients with revision rotator cuff repair are twice as likely to have a retear as those with primary repair.

CUFF TEAR ARTHROPATHY

Reverse total shoulder arthroplasty (RTSA) was developed for the treatment of cuff tear arthropathy. The pathophysiology of the disorder, as well as the technique and outcomes, for RTSA are described in other chapter.

ADHESIVE CAPSULITIS

Much of current understanding of frozen shoulder, or adhesive capsulitis, comes from the work of Neviaser and Lundberg. Neviaser coined the term *adhesive capsulitis* to describe a contracted, thickened joint capsule that seemed to be drawn tightly around the humeral head with a relative absence of synovial fluid and chronic inflammatory changes within the subsynovial layer of the capsule. Evidence suggests that the underlying pathologic changes in adhesive capsulitis are synovial inflammation with subsequent reactive capsular fibrosis. Four stages of disease have been described based on the arthroscopic appearance of the joint capsule. The disease progresses from capsular inflammation to fibrosis. Stage 1, the pre-adhesive stage, consists of a fibrinous inflammatory synovitis reaction without adhesion formation. Patients typically have full motion but report pain, especially at night. Symptoms are nonspecific, and misdiagnosis is common. Stage 2 is marked by acute adhesive synovitis with proliferation of the synovium and early formation of adhesions, most notably in the dependent inferior capsular fold. Pain is a prominent feature, and motion loss is present but typically mild. Stage 3, the maturation stage, involves less synovitis and more fibrosis. The axillary fold is obliterated. Pain may be less severe than in previous stages, but motion is significantly restricted. In stage 4, the chronic stage, adhesions are fully mature, and motion is severely reduced. Patients may have painless, limited range of motion, but pain occurs at the end ranges of motion or when the arm is suddenly moved.

Cytokines, metalloproteinases 2 and 9, and transforming growth factor-beta 1 have been implicated in the process, but the initial triggering event in the cascade is unknown. Using immunohistochemistry, alarmins—endogenous molecules released into the extracellular milieu after infection or tissue injury—have been found to be significantly increased in the frozen shoulder capsules compared to control capsules. The expression of alarmin molecule HMGB1 significantly correlates with the severity of patient-reported pain. The CB1 pathway also has been studied for its role in the pathogenesis of shoulder stiffness. Patients with stiffness had higher messenger RNA expression and immunohistochemistry staining of CB1 in the subacromial bursa and higher CB1 concentration in the subacromial fluid. Hyperlipidemia also has been proposed as a risk factor for primary frozen shoulder, and this association was supported by the findings of a comparative study of 300 patients with frozen shoulder and 900 control subjects. Further research is needed, however, to determine if a nonoptimal serum lipid level is a cause, a related cofactor, or a result of primary frozen shoulder. Increased expression of nerve growth factor receptor and new nerve fibers found in the shoulder capsular tissue of patients with frozen shoulder suggest that neoinnervation and neoangiogenesis in the capsule are important events in the pathogenesis of frozen shoulder and may help explain the often severe pain in patients with this condition. Although it remains a matter of controversy, some authors have suggested that inadequate glycemic control as measured by the glycosylated hemoglobin A1c (HbA1c) level can identify diabetic patients who are at higher risk for developing frozen shoulder. In a series of 1150 diabetic patients with frozen shoulder, no association was found between HbA1c level and the occurrence of frozen shoulder; however, insulin-dependent patients were nearly twice as likely to develop frozen shoulder.

The incidence of frozen shoulder in the general population is approximately 2%, but several conditions are associated with an increased incidence, including female gender, age older than 49 years, diabetes mellitus (five times more), cervical disc disease, prolonged immobilization, hyperthyroidism, stroke or myocardial infarction, the presence of autoimmune diseases, and trauma. Individuals between the ages of 40 and 70 are more commonly affected. Approximately 70% of patients are women. Between 20% and 30% of affected individuals develop adhesive capsulitis in the opposite shoulder. The condition rarely recurs in the same shoulder. Common to almost all patients is a period of immobility, the causes of which are diverse; this probably is the most significant factor related to the development of the condition.

Lundberg developed a classification system of frozen shoulder based on the presence or absence of an inciting event. Frozen shoulders in patients who report no inciting event and with no abnormality on examination (other than loss of motion) or plain radiographs were designated as "primary," and frozen shoulders in patients with precipitant traumatic injuries were designated as "secondary." Patients with shoulder stiffness after a surgical procedure technically have a secondary frozen shoulder, but their clinical course and treatment are different and are not discussed here. These conditions perhaps should be considered more of an arthrofibrosis.

There are no universally accepted criteria for the diagnosis of frozen shoulder. We have noted that internal rotation frequently is lost initially, followed by loss of flexion and external rotation. Most often our patients can internally rotate only to the sacrum, have 50% loss of external rotation, and have less than 90 degrees of abduction. We include these patients in the diagnosis of frozen shoulder, but we have no formal inclusion criteria.

Diagnostic tests in patients with a frozen shoulder (including plain film radiographs) usually are normal, except in patients with medical disorders such as diabetes or thyroid disease. Bone scans have been reported to be positive in some patients, and a positive bone scan has been shown to have positive predictive value for treatment with steroid injections. MRI has shown a contracted inferior capsule and an increased blood flow to the synovium, but its value is in evaluating the other structures in the shoulder to eliminate other pathologic conditions. On dynamic three-dimensional MRI examination, frozen shoulder patients were found to have an abnormal intake of blood flow from the acromial arterial network and the branches of circumflex humeral arteries into the axillary pouch and the rotator interval. This finding has been named the "burning sign."

Arthrograms characteristically show a reduced joint volume with irregular margins. Clinical improvement has been reported after arthrography because of brisement of adhesions from forcefully injecting fluid into the joint. A volume of less than 10 mL and lack of filling of the axillary fold currently are accepted arthrographic findings indicative of a frozen shoulder.

■ PRIMARY FROZEN SHOULDER

The clinical course of primary (idiopathic) frozen shoulder consists of three phases. Secondary frozen shoulders may not exhibit all three phases and may not follow the exact chronology. Although treatment for the two entities often is similar, the cause for the secondary frozen shoulder should be identified and treated as well. The three phases are as follows:

Phase I: Pain. Patients usually have a gradual onset of diffuse shoulder pain, which is progressive over weeks to months. The pain usually is worse at night and is exacerbated by lying on the affected side. As the patient uses the arm less, pain leading to stiffness ensues.

Phase II: Stiffness. Patients seek pain relief by restricting movement. This heralds the beginning of the stiffness phase, which usually lasts 4 to 12 months. Patients describe difficulty with activities of daily living; men have trouble getting to their wallets in their back pockets, and women have trouble with fastening brassieres. As stiffness progresses, a dull ache is present nearly all the time (especially at night), and this often is accompanied by sharp pain during range of motion at or near the new end points of motion.

Phase III: Thawing. This phase lasts for weeks or months, and as motion increases, pain diminishes. Without treatment (other than benign neglect), motion return is gradual in most but may never objectively return to normal, although most patients subjectively feel near normal, perhaps as a result of compensation or adjustment in ways of performing activities of daily living.

▮ TREATMENT

Traditionally, frozen shoulder has been considered a self-limiting condition, lasting 12 to 18 months without long-term sequelae. Approximately 10% of patients have long-term problems, however. In their almost 10-year

average follow-up of 83 patients with frozen shoulder, Vastamäki et al. found that 94% recovered to normal levels of function and motion without treatment; however, only 51% of patients in the untreated group, 44% in the nonoperative treatment group, and 30% in the manipulation group were totally pain-free. Long-term follow-up studies have shown that patients underestimate the amount of objective motion lost and that the duration of symptoms before medical care is sought may be correlated with recovery. Patients seeking care earlier usually recover more quickly. Dominant shoulder involvement has been reported to be predictive of a good result, whereas occupation and treatment programs are not statistically significant. The best treatment of frozen shoulder is prevention (secondary frozen shoulder), but early intervention is paramount; a good understanding of the pathologic process by the patient and the physician also is important.

Treatment options described in the literature include benign neglect, supervised physical therapy, nonsteroidal antiinflammatory medications, oral corticosteroids, intraarticular steroid injections, distention arthrography, hydrodistention, closed manipulation, open surgical release, and arthroscopic capsular release. In two similar groups of patients with frozen shoulders, a home therapy program obtained results equal to those of arthroscopic release. Initial treatment is nonoperative, with emphasis placed on control of pain and inflammation. Intraarticular steroid injections have been shown in a number of studies to obtain more rapid pain relief, better functional outcomes, and higher patient satisfaction than other nonoperative modalities. In a study of nearly 200 patients with adhesive capsulitis, the site of the injection (subacromial, intraarticular, intraarticular combined with subacromial space, or rotator interval) did not affect the effectiveness of treatment, and another comparison study showed no difference in outcomes between glenohumeral and subacromial steroid injections. A prospective randomized study compared three injection techniques—intraarticular, subacromial, and hydrodilatation—and found similar clinical improvement at final follow-up. Hyaluronate intraarticular injections have been shown to be as effective as steroid injections, with fewer side effects. Transcutaneous electrical nerve stimulation and ultrasound may be helpful, combined with passive and active range-of-motion exercises. Extracorporeal shockwave therapy (ESWT) has been shown to result in faster improvement and better final functional scores than those obtained with oral prednisolone. Abduction should be avoided initially to prevent impingement until joint motion becomes suppler. Intraarticular cortisone injections have proved beneficial in phase 1 or early phase 2 of the clinical course.

Although a frozen shoulder usually is self-limiting and resolves in 12 to 18 months, many patients do not wish to wait that long for resolution of symptoms and request active intervention long before 12 months. With appropriate patient selection, significant improvement can be obtained in approximately 70% of patients. Results have been shown to be significantly worse in diabetic patients, even though they may have improvement in function; full range of motion was obtained in only 71% of diabetic patients compared with 90% of nondiabetic patients. We have used closed manipulation under anesthesia with good results over many years and still believe in its efficacy. A systematic review involving 989 patients concluded that the data demonstrated little benefit for a capsular release instead of, or in addition to, manipulation. Failures usually are related to inability to maintain postoperative motion rather than intraoperative complications. For patients in whom closed manipulation fails, arthroscopic release is recommended. If arthroscopic release fails to relieve symptoms, open release of contractures has been recommended, with emphasis on release of the coracohumeral ligament and reestablishment of the interval between the supraspinatus and subscapularis. We have no recent experience with the technique of open release, but it may be appropriate in patients with poor bone stock or recent fractures or in patients who have had surgery recently. For patients who require surgical release, we prefer to do this arthroscopically.

CLOSED MANIPULATION
TECHNIQUE 2.5

- After administering general anesthesia supplemented with an interscalene block for postoperative pain control, manipulate the shoulder using a short lever arm and a fixed scapula.
- The acronym FEAR can be used as a safe sequence for shoulder manipulation-flexion, extension, abduction and adduction, external and internal rotation.
- Audible and palpable release of adhesions is a good prognostic sign.
- We occasionally obtain intraoperative anteroposterior and axillary lateral radiographs after the procedure to check for periarticular fracture or dislocation.

POSTOPERATIVE CARE Rehabilitation after manipulation is crucial in preventing recurrence. We perform manipulations during the earlier part of the week and initiate physical therapy the following day. Supervised physical therapy sessions are performed daily for at least 2 to 4 weeks. The goal of rehabilitation is early full range of motion. In some patients, we recommend an abduction orthosis at night for 3 weeks to prevent significant axial pouch adhesions from returning in the early phase.

▌ COMPLICATIONS

Complications during closed manipulation can occur. The proximal humerus may be fractured during manipulation, or dislocation may occur. Manipulation should be avoided in patients with osteopenia or recently healed fractures and reserved for patients with recalcitrant stiffness unresponsive to conservative management. If dislocation occurs after closed manipulation, rehabilitation should be aggressive, but the abducted, externally rotated position should be avoided.

Arthroscopic release is an option when closed manipulation fails or for patients who have had prolonged, recalcitrant adhesive capsulitis, with marked improvement reported in 80% to 90% of patients. A long-term follow-up study found that motion equal to the contralateral shoulder was maintained or enhanced at 7 years after surgery. For the technique of arthroscopic capsular release, see other chapter.

CALCIFIC TENDINITIS

Calcific tendinitis is a painful, largely self-limited disorder of the rotator cuff in which the tendons are infiltrated with calcium deposits. The most common site of occurrence is within the supraspinatus tendon and at a location 1.5 to 2 cm away from the tendon insertion on the greater tuberosity. Calcific tendinitis usually has its onset in individuals who are older than 30 years, and it affects approximately 10% of the population. An analysis of 1219 patients with and without subacromial pain found calcific deposits in 8% of asymptomatic patients and 43% of those with subacromial pain. Women between the ages of 30 and 60 years were the most frequently affected. Ten percent of patients affected have bilateral deposits. Most individuals with deposits are asymptomatic, but pain can be intense in symptomatic patients.

Although the clinical course and pathologic changes of calcific tendinitis are well delineated, its cause remains unknown. Suggested causes have included a vascular etiology, with degeneration of the tendon fibers preceding calcification, and aging of the tendon, with a general diminishing of the vascularity to the supraspinatus as a normal course of events. Microangiographic studies showed an area of hypovascularity near Codman's "critical zone" just proximal to the supraspinatus insertion into the greater tuberosity. This hypoperfusion is believed to initiate degenerative changes, which subsequently lead to calcification or susceptibility to tearing, as mentioned in the previous section on rotator cuff tears. Other histologic studies, however, showed no evidence of inadequate vascularization, and the supraspinatus, including the critical zone, was found to be well supplied with an anastomosis of vessels. One histologic study demonstrated neovascularization and neoinnervation in calcific tendonitis, with an associated substantial inflammatory response as the cause of pain.

■ CHRONOLOGIC PROGRESSION

Calcific tendinitis follows a definite progression in most patients, and resolution is seen in almost all of them, with the length of time required being the only true variable. The following three-phase chronology described by Sarkar and Uhthoff is useful in planning treatment:

Phase I: Precalcification stage. In the precalcification stage, the site of predilection for calcification (possibly a site with a diminished blood supply) undergoes fibrocartilaginous metaplasia. At this stage, patients generally are asymptomatic.

Phase II: Calcification stage. During this stage, calcium is deposited into matrix vesicles, which are excreted by the cells and coalesce into larger calcium deposits (Fig. 2.19). This initial part of the calcification stage is known as the *phase of formation.* At this time, the deposits on

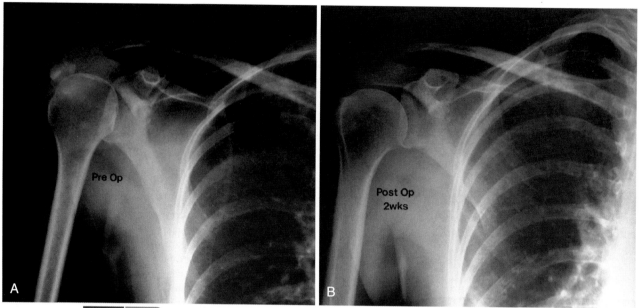

FIGURE 2.19   **A,** Preoperative radiograph showing calcium deposits. **B,** Radiograph taken 2 weeks after surgery.

gross inspection are dry and chalky. As the matrix vesicles coalesce into larger deposits, the fibrocartilage gradually is replaced and eroded. The patient enters a resting phase, during which the pain may be minimal, and the radiographic appearance is one of well-marginated, mature-appearing deposits. This resting phase is of variable length and ends with the beginning of the resorptive phase. During the resorptive phase, vascular channels appear at the periphery of the deposit and calcium resorption ensues. Apatite crystals can also migrate into the subacromial bursa, causing an influx of leukocytes as well as IL-1Beta and Il-18. This stage can, therefore, be exceedingly painful, and many patients seek treatment at this time. The calcium deposits at this time resemble cream or toothpaste. As the calcium is resorbed, the dead space is filled with granulation tissue.

Phase III: Postcalcification phase. During this phase, the granulation tissue matures into mature collagen aligned along stress lines with the longitudinal axis of the tendon, reconstituting the tendon. Pain subsides markedly during this phase.

Although most patients seek treatment during the acutely painful resorptive phase of the calcification stage, in some the calcium deposits are an incidental finding or are part of an impingement syndrome. In these patients, we recommend treatment protocols directed at the particular pathologic condition (e.g., impingement) rather than the calcific deposits.

As noted previously, essentially all patients eventually recover from calcific tendinitis and nonoperative management is the initial treatment of choice. Nonoperative treatment usually includes physical therapy, exercises, antiinflammatory medications, and corticosteroid injections. Although these modalities are generally recommended as effective, there is little high-level supporting evidence. Corticosteroids have been suggested to abort the resorptive phase, returning the

lesion to dormancy and setting into motion the factors necessary for recurrence.

PERCUTANEOUS AND SURGICAL TREATMENT

Gschwend et al. listed the following as indications for operative treatment: (1) symptom progression, (2) constant pain that interferes with activities of daily living, and (3) absence of improvement after conservative therapy.

An ultrasound-guided percutaneous needling technique used in conjunction with subacromial corticosteroid injection was reported to be successful in approximately 70% of patients. Another prospective study showed that initial improvements after ultrasound-guided needle lavage were maintained for at least 2 years. However, although one systematic review found this technique to be as effective as subacromial corticosteroid injection another randomized controlled trial found better results with ultrasound-guided needling and lavage than with corticosteroid injection, while another found no difference in outcomes at 5 years of follow-up. Long-term follow-up studies have confirmed the benign natural history of this disorder; one study with 10 years of follow-up of a randomized controlled trial demonstrated resolution of symptoms and calcific deposits, regardless of whether ultrasound therapy was used. Although treated patients tend to have better results in the short term (1-year follow-up), at longer-term follow-up there are no differences.

Extracorporeal shockwave therapy (ESWT) also has been well studied for the treatment of calcific tendinitis. Several comparative studies have reported greater pain relief with ESWT than with placebo or sham treatment, although in one study half of the patients eventually required surgery. Two systematic reviews concluded it to be a safe and effective treatment for this disorder. Recent investigation has confirmed that high-dose ESWT, with or without use of adjunctive kinesiotaping, continues to be an effective treatment.

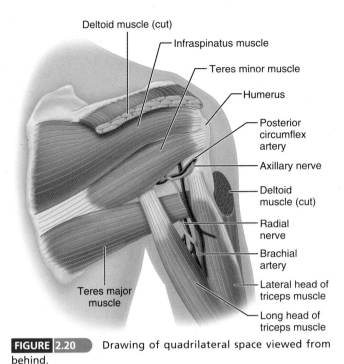

Deltoid muscle (cut)
Infraspinatus muscle
Teres minor muscle
Humerus
Posterior circumflex artery
Axillary nerve
Deltoid muscle (cut)
Radial nerve
Brachial artery
Teres major muscle
Lateral head of triceps muscle
Long head of triceps muscle

FIGURE 2.20 Drawing of quadrilateral space viewed from behind.

QUADRILATERAL SPACE SYNDROME

Quadrilateral space syndrome (QSS) is caused by compression of the axillary nerves and posterior humeral circumflex artery in the quadrilateral space, which is bounded by the teres major and minor muscles, the humeral shaft, and the long head of the triceps (Fig. 2.20). Although the etiology of QSS has not been clearly defined, fibrous bands are the most frequently cited cause. Space-occupying lesions also have been implicated in the development of QSS, including paralabral cysts, bony fracture fragments, and benign tumors such as lipomas, osteochondromas, and schwannomas. Because many symptoms of QSS are nonspecific, the diagnosis, and subsequently treatment, may be delayed. One study documented an average delay from onset of symptoms to surgical decompression of 14.5 months (range, 6 to 24 months). Hangge et al. described a patient who had seven surgical procedures, acupuncture, extensive physical therapy, and steroid injections before the diagnosis of QSS was made.

The syndrome usually affects the dominant arm of young adults, particularly athletes (20 to 35 years of age) involved in overhead sports, and is characterized by poorly localized anterior and lateral shoulder pain and point tenderness over the quadrilateral space near the teres minor insertion. Symptoms are reproduced by holding the arm abducted and externally rotated for 1 minute. Weakness and atrophy are difficult to detect unless significant deltoid involvement is present. Selective atrophy of the teres minor muscle, which is innervated by the axillary nerve, can be seen on MRI and is highly suggestive of QSS. Arteriography shows occlusion of the posterior humeral circumflex artery with the arm in abduction and external rotation, but the artery appears normal with the arm at the side. More recently, ultrasound has been reported to be effective in detecting dilation, occlusion, and stenosis of the posterior humeral circumflex artery and atrophy of the deltoid muscle. Ultrasound also can demonstrate swelling or lesions of the axillary nerve and space-occupying lesion in the quadrilateral space. Color Doppler sonography has been used to compare differences in the posterior humeral circumflex arterial flow between neutral and provocative position.

The lesion seems to consist of oblique fibrous bands that compress the nerve and artery with the shoulder in abduction and external rotation. These bands can be lysed at surgery through a posterior approach with good results. Occasionally, a paralabral cyst from the posterior labrum may cause compression of the nerve. Brown et al. suggested classifying the syndrome into two types—neurogenic and vascular—and provided an algorithm for diagnosis and treatment (Fig. 2.21). According to their system, vascular QSS is caused by repetitive trauma to the posterior circumflex humeral artery during abduction and external rotation and is more likely to occur in professional or collegiate athletes involved in overhead sports. Neurogenic QSS can be caused by various fixed anatomic anomalies, with fibrous bands being the most common.

Nonoperative treatment, including activity modification, NSAIDs, cortisone injections, and physical therapy for rotator cuff muscle strengthening, is indicated initially for all patients. If symptoms persist after 3 to 6 months of nonoperative treatment, a posterior approach to the area with lysis of the fibrous bands usually results in symptom relief.

Recently, there has been a rapid proliferation of high-level studies comparing nonoperative treatments for calcific tendonitis. Several systematic reviews and meta-analyses have agreed that ultrasound-guided needling and ESWT are effective treatments; however, ultrasound-guided needling tends to result in faster resolution of symptoms and calcific deposits. Thus the preponderance of high-level evidence suggests ultrasound-guided needling as the nonoperative treatment of choice for this disorder.

For patients in whom nonoperative treatment fails, we prefer an arthroscopic technique when surgery is warranted. We note, however, that concomitant glenohumeral pathology is uncommon, and an MRI study demonstrated that patients with calcific deposits are not at increased risk for rotator cuff tears, suggesting that they are different disorders arising from different processes. As such, routine diagnostic arthroscopy in patients with calcific tendonitis generally is unnecessary. Removal of calcium deposits is done with a mechanical shaver. Some authors have reported success with using ultrasound intraoperatively to identify the deposits that are not readily seen with arthroscopy. Acromioplasty is done for patients with preoperative evidence of subacromial stenosis. Several authors have reported good results in approximately 90% of patients with arthroscopic removal of calcific deposits, and midterm follow-up studies have demonstrated that these good results are preserved over time. The importance of acromioplasty and the presence of residual calcifications on postoperative radiographs remain unclear. One systematic review found no difference in outcomes of arthroscopic management of calcific tendonitis when comparing three treatment arms: acromioplasty with calcific deposit removal, acromioplasty without deposit removal, and isolated calcific deposit removal. For the operative details of the arthroscopic technique.

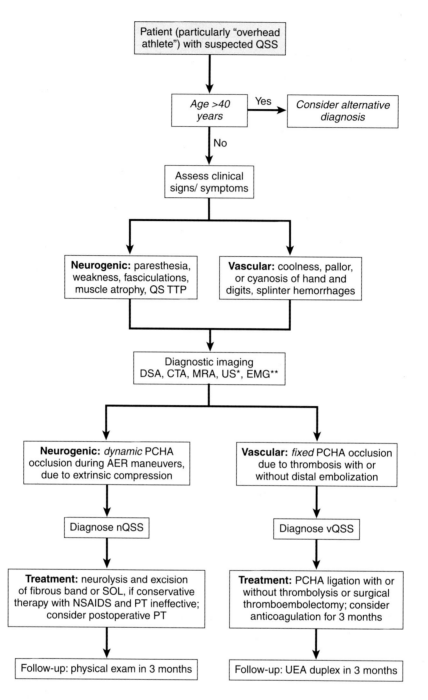

* Ultrasound imaging has been preliminarily studied for the diagnosis of nQSS; there have not yet been studies specifically assessing ultrasound use to diagnose vQSS
** Electromyography has poor sensitivity for nQSS, but can rule out alternative diagnoses

FIGURE 2.21 Diagnosis and treatment algorithm for patients with suspected quadrilateral space syndrome. *AER,* Abduction and external rotation; *CTA,* computed tomography angiography; *DSA,* digital subtraction angiography; *MRA,* magnetic resonance angiography; *nQSS,* neurogenic quadrilateral space syndrome; *NSAID,* nonsteroidal antiinflammatory drug; *overhead athlete,* any patient engaged in elite, college, professional, or dedicated sport or activity involving repetitive abduction and external rotation of the arm above the head; *PCHA,* posterior circumflex humeral artery; *PT,* physical therapy; *QS,* quadrilateral space; *QSS,* quadrilateral space syndrome; *SOL,* space-occupying lesion; *UEA,* upper extremity arterial; *US,* ultrasound; *vQSS,* vascular quadrilateral space syndrome. (From Brown SN, Doolittle DA, Bohanon CJ, et al: Quadrilateral space syndrome: the Mayo Clinic experience with a new classification system and case series, *Mayo Clin Proc* 90[3]:382–394, 2015.)

POSTERIOR SURGICAL APPROACH FOR QUADRILATERAL SPACE SYNDROME

TECHNIQUE 2.6

(CAHILL AND PALMER)

- Make an incision parallel and just inferior to the spine of the scapula and curve it inferiorly over the posterior humerus to allow inferior lateral dissection (Fig. 2.22A). Develop a skin flap, including all subcutaneous tissue.
- Control bleeding, which may be moderately severe, with electrocautery; otherwise, when the deep fascia is opened, the bleeding dissects into the areolar planes and markedly hinders the view of the neurovascular bundle. Hemostasis is necessary before opening the deep fascia.
- Dissect the fascia at the inferior border of the deltoid (Fig. 2.22B), beginning inferolaterally and proceeding superiorly and medially.
- Remove the deltoid from the spine of the scapula by electrocautery, leaving a border of the musculotendinous area for resuture.
- Detach the teres minor at its insertion into the rotator cuff and reflect it medially, leaving a small opening in the posterior glenohumeral capsule. No weakness of external rotation of the humerus has been detected postoperatively if the teres minor has not been reattached.
- Decompress the quadrilateral space by blunt and sharp dissection (Fig. 2.22C). A finger inserted into this space directed anteriorly is tethered and meets resistance before removal of the fibrous bands traversing this space.
- Follow the neurovascular bundle forward to its origin from the main vessel. Avoid injuring any accompanying veins, which are prone to tearing and bleeding.
- After decompression is complete (Fig. 2.22D), place a finger on the posterior circumflex artery. Abduct the arm and test the pulse for adequate decompression.
- Do not reattach the teres minor to the capsule, and approximate only the deltoid.

POSTOPERATIVE CARE A sling is worn until the patient feels comfortable. Early range of motion is encouraged to avoid superimposed adhesive capsulitis.

SUPRASCAPULAR NERVE ENTRAPMENT

Suprascapular neuropathy is a relatively uncommon but well-recognized source of shoulder pain, weakness, and dysfunction. Boykin et al. estimated the prevalence of suprascapular neuropathy to be at least 4.3% in patients with shoulder complaints presenting to an academic referral center. Much higher rates, as high as 33%, have been reported in elite overhead athletes. Suprascapular neuropathy occurs most commonly in young and middle-aged individuals.

The suprascapular nerve is derived from the upper trunk of the brachial plexus formed by the roots of C5 and C6, and occasionally C4 at the Erb point. The nerve passes parallel to the omohyoid muscle dorsal to the brachial plexus and beneath the trapezius to the superior edge of the scapula and through the suprascapular notch, which can assume several configurations.

The transverse scapular ligament forms the roof of the notch. After passing through the notch, the nerve supplies the supraspinatus and the shoulder capsule and the glenohumeral and acromioclavicular joints. The nerve turns around the lateral margin of the scapular spine to innervate the infraspinatus.

Most suprascapular nerve entrapments occur at the suprascapular notch. The nerve can be injured at the suprascapular notch as a result of compression by the overlying transverse scapular ligament. A narrow notch or a calcified ligament has been shown to be associated with an increased risk of injury to the suprascapular nerve. A 3D-CT study of 760 consecutive patients scheduled for shoulder surgery showed that morphologic changes of the scapular notch are related to aging, with the notch narrowing in older individuals.

Lipomas and ganglion cysts have been described compressing the inferior branch of the suprascapular nerve and leading to isolated infraspinatus atrophy. These usually are found at the spinoglenoid notch and can be seen on MRI (Fig. 2.23). The ganglion cyst usually is the result of intraarticular pathology, such as a posterior labral tear. The nerve may be compressed by the spinoglenoid ligament, also known as the inferior transverse scapular ligament, which arises from the lateral aspect of the root of the spine of the scapula and inserts at the margin of the glenoid with fibers to the posterior glenohumeral capsule. This ligament tightens with cross-body adduction and internal rotation, compressing the nerve.

Nerve traction injuries associated with rotator cuff tears have been suggested as a cause of suprascapular neuropathy, as have repetitive overhead activities that may produce muscle and tendon microtrauma with nerve inflammation and compression. Suprascapular nerve injuries have been documented in swimmers, baseball pitchers, volleyball players, and tennis players. In a study of 65 patients with confirmed suprascapular neuropathy, nearly half of the neuropathies were related to trauma; the other two most frequent causes were inflammatory processes, such as brachial neuritis, and cysts; and none were attributed to notch abnormalities. Suprascapular neuropathy has also been described in massive retracted rotator cuff tears. The mechanism is thought to be a traction injury on the nerve by the retracted cuff tendons. Injuries to the nerve also are speculated to occur when massive rotator cuff tears are repaired with excessive tension and subsequent traction on the nerve. In addition, iatrogenic injuries to the nerve have been reported during several procedures that involve drilling and passing sutures and/or placing screws about the glenoid face and rim.

The diagnosis may be confirmed on electromyography as long as the surgeon alerts the electromyographer to the physical findings and proposed diagnosis. Patients usually complain of deep, aching, and diffuse pain and may complain of weakness of external rotation and abduction with overhead activities. An ultrasound-guided diagnostic nerve block may be helpful. Relief of shoulder pain (usually dramatic and of short duration) after an injection of 1% local anesthetic supports the diagnosis, although a negative test does not rule out suprascapular nerve entrapment because the injection may not have been accurately placed. Muscle atrophy may or may not be present. Painless atrophy of the infraspinatus muscle is more common with compression of the nerve at the spinoglenoid notch. Of interest, many athletes with this muscle atrophy appear to have little dysfunction or symptoms and quite frequently are performing successfully at a high level.

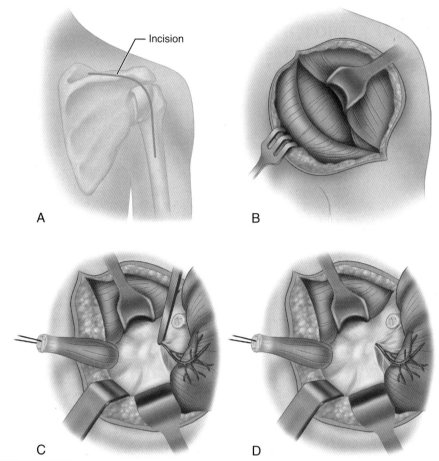

FIGURE 2.22 Cahill and Palmer technique. **A,** Skin incision. **B,** Retractor placed under border of deltoid. **C,** Teres minor is held by suture on left, with circular area on right representing insertion of teres minor. Clamp holds fibrous bands traversing quadrilateral space that tether neurovascular bundle. Deltoid is reflected to right. **D,** Dissection is complete, with fibrous bands dissected away from neurovascular bundle. (Redrawn from Cahill BR, Palmer RE: Quadrilateral space syndrome, *J Hand Surg* 8[1]:65–69, 1983.) **SEE TECHNIQUE 2.6.**

If no structural lesion, such as a cyst, is seen on MRI, activity modification, NSAIDs, and a shoulder rehabilitation program should be the initial treatment. If nonoperative treatment fails, surgery should be considered. In patients with proven compression of the nerve and a space-occupying lesion or cyst, nonoperative treatment may have less favorable results over time, and early surgery generally is recommended. Arthroscopic and open approaches have been described for decompression of the nerve, based on the location and cause of compression. We generally prefer an arthroscopic approach.

POSTERIOR SURGICAL APPROACH FOR SUPRASCAPULAR NERVE ENTRAPMENT

TECHNIQUE 2.7

(POST AND MAYER)
- Place the patient in a semiprone position with the arm draped free.
- Make an incision parallel and slightly cephalad to the spine of the scapula 10 to 12 cm long (Fig. 2.24A). Sharply elevate the trapezius from the scapular spine. Use electrocautery to control bleeding.
- As the fibers of the trapezius and periosteum are elevated, a thin, fatty layer can be seen between the undersurface of the trapezius and supraspinatus muscles. Do not elevate the supraspinatus from its fossa. Retract the trapezius muscle cephalad with a wide blunt retractor.
- Using blunt dissection with a wet, gloved finger, palpate the suprascapular ligament overlying its notch. Only minimal distal retraction of the supraspinatus muscle is required (Fig. 2.24B).
- Use a blunt elevator to clean the suprascapular ligament (Fig. 2.24C). Avoid the suprascapular artery and vein immediately superficial to the ligament.
- Sharply release the ligament, protecting the suprascapular nerve beneath. Further exploration of the nerve or neurolysis is unnecessary.
- Inspect and palpate the surrounding region to rule out any abnormal masses.
- Reattach the trapezius muscle to the spine of the scapula using nonabsorbable sutures placed through several drill holes in the bone.
- Close the wound in the routine manner and apply a sling for immobilization.

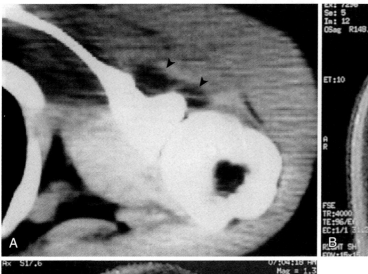
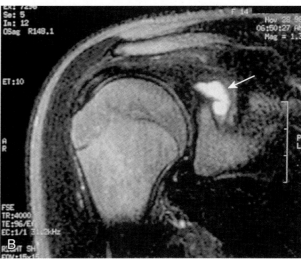
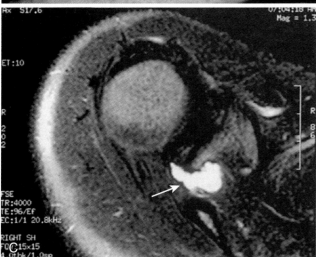

FIGURE 2.23 Magnetic resonance images showing entrapment neuropathy of suprascapular nerve by ganglion. **A,** *Arrowheads* show small, low-density shadow just posterior to neck of glenoid. **B** and **C,** Ganglion cyst *(arrows)* in region of spinoglenoid notch. Cyst appears to originate from posterosuperior aspect of glenohumeral joint. (From Cummins CA, Messer TM, Nuber GW: Suprascapular nerve entrapment, *J Bone Joint Surg* 82A:415–424, 2000.)

SUPRASCAPULAR NOTCH DECOMPRESSION

TECHNIQUE 2.8

- Make a saber or transverse incision along the scapular spine.
- Split the trapezius along its fibers and retract the supraspinatus posteriorly.
- Locate and release the transverse ligament, taking care to preserve the vascular structures running above and the nerve running below the ligament.
- In addition to ligament release, the notch can be widened with a burr if indicated.

SPINOGLENOID NOTCH DECOMPRESSION

TECHNIQUE 2.9

- Make a posterior incision, with a longitudinal incision 3 cm medial to the posterolateral corner of the acromion or with a vertical incision in the skin lines (Fig. 2.25A).
- Divide the deltoid in line with its fibers, taking care not to split it too distally to avoid injury to the axillary nerve.
- Identify the infraspinatus fascia and incise it; retract the infraspinatus muscle inferiorly.
- Carry dissection down the lateral aspect of the scapular spine; identify and release the spinoglenoid ligament (Fig. 2.25B and C).

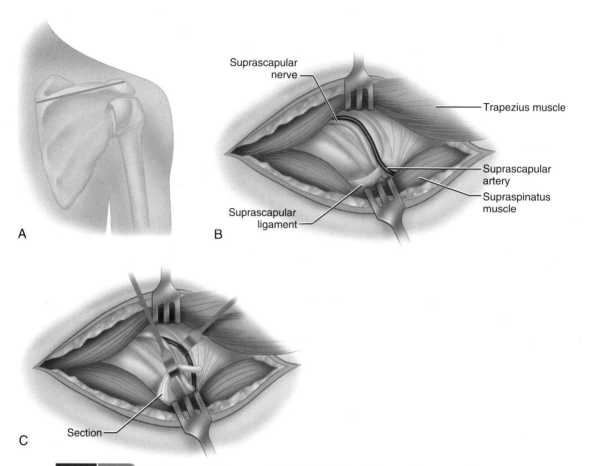

A

B

Suprascapular nerve

Trapezius muscle

Suprascapular artery

Supraspinatus muscle

Suprascapular ligament

C

Section

FIGURE 2.24 Posterior surgical approach. **A,** Skin incision. **B,** Supraspinatus muscle retracted downward to bring into view suprascapular artery and nerve. **C,** Suprascapular artery and transverse scapular ligament are isolated, permitting easy removal of ligament. **SEE TECHNIQUE 2.7.**

REMOVAL OF A GANGLION FROM THE INFERIOR BRANCH OF THE SUPRASCAPULAR NERVE

TECHNIQUE 2.10

(THOMPSON ET AL.)

- Detach the infraspinatus muscle and reflect it toward the vertebral border of the scapula to expose the posterior shoulder capsule and the posterior neck of the glenoid (Fig. 2.26).
- Identify and dissect the ganglion, leaving the nerve intact.

POSTOPERATIVE CARE Active motion is allowed within 10 to 14 days after surgery and is increased as pain permits.

More recently, arthroscopic treatment has become our preferred method for suprascapular nerve entrapment at the spinoglenoid notch owing to a ganglion cyst. Usually the cyst results from some intraarticular pathology, such as a posterior labral tear, and arthroscopic treatment of the pathology with internal cyst decompression has been successful. This technique is described in other chapter.

ELBOW INJURIES

ELBOW TENOPATHIES

■ LATERAL EPICONDYLITIS (TENNIS ELBOW)

Lateral epicondylitis (tennis elbow), a familiar term used to describe myriad symptoms around the lateral aspect of the elbow, occurs more frequently in nonathletes than athletes, with a peak incidence in the early fifth decade and has a nearly equal gender incidence. Lateral epicondylitis can occur during activities that require repetitive supination and pronation of the forearm with the elbow in near full extension. Runge first described the clinical entity in 1873, and since then almost 30 different conditions have been proposed as causes. Studies have suggested that some individuals may have a genetic predisposition to develop tennis elbow. Although originally described as an inflammatory process, the current consensus is that lateral epicondylitis is initiated as a microtear, most often within the origin of the extensor carpi radialis brevis. Microscopic findings show immature reparative tissue that resembles angiofibroblastic hyperplasia. The pathologic process mainly involves the origin of the extensor carpi radialis brevis but can involve the tendons of the extensor carpi radialis longus and the extensor digitorum communis.

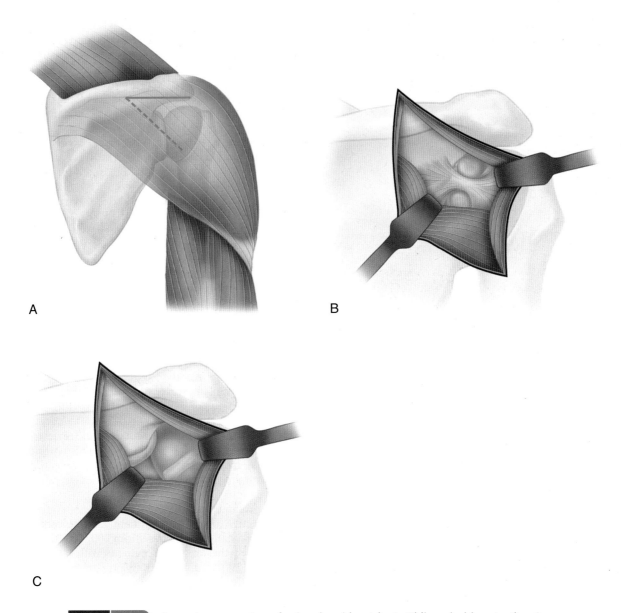

A

B

C

FIGURE **2.25**   Open decompression of spinoglenoid notch. **A,** Oblique incision starting 4 cm medial to posterolateral corner of acromion. **B,** Exposure of notch after splitting deltoid and retracting the infraspinatus inferiorly. **C,** Spinoglenoid ligament is released. (Redrawn from Piasecki DP, Romeo AA, Bach BR Jr, Nicholson GP: Suprascapular neuropathy, *J Am Acad Orthop Surg* 17[11]:665–676, 2009.) **SEE TECHNIQUE 2.9.**

The diagnosis of tennis elbow is made by localizing discomfort to the origin of the extensor carpi radialis brevis. Tenderness typically is present over the lateral epicondyle approximately 5 mm distal and anterior to the midpoint of the condyle. Pain usually is exacerbated by resisted wrist dorsiflexion and forearm supination, and there is pain when grasping objects. Plain radiographs usually are negative; occasionally, calcific tendinitis may be present. MRI shows tendon thickening with increased T1 and T2 signal intensity. One study showed that excellent surgical results corresponded with a high-signal intensity focus on T2-weighted images of the extensor carpi radialis brevis at the lateral epicondyle.

Other entities that can produce pain in this general vicinity are osteochondritis dissecans of the capitellum, lateral compartment arthrosis, varus instability, and, perhaps most commonly, radial tunnel syndrome. Radial tunnel syndrome is a compressive neuropathy of the posterior interosseous nerve caused by any of four different anatomic structures in the radial tunnel, including a fibrous band near the anterior aspect of the radial head, a vascular leash of the recurrent radial artery, the distal extensor carpi radialis brevis tendon margin, or the supinator margin at the arcade of Frohse. The pain of radial tunnel syndrome is located 3 to 4 cm distal to the lateral epicondyle and may be reproduced with long finger extension against resistance. The latter finding is inconsistent, as are abnormalities on electromyography. True lateral epicondylitis and radial tunnel syndrome may coexist in 5% of patients.

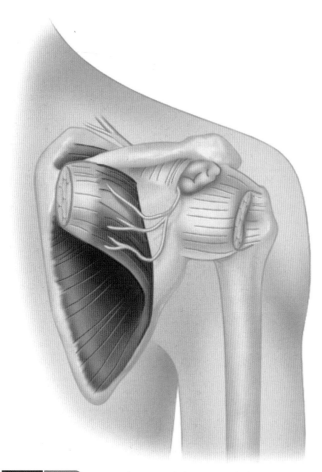

FIGURE 2.26   Surgical approach for removal of ganglion. **SEE TECHNIQUE 2.10.**

TREATMENT

Regardless of the underlying cause, nonoperative treatment is successful in 95% of patients with tennis elbow. Initial nonoperative treatment includes rest, ice, injections, and physical therapy with ultrasound, iontophoresis, electrical stimulation, manipulation, soft-tissue mobilization, friction massage, stretching and strengthening exercises, and counterforce bracing.

In some patients, one or two local injections of a steroid preparation to the area of maximal tenderness are helpful. Early studies were promising for ESWT, but more recent studies have shown conflicting results. One study did not find a meaningful difference between treatment of lateral epicondylitis with ESWT combined with forearm stretching and treatment with forearm stretching alone. A double-blind, randomized, placebo-controlled trial found that radial ESWT was not more effective in reducing pain or improving function or grip strength than sham treatment. However, two other studies reported that ESWT was effective in the treatment of acute and chronic lateral epicondylitis.

From the current literature, no firm conclusions can be drawn about the effectiveness of PRP or autologous blood injections or the superiority of one method over the other. Autologous blood injection has been shown to be beneficial in certain patients. Edwards and Calandruccio achieved 79% success in relieving pain in patients in whom all other nonoperative treatments failed. Several meta-analyses have reported PRP injections to be more effective in relieving pain and improving function at long-term follow-up than corticosteroid injections, although corticosteroid injections were more effective at short-term follow-up. In a meta-analysis, Tang et al. compared PRP, autologous blood, and corticosteroid injections in a meta-analysis of randomized controlled trials and determined that corticosteroid ranked first for visual analog score (VAS), modified Nirschl score, maximal grip strength, modified Mayo score (MMS), and Patient-Related Tennis Elbow Evaluation (PRTEE) score for the short-term period. For the long-term period, PRP ranked first for VAS, pressure pain threshold, Disabilities of Arm Shoulder and Hand (DASH) score, MMS, and PRTEE score. Houck et al. came to the same conclusion in their systematic review: the current best available evidence suggests that corticosteroid injection improves functional outcomes and pain relief in the short term, while autologous blood and PRP injections are more effective treatments in the intermediate term.

Despite claims of success of a multitude of nonoperative treatment methods, a meta-analysis involving 2280 patients reported in randomized controlled trials concluded that there is no intermediate-term to long-term clinical benefit after nonoperative treatment compared with observation only or placebo. Another systematic review of randomized controlled trials, however, did not report a lack of benefit but noted that the existing literature provides no conclusive evidence of superiority of any one nonoperative treatment method. More recently, Bateman et al. reviewed 12 studies of admittedly poor methodology and reported that the available data suggest that operative interventions for tennis elbow are no more effective than nonoperative and sham interventions.

If prolonged (6 to 12 months) nonoperative treatment is ineffective, operative treatment may be considered. In a review of a national database from 2007 to 2014, Degen et al. determined that of 85,318 patients with lateral epicondylitis, 1694 (2%) required operative treatment. Operative treatment is effective in approximately 90% of properly selected patients. In a study of 580 patients with lateral epicondylitis, Knutsen et al. reported 84% success with nonoperative treatment. Factors identified as predictive of the need for surgical treatment included a worker's compensation claim, prior injection, presence of radial tunnel syndrome, previous orthopaedic surgery, and duration of symptoms of more than 12 months. Numerous surgical procedures have been described for the treatment of tennis elbow. Formerly, we used the technique popularized by Boyd and McLeod, which was an effort to eliminate all possible causes of lateral epicondylitis. This procedure included excision of the proximal portion of the annular ligament, release of the entire extensor origin, excision of an adventitious bursa (if found), and resection of hypertrophic synovium in the radiocapitellar articulation. Currently, we favor a more limited approach, which consists of exposure of the diseased extensor carpi radialis brevis origin, resection of degenerative tissue, and possibly direct repair to bone.

Arthroscopic debridement has become increasingly popular as a less invasive alternative to open debridement. Several systematic reviews have compared open and arthroscopic techniques and found no clinically significant differences in DASH scores, pain intensity, and patient satisfaction. Lai et al. reported that arthroscopic approaches may result in faster recovery and earlier return to work. Riff et al., on the other hand, reported that more patients were pain free after open surgery than arthroscopic surgery and recommended open debridement as more likely to obtain a pain-free outcome. More recently, Wang et al.'s meta-analysis determined that arthroscopic and open debridement had similar effectiveness in relieving pain and improving self-function, with no significant difference in failure rates, functional outcome scores, and complication rates, a finding collaborated by Clark et al. in a prospective randomized controlled trial. Suggested advantages of arthroscopy include treatment of the lesion without sacrifice of the common extensor origin. Arthroscopy allows intraarticular examination for other pathologic processes and may permit a shorter postoperative rehabilitation period and an earlier return to work. Three distinct patterns of pathologic changes have been identified in the lateral capsule and at the undersurface of the extensor carpi radialis brevis. Type I lesions appear arthroscopically with intact capsules, type II are linear tears at the undersurface of the capsule, and type III are complete tears of the capsule with partial or complete avulsion of the extensor carpi radialis brevis tendon. For the arthroscopic technique.

Manipulation under anesthesia, especially in patients with concomitant flexion contractures, has been advocated. The technique involves sudden, forcible, full extension of the elbow with the wrist and fingers flexed and the forearm pronated to place the extensor carpi radialis brevis and extensors under tension. An audible, palpable snap frequently can be elicited, and the results can be excellent. We have no experience with this particular technique, but it seems to be a more aggressive form of a manipulative attempt at completion of the lesion.

Only a few patients with lateral epicondylitis (1% to 2%) cannot be treated successfully by either nonoperative or operative methods. Morrey divided operative failures into two groups based on postoperative symptoms. Patients in the first group had symptoms similar to those experienced before surgery, whereas patients in the second group reported a different symptom complex after surgery. Treatment failed in patients in the first group because of inadequate release or incorrect initial diagnosis, most often related to radial tunnel syndrome; in the second group, treatment failed because of capsular or ligamentous insufficiency that resulted in either a capsular fistula or posterolateral instability. Elbow instability can occur in patients in either group (especially patients with traumatic origins for lateral elbow pain) after overzealous release that includes the anterior band of the lateral collateral ligament. It is important to obtain a thorough history to determine if the patient's symptoms have changed and a careful physical examination to identify instability, pain in the region of the epicondyle, or radial tunnel syndrome. These should be supplemented with arthrograms to detect synovial fistula and capsular insufficiency or with arthroscopy and examination with the use of anesthesia to detect instability or arthrosis.

According to most authors, patients who will improve after surgery do so within 3 to 4 months. We believe that 1 year is a reasonable period to consider repeat intervention if symptoms have not improved.

CORRECTION OF TENNIS ELBOW
TECHNIQUE 2.11

(NIRSCHL, MODIFIED)
- Make a gently curved incision 5 cm long centered over the lateral epicondyle (Fig. 2.27A).
- Incise the deep fascia in line with the incision and retract it. Identify the extensor carpi radialis longus and the origin of the extensor digitorum communis, which partially obscures the origin of the deeper extensor carpi radialis brevis (Fig. 2.27B and C).
- Elevate the brevis portion of the conjoined tendon at the midportion of the lateral epicondyle toward the elbow joint.
- Because normal-appearing Sharpey fibers are elevated, excise abnormal-appearing tendon. The diseased tissue may appear fibrillated and discolored and may contain calcium deposits.
- Occasionally, the disease process will have spread to the origin of the extensor digitorum communis, and a portion of this can be excised. We see no reason to enter the joint itself, unless preoperative evaluation indicates intraarticular processes, such as a loose body, degenerative joint disease, effusion, or synovial thickening.
- Decorticate a small area of the lateral epicondyle with a rongeur or osteotome, taking care not to enter the joint and damage the articular cartilage (Fig. 2.27D).
- Consider suturing the remaining normal tendon to the fascia or periosteum, or attach it with nonabsorbable sutures through drill holes in the epicondyle. Suture anchors can be used at the discretion of the surgeon.
- Close the extensor carpi radialis longus and extensor digitorum communis interval with absorbable sutures (which cover the knots made for the extensor carpi radialis brevis repair to bone if anchors are used).
- Close the skin incision with absorbable 4-0 sutures and adhesive strips.

POSTOPERATIVE CARE The splint is removed within the first week of surgery, and range-of-motion exercises are begun. After the wound has healed (10 to 14 days), therapy is continued, including edema control and range-of-motion exercises, followed by strengthening exercises. Strenuous activity can be resumed within the limits of pain in 8 to 10 weeks, and full power should return in approximately 3 months. The rehabilitation protocol is not time dependent, but rather goal dependent, with patients passing from one phase to the next after certain goals have been met (Box 2.3).

Percutaneous lateral release has been reported to be as effective as open release. We have no experience with this technique; it does not remove diseased tendon, but it may trigger the inflammatory cascade, which leads to the resolution of symptoms.

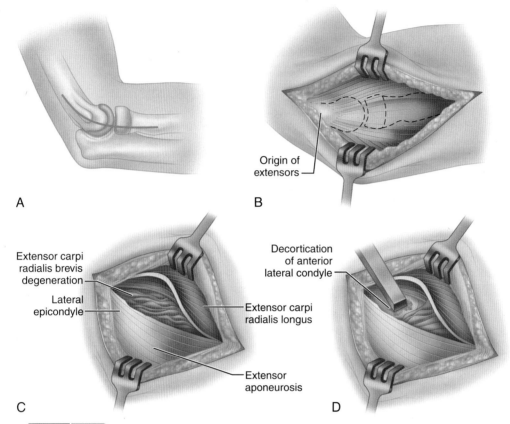

FIGURE 2.27 Surgical technique for correction of tennis elbow. **A,** Skin incision. **B,** Origins of extensor carpi radialis longus and extensor digitorum communis are identified. **C,** Reflection of conjoined extensor tendon. **D,** Osteotome decortication. **SEE TECHNIQUE 2.11.**

▮ MEDIAL EPICONDYLITIS

Medial epicondylitis is similar to lateral epicondylitis, although much less common and more difficult to treat. The origin of the flexor carpi radialis and pronator teres (flexor pronator mass) are commonly involved and, less typically, the flexor digitorum superficialis and flexor carpi ulnaris. This entity must be differentiated from ulnar nerve neuropathy and medial collateral ligament instability.

Medial epicondylitis frequently occurs with repetitive overhead motion and affects athletes involved in racket sports and others who participate in activities that create a valgus force at the elbow. Physical examination usually reveals pain along the medial elbow that becomes worse on resisted forearm pronation and wrist flexion. The area of maximal tenderness is approximately 5 mm distal and anterior to the midpoint of the medial epicondyle. Loss of range of motion and a flexion contracture may be present. Radiographs usually are normal, but medial ulnar traction spurs and medial collateral ligament calcifications may be seen and may be associated with a chronic ulnar collateral ligament injury.

Conservative treatment is the mainstay of management. Antiinflammatory medication, splinting, and an occasional steroid injection, which can be more precisely administered under ultrasound guidance technology, provide sustained relief in most patients. If nonoperative treatment fails, excision of the diseased tendon origin and reattachment usually are successful. Techniques range from a percutaneous release to open debridement with or without release of the flexor pronator origin. Vangsness and Jobe described

release of the flexor pronator origin, excision of the pathologic tissue, and reattachment of the flexor pronator origin to bleeding bone. Nirschl preferred excising the pathologic tissue of the flexor-pronator origin in a manner that leaves normal tissue intact and repairing the subsequent defect (Fig. 2.28). The ulnar nerve should be decompressed and transposed in patients who have ulnar nerve symptoms preoperatively. Epicondylectomy also can be done, but no more than 20% to 25% of the epicondyle should be removed to avoid damage to the ulnar collateral ligament. Overall, the results are not as successful as with lateral epicondylar procedures.

CORRECTION OF MEDIAL EPICONDYLITIS

TECHNIQUE 2.12

(NIRSCHL)

- Make a slightly curved 5-cm incision starting approximately 1 cm proximal and just posterior to the medial epicondyle (Fig. 2.28A). Placement of the incision posteriorly avoids sensory branches of the medial antebrachial cutaneous nerve anterior and distal to the epicondyle.

BOX 2.3

Rehabilitation Protocol for Epicondylitis

Phase 1: Acute

Goals

1. Reduce inflammation and pain
2. Promote tissue healing
3. Retard muscular atrophy

Treatment Regimen

- Cryotherapy
- Whirlpool
- Stretching to increase flexibility
- Wrist extension and flexion
- Elbow extension and flexion
- Forearm supination and pronation
- High-voltage galvanic stimulation
- Phonophoresis
- Friction massage
- Iontophoresis (with an antiinflammatory drug such as dexamethasone)
- Avoiding painful movements (e.g., gripping)

Phase 2: Subacute

Goals

1. Improve flexibility
2. Increase muscular strength and endurance
3. Increase functional activities and return to function

Treatment Regimen

- Emphasize concentric and eccentric strengthening
- Concentrate on involved muscle group or groups

- Wrist extension and flexion
- Forearm pronation and supination
- Initiate shoulder strengthening (if deficiencies are noted)
- Continue flexibility exercises
- May use counterforce brace
- Continue use of cryotherapy after exercise or function
- Initiate gradual return to stressful activities
- Gradually reintroduce previously painful movements

Phase 3: Chronic

Goals

1. Improve muscular strength and endurance
2. Maintain and enhance flexibility
3. Gradually return patient to sport or high-level activities

Treatment Regimen

- Continue strengthening exercises (emphasize eccentric and concentric exercises)
- Continue to emphasize deficiencies in shoulder and elbow strength
- Continue flexibility exercises
- Gradually diminish use of counterforce brace
- Use cryotherapy as needed
- Initiate gradual return to sport activity
- Recommend equipment modifications (e.g., grip size, string tension, playing surface)
- Emphasize maintenance program

From Wolk KE, Arrigo C, Andrews JR: Rehabilitation of the elbow in the throwing athlete, *J Orthop Sports Phys Ther* 17(6):305–317, 1993.

- Retract the subcutaneous tissue and skin over the medial epicondyle to expose the common flexor origin.
- Make a longitudinal incision in the tendon origins, beginning at the tip of the medial epicondyle, distally for 3 to 4 cm to expose the pathologic tissue (Fig. 2.28B).
- Excise the pathologic tissue elliptically, including the joint capsule if necessary, while leaving the normal tissue of the attachment to the medial epicondyle intact (Fig. 2.28C and D).
- Close the elliptical defect with absorbable suture (Fig. 2.28E).
- Transpose the ulnar nerve in patients with symptoms or pathologic anatomy found at the time of surgery.
- Close the subcutaneous tissue with absorbable suture and the skin with a running subcuticular suture.
- Apply a dressing and a posterior splint with the elbow in 90 degrees of flexion.

POSTOPERATIVE CARE The splint is removed 1 week after surgery, and elbow range-of-motion exercises are initiated. Strengthening exercises are started when full range of motion is achieved, typically 3 weeks after surgery. Strenuous activity can resume when the patient achieves normal strength without pain, which is typically 3 months after surgery. A longer period of immobilization and slower progression of rehabilitation are indicated in patients who had ulnar nerve transposition.

ELBOW CONTRACTURES

A normal range of elbow motion is 0 to 150 degrees. Some loss of motion is associated with all but the most trivial of elbow injuries, but a full range of elbow motion is unnecessary for most activities of daily living. A functional range of motion generally is considered to be 30 to 130 degrees, with 50 degrees of pronation and supination each. A flexion contracture that exceeds 45 degrees markedly impairs the ability to position the hand in space. Elbow contractures result from a variety of causes, including trauma, heterotopic ossification, burns, spasticity, postoperative scarring, and prolonged immobilization. Of these, only the last can be effectively prevented. Recent investigation into the molecular pathogenesis has revealed the involvement of neuroinflammatory mechanisms, including mast cell activation and aberrant growth factor expression.

Contractures can be initially managed effectively with physical therapy and splinting. Ulrich et al. described a static progressive stretching orthosis using stress relaxation principles that resulted in a mean increase of 26 degrees in flexion arc. Our goal is to restore a functional range of motion (30 to 130 degrees). Surgery should be considered for patients with a flexion arc of less than 100 degrees after nonoperative treatment, especially patients with flexion contractures of more than 45 degrees.

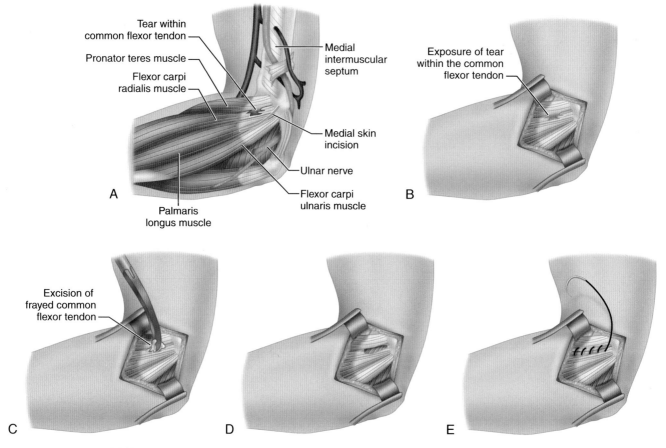

FIGURE 2.28 Nirschl technique for medial epicondylitis. **A,** Skin incision. **B,** Longitudinal exposure of tissue of flexor-pronator origin. **C,** Excision of pathologic tissue. **D,** Normal tissue of pronator origin left intact. **E,** Closure of defect in flexor-pronator origin with absorbable suture. (Redrawn from Dlabach JA, Baker CL: Lateral and medial epicondylitis in the overhead athlete, *Oper Tech Orthop* 11[1]:46–54, 2001.) **SEE TECHNIQUE 2.12.**

Causes of motion loss are classified as intrinsic or extrinsic. Extrinsic causes include contractures of the capsule or collateral ligaments, extraarticular malunions, and heterotopic ossification. Intrinsic causes include the sequelae of intraarticular fractures, such as cartilage damage, articular incongruity, and adhesions. Contracture resulting from primarily extrinsic causes can be treated with resection of the contracted structures. In contrast, contractures resulting from intrinsic causes may require alteration of the articular anatomy. Extrinsic causes (capsular contracture) are almost always present when intrinsic causes are primary.

A history and physical examination, plain radiographs, MRI, and CT with three-dimensional reconstruction can be used to determine the type of contracture. If joint surfaces are normal and contractures are secondary to capsular problems, a simple arthroscopic or open release is performed. If intraarticular surfaces have been altered or destroyed total elbow arthroplasty is our preferred procedure in appropriate patients. These procedures are described in detail in other chapter.

Although elbow manipulation under anesthesia has been reported to improve range of motion, we do not recommend isolated manipulation in patients with long-standing contractures because it may predispose to fracture, hematoma formation, scarring, and heterotopic ossification. Rather,

manipulation after operative contracture release has been found to be a useful adjunct.

A variety of surgical release procedures have been described for treatment of elbow contractures. Anterior release without biceps lengthening works best in patients with flexion contractures but is unlikely to improve function in patients with concomitant articular surface damage. Candidates for this treatment have a relatively well-preserved ulnohumeral joint and minimal or no osteophytes in the olecranon fossa. Combined anterior and posterior releases, as well as combined medial and lateral approaches, also have been described for treatment of elbow contractures. All approaches have similar reported success rates in improving elbow flexion arc. In addition to improving elbow motion, such releases have been found to improve general health status measures, although the scores do not necessarily correlate with range of motion gains.

For the open treatment of elbow contractures, some authors prefer an olecranon osteotomy to improve visualization or a mini-open technique; however, an extensile lateral approach (the so-called column procedure) is our preferred technique for this disorder. Anterior and posterior capsulectomy can be performed, and additional extension can be obtained by removing debris from the olecranon fossa. Similarly, flexion can be increased by triceps tenolysis and/or "pie-crusting" posteriorly. Skin problems also are less likely if constant passive motion is used. Reported increases in total arc of motion average 40 to 50 degrees. Although reliable for posttraumatic contractures, open surgical release is less reliable for adolescents and patients with traumatic brain injuries. In posttraumatic patients where fracture fixation constructs are removed, risk of refracture must be considered. We typically recommend release of any constricting adhesions around the fixation implants but reserve removal for a staged procedure, if necessary.

Hinged external fixation can be used as an adjunct after contracture release, particularly if the lateral ligamentous complex is violated as part of the procedure. However, because the range of motion is not markedly improved, complications are frequent, and the device is expensive, we reserve hinged external fixation for instances where elbow stability would be otherwise compromised without the device.

We usually approach elbow contractures arthroscopically as a primary procedure. Open techniques are described here for elbow contractures that cannot be treated arthroscopically. We approach open release of elbow contractures using the method outlined by Morrey.

ANTERIOR AND POSTERIOR RELEASE OF ELBOW CONTRACTURE
TECHNIQUE 2.13

(MORREY)
- Place the patient supine on the operating table with a sandbag under the ipsilateral shoulder. Drape the extremity free and bring the forearm across the abdomen.
- Extend the Kocher approach by making an extensive skin incision (15 cm) proximally along the supracondylar ridge; continue it distally to the lateral epicondyle, ending over the subcutaneous border of the ulna (Fig. 2.29A).
- Proximally carry the dissection onto the supracondylar ridge.
- Carefully elevate the brachialis from the anterior joint capsule (Fig. 2.29B and C).
- Place retractors deep to the brachioradialis and brachialis to expose the underlying joint capsule (Fig. 2.29D).
- Perform an anterior capsulectomy from lateral to medial (Fig. 2.29E). Preserve the lateral collateral ligament and stay anterior to its origin.
- Then elevate the triceps from the posterior aspect of the humerus, taking care to stay posterior to the lateral collateral ligament origin.
- Retract the triceps to expose the underling joint capsule.
- To improve flexion, perform a posterior capsulectomy proceeding from lateral to medial. Take care not to venture too far medially so as to injure the ulnar nerve.
- Completely extend the elbow. If extension is incomplete, debride the olecranon fossa and the tip of the olecranon, along with any enlargement of its margins. If flexion to 135 degrees is impossible, look for a source of anterior

impingement. If necessary, remove scar tissue or any osteophytes in or around the coronoid fossa.
- Examine the elbow to ensure that a functional range of motion has been achieved.
- Carefully repair the entire lateral tissue sleeve. Apply a splint with the elbow in full extension.

POSTOPERATIVE CARE A continuous passive motion machine can be used 12 hours a day for 1 week, but this is somewhat controversial, with one study suggesting no benefit to use of continuous passive motion after open contracture release. After this first phase, active and passive range-of-motion exercises are done hourly, with the elbow splinted between exercise sessions and at night. Supervised physical therapy visits continue for 6 weeks, two or three times a week. At 6 weeks, daytime splinting is discontinued, although splinting at night is continued for another 6 weeks.

Complications after elbow contracture release include wound healing problems, infection, and recurrent stiffness. Because range of motion can continue to improve for up to 1 year after initial release, we encourage patience in postoperative management. In patients with a recurrent contracture unresponsive to conservative management, repeat surgical excision has resulted in good reported outcomes. One of the unique complications after elbow contracture release is delayed onset ulnar neuritis (DOUN), which has been reported in 11% of patients undergoing arthroscopic contracture release, but this complication is more common in patients with more severe contractures. Prophylactic ulnar nerve decompression and/or transposition at the time of contracture release is recommended to prevent this complication.

HETEROTOPIC OSSIFICATION
Heterotopic ossification around the elbow remains a challenging problem seen most commonly in association with trauma, burns, and head injuries (Box 2.4). Although the precise mechanism at the histologic level has yet to be elucidated, a complex interaction of factors results in the conversion of progenitor cells to osteogenic cells with subsequent bone formation. Furthermore, the character and location of heterotopic ossification tend to vary with the associated pathology (Box 2.5), rendering generalized statements about this disorder difficult to make. However, most authors agree that if ectopic bone around the elbow is causing or contributing to a loss of functional elbow motion (including pronosupination), then an operative procedure is warranted to remove the offending bone and release the joint capsule. This principle applies whether the motion limitation is partial or complete (ankylosis).

Much investigation has focused on the risk factors relevant to the formation of clinically significant heterotopic ossification. The preponderance of evidence identifies more complex trauma (fracture-dislocations), delay in fracture fixation, multiple attempts at closed reduction, use of adjunctive bone grafts, concomitant head injuries, and prolonged immobilization to be associated with ectopic bone formation after elbow injuries. In particular, more severe injuries and delay in surgical management are most commonly cited as important associations. We therefore

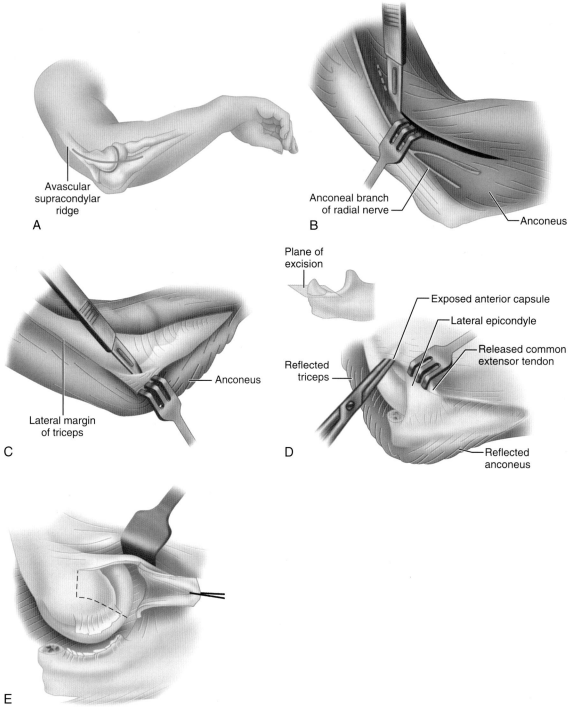

A

Avascular
supracondylar
ridge

B

Anconeal branch
of radial nerve

Anconeus

C

Lateral margin
of triceps

Anconeus

Plane of
excision

Reflected
triceps

D

Exposed anterior capsule

Lateral epicondyle

Released common
extensor tendon

Reflected
anconeus

E

FIGURE 2.29 Lateral approach (Morrey). **A,** Skin incision for extensile Kocher approach. **B,** Deep fascia is incised along lateral margin of triceps proximally and along interval between anconeus and extensor carpi ulnaris distally. **C,** To preserve periosteal continuity, triceps tendon is reflected subperiosteally from tip of olecranon. **D,** Extensor mechanism of elbow is reflected medially, tip of olecranon is removed *(inset),* and common origin of extensors of forearm is released from lateral epicondyle and adjacent structures. Extensor muscles are elevated to expose anterior part of capsule of elbow in interval between brachialis and capsule. **E,** Lateral collateral ligament is identified and released as distally based flap that can be reattached later to anatomic site of its proximal attachment on humerus. With lateral collateral ligament carefully retracted, anterior part of capsule now can be exposed and resected way across to medial site. (Redrawn from Morrey BF: Post-traumatic contracture of the elbow: operative treatment, including distraction arthroplasty, *J Bone Joint Surg* 72[4]:601–618, 1990.) **SEE TECHNIQUE 2.13.**

BOX 2.4

Risk Factors for Developing Heterotopic Ossification About the Elbow

Trauma
- Open elbow dislocation requiring extensive or multiple debridements
- Elbow dislocation associated with fractures that require open reduction internal fixation
- Radial head fractures treated with surgery >24 h after injury

Surgery
- Distal biceps tendon repair
- Repeated procedures with an improper exposure in the first 2 weeks
- Central nervous system injury
  - Traumatic brain injury
  - Elbow trauma in patients with traumatic brain injury

Burns
- Third-degree burns over 20% of total body area
- Third-degree burns over the elbow
- Long periods of bed confinement

Genetic Conditions
- Fibrodysplasia ossificans progressiva
- History of heterotopic bone formation

Modified from Morrey BF, Harter GD: Ectopic ossification about the elbow. In Morrey BF, Sanchez-Sotelo J, editors: *The elbow and its disorders*, ed 4, Philadelphia, 2009, Elsevier.

BOX 2.5

Location of Heterotopic Ossification Related to Associated Pathologic Process

Traumatic
- Most often posterolateral elbow
  - Bone bridge between lateral humeral condyle and posterolateral olecranon
  - Bone may fill olecranon fossa
- Anterolateral compartment second most common location
  - Bone may extend from distal humerus to radius and ulna at level of bicipital tuberosity
  - Coronoid frequently enlarged, blocking elbow flexion

Burn-Related
- Most often posteromedial
- Cubital tunnel often obliterated
- Ulnar nerve may be completely encased in bone

Neurogenic
- Most common anteriorly in flexor muscles or posteriorly in extensors
- Ossification tends to occur within the muscle and follow a single plane
- Forearm and proximal radioulnar joint also may be involved

Modified from Morrey BF, Harter GD: Ectopic ossification about the elbow. In Morrey BF, Sanchez-Sotelo J, editors: *The elbow and its disorders*, ed 4, Philadelphia, 2009, Elsevier.

recommend early surgical management of complex elbow trauma in an attempt to limit ectopic bone formation. Total elbow arthroplasty was not associated with an increased risk of clinically significant heterotopic ossification in a systematic review; however, it is more likely to develop when total elbow arthroplasty is performed for a traumatic indication. Heterotopic ossification has been reported after ulnar collateral ligament reconstruction as well, but it is relatively uncommon (5%); it can be associated with a higher rate of ulnar nerve symptoms.

Although the timing of excision of heterotopic ossification around the elbow remains a matter of debate, the current trend is for early surgical excision. One study suggested that the average area of heterotopic ossification does not tend to expand following initial identification. Other studies have shown no evidence of increased recurrence rates with early excision, and there is evidence that delay in excision may predispose to worse outcomes. Criteria suggested for early excision (3 to 6 months after injury) include union of all fractures, healing of all initial wounds, and resolution of inflammation. Excision of heterotopic ossification around the elbow is typically done through a limited or extended Kocher approach; a multiple incision technique also has been described for heterotopic ossification excision after burn injuries, in which soft-tissue preservation is paramount to avoid skin breakdown and infection. Preoperative CT scanning is recommended to identify the precise location of the ectopic bone and the position of the median, radial, and ulnar nerves.

EXCISION OF HETEROTOPIC OSSIFICATION

TECHNIQUE 2.14

(MORREY AND HARTER)
- Usually a posterior skin incision is made to provide circumferential access to the elbow, and subcutaneous dissection is carried laterally or medially depending on the location of the heterotopic ossification. Care must be taken to identify and protect the ulnar nerve.

POSTEROLATERAL EXCISION
- For posterolateral resection, retract the triceps mechanism medially without disturbing its insertion and expose the ectopic bone subperiosteally. Resect the central portion of the bony bridge.
- Flex the elbow and remove the attachments of the ectopic bone to the humerus and olecranon. Anterior capsular release is not necessary.
- Excise any ectopic bone in the olecranon fossa to reduce olecranon impingement.

MEDIAL EXCISION
- When the posterior ectopic bone extends to the medial aspect of the elbow, ulnar nerve transposition is necessary.

- Identify the ulnar nerve, which may be completely surrounded by bone. A Kerrison rongeur is helpful to remove the encasing bone while also protecting the nerve.
- Expose the triceps expansion and incise it distal to its insertion.
- Expose the ectopic bone subperiosteally and resect it.
- If the ectopic bone interferes with ulnar nerve function, decompress the nerve or transfer it anteriorly if necessary.

ANTERIOR EXCISION

- If anterior excision is necessary, elevate the origins of the brachioradialis and brachialis muscles from the lateral supracondylar ridge to expose the ectopic bone.
- Identify the radial nerve and retract it laterally.
- Resect the bone subperiosteally.

CLOSURE

- Deflate the tourniquet and obtain hemostasis before routine layered closure over a suction drain. Do not close the capsule. Apply a soft dressing that will allow immediate postoperative range of motion.

POSTOPERATIVE CARE Indomethacin is prescribed for 6 weeks after surgery. Although low-dose radiation has been used for prophylaxis against recurrence, evidence to support its use is weak. Intensive physical therapy and adjunctive progressive splinting are initiated to preserve the gains in range of motion. If motion goals are not met, manipulation under anesthesia can be done at about 6 weeks after surgery.

Outcomes following ectopic bone excision are generally improved. Studies have reported an average gain in flexion arc of approximately 50 to 70 degrees, and clinical results do not vary by etiology (traumatic brain injury, burns, or direct elbow trauma). Patients with preoperative ankylosis can expect more improvement than those with partial motion restriction; however, recurrence is more common in patients with central nervous system injuries.

REFERENCES

SHOULDER INJURIES
ANATOMY, CLINICAL PRESENTATION, AND PHYSICAL EXAMINATION

Bakhsh W, Nicandri G: Anatomy and physical examination of the shoulder, *Sports Med Arthrosc Rev* 26:e10, 2018.

Chalmers PN, Cvetanovich GL, Kupfer N, et al.: The champagne toast position isolates the supraspinatus better than the Jobe test: an electromyographic study of shoulder physical examination tests, *J Shoulder Elbow Surg* 25:322, 2016.

Collin P, Treseder T, Denard PJ, et al.: What is the best clinical test for assessment of the teres minor in massive rotator cuff tears? *Clin Orthop Relat Res* 473:2959, 2015.

Gismervik SØ, Drogset JO, Granviken F, et al.: Physical examination tests of the shoulder: a systematic review and meta-analysis of diagnostis test performance, *BMC Musculoskelet Disord* 18:41, 2017.

Haley CA: History and physical examination for shoulder instability, *Sports Med Arthrosc Rev* 25:150, 2017.

Hegedus EJ, Goode AP, Cook CE, et al.: Which physical examination tests provide clinicians with the most value when examining the shoulder? Update of a systematic review with meta-analysis of individual tests, *Br J Sports Med* 46:964, 2012.

Hegedus EJ: Which physical examination tests provide clinicians with the most value when examining the shoulder? Update of a systematic review with meta-analysis of individual tests, *Br J Sports Med* 46:964, 2012.

Hippensteel KJ, Brophy R, Smith MV, et al.: Comprehensive review of provocative and instability physical examination tests of the shoulder, *J Am Acad Orthop Surg* 27:395, 2019.

Huri G, Kaymakoglu M, Garbis N: Rotator cable and rotator interval: anatomy, biomechanics and clinical importance, *EFORT Open Rev* 4:56, 2019.

Kappe T, Sgroi M, Reichel H, et al.: Diagnostic performance of clinical tests for subscapularis tendon tears, *Knee Surg Sports Traumatol Arthrosc* 26:176, 2018.

Kibler WB, O'Driscoll S: Dynamic labral shear test in diagnosis of SLAP lesions: letter to the editor, *Am J Sports Med* 41(7):NP36–NP37, 2013.

Penning LI, De Bie RA, Leffers P, et al.: Empty can and drop arm tests for cuff rupture: improved specificity after subacromial injection, *Acta Orthop Belg* 82:166, 2016.

Somerville LE, Willits K, Johnson AM, et al.: Clinical assessment of physical examination maneuvers for rotator cuff lesions, *Am J Sports Med* 42:1911, 2014.

Williams MD, Edwards TB, Walch G: Understanding the importance of the teres minor for shoulder function: functional anatomy and pathology, *J Am Acad Orthop Surg* 26:150, 2018.

IMAGING

Gupta H, Robinson P: Normal shoulder ultrasound: anatomy and technique, *Semin Musculoskelet Radiol* 19:203, 2015.

IMPINGEMENT SYNDROME

Balke M, Liem D, Greshake O, et al.: Differences in acromial morphology of shoulders in patients with degenerative and traumatic supraspinatus tendon tears, *Knee Surg Sports Traumatol Arthrosc* 24:2200, 2016.

Balke M, Schmidt C, Dedy N, et al.: Correlation of acromial morphology with impingement syndrome and rotator cuff tears, *Acta Orthop* 84:178, 2013.

Bouchard A, Garret J, Favard L, et al.: Failed subacromial decompression. Risk factors, *Orthop Traumatol Surg Res* 100(Suppl 8):S365, 2014.

Ertan S, Ayhan E, Güven MF, et al.: Medium-term natural history of subacromial impingement syndrome, *J Shoulder Elbow Surg* 24:1512, 2015.

Escamilla RF, Hooks TR, Wilk KE: Optimal management of shoulder impingement syndrome, *Open Access J Sports Med* 5:13, 2014.

Farfaras S, Sernert N, Hallström E, et al.: Comparison of open acromioplasty and physiotherapy in patients with subacromial impingement syndrome: a prospective randomised study, *Knee Surg Sports Traumatol Arthrosc* 24:2181, 2016.

Gumina S, Arceri V, Fagnani C, et al.: Subacromial space width: does overuse or genetics play a greater role in determining it? An MRI study on elderly twins, *J Bone Joint Surg Am* 97:1647, 2015.

Harrison AK, Flatow EL: Subacromial impingement syndrome, *J Am Acad Orthop Surg* 19:701, 2011.

Jacobsen JR, Jensen CM, Deutch SR: Acromioplasty in patients selected for operation by national guidelines, *J Shoulder Elbow Surg* 26:1854, 2017.

Kappe T, Knappe K, Elsharkawi M, et al.: Predictive value of preoperative clinical examination for subacromial decompression in impingement syndrome, *Knee Surg Sports Traumatol Arthrosc* 23:443, 2015.

Ketola S, Lehtinen J, Elo P, et al.: No difference in long-term development of rotator cuff rupture and muscle volumes in impingement patients with or without decompression, *Acta Orthop* 87:351, 2016.

Ketola S, Lehtinen JT, Arnala I: Arthroscopic decompression not recommended in the treatment of rotator cuff tendinopathy: a final review of randomised controlled trial at a minimum follow-up of ten years, *Bone Joint Lett J* 99-B:799, 2017.

Ketola S, Lehtinen J, Rousi T, et al.: Which patients do not recover from shoulder impingement syndrome, either with operative treatment or with nonoperative treatment? *Acta Orthop* 86:641, 2015.

Koh KH, Laddha MS, Lim TK, et al.: A magnetic resonance imaging study of 100 cases of arthroscopic acromioplasty, *Am J Sports Med* 40:352, 2012.

Kolk A, Thomassen BJW, Hund H, et al.: Does acromioplasty result in favorable clinical and radiologic outcomes in the management of chronic subacromial pain syndrome? A double-blinded randomized clinical trial with 9 to 14 years' follow-up, *J Shoulder Elbow Surg* 26:1407, 2017.

Mauro CS, Jordan SS, Irrgang JJ, Harner CD: Practice patterns for subacromial decompression and rotator cuff reapir: an analysis of the American Board of Orthopaedic Surgery database, *J Bone Joint Surg* 94A:1492, 2012.

Mihata T, Gates J, McGarry MH, et al.: Effect of posterior shoulder tightness on internal impingement in a cadaveric model of throwing, *Knee Surg Sports Traumatol Arthrosc* 23:548, 2015.

Mihata T, Jun BJ, Bui CN, et al.: Effect of scapular orientation on shoulder internal impingement in a cadaveric model of the cocking phase of throwing, *J Bone Joint Surg* 94A:1576, 2012.

Mihata T, McGarry MH, Neo M, et al.: Effect of anterior capsular laxity on horizontal abduction and forceful internal impingement in a cadaveric model of the throwing shoulder, *Am J Sports Med* 43:1758, 2015.

Misirlioglu M, Aydin A, Yildiz V, et al.: Prevalence of the association of subacromial impingement with subcoracoid impingement and their clinical effects, *J Int Med Res* 40:810, 2012.

Nejati P, Ghahremaninia A, Naderi F, et al.: Treatment of subacromial impingement syndrome: platelet-rich plasma or exercise therapy? A randomized controlled trial, *Orthop J Sports Med* 5: 2325967117702366,2017 .

Otoshi K, Takegami M, Sekiguchi M, et al.: Association between kyphosis and subacromial impingement syndrome: LOHAS study, *J Shoulder Elbow Surg* 23:e300, 2014.

Paavola M, Malmivaara A, Taimela S, et al.: Subacromial decompression versus diagnostic arthroscopy for shoulder impingement: randomised, placebo surgery controlled clinical trial, *BMJ* 362:k2860, 2018.

Paavola M, Malmivaara PM, Taimela S, et al.: In shoulder impingement syndrome, subacromial decompression did not differ from diagnostic arthroscopy for shoulder pain at 24 months, *J Bone Joint Surg Am* 101:369, 2019.

Papadonikolakis A, McKenna M, Warme W, et al.: Published evidence relevant to the diagnosis of impingement syndrome of the shoulder, *J Bone Joint Surg* 93A:1827, 2011.

Park I, Lee HJ, Kim SE, et al.: Which shoulder motions cause subacromial impingement? Evaluating the vertical displacement and peak strain of the coracoacromial ligament by ultrasound speckle tracking imaging, *J Shoulder Elbow Surg* 24:1801, 2015.

Park JY, Lhee SH, Oh KS, et al.: Is arthroscopic coracoplasty necessary in subcoracoid impingement syndrome? *Arthroscopy* 28:1766, 2012.

Penning LI, de Bie RA, Walenkamp GH: The effectiveness of injections of hyaluronic acid or corticosteroid in patients with subacromial impingement: a three-arm randomised controlled trial, *J Bone Joint Surg* 94B:1246, 2012.

Saltychev M, Äärimaa V, Virolainen P, Laimi K: Conservative treatment or surgery for shoulder impingement: systematic review and meta-analysis, *Disabil Rehabil* 37:1, 2015.

Sasiponganan C, Dessouky R, Ashikyan O, et al.: Subacromial impingement anatomy and its association with rotator cuff pathology in women: radiograph and MRI correlation, a retrospective evaluation, *Skeletal Radiol* 48:781, 2019.

Tashjian RZ: Is there evidence in favor of surgical interventions for the subacromial impingement syndrome? *Clin J Sport Med* 23:406, 2013.

Worsley P, Warner M, Mottram S, et al.: Motor control retraining exercises for shoulder impingement: effects on function, muscle activitation, and biomechanics in young adults, *J Shoulder Elbow Surg* 22:e11, 2013.

ROTATOR CUFF TEAR

Acevedo DC, Shore B, Mirzayan R: Orthopedic applications of acellular human dermal allograft for shoulder and elbow surgery, *Orthop Clin North Am* 46:377, 2015.

Aurora A, Gatica JE, van den Bogert AJ, et al.: An analytical model for rotator cuff repairs, *Clin Biomech* 25:751, 2010.

Baumgarten KM, Gerlach D, Galatz LM, et al.: Cigarette smoking increases the risk for rotator cuff tears, *Clin Orthop Relat Res* 468:1534, 2010.

Bektaser B, Ocgüder A, Solak S, et al.: Free coracoacromial ligament graft for augmentation of massive rotator cuff tears treated with mini-open repair, *Acta Orthop Traumatol Turc* 44:426, 2010.

Bhatia S, Greenspoon JA, Horan MP, et al.: Two-year outcomes after arthroscopic rotator cuff repair in recreational athletes older than 70 years, *Am J Sports Med* 43:1737, 2015.

Castricini R, Longo UG, De Benedetto M, et al.: Platelet-rich plasma augmentation for arthroscopic rotator cuff repair: a randomized controlled trial, *Am J Sports Med* 39:258, 2011.

Chen M, Xu W, Dong Q, et al.: Outcomes of single-row versus double-row arthroscopic rotator cuff repair: a systematic review and meta-analysis of current evidence, *Arthroscopy* 29:1437, 2013.

Cheung EV, Silverio L, Sperling JW: Strategies in biologic augmentation of rotator cuff repair: a review, *Clin Orthop Relat Res* 468:1476, 2010.

Cho CH, Lee SM, Lee YK, Shin HK: Mini-open suture bridge repair with procine dermal patch augmentation for massive rotator cuff tear: surgical technique and preliminary results, *Clin Orthop Surg* 6:329, 2014.

Connelly TM, Shaw A, O'Grady P: Outcome of open massive rotator cuff repairs with double-row suture knotless anchors: case series, *Int Orthop* 39:1109, 2015.

Craig EV, Galantz LM, Sperling JW: From platelet-rich plasma to the reverse prosthesis: controversies in treating rotator cuff pathology, *Instr Course Lect* 63:63, 2014.

Derwin KA, Badylak SF, Steinmann SP, Iannotti JP: Extracellular matrix scaffold devices for rotator cuff repair, *J Shoulder Elbow Surg* 19:467, 2010.

Familiari F, Gonzalez-Zapata A, Ianno B, et al.: Is acromioplasty necessary in the setting of full-thickness tears? A systematic review, *J Orthop Traumatol* 16:167, 2015.

Fehringer EV, Sun J, Cotton J, et al.: Healed cuff repairs impart normal shoulder scores in those 65 years of age and older, *Clin Orthop Relat Res* 468:1521, 2010.

Franceschi F, Papalia R, Vasta S, et al.: Surgical management of irreparable rotator cuff tears, *Knee Surg Sports Traumatol Arthrosc* 23:494, 2015.

Gerber C, Rahm SA, Catanzaro S, et al.: Latissimus dorsi tendon transfer for treatment of irreparable posterosuperior rotator cuff tears: long-term results at a minimum follow-up of ten years, *J Bone Joint Surg* 95A:1920, 2013.

Gilot GJ, Alvarez-Pinzon AM, Barcksdale L, et al.: Outcome of large to massive rotator cuff tears repaired with and without extracellular matrix augmentation: a prospective comparative study, *Arthroscopy* 31:1459, 2015.

Grimberg J, Kany J, Valenti P, et al.: Arthroscopic-assisted latissimus dorsi tendon transfer for irreparable posterosuperior cuff tears, *Arthroscopy* 31:599, 2015.

Gulotta LV, Kovacevic D, Montgomery S, et al.: Stem cells genetically modified with the developmental gene MT1-MMP improve regeneration of the supraspinatus tendon-to-bone insertion site, *Am J Sports Med* 38:1429, 2010.

Gulotta LV, Kovacevic D, Packer JD, et al.: Adenoviral-mediated gene transfer of human bone morphogenetic protein-13 does not improve rotator cuff healing in a rat model, *Am J Sports Med* 39:180, 2011.

Hartzler RU, Sperling JW, Schleck CD, Cofield RH: Clinical and radiographic factors influencing the results of revision rotator cuff repair, *Int J Shoulder Surg* 7:41, 2013.

Henseler JF, Kolk A, van der Zwall P, et al.: The minimal detectable change of the Constant score in impingement, full-thickness tears, and massive rotator cuff tears, *J Shoulder Elbow Surg* 24:376, 2015.

Hernigou P, Flouzat Lachaniette CH, Delambre J, et al.: Biologic augmentation of rotator cuff repair with mesenchymal stem cells during arthroscopy improves healing and prevents further tears: a case controlled study, *Int Orthop* 38(9):1811–1818, 2014.

Hinsley H, Nicholls A, Daines M, et al.: Classification of rotator cuff tendinopathy using high definition ultrasound, *Muscles Ligaments Tendons J* 4:391, 2014.

Hoppe S, Alini M, Benneker LM, et al.: Tenocytes of chronic rotator cuff tendon tears can be stimulated by platelet-released growth factors, *J Shoulder Elbow Surg* 22:340, 2013.

Iagulli ND, Field LD, Hobgood ER, et al.: Comparison of partial versus complete arthroscopic repair of massive rotator cuff tears, *Am J Sports Med* 40:1022, 2012.

Inderhaug E, Kollevoid KH, Kalsvik M, et al.: Preoperative NSAIDs, non-acute onset and long-standing symptoms predict inferior outcome at long-term follow-up after rotator cuff repair, *Knee Surg Sports Traumatol Arthrosc* 25:2067, 2017.

Ji X, Bi C, Wang F, Wang Q: Arthroscopic versus mini-open rotator cuff repair; an up-to-date meta-analysis of randomized controlled trials, *Arthroscopy* 31:118, 2015.

Jo CH, Shin JS, Lee YG, et al.: Platelet-rich plasma for arthroscopic repair of large to massive rotator cuff tears: a randomized, single-blind, parallel-group trial, *Am J Sports Med* 41:2240, 2013.

Jones CR, Snyder SJ: Massive irreparable rotator cuff tears: a solution that bridges the gap, *Sports Med Arthrosc* 23:130, 2015.

Kenner JD, Galatz LM, Teefey SA, et al.: A prospective evaluation of survivorship of asymptomatic degenerative rotator cuff tears, *J Bone Joint Surg* 97A:89, 2015.

Kovacevic D, Fox M, Bedi A, et al.: Calcium-phospate matrix with or without TGF-beta 3 improves tendon-bone healing after rotator cuff repair, *Am J Sports Med* 39:811, 2011.

Kowalsky MS, Keener JD: Revision arthroscopic rotator cuff repair: repair integrity and clinical outcome: surgical technique, *J Bone Joint Surg* 93A(Suppl 1):62, 2011.

Lädermann A, Denard PJ, Collin P: Massive rotator cuff tears: definition and treatment, *Int Orthop* 39:2403, 2015.

Lambers Heerspink FO, van Raay JJ, Koorevaar RC, et al.: Comparing surgical repair with conservative treatment for degenerative rotator cuff tears: a randomized controlled trial, *J Shoulder Elbow Surg* 24:1274, 2015.

Lazarides AL, Alentorn-Geli E, Choi JH, et al.: Rotator cuff tears in young patients: a different disease than rotator cuff tears in elderly patients, *J Shoulder Elbow Surg* 24:1834, 2015.

Lenart BA, Martens KA, Kearns KA, et al.: Treatment of massive and recurrent rotator cuff tears augmented with a poly-l-lactide graft, a preliminary study, *J Shoulder Elbow Surg* 24:915, 2015.

Longo UG, Lamberti A, Maffulli N, Denaro V: Tendon augmentation grafts: a systematic review, *Br Med Bull* 94:165, 2010.

Longo UG, Lamberti A, Maffuli N, Denaro V: Tissue engineered biological augmentation for tendon healing: a systematic review, *Br Med Bull* 98:31, 2011.

MacKechnie MA, Chalal J, Wasserstein D, et al.: Repair of full-thickness rotator cuff tears in patients aged younger than 55 years, *Arthroscopy* 30:1366, 2014.

Mall NA, Tanaka MJ, Choi LS, Paletta Jr GA: Factors affecting rotator cuff healing, *J Bone Joint Surg* 96A:778, 2014.

Melis B, DeFranco MJ, Chuinard C, Walch G: Natural history of fatty infiltration and atrophy of the supraspinatus muscle in rotator cuff tears, *Clin Orthop Relat Res* 468:1498, 2010.

Merolla G, Chillemi C, Franceschini V, et al.: Tendon transfer for irreparable rotator cuff tears: indications and surgical rationale, *Muscles Tendons Ligaments J* 4:425, 2015.

Millett PJ, Horan MP, Maland KE, Hawkins RJ: Long-term survivorship and outcomes after surgical repair of full-thickness rotator cuff tears, *J Shoulder Elbow Surg* 20:591, 2011.

Moraiti C, Valle P, Magdes A, et al.: Comparison of functional gains after arthroscopic rotator cuff repair in patients over 70 years of age versus patients under 50 years of age: a prospective multicenter study, *Arthroscopy* 31(2):184–190, 2015.

Nakamura Y, Yokoya S, Mochizuki Y, et al.: Monitoring of progression of nonsurgically treated rotator cuff tears by magnetic resonance imaging, *J Orthop Sci* 20:314, 2015.

Namdari S, Voleti P, Baldwin K, et al.: Latissimus dorsi tendon transfer for irreparable rotator cuff tears: a systematic review, *J Bone Joint Surg* 94A:891, 2012.

Nho SJ, Delos D, Yadav H, et al.: Biomechanical and biologic augmentation for the treatment of massive rotator cuff tears, *Am J Sports Med* 38:619, 2010.

Olivia F, Via AG, Maffulli N: Role of growth factors in rotator cuff healing, *Sports Med Arthrosc* 19:218, 2011.

Orr SB, Chainani A, Hippensteel KJ, et al.: Aligned multilayered electrospun scaffolds for rotator cuff tendon tissue engineering, *Acta Biomater* 24:117, 2015.

Owens BD, Williams AE, Wolf JM: Risk factors for surgical complications in rotator cuff repair in a veteran population, *J Shoulder Elbow Surg* 24:1707, 2015.

Pauly S, Stahnke K, Klatte-Schulz F, et al.: Do patient age and sex influence tendon cell biology and clinical/radiographic outcomes after rotator cuff repair? *Am J Sports Med* 43:549, 2015.

Rhee YG, Cho NS, Yoo JH: Clinical outcome and repair integrity after rotator cuff repair in patients older than 70 years versus patients younger than 70 years, *Arthroscopy* 30:546, 2014.

Roy JS, Braën C, Leblond J, et al.: Diagnostic accuracy of ultrasonography, MRI and MR arthrography in the characterisation of rotator cuff disorders: a meta-analysis, *Br J Sports Med* 49:1316, 2015.

Schmidt CC, Morrey BF: Management of full-thickness rotator cuff tears: appropriate use criteria, *J Shoulder Elbow Surg* 24:1860, 2015.

Sears BW, Choo A, Yu A, et al.: Clinical outcomes in patients undergoing revision rotator cuff repair with extracellular matrix augmentation, *Orthopedics* 38: e292, 2015.

Shamsudin A, Lam PH, Peters K, et al.: Revision versus primary arthroscopic rotator cuff repair: a 2-year analysis of outcomes in 360 patients, *Am J Sports Med* 43:557, 2015.

Skoff HD: Revision rotator cuff reconstruction for large tears with retraction: a novel technique using autogenous tendon and autologous marrow, *Am J Orthop (Belle Mead NJ)* 44:326, 2015.

Taniguchi N, Suenaga N, Oizumi N, et al.: Bone marrow stimulation at the footprint of arthroscpic surface-holding repair advances cuff repair integrity, *J Shoulder Elbow Surg* 24:860, 2015.

van deer Zwaal P, Thomassen BJ, Nieuwenhuijse MJ, et al.: Clinical outcome in all-arthroscopic versus mini-open rotator cuff repair in small to medium-sized tears: a randomized controlled trial in 100 patients with 1-year follow-up, *Arthroscopy* 29:266, 2013.

Vavken P, Sadoghi P, Palmer M, et al.: Platelet-rich plasma reduces retear rates after arthroscopic repair of small- and medium-sized rotator cuff tears but is not cost-effective, *Am J Sports Med* 43:3071, 2015.

Walton JR, Murrell GA: A two-year clinical outcomes study of 400 patients, comparing open surgery and arthroscopy for rotator cuff repair, *Bone Joint Res* 1:210, 2012.

Williams Jr G, Kraeutler MJ, Zmistowski B, Fenlin Jr M: No difference in postoperative pain after arthroscopic versus open rotator cuff repair, *Clin Orthop Relat Res* 472:2759, 2014.

Xiao J, Cui G: Clinical and structural results of arthroscopic repair of bursal-side partial-thickness rotator cuff tears, *J Shoulder Elbow Surg* 24:e41, 2015.

Yamaguchi H, Suenaga N, Oizumi N, et al.: Open repair for massive rotator cuff tear with a modified transosseous equivalent procedure: preliminary results at short-term follow-up, *J Orthop Sci* 16:398, 2011.

CUFF TEAR ARTHROPATHY

Aumiller WD, Kleuser TM: Diagnosis and treatment of cuff tear arthropathy, *JAAPA* 28:33, 2015.

Eajazi A, Kussman S, LeBedis C, et al.: Rotator cuff tear arthropathy: pathophysiology, imaging characteristics, and treatment options, *AJR Am J Roentgenol* 205:W502, 2015.

Urita A, Funakoshi T, Suenaga N, et al.: A combination of subscapularis tendon transfer and small-head hemiarthroplasty for cuff tear arthropathy: a pilot study, *Bone Joint Lett J* 97-B:1090, 2015.

ADHESIVE CAPSULITIS

Barnes CP, Lam PH, Murrell GA: Short-term outcome after arthroscopic capsular release for adhesive capsulitis, *J Shoulder Elbow Surg* 25:e256, 2016.

Chen CY, Hu CC, Weng PW, et al.: Extracorporeal shockwave therapy improves short-term functional outcomes of shoulder adhesive capsulitis, *J Shoulder Elbow Surg* 23:1843, 2014.

Cher JZB, Akbar M, Kitson S, et al.: Alarmins in frozen shoulder. A molecular association between inflammation and pain, *Am J Sports Med* 46:671, 2017.

Cho CH, Lho YM, Hwang I, et al.: Role of matrix metalloproteinases 2 and 9 in the development of frozen shoulder: human data and experimental analysis in a rat contracture model, *J Shoulder Elbow Surg* 28:1265, 2019.

Chuang TY, Ho WP, Chen CH, et al.: Arthroscopic treatment of rotator cuff tears with shoulder stiffness: a comparison of functional outcome with and without capsular release, *Am J Sports Med* 40:2121, 2012.

Ebrahimzadeh MH, Moradi A, Pour MK, et al.: Clinical outcomes after arthroscopic release for recalcitrant frozen shoulder, *Arch Bone Jt Surg* 2:220, 2014.

Eljabu W, Klinger HM, von Knoch M: Prognostic factors and therapeutic options for treatment of frozen shoulder: a systematic review, *Arch Orthop Trauma Surg* 136(1):1–7, 2016.

Grant JA, Schroeder N, Miller BS, Carpenter JE: Comparison of manipulation and arthroscopoic capsular release for adhesive capsulitis: a systematic review, *J Shoulder Elbow Surg* 22:1135, 2013.

Harris JD, Griesser MJ, Copelan A, Jones GL: Treatment of adhesive capsulitis with intra-articular hyaluronate: a systematic review, *Int J Shoulder Surg* 5:31, 2011.

Jenkins EF, Thomas WJ, Corcoran JP, et al.: The outcome of manipulation under general anesthesia for the management of frozen shoulder in patients with diabetes mellitus, *J Shoulder Elbow Surg* 21:1492, 2011.

Kitridis D, Tsikopoulos K, Bisbinas I, et al.: Efficacy of pharmacological therapies for adhesive capsulitis of the shoulder: a systematic review and network meta-analysis, *Am J Sports Med*, 2019 Feb 8, [Epub ahead of print].

Kuo SJ, Wang FS, Ko JY, et al.: Increased expression of type 1 cannabinoid (CB1) receptor among patients with rotator cuff lesions and shoulder stiffness, *J Shoulder Elbow Surg* 27:333, 2018.

Lee SY, Lee KJ, Kim W, Chung SG: Relationships between capsular stiffness and clinical features in adhesive capsulitis of the shoulder, *Pharm Manag PM R* 7:1226, 2015.

Le Lievre HM, Murrell GA: Long-term outcomes after arthroscopic capsular release for idiopathic adhesive capsulitis, *J Bone Joint Surg* 94A:1208, 2012.

Lho YM, Ha E, Cho CH, et al.: Inflammatory cytokines are overexpressed in the subacromial bursa of frozen shoulder, *J Shoulder Elbow Surg* 22:666, 2013.

Lubis AM, Lubis VK: Matrix metalloproteinase, tissue inhibitor of metalloproteinase and transforming growth factor-beta 1 in frozen shoulder, and their changes as response to intensive stretching and supervised neglect exercises, *J Orthop Sci* 18:519, 2013.

Mehta SS, Singh HP, Pandey R: Comparative outcome of arthroscopic release for frozen shoulder in patients with and without diabetes, *Bone Joint Lett J* 96B:1355, 2014.

Neviaser AS, Hannafin JA: Adhesive capsulitis: a review of current treatment, *Am J Sports Med* 38:2346, 2010.

Neviaser AS, Neviaser RJ: Adhesive capsulitis of the shoulder, *J Am Acad Orthop Surg* 19:536, 2011.

Oh JH, Oh CH, Choi JA, et al.: Comparison of glenohumeral and subacromial steroid injection in primary frozen shoulder: a prospective, randomized short-term comparison study, *J Shoulder Elbow Surg* 20:1034, 2011.

Park KD, Nam HS, Lee JK, et al.: Treatment effects of ultrasound-guided capsular distension with hyaluronic acid in adhesive capsulitis of the shoulder, *Arch Phys Med Rehabil* 94:264, 2013.

Paul A, Rajkumar JS, Peter S, Lambert L: Effectiveness of sustained stretching of the inferior capsule in the management of a frozen shoulder, *Clin Orthop Relat Res* 472:2262, 2014.

Ranalletta M, Rossi LA, Bongiovanni SL, et al.: Corticosteroid injections accelerate pain relief and recovery of function compared with oral NSAIDs in patients with adhesive capsulitis: a randomized controlled trial, *Am J Sports Med* 44:474, 2015.

Rill BK, Fleckenstein CM, Levy MS, et al.: Predictors of outcome after nonoperative and operative treatment of adhesive capsulitis, *Am J Sports Med* 39:567, 2011.

Sasanuma H, Sugimoto H, Fujita A, et al.: Characteristics of dynamic magnetic resonance imaging of idiopathic severe frozen shoulder, *J Shoulder Elbow Surg* 26:e52, 2017.

Sasanuma H, Sugimoto H, Kanaya Y, et al.: Magnetic resonance imaging and short-term clinical results of severe frozen shoulder treated with manipulation under ultrasound-guided cervical nerve root block, *J Shoulder Elbow Surg* 25:e13, 2016.

Shin SJ, Lee SY: Efficies of corticosteroid injection at different sites of the shoulder for the treatment of adhesive capsulitis, *J Shoulder Elbow Surg* 22:521, 2013.

Smitherman JA, Struk AM, Cricchio M, et al.: Arthroscopy and manipulation versus home therapy program in treatment of adhesive capsulitis of the shoulder: a prospective randomized study, *J Surg Orthop Adv* 24:69, 2015.

Sun Y, Liu S, Chen S, et al.: The effect of corticosteroid injection into rotator interval for early frozen shoulder: a randomized controlled trial, *Am J Sports Med* 46:663, 2016.

Sun Y, Zhang P, Liu S, et al.: Intra-articular steroid injection for frozen shoulder: a systematic review and meta-analysis of randomized controlled trials with trial sequential analysis, *Am J Sports Med* 45:2171, 2016.

Sung CM, Jung TS, Park HB: Are serum lipids involved in primary frozen shoulder? A case-control study, *J Bone Joint Surg* 96A:1828, 2014.

Ueda Y, Sugava H, Takahashi N, et al.: Rotator cuff lesions in patients with stiff shoulders: a prospective analysis of 379 shoulders, *J Bone Joint Surg* 97A:1233, 2015.

Vastamäki H, Kettunen J, Vastamäki M: The natural history of idiopathic frozen shoulder: a 2- to 27-year followup study, *Clin Orthop Relat Res* 470:1133, 2012.

Wu CH, Chen WS, Wang TG: Elasticity of the coracohumeral ligament in patients with adhesive capsulitis of the shoulder, *Radiology* 278:458, 2016.

Xu Y, Bonar F, Murrell GA: Enhanced expression of neuronal proteins in idiopathic frozen shoulder, *J Shoulder Elbow Surg* 21:1391, 2012.

Yian EH, Contreras R, Sodl JF: Effects of glycemic control on prevalence of diabetic frozen shoulder, *J Bone Joint Surg* 94A:919, 2012.

Yoon JP, Chung SW, Kim JE, et al.: Intra-articular injection, subacromial injection, and hydrodilation for primary frozen shoulder: a randomized clinical trial, *J Shoulder Elbow Surg* 25:376, 2016.

Yoon JP, Chung SW, Lee BJ, et al.: Correlations of magnetic resonance imaging findings with clinical symptom severity and prognosis of frozen shoulder, *Knee Surg Sports Traumatol Arthrosc* 25:3242, 2017.

Zhang K, de Sa D, Kanakamedala A, et al.: Management of concomitant preoperative rotator cuff pathology and adhesive capsulitis: a systematic review of indications, treatment approaches, and outcomes, *Arthroscopy* 35:979, 2019.

CALCIFIC TENDINITIS

Arirachakaran A, Boonard M, Yamaphai S, et al.: Extracorporeal shock wave therapy, ultrasound-guided percutaneous lavage, corticosteroid injection and combined treatment for the treatment of rotator cuff calcific tendinopathy: a network meta-analysis of RCTs, *Eur J Orthop Surg Traumatol* 27:381, 2017.

Beckman NM, Tran MQ, Cai C: Incidence of rotator cuff tears in the setting of calcific tendinopathy on MRI: a case controlled comparison, *Skeletal Radiol* 48:245, 2019.

Darrieutort-Laffite C, Blanchard F, Le Goff B: Calcific tendonitis of the rotator cuff: from formation to resorption, *Joint Bone Spiine* 85:687, 2018.

De Boer FA, Mocking F, Nelissen EM, et al.: Ultrasound guided needling vs radial shockwave therapy in calcific tendinitis of the shoulder: a prospective randomized trial, *J Orthop* 14:466, 2017.

Del Castillo-González F, Ramos-Alvarez JJ, et al.: Extracorporeal shockwaves versus ultrasound-guided percutaneous lavage for the treatment of rotator cuff calcific tendinopathy: a randomized controlled trial, *Eur J Phys Rehabil Med* 52:145, 2016.

de Witte PB, Kolk A, Overes F, et al.: Rotator cuff calcific tendinitis: ultrasound-guided needling and lavage versus subacromial corticosteroids: five-year outcomes of a randomized controlled trial, *Am J Sports Med* 45:3305, 2017.

de Witte PB, Selten JW, Navas A, et al.: Calcific tendinitis of the rotator cuff: a randomized controlled trial of ultrasound-guided needling and lavage versus subacromial corticosteroids, *Am J Sports Med* 41:1665, 2013.

ElShewy MT: Calcific tendinitis of the rotator cuff, *World J Orthop* 7:55, 2016.

Frassanito P, Cavalieri C, Maestri R, et al.: Effectiveness of extracorporeal shock wave therapy and kinesio taping in calcific tendinopathy of the shoulder: a randomized controlled trial, *Eur J Phys Rehabil Med* 54:333, 2018.

Greis AC, Derringtonn SM, McAuliffe M: Evaluation and nonsurgical management of rotator cuff calcific tendinopathy, *Orthop Clin North Am* 46:293, 2015.

Hackett L, Millar NL, Lam P, et al.: Are the symptoms of calcific tendinitis due to neoinnervation and/or neovascularization? *J Bone Joint Surg Am* 98:186, 2016.

Kim JW, Kim YN, Lee DK: The effect of combined exercise with slings and a flexi-bar on muscle activity and pain in rotator cuff repair patients, *J Phys Ther Sci* 28:2890, 2016.

Kim YS, Lee HJ, Kim YV, Kong CG: Which method is more effective in treatment of calcific tendinitis in the shoulder? Prospective randomized comparison between ultrasound-guided needling and extracorporeal shock wave therapy, *J Shoulder Elbow Surg* 23:1640, 2014.

Lafrance S, Doiron-Cadrin P, Saulnier M, et al.: Is ultrasound-guided lavage an effective intervention for rotator cuff calcific tendinopathy? A systematic review with a meta-analysis of randomised controlled trials, *BMJ Open Sport Exerc Med* 5:e000506, 2019.

Lang G, Izadpanah K, Kubosch EJ, et al.: Examination of concomitant glenohumeral pathologies in patients treated arthroscopically for calcific tendinitis of the shoulder and implications for routine diagnostic joint exploration, *BMC Musculoskelet Disord* 18:476, 2017.

Louwerens JK, Sierevelt IN, van Hove RP, et al.: Prevalence of calcific deposits within the rotator cuff tendons in adults with and without subacromial pain syndrome: clinical and radiologic analysis of 1219 patients, *J Shoulder Elbow Surg* 24:1588, 2015.

Louwerens JK, Sierevelt IN, van Noort A, van den Bekerom MP: Evidence for minimally invasive therapies in the management of chronic calcific tendinopathy of the rotator cuff: a systematic review and meta-analysis, *J Shoulder Elbow Surg* 23:1240, 2014.

Louwerens JK, Veltman ES, van Noort A, van den Bekerom MP: The effectiveness of high-energy extracorporeal shockwave therapy versus ultrasound-guided needling versus arthroscopic surgery in the management of chronic calcific rotator cuff tendinopathy: a systematic review, *Arthroscopy* 32:165, 2016.

Malliaropoulos N, Thompson D, Meke M, et al.: Individualised radial extracorporeal shock wave therapy (rESWT) for symptomatic calcific shoulder tendinopathy: a retrospective clinical study, *BMC Musculoskelet Disrod* 18:513, 2017.

Merolla G, Singh S, Paladini P, Porcellini G: Calcific tendinitis of the rotator cuff: state of the art in diagnosis and treatment, *J Orthop Traumatol* 17:7, 2015.

Pieber K, Grim-Stieger M, Kainberger F, et al.: Long-term course of shoulders after ultrasound therapy for calcific tendinitis: results of the 10-year follow-up of a randomized controlled trial, *Am J Phys Med Rehabili* 97:651, 2018.

Sabeti-Aschraf M, Gonano C, Nemecek E, et al.: Intra-operative ultrasound facilitates the localization of the calcific deposit during arthrosopic treatment of calcifying tendinitis, *Knee Surg Sports Traumatol Arthrosc* 18:1792, 2010.

Suzuki K, Potts A, Anakenze O, Ssingh A: Calcific tendinitis of the rotator cuff: management options, *J Am Acad Orthop Surg* 22:707, 2014.

Verstraelen FU, Fievez E, Janssen L, et al.: Surgery for calcifying tendinitis of the shoulder: a systematic review, *World J Orthop* 8:424, 2017.

Wu KT, Chou WY, Wang CJ, et al.: Efficacy of extracorporeal shockwave therapy on calcified and noncalcified shoulder tendinosis: a propensity score matched analysis, *BioMed Res Int* 2019: 2958251, 2019.

Wu YC, Tsai WC, Tu YK, et al.: Comparative effectiveness of nonoperative treatments for chronic calcific tendinitis of the shoulder: a systematic review and network meta-analysis of randomized controlled trials, *Arch Phys Med Rehabil* 98:1678, 2017.

Yoo JC, Koh KH, Park WH, et al.: The outcome of ultrasound-guided needle decompression and steroid injection in calcific tendinitis, *J Shoulder Elbow Surg* 19:596, 2010.

Zhang T, Duan Y, Chen P, et al.: Efficacy of ultrasound-guided percutaneous lavage for rotator cuff calcific tendinopathy: a systematic review and meta-analysis, *Medicine (Baltim)* 98:e15552, 2019.

QUADRILATERAL SPACE SYNDROME

Bourget-Murray J, Davison E, Frizzell B, et al.: Fluoroscopic-guided quadrilateral space block for the treatment of quadrilateral space syndrome—a case report, *J Clin Orthop Trauma* 10:655, 2019.

Brown SA, Doolittle DA, Bohanon CJ, et al.: Quadrilteral space syndrome: the Mayo Clinic experience with a new classification system and case service, *Mayo Clin Proc* 90:382, 2015.

Chen H, Narvaez VR: Ultrasound-guided quadrilateral space block for the diagnosis of quadrilateral syndrome, *Case Rep Orthop* 2015: 378627, 2015.

de Mooij T, Duncan AA, Kakar S: Vascular injuries in the upper extremity in athletes, *Hand Clin* 31:39, 2015.

Feng SH, Hsiao MY, Wu CH, et al.: Ultrasound-guided diagnosis and management for quadrilateral space syndrome, *Pain Med* 184, 2017.

Flynn LS, Wright TW, King JJ: Quadrilateral space syndrome: a review, *J Shoulder Elbow Surg* 27:950, 2018.

Hangge PT, Breen I, Albadawi H, et al.: Quadrilateral space syndrome: diagnosis and clinical management, *J Clin Med* 7:E86, 2018.

Hong CC, Thambiah MD, Manohara R: Quadrilatral space syndrome: the forgotten differential, *J Orthop Surg* 27:2309499019847145, 2019.

Rollo J, Rigberg D, Gelabert H: Vascular quadrilateral space syndrome in 3 overhead throwing athletes: an undiagnosied cause of digital ischemia, *Ann Vasc Surg* 63:e1, 2017.

Zurkiya O, Walker TG: Quadrilateral space syndrome, *J Vasc Interv Radiol* 25:229, 2014.

SUPRASCAPULAR NERVE ENTRAPMENT

Arriaza R, Ballesteros J, López-Vidriero E: Suprascapular neuropathy as a cause of swimmer's shoulder: results after arthroscopic treatment in 4 patients, *Am J Sports Med* 41:887, 2013.

Boykin RE, Friedman DJ, Higgins LD, Warner JJ: Suprascapular neuropathy, *J Bone Joint Surg* 92A:2348, 2010.

Boykin RE, Friedman DJ, Zimmer ZR, et al.: Suprascapular neuropathy in a shoulder referral practice, *J Shoulder Elbow Surg* 20:983, 2011.

Brand JC: *Editorial Commentary*: mounting evidence for a landmark-based approach to suprascapular nerve block, *Arthroscopy* 35:2282, 2019.

Denard PJ: *Editorial Commentary*: suprascapular neuropathy in overhead athletes: to release or not to release, *Arthroscopy* 35:2558, 2018.

Duparc F, Coquerel D, Ozeel J, et al.: Anatomical basis of the suprascapular nerve entrapment, and clinical relevance of the supraspinatus fascia, *Surg Radiol Anat* 32:277, 2010.

Freehill MT, Shi LL, Tompson JD, Warner JJ: Suprascapular neuropathy: diagnosis and management, *Phys Sportsmed* 40:72, 2012.

Hill LJ, Jelsing EJ, Terry MJ, Stormmen JA: Evaluation, treatment, and outcomes of suprascapular neuropathy: a 5-year review, *Pharm Manag PM R* 6:774, 2014.

Laumonerie P, Blasco L, Tibbo ME, et al.: Ultrasound-guided versus landmark-based approach to the distal suprascapular nerve block: a comparative cadaveric study, *Arthroscopy* 35:2274, 2019.

Mall NA, Hammond JE, Lenart BA, et al.: Suprascapular nerve entrapment isolated to the spinoglenid notch: surgical technique and results of open decompression, *J Shoulder Elbow Surg* 22:e1, 2013.

McFarland E, Bernard J, Dein E, et al.: Diagnostic injections about the shoulder, *J Amer Acad Orthop Surg* 25:799, 2017.

Polguj M, Jedrzejewski K, Podgorski M, et al.: A proposal for classification of the superior transverse scapular ligament: variable morphology and its potential influence on suprascapular nerve entrapment, *J Shoulder Elbow Surg* 22:1265, 2013.

Scully WF, Wilson DJ, Parada SA, et al.: Iatrogenic nerve injuries in shoulder surgery, *J Amer Acad Orthop Surg* 21:717, 2013.

Shah AA, Butler RB, Sung SY, et al.: Clinical outcomes of suprascapular nerve decompression, *J Shoulder Elbow Surg* 20:975, 2011.

Shi LL, Boykin RE, Lin A, Warner JJ: Association of suprascapular neuropathy with rotator cuff tendon tears and fatty degeneration, *J Shoulder Elbow Surg* 23:339, 2014.

Tsikouris GD, Bolia IK, Vlaserou P, et al.: Shoulder arthroscopy with versus without suprascapular nerve releae: clinical outcomes and return to sport rate in elite overhead athletes, *Arthroscopy* 34:2552, 2018.

Tubbs RS, Nechtman C, D'Antoni AV, et al.: Ossification of the suprascapular ligament: a risk factor for suprascapular nerve compression? *Int J Shoulder Surg* 7:19, 2013.

Yamakado K: The suprascapular notch narrows with aging: a preliminary solution of the old conjecture based on a 3D-CT evaluation, *Surg Radiol Anat* 38:693, 2016.

ELBOW INJURIES

ELBOW TENOPATHIES (LATERAL AND MEDIAL EPICONDYLITIS)

Altiniski J, Meric G, Erduran M, et al.: The BstUI and DpnII variants of the COL5A1 gene are associated with tennis elbow, *Am J Sports Med* 43:1784, 2015.

Amin NH, Kumar NS, Schickendantz MS: Medial epicondylitis: evaluation and management, *J Am Acad Orthop Surg* 23:348, 2015.

Bateman M, Littlewood C, Rawson B, et al.: Surgery for tennis elbow: a systematic review, *Shoulder Elbow* 11:35, 2019.

Ben-Nafa W, Munro W: The effect of corticosteroid versus platelet-rich plasma injection therapies for the management of lateral epicondylitis: a systematic review, *SICOT J* 4:11, 2018.

Buchbinder R, Johnston RV, Barnsley L, et al.: Surgery for lateral elbow pain, *Cochrane Database Syst Rev* 3:CD003525, 2011.

Clark T, McRae S, Leiter J, et al.: Arthroscopic versus open lateral release for the treatment of lateral epicondylitis: a prospective randomized controlled trial, *Arthroscopy* 34:3177, 2018.

Clarke AW, Ahmad M, Curtis M, Connell DA: Lateral elbow tendinopathy: correlation of ultrasound findings with pain and functional disability, *Am J Sports Med* 38:1209, 2010.

Coombes BK, Bisset L, Vicenzino B: Efficacy and safety of corticosteroid injections and other injection for management of tendinopathy: a systematic review of randomized controlled trials, *Lancet* 376:1751, 2010.

Creaney L, Wallace A, Curtis M, Connell D: Growth factor–based therapies provide additional benefit beyond physical therapy in resistant elbow tendinopathy: a prospective, single-blind, randomised trial of autologous blood injections versus platelet-rich plasma injections, *Br J Sports Med* 45:966, 2011.

Degen RM, Conti MS, Camp CL, et al.: Epidemiology and disease burden of lateral epicondylitis in the USA: analysis of 85,318 patients, *HSS J* 14:9, 2018.

Ford RD, Schmitt WP, Lineberry K, Luce P: A retrospective comparison of the management of recalcitrant lateral elbow tendinosis: platlet-rich plasma injections versus surgery, *Hand (N Y)* 10:285, 2015.

Galvin R, Callaghan C, Chan WS, et al.: Injection of botulinum toxin for treatment of chronic lateral epicondylitis: systematic review and meta-analysis, *Semin Arthritis Rheum* 40:585, 2011.

Gosens T, Peerbooms JC, van Laar W, den Oudsten BL: Ongoing positive effect of platelet-rich plasma versus corticosteroid injection in lateral epicondylitis: a double-blind randomzed controlled trial with 2-year follow-up, *Am J Sports Med* 39:1200, 2011.

Gupta PK, Acharya A, Khanna V, et al.: PRP versus steroids in a deadlock for efficacy: long-term stability versus short-term intensity-results from a randomised trial, *Musculoskelet Surg*, 2019 Aug 26, [Epub ahead of print].

Houck DA, Kraeutler MJ, Thornton LB, et al.: Treatment of lateral epicondylitis with autologous blood, platelet-rich plasma, or corticosteroid injections: a systematic review of overlapping meta-analyses, *Orthop J Sports Med* 7:2324967119831052, 2019.

Judson CH, Wolf JM: Lateral epicondylitis: review of injection therapies, *Orthop Clin North Am* 44:615, 2013.

Kazemi M, Azma K, Tavana B, et al.: Autologous blood versus corticosteroid local injection in the soft-term treatment of lateral elbow tendinopathy: a randomized clinical trial of efficacy, *Am J Phys Med Rehabil* 89:660, 2010.

Knutson EJ, Calfee RP, Chen RE, et al.: Factors associated with failure of non-operative treatment in lateral epicondylitis, *Am J Sports Med* 43:2133, 2015.

Krogh TP, Bartels EM, Ellingsen T, et al.: Comparative effectiveness of injection therapies in lateral epicondylitis: a systematic review and network meta-analysis of randomized controlled trials, *Am J Sports Med* 41:1435, 2013.

Lai WC, Erickson BJ, Mlynarek RA, et al.: Chronic lateral epicondylitis: challenges and solutions, *Open Access J Sports Med* 9:243, 2018.

Lebiedzinski R, Snydeer M, Buchcic P, et al.: A randomized study of autologous conditioned plasma and steroid injections in the treatment of lateral epicondylitis, *Int Orthop* 39:2199, 2015.

Li A, Wang H, Yu Z, et al.: Platelet-rich plasma vs corticosteroids for elbow epicondylitis: a systematic review and meta-analysis, *Medicine (Baltim)* 98:e18358, 2019.

Mishra AK, Skrepnik NV, Edwards SG, et al.: Efficacy of platelet-rich plasma for chronic tennis elbow: a double-blind prospective multicenter, randomized controlled trial of 230 patients, *Am J Sports Med* 42:463, 2014.

Ozturan KE, Yucel I, Cakici H, et al.: Autologous blood and corticosteroid injection and extracorporeal shock wave therapy in the treatment of lateral epicondylitis, *Orthopedics* 33:84, 2010.

Peerbooms JC, Sluimer J, Bruijn DJ, Gosens T: Positive effect of an autologous platelet concentrate in lateral epicondylitis in a double-blind randomized controlled trial: platelet-rich plasma versus corticosteroid injection with a 1-year follow-up, *Am J Sports Med* 38:255, 2010.

Raeissadat SA, Rayegani SM, Hassanabadi H, et al.: Is platelet-rich plasma superior to whole blood in the management of chronic tennis elbow: one-year randomized clinical trial, *BMC Sports Sci Med Rehabil* 6:12, 2014.

Reddy VR, Satheesan KS, Bayliss N: Outcome of Boyd-McLeod procedure for recalcitrant lateral epicondylitis of the elbow, *Rheumatol Int* 31:1081, 2011.

Riff AJ, Saltzman BM, Cvetanovich G, et al.: Open vs percutaneous vs arthroscopic surgical treatment of lateral epicondyltis: an updated systematic review, *Am J Orthop (Belle Mead NJ)* 47:6, 2018.

Ruch DS, Orr SB, Richard MJ, et al.: A comparison of debridement with and without anconeus muscle flap for treatment of refractory lateral epicondylitis, *J Shoulder Elbow Surg* 24:236, 2015.

Saccomanni B: Corticosteroid injection for tennis elbow or lateral epicondylitis: a review of the literature, *Curr Rev Musculoskelet Med* 3:38, 2010.

Savoie 3rd FH, O'Brien MJ: Arthroscopic tennis elbow release, *Instr Course Lect* 64:225, 2015.

Sayegh ET, Strauch RJ: Does nonsurgical treatment improve longitudinal outcomes of lateral epicondylitis over no treatment? A meta-analysis, *Clin Orthop Relat Res* 473:1093, 2015.

Schipper ON, Dunn JH, Ochiai DH, et al.: Nirschl surgical technique for concomitant lateral and medial elbow tendinosis: a retrospective review of 53 elbows with a mean follow-up of 11.7 years, *Am J Sports Med* 39:972, 2011.

Sims SE, Miller K, Elfar JC, Hammert WC: Non-surgical treatment of lateral epicondylitis: a systematic review of randomized controlled trials, *Hand (N Y)* 9:419, 2014.

Solheim E, Hegna J, Øyen J: Arthroscopic versus open tennis elbow release: 3- to 6-year results of case-control series of 305 elbows, *Arthroscopy* 29:854, 2013.

Solheim E, Hegna J, Oyen J: Extensor tendon release in tennis elbow: results and prognostic factors in 80 elbows, *Knee Surg Sports Traumatol Arthrosc* 19:1023, 2011.

Tang S, Wang X, Wu P, et al.: Platelet-rich plasma vs autologous blood vs corticosteroid injections in the treatment of lateral epicondylitis: a systematic review, pairwise and network meta-analysis of randomized controlled trials, *Pharm Manag PM R*, 2019 Nov, 17. [Epub ahead of print].

Titchener AG, Fakis A, Tambe AA, et al.: Risk factors in lateral epicondylitis (tennis elbow): a case-control study, *J Hand Surg Eur* 38:159, 2013.

Trentini R, Mangano T, Repetto I, et al.: Short- to mid-term follow-up effectiveness of US-guided focal extracorporeal shock wave therapy in the treatment of elbow lateral epicondylitis, *Musculoskelet Surg* 99(Suppl 1):S91, 2015.

Van Hofwegen C, Baker 3rd CL, Baker Jr CL: Epicondylitis in the athlete's elbow, *Clin Sports Med* 29:5767, 2010.

Vinod AV, Ross G: An effective approach to diagnosis and surgical repair of refractory medial epicondylitis, *J Shoulder Elbow Surg* 24:1172, 2015.

Walton MJ, Mackie K, Fallon M, et al.: The reliability and validity of magnetic resonance imaging in the assessment of chronic lateral epicondylitis, *J Hand Surg Am* 36:475, 2011.

Walz DM, Newman JS, Konin GP, Ross G: Epicondylitis: pathogenesis, imaging, and treatment, *Radiographics* 30:167, 2010.

Wang A, Mackie K, Breidahl W, et al.: Evidence for the durability of autologous tenocyte injection for treatment of chronic resistant lateral epicondylitis: mean 4.5-year clinical follow-up, *Am J Sports Med* 43:1775, 2015.

Wang W, Chen J, Lou J, et al.: Comparison of arthroscopic debridement and open debridement in the management of lateral epicondylitis: a systematic review and meta-analysis, *Medicine (Baltim)* 98:17668, 2019.

Wolf JM, Ozer K, Scott F, et al.: Comparison of autologous blood, corticosteroid, and saline injection in the treatment of lateral epicondylitis: a prospective, randomized, controlled multicenter study, *J Hand Surg Am* 36:1269, 2011.

Xu Q, Chen J, Cheng L: Comparison of platelet rich plasma and corticosteroids in the management of lateral epicondylitis: a meta-analysis of randomized controlled trials, *Int J Surg* 67:37, 2019.

Yoon JP, Chung SW, Yi JH, et al.: Prognostic factors of arthroscopic extensor carpi radialis brevis release for lateral epicondylitis, *Arthroscopy* 31:1232, 2015.

ELBOW CONTRACTURES

Araghi A, Celli A, Adams R, Morrey B: The outcome of examination (manipulation) under anesthesia on the stiff elbow after surgical contracture release, *J Shoulder Elbow Surg* 19:202, 2010.

Blonna D, Huffmann GR, O'Driscoll SW: Delayed-onset ulnar neuritis after release of elbow contractures: clinical presentation, pathological findings, and treatment, *Am J Sports Med* 42:2113, 2014.

Breborowicz M, Lubiatowski P, Dlugosz J, et al.: The outcome of open elbow arthrolysis: comparison of four different approaches based on one hundred cases, *Int Orthop* 38:561, 2014.

Edwards SG, Rhodes DA, Jordan TW, et al.: The olecranon osteotomy-facilited elbow release (OFER), *J Bone Joint Surg Am* 99:1859, 2017.

Ehsan A, Huang JI, Lyons M, Hanel DP: Surgical management of posttraumatic elbow arthrofibrosis, *J Trauma Acute Care Surg* 72:1399, 2012.

Haglin JM, Kugelman DN, Christiano A, et al.: Open surgical elbow contracture release after trauma: results and recommendations, *J Shoulder Elbow Surg* 27:418, 2018.

Hildebrand KA: Posttraumatic elbow joint contractures: defining pathologic capsular mechanisms and potential future treatment paradigms, *J Hand Surg Am* 38:2227, 2013.

Koh KH, Lim TK, Lee HI, Park MJ: Surgical release of elbow stiffness after internal fixation of intercondylar fracture of the distal humerus, *J Shoulder Elbow Surg* 22:268, 2013.

Kruse KK, Papatheodorou LK, Weiser RW, et al.: Release of the stiff elbow with mini-open technique, *J Shoulder Elbow Surg* 25:355, 2016.

Lindenhovius AL, Doornberg JN, Ring D, Jupiter JB: Health status after open elbow contracture release, *J Bone Joint Surg* 92A:2187, 2010.

Monument MJ, Hart DA, Salo PT, et al.: Posttraumatic elbow contractures: targeting neuroinflammatory fibrogenic mechanisms, *J Orthop Sci* 18:869, 2013.

Myden C, Hildebrand K: Elbow joint contracture after traumatic injury, *J Shoulder Elbow Surg* 20:39, 2011.

Streubel PN, Cohen MS: Open surgical release for contractures of the elbow, *J Am Acad Orthop Surg* 23:328, 2015.

Ulrich SD, Bonutti PM, Seyler TM, et al.: Restoring range of motion via stress relaxation and static progressive stretch in posttraumatic elbow contractures, *J Shoulder Elbow Surg* 19:196, 2010.

Wang W, Zhan YL, Yu SY, et al.: Open arthrolysis with pie-crusting release of the triceps tendon for treating post-traumatic contracture of the elbow, *J Shoulder Elbow Surg* 25:816, 2016.

Williams BG, Sotereanos DG, Baratz ME, et al.: The contracted elbow: is ulnar nerve release necessary? *J Shoulder Elbow Surg* 21:1632, 2012.

HETEROTOPIC OSSIFICATION

Bachman DR, Kamaci S, Thaveepunsan S, et al.: Preoperative nerve imaging using computed tomography in patients with heterotopic ossification of the elbow, *J Shoulder Elbow Surg* 24:1149, 2015.

Baldwin K, Hosalkar HS, Donegan DJ, et al.: Surgical resection of heterotopic bone about the elbow: an institutional experience with traumatic and neurologic etiologies, *J Hand Surg Am* 36:798, 2011.

Bauer AS, Lawson BK, Bliss RL, Dyer GS: Risk factors for posttraumatic heterotopic ossification of the elbow: case-control study, *J Hand Surg Am* 37:1422, 2012.

Brouwer KM, Lindenhovius AL, de Witte PB, et al.: Resection of heterotopic ossification of the elbow: a comparison of ankylosis and partial restriction, *J Hand Surg Am* 35:1115, 2010.

Chen S, Liu J, Cai J, et al.: Results and outcome predictors after open release of complete ankylosis of the elbow caused by heterotopic ossification, *Int Orthop* 41:1627, 2017.

Chen S, Yu SY, Yan H, et al.: The time point in surgical excision of heterotopic ossification of post-traumatic stiff elbow: recommendation for early excision followed by early exercise, *J Shoulder Elbow Surg* 24:1165, 2015.

Douglas K, Cannada LK, Archer KR, et al.: Incidence and risk factors of heterotopic ossification following major elbow trauma, *Orthopedics* 35: e815, 2012.

Foruria AM, Lawrence TM, Augustin S, et al.: Heterotopic ossification after surgery for distal humeral fractures, *Bone Joint Lett J* 96B:1681, 2014.

Hong CC, Nashi N, Hey HW, et al.: Clinically relevant heterotopic ossification after elbow fracture surgery: a risk factors study, *Orthop Traumatol Surg Res* 101:209, 2015.

Koh KH, Lim TK, Lee HI, Park MJ: Surgical treatment of elbow stiffness caused by post-traumatic heterotopic ossification, *J Shoulder Elbow Surg* 22:1128, 2013.

Lee EK, Namdari S, Hosalkar HS, et al.: Clinical results of the excision of heterotopic bone around the elbow: a systematic review, *J Shoulder Elbow Surg* 22:716, 2013.

Liu EY, Hildebrand A, Horner NS, et al.: Heterotopic ossification after total elbow arthroplasty: a systematic review, *J Shoulder Elbow Surg* 28:587, 2019.

Maender C, Sahajpal D, Wright TW: Treatment of heterotopic ossification of the elbow following burn injury: recommendations for surgical excision and perioperative prophylaxis using radiation therapy, *J Shoulder Elbow Surg* 19:1269, 2010.

Park JY, Seo BH, Hong KH, et al.: Prevalence and clinical outcomes of heterotopic ossification after ulnar collateral ligament reconstruction, *J Shoulder Elbow Surg* 27:427, 2018.

Ploumis A, Belbasis L, Ntzani E, et al.: Radiotherapy for prevention of heterotopic ossification of the elbow: a systematic review of the literature, *J Shoulder Elbow Surg* 22:1580, 2013.

Ranganathan K, Loder S, Agarwal S, et al.: Heterotopic ossification: basic-science principles and clinical correlates, *J Bone Joint Surg* 97A:1101, 2015.

Robinson PM, MacInnes SJ, Stanley D, et al.: Heterotopic ossification following total elbow arthroplasty: a comparison of the incidence following elective and trauma surgery, *Bone Joint Lett J* 100-B:767, 2018.

Salazar D, Golz A, Israel H, Marra G: Heterotopic ossification of the elbow treated with surgical resection: risk factors, bony ankylosis, and complications, *Clin Orthop Relat Res* 472:2269, 2014.

Shukla DR, Pillai G, McAnay S, et al.: Heterotopic ossification formation after fracture-dislocations of the elbow, *J Shoulder Elbow Surg* 24:333, 2015.

Ter Meulen DP, Nota SP, Hageman MG, et al.: Progression of heterotopic ossification around the elbow after trauma, *Arch Bone Jt Surg* 4:228, 2016.

Vasileiadis GI, Ramazanian T, Kamaci S, et al.: Loss of pronation-supination in patients with heterotopic ossification around the elbow, *J Shoulder Elbow Surg* 28:1406, 2019.

Wiggers JK, Helmerhorst GT, Brouwer KM, et al.: Injury complexity factors predict heterotopic ossification restricting motion after elbow trauma, *Clin Orthop Relat Res* 472:2162, 2014.

The complete list of references is available online at ExpertConsult.com.

RECURRENT DISLOCATIONS

Barry B. Phillips

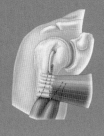

Recurrent instability can result from congenital, developmental, or traumatic ligamentous or bony containment deficiencies or from deformities caused by muscular imbalance, joint incongruity, or joint malalignment in one or more planes. Proper treatment begins with knowledge and skillful evaluation of deformities before initiating a specific treatment plan.

PATELLA

Patellar instability results from a direct or indirect valgus-producing force. When significant force results in dislocation, a tear of medial soft-tissue restraints, as well as an osteochondral defect in the medial facet of the patella or lateral femoral condyle, may result. Dislocations in skeletally immature individuals tend to recur as in other joints, with recurrences in two thirds of patients.

The amount of trauma necessary to result in patellar instability depends on soft-tissue restraints both static (medial patellofemoral ligament [MPFL]) and dynamic (vastus medialis obliquus [VMO]), bony restraints, trochlear and patellar morphology, and extremity alignment in the axial and coronal planes. Normally, the MPFL and VMO maintain patellar stability in 0 to 20 degrees of flexion. At 30 degrees, the patella is centered and stabilized by the bony contour of the trochlea. When patella alta or trochlear or patellar dysplasia is present, bony stability is compromised. Genu valgus or rotational deformities from femoral anteversion or external tibial torsion increase the quadriceps angle and result in valgus-directed force on the patella. These factors must all be considered when conservative or operative management is indicated.

CLINICAL FEATURES

In patients with recurrent dislocation or subluxation of the patella, an accurate history is still one of the most important diagnostic tools. Patellar problems can mimic various "internal derangements" of the knee. An accurate history of the mechanism of injury and the type and area of pain is important. Patients with patellar instability frequently report diffuse pain around the knee that is aggravated by going up and down stairs or hills. The pain usually is located anterior in the knee and often is described as an aching pain with intermittent episodes of sharp, severe pain. A feeling of insecurity in the knee and occasionally of "giving way" or "going out" of the knee may be present. Patellar crepitation and swelling of the knee are common. Physical findings include the previously cited factors that contribute to increasing the Q angle.

The examination begins by observing the patient's patellar height, with the patient in the seated position. An upward tilt indicates patella alta. Dynamic patellar tracking is evaluated with the examiner standing in front of the seated patient while the patient slowly extends the knee. A positive J sign (slight lateral subluxation of the patella as the knee approaches full extension) indicates some degree of maltracking. Active patellar tracking also should be examined with the knee relaxed in the extended position. When the quadriceps muscle is tightened, motion of the patella is examined. Normally, the patella should move more superiorly than laterally. With the patient supine and the knee flexed 30 degrees with a bolster behind the knee, the Q angle is measured. Insufficiency of the femoral sulcus and the MPFL, which provide 60% of the medial stabilization, is tested by applying an inferolaterally directed stress while palpating the ligament. Displacement of more than two quadrants and a soft end point generally indicate MPFL insufficiency. The patellar grind test is done by applying pressure to the patella and manually displacing it medially, laterally, superiorly, and inferiorly in the trochlear groove. This test reproduces anterior knee pain when a patellofemoral pathologic condition is present.

For the "apprehension test," the examiner holds the relaxed knee in 20 to 30 degrees of flexion and manually subluxes the patella laterally. When the test is positive, the patient suddenly complains of pain and resists any further lateral motion of the patella. The active apprehension test is more accurate: the same controlled maneuver is done while slowly flexing and extending the patient's knee. Patella laxity is evaluated by visually dividing the patella into four quadrants and passively moving the patella medially and then laterally, measuring the amount of excursion in the patellar quadrants. This is done with the knee at 0 degrees and at 20 degrees of flexion. Normally, passive patellar glide is one to two quadrants medially and laterally; motion of more than two quadrants indicates soft-tissue laxity. Excessive lateral retinacular tightness is indicated by limited medial passive patellar glide and by a negative patellar tilt. The patellar tilt test is done with the knee in 20 degrees of flexion. The examiner's fingers are placed along the medial side of the patella with the thumb on the lateral aspect. Inability to raise the lateral facet to the horizontal plane or slightly past indicates excessive lateral retinacular tightness. Tenderness along the MPFL, medial patellar facet, and lateral condyle are common with stability.

Thigh circumferences measured proximal to the patella often show quadriceps atrophy on the involved side. With the patient sitting and the knees flexed 90 degrees, a lateral or superior position of the patella sometimes can be seen. After careful examination of the uninvolved and injured knees, other joints should be examined for hyperlaxity. Hyperextension of the knees or elbows past 10 degrees,

ability to touch the thumb passively to the forearm, hyperextension of the metacarpophalangeal joint of the index finger, and multidirectional laxity of the shoulder joint all are indicative of generalized ligamentous laxity. Patients with generalized ligamentous laxity have been found to have fewer articular lesions associated with dislocations than patients without ligamentous laxity. The thigh-foot angle is measured with the patient prone and the knee flexed 90 degrees. An angle of more than 30 degrees indicates significant rotational deformity of the lower extremity. The final part of the examination is done with the patient standing and consists of observation for malalignment (i.e., femoral anteversion, genu valgum, external tibial torsion, and pes planus) and core condition.

RADIOGRAPHIC FEATURES (TABLE 3.1)

The anteroposterior view of the knee can be used to confirm valgus alignment and lateral position of the patella and to look for osteochondral damage. The lateral view of the knee is helpful in determining patella alta. Blumensaat showed that with the knee flexed 30 degrees, a line extending through the intercondylar notch should just touch the lower pole of the patella (Fig. 3.1).

Patellar height is more accurately evaluated by the Insall, Clanton, or Blackburn-Peel index (see Table 3.1). The crossover sign is the best indicator of trochlear dysplasia—the earlier the crossover, the more dysplasia present. A trochlear depth of less than 3 mm or trochlear bump of more than 4 mm indicates significant dysplasia.

TABLE 3.1

Radiographic Measurements of the Patella

TECHNIQUE	MEASUREMENT	CHARACTERISTICS
Blumensaat line (Fig. 3.1), lateral radiograph, to determine patella alta	With knee flexed 30 degrees, line is drawn through intercondylar notch	Should approximate the lower pole of the patella
Insall-Salvati index lateral radiograph	LT:LP = 1.0	Patella alta if ratio ≤1.2
Trochlear depth (Dejour) lateral radiograph	Trochlear depth measured 1 cm from top of groove	Should be ≥5 mm
Patellar height (Caton-Deschamps), lateral radiograph	Ratio between articular facet length of patella (AP) and distance between articular facet of patella and anterior corner of superior tibial epiphysis (AT). Knee flexed 30 degrees.	AP/AT ratio—normal 0.6-1.3 Patella infera—ratio <0.6 Patella alta—ratio >1.3
Blackburne-Peel ratio	Length of articular surface of patella to length measured from articular surface of tibia to inferior pole of patella	Normal ratio 0.54-1.06
Patellar tilt (CT scan)	Angle formed by intersection of the tangent of the posterior condyles and the major axis of the patella on 20-degree flexion scan	Normal angle: <20 degrees Angle >20 degrees: dysplasia
TT-TG (axial radiograph, CT scan)	Two lines drawn perpendicular to posterior bicondylar line, one line through middle of trochlear groove and second through tibial tuberosity. Distance between the lines is measured	>20 mm = malalignment
Crossing sign	Anterior cortical outline of condyle intersects trochlear outline	Dysplastic sulcus
Trochlear bump	Trochlear line extends anterior to femoral cortex	Dysplastic sulcus

CT, Computed tomography; LP, length of the patella; LT, length of the patellar tendon; TT-TG, tibial tubercle-trochlear groove.

The most important routine view of the patellofemoral joint is the axial view of the patella. Several methods have been described for taking this axial view (Fig. 3.2B). For this radiograph to be meaningful, both knees should be exposed at the same time for comparison. The plane of the film should be perpendicular to the x-ray beam to avoid distortion, the legs should be held vertical to prevent rotation that might simulate low lateral femoral condyles, the quadriceps muscles should be relaxed to prevent the patella from being reduced at the time the radiograph is made, and the knee should be flexed in the range of 20 to 45 degrees because more flexion generally reduces most patellofemoral abnormalities.

When the axial view has been obtained, the shape of the patella should be evaluated, along with the shape of the femoral trochlea and the relationship of the patella to the femur. Normally, the patella appears evenly seated within the trochlear groove of the femur, with an equal distance between both patellar facets and the adjacent femoral surfaces. Abnormalities include tilting of the patella or subluxation and complete dislocation of the patella (Fig. 3.3). The trochlea is evaluated on the Merchant view for dysplasia, sulcus angle greater than 145 degrees, and congruence—normally 60 ± 11 degrees (Figs. 3.4 and 3.5). For most dislocations or first-time dislocations, particularly in athletes, MRI or three-dimensional (3D) CT examination may be indicated to evaluate for chondral damage, loose bodies, dysplasia, and malalignment. An axial view at the superior trochlear groove is used to evaluate dysplasia; superimposed views are used to evaluate malalignment. Tibial tubercle–trochlear groove (TT-TG) distance of more than 20 mm on

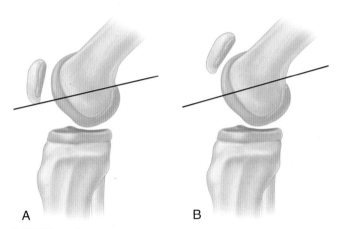

FIGURE 3.1   A, Normal knee. Lower pole of patella at Blumensaat line at 30 degrees of flexion of knee. **B,** Patella alta. Patella significantly proximal to Blumensaat line.

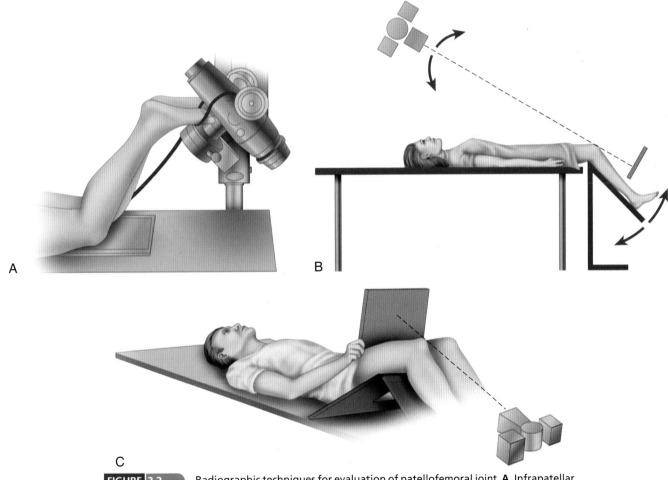

FIGURE 3.2   Radiographic techniques for evaluation of patellofemoral joint. **A,** Infrapatellar view. **B,** Axial view. **C,** Skyline view.

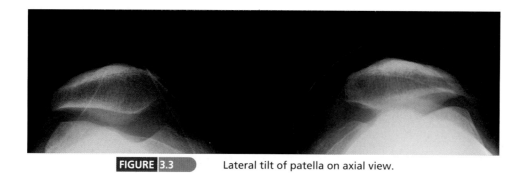

FIGURE 3.3   Lateral tilt of patella on axial view.

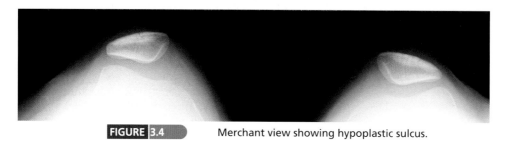

FIGURE 3.4   Merchant view showing hypoplastic sulcus.

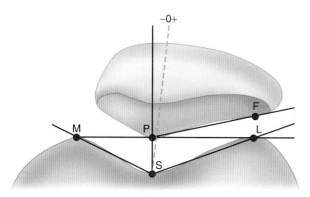

FIGURE 3.5   Measurements of patellofemoral congruence described by Merchant et al. *F,* Facet; *L,* lateral condyle; *M,* medial condyle; *P,* patellar ridge; *S,* sulcus. Angle *MSL* is sulcus angle (average, 137 degrees; standard deviation, 6 degrees). Line *SO* is zero reference line bisecting sulcus angle. Angle *PSO* is congruence angle (average, −8 degrees; standard deviation, 6 degrees). Line *PF* (lateral facet) and line *ML* form patellofemoral angle that should diverge laterally.

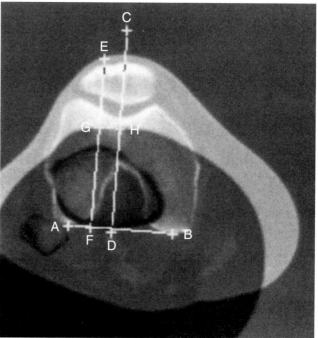

FIGURE 3.6   Lines used to calculate tibial tubercle lateralization using CT. Line is drawn on superimposed image between posterior margins of femoral condyles *(AB).* Two lines are drawn perpendicular to this, one bisecting femoral trochlear groove *(CD)* and one bisecting anterior tibial tuberosity through chosen point in center of patellar tendon insertion *(EF).* Distance between these two lines *(GH)* is measured in millimeters. (From Jones RB, Barletta EC, Vainright JR, et al: CT determination of tibial tubercle lateralization in patients presenting with anterior knee pain, *Skeletal Radiol* 24:505–509, 1995.)

CT (Fig. 3.6) or MRI may indicate malalignment and may necessitate distal realignment.

CONSERVATIVE TREATMENT
▮ ACUTE PATELLAR DISLOCATION OR SUBLUXATION

After an acute dislocation or subluxation of the patella, the knee is immobilized in a commercial immobilizer with a Jones-type compressive dressing and crutches are used for ambulation. If hemarthrosis is present, causing significant pain and tightness, aspiration under sterile conditions is indicated before the extremity is immobilized.

Quadriceps-setting exercises and three sets of 15 to 20 straight-leg raises are done four or five times a day during the acute period. Ice is applied for 20 minutes every 2 to 3 hours to reduce swelling. The knee immobilizer and compressive wrap are discontinued at 3 to 5 days, after the acute reaction has resolved. The crutches are discontinued when the patient is able to do straight-leg raises with a 5-lb ankle weight and is able to walk with a near-normal gait.

Rehabilitation should emphasize closed-chain exercises, including wall sets, in which the patient squats to approximately 40 degrees while keeping the back flat against the wall for 15 to 20 seconds, for a total of 10 to 15 repetitions. Side and forward step-up exercises using a 6- to 8-inch platform should be performed after the acute inflammatory reaction has resolved. These are followed by short-arc leg presses and endurance-type strengthening using a stationary bike and Stairmaster. Core, hip, knee, and ankle exercises all are important to success. The patient can return to sports activity when quadriceps and hamstring muscle strength is at least 85% normal and sport-specific agility has been regained. In general, a patellar stabilizing brace is prescribed for the first 6 to 8 weeks during rehabilitation and long-term for sports activity.

SURGICAL TREATMENT OF PATELLAR INSTABILITY

First-time dislocations generally are treated conservatively with good results, except for patients with open physes and trochlear dysplasia, two thirds of whom will have a recurrence. These patients and those who have recurrent instability of the contralateral patella may require more aggressive treatment (Table 3.2).

Choosing treatment for malalignment requires thorough evaluation, imaging, and planning. Many instabilities are multifactorial and must be treated as such. Containment issues are most commonly treated by reconstruction of the medial quadriceps tendon–femoral ligament (MQTFL) or the MPFL. Avulsion from the patella can be repaired with some success. Severe dysplasia can be directly treated with trochleoplasty, with good stability results, but often with persistent pain and swelling and the potential for chondral damage.

Malalignment measured by a tibial tubercle–to–trochlear groove (TT-TG) distance of 20 mm with a normal trochlea or a TT-TG of more than 15 mm with a dysplastic trochlea is treated with tibial tuberosity osteotomy.

When patellar chondral damage is distal and lateral, an anterior medialization of the tuberosity can stabilize and unload the cartilage defect. Medialization procedures are contraindicated for proximal and medial chondral defects. It has been noted that an oblique tuberosity osteotomy of 30 degrees produces 1 mm of anterior elevation for each 2 mm of medial displacement. A 45-degree oblique osteotomy produces 1 mm anterior to 1 mm medial displacement. Rarely, for severe angulation deformities, distal femoral rotational osteotomy is indicated.

Patellar instability in patients with open physes can be treated by MPFL reconstruction avoiding the physis or, occasionally, soft-tissue distal patellar tendon realignment. For angular deformities, epiphysiodesis can be used to aid realignment; soft-tissue repairs have a high failure rate.

A number of factors may contribute to patellar instability, and all must be corrected for optimal results (Table 3.3). For instability with normal alignment and Dejour type A or B dysplasia, MQTFL reconstruction is indicated. Distal realignment may be indicated for dysplasia for a TT-TG distance of 15 mm. Lateral release is not an operation for instability but is indicated as an additional procedure only if the tight tissues

TABLE 3.2

Treatment of Patellofemoral Instability

PATHOLOGY	DIAGNOSTIC FINDINGS	PROCEDURE
CONTAINMENT		
Patella alta	Insall index >1:3	Distalization*
Trochlear dysplasia	Crossing sign Trochlear bump Sulcus angle >145 degrees, depth ≥3 mm	MPFL reconstruction Trochleoplasty†
Patellar dysplasia	Wiberg type C	MPFL reconstruction
ALIGNMENT		
Tibial tubercle	Q angle >20 degrees, TT-TG >20 mm, >15 mm with trochlear dysplasia	Anteromedialization of tuberosity
Femoral anteversion Severe genu valgum	Thigh-foot angle >30 degrees	Rotational osteotomy‡/ epiphysiodesis
External tibial torsion, genu valgum, hyperpronation	Observation for malalignment	Orthotics and rehabilitation
SOFT-TISSUE IMBALANCE		
Dynamic (VMO dysfunction)	TT-TG <20 mm	Rehabilitation
Static		
Incompetent MPFL or generalized hyperlaxity	Lateral glide 3 quadrants	MPFL reconstruction‡
Overconstraint	Lateral tilt (excessive lateral pressure syndrome)	Lateral release

*Distalization can result in loss of motion or of fixation.
†Trochleoplasty: risk/benefit excessively high.
‡Rotational osteotomy: high risk/benefit.
MPFL, Medial patellofemoral ligament; *TG*, trochlear groove; *TT*, anterior tibial tuberosity; *VMO*, vastus medialis oblique.

TABLE 3.3	
Surgical Procedures for Treatment of Patellar Instability	
LOW RISK—LOW REWARD	
Medial repair/imbrication	30% failure rate, approximately the same as conservative treatment Indication: first dislocation + repairable chondral defect Instability in skeletally mature? In combination with distal realignment
Lateral release	Excessive lateral pressure syndrome In combination with realignment procedure when excessive tightness prevents patellar centering May increase risk for both medial and lateral patellar subluxation
LOW RISK—HIGH REWARD	
MPFL reconstruction	Indicated for recurrent MPFL deficiency ± trochlear dysplasia Proximal or anterior femoral placement or overtightening results in medial facet overload May combine with distal realignment
Elmslie-Trillat procedure	Indicated for instability, TT-TG >20 mm + strong repairable medial structures Healing time and risk for stress or contact fracture of proximal tibia much less than Fulkerson procedure
Fulkerson distal realignment	Indicated for symptomatic lateral facet or distal pole arthritis + TT-TG >20 mm, >15 mm with dysplasia Contraindicated with proximal/medial facet arthritis Long healing time, increased risk of proximal tibial fracture with sports
HIGH RISK—HIGH REWARD*	
Rotational high tibial osteotomy Distal femoral osteotomy	Indicated for instability + severe rotational deformity More normalized gait compared with distal realignment
Trochleoplasty	Indicated for dysplastic trochlea Low recurrence rate Increased risk for osteonecrosis, DJD, arthrofibrosis Lateral condyle: increased pressure; increased DJD of lateral facet
Grooveplasty	Increased DJD Good results with less risk reported with MPFL reconstruction
3-in-1 procedure—extensor mechanism realignment + VMO advancement + transfer of the medial third of the patellar tendon to the MCL	Recurrent instability, TT-TG >20 mm Open physes Not as effective as MQTFL reconstruction avoiding physis

*Indicated in special circumstances when risk/benefit ratio is acceptable.
DJD, Degenerative joint disease; *MCL,* medial collateral ligament; *MPFL,* medial patellofemoral ligament; *TT-TG,* tibial tubercle–trochlear groove; *VMO,* vastus medialis oblique.

prevent the patella from relocating. Routine lateral release should not be done because it may create more instability.

RECONSTRUCTION OF THE MEDIAL PATELLOFEMORAL LIGAMENT

The MPFL can be repaired by making a 3-cm incision over the site of injury as shown by MRI. An incompetent ligament with damage limited to the femoral attachment can be repaired and reinforced by use of the adductor magnus tendon (Fig. 3.7). Chronic instability with a Q angle of less than 20 degrees or an extensively damaged MPFL should be treated using a semitendinosus hamstring tendon graft technique. Nelitz et al. reported no growth abnormalities or recurrences in 21 skeletally immature patients treated

with MPFL reconstruction. Two patients with severe dysplasia had persistence of apprehension. In their systematic review, Vavken et al. also found no growth abnormalities or recurrences in the 425 patients (456 knees) reported. Hopper et al. found that severe dysplasia reduced satisfactory results from 83% to 57%.

Numerous techniques have been described for MPFL reconstruction, most using autogenous doubled semitendinosus-hamstring grafts placed in a physiometric position confirmed by palpation of landmarks and imaging, and tested for isometry. The technique we have been using for over a decade involves appropriate placement of a strong, physiologically tensioned graft through the quadriceps tendon, thus reproducing the MQTFL. This technique has resulted in low recurrence rates, no risk of patellar fracture, and minimal risk of loss of motion.

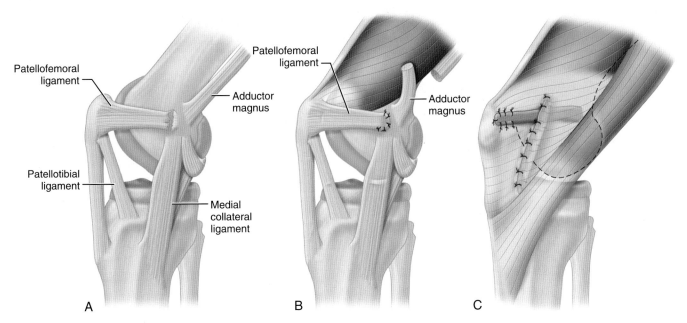

FIGURE 3.7   **A,** Medial patellofemoral ligament detached from medial femoral epicondyle after acute patellar dislocation. **B,** Medial patellofemoral ligament with firm edge of vastus medialis obliquus muscle reinserted to periosteum of medial femoral epicondyle, and adductor magnus tendon harvested. **C,** Adductor magnus tendon fixed near medial border of patella, and retinaculum duplicated.

MEDIAL QUADRICEPS TENDON-FEMORAL LIGAMENT RECONSTRUCTION

TECHNIQUE 3.1

(PHILLIPS)

- With the patient supine, place a tourniquet on the upper thigh. Use a lateral post on the operating table to assist with arthroscopic examination.
- After sterile preparation and draping, arthroscopically examine the knee through standard medial and lateral portals to evaluate patellar tracking and look for intraarticular damage. This evaluation is essential for determining appropriate treatment.
- Make a 3-cm incision 3 cm medial to the inferior portion of the patellar tuberosity and harvest the semitendinosus tendon in standard fashion. Size the folded graft so that the appropriately sized tunnel can be reamed later. Place a 0 Vicryl Krakow suture in each tail of the semitendinosus graft (Fig. 3.8A).
- Make two 2-cm incisions, the first just medial to the superior border of the patella and the second starting at the adductor tubercle and extending just distal to the medial epicondyle of the femur, to expose the patellofemoral ligament.
- Dissect subcutaneously to expose the proximal medial retinaculum at its insertion into the proximal portion of the patella. Make a 1.5-cm incision in the retinaculum adjacent to the quadriceps insertion.

- Make a second 1-cm vertical incision 1.5 cm lateral to the first incision through the quadriceps at its insertion into the patella. Use a Kelly clamp to spread the soft tissues and pass a looped no. 2 suture to use as a shuttle for the graft.
- Use blunt dissection to spread between layers 2 and 3 (between the MPFL and the capsular layer), staying extrasynovial and developing the plane with a curved Kelly clamp directed toward the medial epicondyle, spreading between the layers to create a soft-tissue tunnel. Use the Kelly clamp to pass a looped suture to use as a shuttle for the tunnel thus created (Fig. 3.8B).
- Shuttle one tail of the graft through the slit in the quadriceps, and then shuttle both tails through the MPFL tunnel to the femoral insertion site.
- Select the site for the femoral tunnel approximately 4 mm distal and 2 mm anterior to the adductor tubercle, in the "saddle" region between the tubercle and the medial epicondyle. Confirm correct position with imaging (Figs. 3.8C and 3.9).
- Place a Beath-tip guidewire at the chosen spot, and pass two suture tails from the graft around the wire. Mark the sutures so that pistoning of the graft can be identified with range of motion of the knee.
- Move the knee through a range of motion and observe the sutures, which should have minimal motion between 0 and 70 degrees of flexion and slight laxity above 70 degrees. If tension increases with flexion, the femoral tunnel site is too far proximal (most commonly) or possibly too far anterior. If the sutures tighten excessively in extension, the tunnel is too far distal or too far posterior. If necessary, correct the guidewire position and repeat the evaluation.

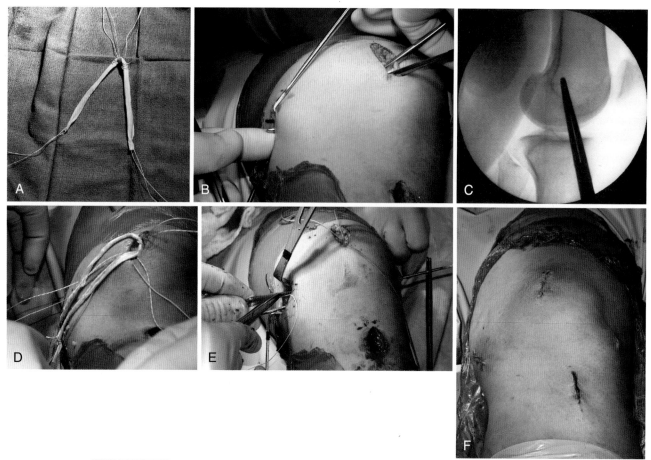

FIGURE 3.8   Phillips reconstruction of the medial patellofemoral ligament. **A,** Semitendinosus tendon graft. **B,** Creation of soft-tissue tunnel. **C,** Correct position confirmed radiographically. **D,** Whip stitch placed in each end of graft. **E,** Graft tails passed through soft-tissue tunnel. **F,** Closure. **SEE TECHNIQUE 3.1.**

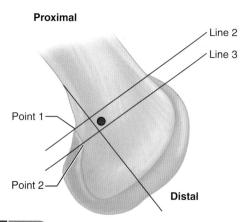

FIGURE 3.9   Schöttle and colleagues' radiographic landmark for femoral tunnel placement in medial patellofemoral ligament reconstruction. Two perpendicular lines to line 1 are drawn, intersecting the contact point of the medial condyle and posterior cortex (point 1, line 2) and intersecting the most posterior point of the Blumensaat line (point 2, line 3). For determination of vertical position, distance between line 2 and the lead ball center is measured as is the distance between line 2 and line 3. **SEE TECHNIQUE 3.1.**

- At the selected femoral tunnel site, ream a 30-mm tunnel the diameter of the doubled tendon.
- Pull the graft taut, and stress the patella so as to allow for one to two quadrants of lateral passive glide. When the physiologic amount of tension on the graft is determined, make a mark on the graft, which will correspond to the aperture of the femoral tunnel (Fig. 3.8D).
- Cut the graft 20 mm distal to this mark to allow 20 mm of graft to be placed into the tunnel.
- Place absorbable whip sutures into the tails of the graft (see Fig. 3.8D), place them into the tip of a Beath pin, and pull them out laterally (Fig. 3.8E).
- Before fixation with a biocomposite screw, move the knee through a range of motion, once again making sure that the tendons do not become taut in flexion and that the tendon length is appropriate to allow one to two quadrants of passive glide at 30 degrees of flexion so as not to overconstrain the patella.
- With the knee held in 60 degrees of flexion, maintain this graft length while it is secured with a biocomposite screw equal to the tunnel size chosen. Again, move the knee through a range of motion to make sure motion is not inhibited.

- Repair the retinaculum and place a stay suture in the quadriceps tendon just proximal to the split. Close the subcutaneous tissues with 2-0 Vicryl and the skin with absorbable monofilament suture (Fig. 3.8F). Apply a postoperative dressing and a knee brace.

POSTOPERATIVE CARE The knee joint is immobilized in extension with a simple knee brace for 3 days after surgery. Range-of-motion exercises and gait with weight bearing on two crutches are started and gradually progressed. Weight bearing is allowed as tolerated immediately after surgery. Walking with full weight bearing is usually possible 2 or 3 weeks after surgery. Achieving at least 90 degrees knee flexion by the end of postoperative week 3 is encouraged. Jogging is allowed after 3 months, and participation in the original sporting activity is allowed 4 to 6 months after surgery, depending on the patient's rehabilitation progress.

- If tracking is acceptable and the transferred tubercle fits flush with the underlying tibia, fix it with one or two AO 4-mm cancellous lag screws. Use a 2.7-mm bit to drill through the tubercle and tibia. Angle the drill toward the joint and advance it until the posterior cortex is felt. Angling the drill proximally allows fixation to be placed in cancellous bone near the proximal tibia. Bicortical fixation is not used, and the screw should be long enough (usually 40-50 mm) to come near, but not penetrate, the posterior cortex.

POSTOPERATIVE CARE Weight bearing is allowed to tolerance using a straight-leg splint for ambulation for the first 6 weeks after surgery. At 1 week after surgery, closed chain kinetic strengthening is begun, with a goal of achieving 70% strength by 6 weeks. A functional progression program that allows the patient to return to unrestricted sports is begun 12 weeks after surgery. Most athletes can return to sport at 6 to 9 months.

DISTAL REALIGNMENT

Indications for distal realignment include patellar instability secondary to malalignment indicated by a Q angle of more than 20 degrees and anterior TT-TG distance of more than 20 mm. When trochlear dysplasia is present, less malalignment is tolerated, and a TT-TG distance of as little as 15 mm may require realignment procedures. If chondral damage is present distal and lateral on the patella, an oblique osteotomy helps unload these areas and transfer weight bearing proximal and medial. Bony distal realignment procedures are contraindicated in skeletally immature patients.

We recommend the Trillat procedure for dislocations due to malalignment with an Insall index of less than 1:3 and grade 2 or less chondromalacia noted at arthroscopy. We have found the modification described by Shelbourne, Porter, and Rozzi to be an effective technique.

TECHNIQUE 3.2

(MODIFIED BY SHELBOURNE, PORTER, AND ROZZI)
- Make a 6-cm lateral parapatellar incision approximately 1 cm lateral to the patellar tendon.
- Perform a lateral release from the tibial tubercle to the level of the insertion of the vastus lateralis tendon on the proximal patella. The release is considered adequate when the patellar articular surface can be everted 90 degrees laterally.
- Approach the tibial tubercle through the same parapatellar incision, and identify the patellar tendon insertion. Using a 2.5-cm flat osteotome, raise a flat, 6-cm long, 7-mm thick osteoperiosteal flap, tapering anteriorly and hinged distally with periosteum. Do not violate the soft tissues.
- Rotate the bone flap medially, cracking the cortex distally, and hold it in place with a Kirschner wire while the knee is moved through a full passive range of motion to evaluate patellar tracking.

OBLIQUE OSTEOTOMY OF THE TUBEROSITY

We generally prefer a slightly oblique osteotomy of the tuberosity, such as that described by Fulkerson and by Brown et al. that transfers the tuberosity anteriorly and medially. This procedure is indicated when grade 3 or 4 chondromalacia is associated with recurrent dislocations. A guide can be used to cut a flat osteotomy surface that angled from anteromedial just deep to the anterior crest of the tibia in a posterolateral direction. Increased obliquity of the cut increases anterior translation; however, the more superficial cut avoids a stress riser effect and reduces the risk of later fracture through the osteotomy. It is important to taper the osteotomy distally to prevent a stress riser.

Although this technique has been reported to produce 86% good to excellent results, complications have included stress risers and stress fractures through the area months after clinical and radiographic healing are present. Mechanical testing showed that a flat (Elmslie-Trillat) osteotomy had significantly higher mean load-to-failure and total energy-to-failure rates than the oblique osteotomy technique. In general, this procedure is not indicated for athletes and should be reserved for patients with patellofemoral degenerative changes.

For recurrent patellar dislocation and significant patella alta with an Insall index of more than 1.3, medial and distal transfer of the tuberosity occasionally is indicated. Preoperative radiographs are used to determine the amount of distal transfer necessary and to ensure the inferior pole of the patella is not placed distal to the Blumensaat line, creating patella baja. The tuberosity is detached distally, and 5 to 10 mm of bone is resected from the distal tip of the tuberosity to allow distal transfer before secure fixation. Because loss of flexion or loss of fixation may occur, distalization is not routinely done.

FULKERSON OSTEOTOMY

TECHNIQUE 3.3

- Make a 9-cm lateral parapatellar incision extending from the inferior pole of the patella distally. Exposure is similar to the Elmslie-Trillat procedure, with the difference being in the oblique osteotomy of the tuberosity.
- Extend the cut distally about 6 cm with the medial tip of the cut being more superficial.
- Drill holes to perforate the cortex distally so that the fragment can be hinged.
- Using an osteotome, complete the osteotomy deep and just proximal to the insertion of the patellar tendon and pry the tuberosity medially so that the Q angle is corrected to between 10 and 15 degrees. This usually requires moving the tuberosity anteriorly 8 to 10 mm. Obliquity of the osteotomy determines the amount of anterior displacement. A 30-degree osteotomy produces 1 mm of anteriorization for each 2 mm of medialization, whereas a 45-degree cut produces a 1 mm to 1 mm translation.
- Secure the transferred tuberosity by placing a drill bit proximally through the tuberosity and tibia with the knee in 90 degrees of flexion to decrease risk to neurovascular structures.
- Move the knee through a range of motion, and evaluate patellar tracking.
- If tracking is satisfactory, secure the tuberosity with two countersunk, low-profile, cancellous screws (Fig. 3.10) or bicortical screws.
- Close the medial retinaculum in a pants-over-vest fashion, plicating the medial side. Do not close the lateral retinaculum.

POSTOPERATIVE CARE Weight bearing is allowed as tolerated after surgery. Immobilization is continued 4 to 6 weeks, at which time range-of-motion and strengthening exercises are instituted. Return to sports usually is allowed at 6 to 9 months after surgery. In our opinion, there is some long-term risk for fracture after this procedure if an osteotomy of more than 30 degrees is done.

For severe rotational deformities, a distal femoral rotational osteotomy or proximal tibial osteotomy rarely may be indicated. Epiphysiodesis can be done for severe coronal malalignment deformities in immature patients. Most recurrent instability problems in skeletally immature patients are treated with MQTFL procedures, with the femoral fixation looped around the adductor tendon insertion or in a carefully placed tunnel distal to the physis.

TROCHLEOPLASTY

Sulcus-deepening trochleoplasty is a technically demanding procedure with precise indications: high-grade trochlear dysplasia with patellar instability and/or abnormal tracking. The primary goal is to improve patellar tracking by decreasing the prominence of the trochlea and creating a new groove with normal depth. Associated abnormalities should be evaluated and corrected (Box 3.1).

TECHNIQUE 3.4

- After administration of regional anesthesia, supplemented with patient sedation, position the patient supine and prepare and drape the extremity.

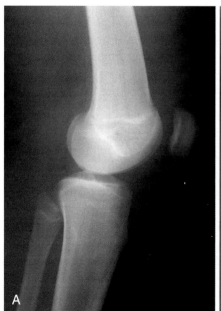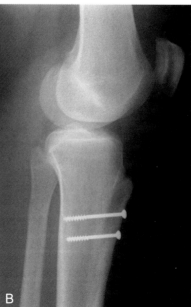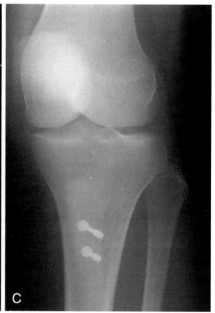

FIGURE 3.10 Fulkerson procedure. **A,** Preoperative lateral radiograph. **B,** Postoperative lateral radiograph. **C,** Anteroposterior radiograph. **SEE TECHNIQUE 3.3.**

- With the knee flexed to 90 degrees, make a straight midline skin incision from the superior patellar margin to the tibiofemoral articulation.
- Move the knee into extension and develop a medial full-thickness skin flap.
- Make a modified midvastus approach with sharp dissection of the medial retinaculum starting over the 1 to 2

cm medial border of the patella and blunt dissection of the vastus medialis oblique (VMO) fibers starting distally at the patellar superomedial pole and extending approximately 4 cm into the muscle belly.
- Evert the patella for inspection and treatment of chondral injuries if needed, and then retract it laterally.
- Expose the trochlea by incising the peritrochlear synovium and periosteum along their osteochondral junction and reflecting them from the field with a periosteal elevator. The anterior femoral cortex should be visible to orientate the amount of deepening. Changing the degree of flexion/extension allows a better view of the complete operative field and avoids extending the incision.
- Once the trochlea is fully exposed, draw the new trochlear limits with a sterile pen. Use the intercondylar notch as a starting point to draw the new trochlear groove. From there, draw a straight line directed proximally and 3 to 6 degrees laterally; the superior limit is the osteochondral edge. Draw two divergent lines, starting at the notch and passing proximally through the condyle-trochlear grooves, representing lateral and medial facet limits; these lines should not enter the tibiofemoral joint (Fig. 3.11A).
- To access the undersurface of the femoral trochlea, remove a thin strip of cortical bone from the osteochondral

---

BOX 3.1

Associated Abnormalities That May Require Correction in Addition to Trochleoplasty

- Tibial tubercle-trochlear groove (TT-TG) >20 mm: tibial tuberosity medializing osteotomy to obtain TT-TG distance between 10 and 15 mm.
- Patella alta (Canton-Deschamps index >1.2): distalization osteotomy to obtain normal patellar index of 1.0.
- Lateral patellar tilt >20 degrees: VMO plasty or reconstruction of the MPFL with a double-looped gracilis tendon graft.

MPFL, Medial patellofemoral ligament; *VMO,* vastus medialis obliquus.

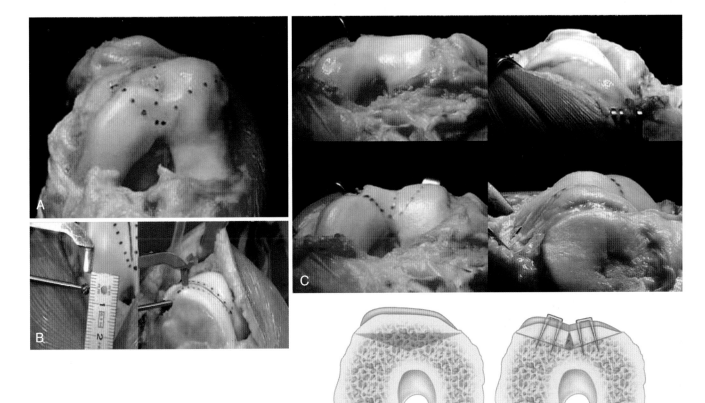

FIGURE 3.11 DeJour sulcus-deepening trochleoplasty. **A,** Drawing of the new trochlear limits. **B,** Removal of subchondral bone under the trochlea to correct the prominence and reshape the groove. **C,** Shape of the trochlea before (above) and after (below) sulcus-deepening trochleoplasty. **D,** Fixation of new trochlea with two staples after restoration of trochlear sulcus and more "anatomic" shape. (From DeJour D, Saggin P: The sulcus deepening trochleoplasty—the Lyon's procedure, *Int Orthop* 34:311–316, 2010.) **SEE TECHNIQUE 3.4.**

edge. The width of the strip is similar to the prominence of the trochlea from the anterior femoral cortex (the bump). Gently tap with a sharp osteotome and then use a rongeur to remove the bone.

- To remove cancellous bone from the undersurface of the trochlea, use a drill with a depth guide set at 5 mm to ensure uniform thickness of the osteochondral flap and maintain an adequate amount of bone attached to the cartilage (Fig. 3.11B). The guide also avoids injuring the cartilage or getting too close to it and causing thermal injury. The shell produced must be sufficiently compliant to allow modeling without being fractured.
- Extend cancellous bone removal up to the notch; remove more bone from the central portion where the new trochlear groove will lie (Fig. 3.11C).
- Use light pressure to mold the flap to the underlying cancellous bone bed in the distal femur. If needed, cut the bottom of the groove and the external margin of the lateral facet to allow further modeling by gently tapping over a scalpel.
- If the correction obtained is satisfactory, fix the new trochlea with two staples, one in each side of the groove, with one arm in the cartilaginous upper part of each facet and the other arm in the anterior femoral cortex (Fig. 3.11D).
- Test patellar tracking. Suture the periosteum and synovial tissue to the osteochondral edge and anchor them in the staples.

POSTOPERATIVE CARE Immediate weight bearing is permitted, and no limitation is placed on range of motion. Continuous passive motion is indicated to model the trochlea and patella, and frequent knee movement is encouraged to help ensure cartilage nutrition and further molding of the trochlea by the tracking patella. Because trochleoplasty is rarely done as an isolated procedure, postoperative care must consider associated procedures. Radiographs, including anteroposterior and lateral views and an axial view in 30 degrees of flexion, are reviewed at 6 weeks. At 6 months, a CT scan is obtained to document correction.

IATROGENIC MEDIAL PATELLAR INSTABILITY

Iatrogenic medial patellar instability is diagnosed when manual medial subluxation re-creates a patient's symptoms. Treatment consists of repairing the vastus lateralis if previously released and revising a distal realignment to a more lateral position. If the initial procedure was proximal and inadequate tissues remain, repair or reconstruction using the lateral portion of the patellar tendon is done (Fig. 3.12).

HIP

With the evolution of hip arthroscopy and MR arthrography of the hip, the diagnosis and treatment of hip instability have greatly improved. The diagnosis is indicated by recurrent "giving way," pain, or popping with hip extension and external rotation during activities, such as getting out of a car or kicking or pivoting maneuvers during sports. The physical examination should include evaluation for generalized ligamentous

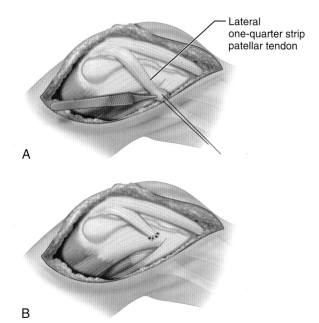

FIGURE 3.12 Reconstruction using patellar tendon. **A,** Lateral one-quarter strip of patellar tendon is developed. **B,** Strip is attached at lateral tibial tubercle by suture to periosteum or through bony tunnel.

laxity, as well as examination of the uninvolved hip for comparison. Tests that may indicate pathologic laxity include the dial test, passive external rotation of the more than 45 degrees, particularly if symptoms are reproduced. Other tests to reproduce symptoms of instability are the Ganz test, in which hip extension and external rotation produce anterior capsular pain. Finally, direct axial traction may produce apprehension. Moving the hip from flexion, abduction, and external rotation into extension, adduction, and internal rotation may re-create catching or popping associated with labral pathology.

Plain anteroposterior and lateral radiographs are helpful in evaluating acetabular dysplasia and impingement. A center-edge (CE) angle of less than 20 degrees, a crossover sign, and a Sharp angle of more than 42 degrees also are indicative of dysplasia. MR arthrography is used to evaluate for labral tears or capsular redundancy that may be related to recurrent instability.

Hip instability may be categorized as loss of bony acetabular containment, disruption of the capsulolabral complex, or a combination of the two. Recurrent trauma from stress at extremes of motion may result in capsulolabral deficiency and instability. Bony development problems can cause containment issues resulting in impingement or straight-forward instability. Finally, hyperlax joints from collagen deficiencies, Ehlers-Danlos and Marfan syndromes, and generalized joint laxity can result in symptomatic hip instability.

Treatment of these conditions must be tailored to the pathology, as in any other joint. Many of these procedures are now done arthroscopically and are described in other chapter.

STERNOCLAVICULAR JOINT

Most recurrent dislocations of the sternoclavicular joint are anterior and require only conservative treatment; posterior dislocations, although uncommon, require reduction because of the proximity and potential compromise of the subclavian vessels, esophagus, and trachea. A complete discussion of acute dislocations and their treatment is presented in other chapter.

Recurrent atraumatic anterior subluxation of the sternoclavicular joint with shoulder abduction and extension usually occurs in young girls. Often it is associated with laxity of other joints and generally is a self-limiting condition. Most patients with recurrent anterior sternoclavicular joint dislocation should be treated with a generalized upper extremity strengthening program and avoidance of activities that produce stress on the sternoclavicular joint. Surgery is recommended only if severe symptoms limit activities of daily living. The surgical procedures, which include open repair of the sternoclavicular capsule, reconstruction of the sternoclavicular joint, and resection of the medial end of the clavicle and securing of the clavicle to the first rib, all are fraught with potentially severe complications, including injury to major vessels, persistent pain, unsightly scar formation, and recurrence of dislocation.

A strong semitendinosus graft is recommended for reconstruction of the joint. A figure-of-eight configuration through drill holes in the manubrium and midclavicle produces a strong, stable configuration that was shown in mechanical testing to restore native joint stiffness better than resection arthroplasty (Fig. 3.13). The reconstruction should be reinforced with local tissue repair, in particular the important posterior capsular tissue. It is wise to have a thoracic surgeon available for the procedure because of the potential complications associated with the procedure. Because of the possibility of pin migration and potentially severe complications, pins or wires should not be placed across the joint.

After reconstruction, the shoulder is immobilized in a sling for 6 weeks. On the second day, the patient is allowed to perform gentle pendulum exercises but is cautioned against active flexion or abduction of the shoulder above 90 degrees. Pushing, pulling, and lifting are avoided for 3 months. Strengthening exercises are started at 8 to 12 weeks. The patient is restricted from returning to strenuous manual labor for a minimum of 3 months.

SHOULDER

The shoulder, by virtue of its anatomy and biomechanics, is one of the most unstable and frequently dislocated joints in the body, accounting for nearly 50% of all dislocations, with a 2% incidence in the general population. Factors that influence the probability of recurrent dislocations are age, return to contact or collision sports, hyperlaxity, and the presence of a significant bony defect in the glenoid or humeral head. In a study of 101 acute dislocations, recurrence developed in 90% of the patients younger than 20 years old, in 60% of patients 20 to 40 years old, and in only 10% of patients older than 40 years old. Contact and collision sports increase the recurrence rate to near 100% in skeletally immature athletes. The duration of immobilization also does not seem to affect stability; a recent meta-analysis determined that there is no benefit for conventional sling immobilization longer than 1 week for primary anterior dislocation. Immobilization in external rotation is thought to decrease recurrence rates, but this has not been proven; meta-analyses found a recurrence risk of 36% with immobilization in internal rotation compared with 25% with external rotation bracing, but the numbers were small and the difference was not significant. Burkhart and DeBeer, Sugaya

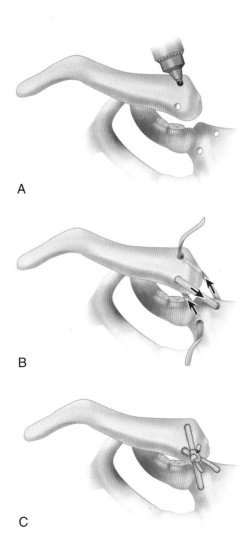

A

B

C

FIGURE 3.13 Semitendinosus figure-of-eight reconstruction. **A,** Drill holes passed anterior to posterior through medial part of clavicle and manubrium. **B,** Free semitendinosus tendon graft woven through drill holes so tendon strands are parallel to each other posterior to the joint and cross each other anterior to the joint. **C,** Tendon tied in square knot and secured with suture.

et al., and Itoi et al. have shown that glenoid bone loss of more than 20% results in bony instability and increased recurrence rates. This is because the "safe arc" that the glenoid provides for humeral rotation is diminished, resulting in instability when the deficient edge is loaded at extremes of motion (Fig. 3.14).

NORMAL FUNCTIONAL ANATOMY

An understanding of the normal functional anatomy of the shoulder is necessary to understand the factors influencing the stability of the joint. The bony anatomy of the shoulder joint does not provide inherent stability. The glenoid fossa is a flattened, dish-like structure. Only one fourth of the large humeral head articulates with the glenoid at any given time. This small, flat glenoid does not provide the inherent stability for the humeral head that the acetabulum does for the hip. The glenoid is deepened by 50% by the presence of the glenoid labrum. The labrum increases the humeral contact to 75%. Integral to the glenoid labrum is the insertion of the tendon of the long head of the biceps, which inserts on the superior aspect of the joint and blends to become indistinguishable from the posterior glenoid labrum. Matsen et al. suggested that the labrum may serve as a "chock block" to

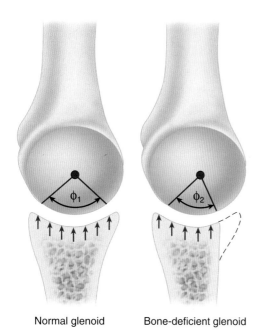

Normal glenoid   Bone-deficient glenoid

FIGURE 3.14 Glenoid bone loss shortens "safe arc" through which glenoid can resist axial forces. Φ_2 (bone-deficient condition) is less than Φ_1.

prevent excessive humeral head rollback. The shoulder joint capsule is lax and thin and, by itself, offers little resistance or stability. Anteriorly, the capsule is reinforced by three capsular thickenings or ligaments that are intimately fused with the labral attachment to the glenoid rim.

The superior glenohumeral ligament attaches to the glenoid rim near the apex of the labrum conjoined with the long head of the biceps (Fig. 3.15). On the humerus, it is attached to the anterior aspect of the anatomic neck of the humerus (Fig. 3.16). The superior glenohumeral ligament is the primary restraint to inferior humeral subluxation in 0 degrees of abduction and is the primary stabilizer to anterior and posterior stress at 0 degrees of abduction. Tightening of the rotator interval (which includes the superior glenohumeral ligament) decreases posterior and inferior translation; external rotation also may be decreased. The middle glenohumeral ligament has a wide attachment extending from the superior glenohumeral ligament along the anterior margin of the glenoid down as far as the junction of the middle and inferior thirds of the glenoid rim. On the humerus, it also is attached to the anterior aspect of the anatomic neck. The middle glenohumeral ligament limits external rotation when the arm is in the lower and middle ranges of abduction but has little effect when the arm is in 90 degrees of abduction. The inferior glenohumeral ligament attaches to the glenoid margin from the 2- to 3-o'clock positions anteriorly to the 8- to 9-o'clock positions posteriorly. The humeral attachment is below the level of the horizontally oriented physis into the inferior aspect of the anatomic and surgical neck of the humerus. The anterosuperior edge of this ligament usually is quite thickened. There is a less distinct posterior thickening, a hammock-type model consisting of thickened anterior and posterior bands and a thinner axillary pouch. With external rotation, the hammock

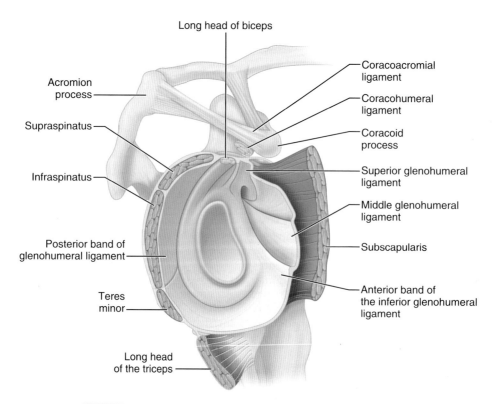

Long head of biceps

Acromion process

Supraspinatus

Infraspinatus

Posterior band of glenohumeral ligament

Teres minor

Long head of the triceps

Coracoacromial ligament

Coracohumeral ligament

Coracoid process

Superior glenohumeral ligament

Middle glenohumeral ligament

Subscapularis

Anterior band of the inferior glenohumeral ligament

FIGURE 3.15 Glenoid and surrounding capsule, ligaments, and tendons.

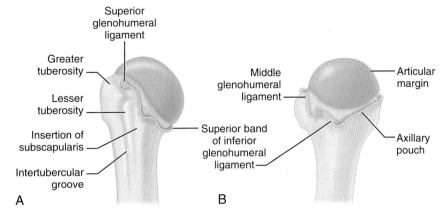

FIGURE 3.16 Upper part of left humerus showing attachments of glenohumeral ligaments on anterior **(A)** and medial **(B)** aspects of surgical and anatomic neck.

slides anteriorly and superiorly. The anterior band tightens, and the posterior band fans out. With internal rotation, the opposite occurs. The anteroinferior glenohumeral ligament complex is the main stabilizer to anterior and posterior stresses when the shoulder is abducted 45 degrees or more. The ligament provides a restraint at the extremes of motion and assists in the rollback of the humeral head in the glenoid.

The muscles around the shoulder also contribute significantly to its stability. The action of the deltoid (the principal extrinsic muscle) produces primarily vertical shear forces, tending to displace the humeral head superiorly. The intrinsic muscle forces from the rotator cuff provide compressive or stabilizing forces. Concavity compression is produced by dynamic rotator cuff muscular stabilization of the humeral head when the concavity of the glenoid and labral complex is intact. Loss of the labrum can reduce this stabilizing effect by 20%. In the concavity of the glenoid-labral complex, synchronous eccentric deceleration, and concentric contraction of the rotator cuff and biceps tendon are necessary for humeral stability during mid-ranges of humeral motion. Asynchronous fatigue of the rotator cuff from overuse or incompetent ligamentous support can result in further damage to the static and dynamic supports. MRI studies have shown fatty infiltration and thinning of the subscapularis tendon in recurrent anterior instability.

Several authors have noted the importance of synchronous mobility of the scapula and glenoid to shoulder stability and emphasized the importance of this dynamic balance to appropriate positioning of the glenoid articular surface so that the joint reaction force produced is a compressive rather than a shear force. With normal synchronous function of the scapular stabilizers, the scapula and the glenoid articular structures are maintained in the most stable functional position. Strengthening rehabilitation of the scapular stabilizers (serratus anterior, trapezius, latissimus dorsi, rhomboids, and levator scapulae) is especially important in patients who participate in upper extremity-dominant sports. Although the glenoid is small, it has the mobility to remain in the most stable position in relation to the humeral head with movement. Rowe compared this with a seal balancing a ball on its nose. The glenoid also has the ability to "recoil" when a sudden force is applied to the shoulder joint, such as in a fall on the outstretched hand. This ability to "recoil" lessens the impact on the shoulder as the scapula slides along the chest wall.

Scapular dyskinesis is an alteration of the normal position or motion of the scapula during coupled scapulohumeral movements and can occur after overuse of and repeated injuries to the shoulder joint. A particular overuse muscle fatigue syndrome has been designated the SICK scapula: scapular malposition, inferior medial border prominence, coracoid pain and malposition, and dyskinesis of scapular movement.

The demonstration of Ruffini end organs and Pacinian corpuscles in the shoulder capsule helps solidify the concept of proprioceptive neuromuscular training as an important part of shoulder stabilization. Another force that has a lesser effect on glenohumeral stability is glenoid version. Glenoid version probably is not a significant contributor to instability except in a severely deformed shoulder. Cohesion produced by joint fluid and the vacuum effect produced by negative intraarticular pressure in normal shoulders play lesser roles in joint stability.

PATHOLOGIC ANATOMY

No essential pathologic lesion is responsible for every recurrent subluxation or dislocation of the shoulder. In 1906, Perthes considered detachment of the labrum from the anterior rim of the glenoid cavity to be the "essential" lesion in recurrent dislocations and described an operation to correct it. In 1938, Bankart published his classic paper in which he recognized two types of acute dislocations. In the first type, the humeral head is forced through the capsule where it is the weakest, generally anteriorly and inferiorly in the interval between the lower border of the subscapularis and the long head of the triceps muscle. In the second type, the humeral head is forced anteriorly out of the glenoid cavity and tears not only the fibrocartilaginous labrum from almost the entire anterior half of the rim of the glenoid cavity but also the capsule and periosteum from the anterior surface of the neck of the scapula. This traumatic detachment of the glenoid labrum has been called the *Bankart lesion.* Most authors agree that the Bankart lesion is the most commonly observed pathologic lesion in recurrent subluxation or dislocation of the shoulder, but it is not the "essential" lesion.

Excessive laxity of the shoulder capsule also causes instability of the shoulder joint. Excessive laxity can be caused by a congenital collagen deficiency, shown by hyperlaxity of other joints, or by plastic deformation of the capsuloligamentous complex from a single macrotraumatic event or repetitive microtraumatic events. Hyperlaxity has been implicated as a cause of failure in surgical correction of chronic shoulder instability. An arthroscopic study of anterior shoulder dislocations found that 38% of the acute injuries were intrasubstance ligamentous failures, and 62% were disruptions of the capsuloligamentous insertion into the glenoid neck. The "circle concept" of structural damage to the capsular structures was suggested by cadaver studies that showed that humeral dislocation does not occur unless the posterior capsular structures are disrupted, in addition to the anterior capsular structures. Posterior capsulolabral changes associated with recurrent anterior instability often are identified by arthroscopy.

A humeral head impaction fracture can be produced as the shoulder is dislocated, and the humeral head is impacted against the rim of the glenoid at the time of dislocation. This Hill-Sachs lesion is a defect in the posterolateral aspect of the humeral head. Instability results when the defect engages the glenoid rim in the functional arc of motion at 90 degrees abduction and external rotation. In a cadaver model, humeral head defects of 35% to 40% were shown to decrease stability, whereas glenoid defects of as little as 13% were found to decrease stability. Glenoid rim fractures or attrition also can occur with an anterior or posterior dislocation. If these lesions involve more than 20% to 25% of the glenoid, they can result in recurrent instability despite having an excellent soft-tissue repair. These lesions are difficult to see on plain radiographs; if a defect is visible in an acute dislocation or one is evaluating recurrent instability, (3D) CT is the best method for evaluating the extent of the defect (Fig. 3.17).

It seems that no single "essential" lesion is responsible for all recurrent dislocations of the shoulder. Stability of this inherently unstable joint depends on a continuing balance between the static and dynamic mechanisms influencing motion and stability. In addition to the various possible primary deficiencies influencing instability, secondary deficiencies can be caused by repeated dislocations. Erosion of the anterior glenoid rim, stretching of the anterior capsule and subscapularis tendon, and fraying and degeneration of the glenoid labrum all can occur with repeated dislocation. The primary deficiency and the secondary deficiencies need to be considered at the time of surgery and in postoperative rehabilitation to correct the instability. Because no single deficiency is responsible for all recurrent dislocations of the shoulder, no single operative procedure can be applied to every patient. The surgeon must search carefully for and identify the deficiencies present to choose the proper procedure.

CLASSIFICATION

Successful treatment of shoulder instability is based on a thorough understanding of the various posttraumatic lesions that can be associated with a deficient capsulolabral complex and on correct classification of the patient's primary and secondary lesions. Classification and treatment of shoulder instability are based on the direction, degree, and duration of symptoms; the trauma that resulted in instability; and the patient's age, mental set, and associated conditions, such as seizures, neuromuscular disorders, collagen deficiencies, and congenital disorders.

The direction of instability should be categorized as unidirectional, bidirectional, or multidirectional. Anterior dislocations account for 90% to 95% of recurrent dislocations, and posterior dislocations account for approximately 5% to 10%.

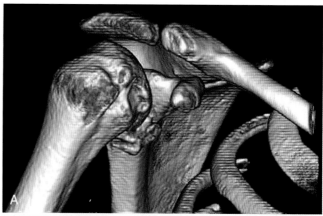

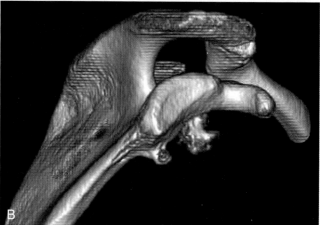

FIGURE 3.17   **A,** Three-dimensional CT showing large Hill-Sachs lesion and deficient glenoid. **B,** Three-dimensional CT with humeral head subtracted showing loss of anterior glenoid surface.

Despite increased understanding of shoulder instability, 50% of posterior shoulder dislocations can be missed unless an adequate examination and appropriate radiographs are done. Inferior and superior dislocations are rare. Superior instability generally arises secondary to severe rotator cuff insufficiency.

Instability is categorized as subluxation with partial separation of the humeral head from the glenoid or dislocation with complete separation of the humeral head from the glenoid concavity. The duration of the symptoms should be recorded as acute, subacute, chronic, or recurrent. The dislocation is classified as chronic if the humeral head has remained dislocated longer than 6 weeks.

The type of trauma associated with the dislocation is important in determining whether conservative or operative treatment is appropriate. Instability should be categorized as *macrotraumatic*, in which a single traumatic event results in dislocation, or *microtraumatic* (acquired), in which repetitive trauma at the extremes of motion results in plastic deformation of the capsulolabral complex. Secondary trauma to the rotator cuff and biceps tendon may cause asynchronous rotator cuff function. These injuries most commonly occur in pitchers, batters, gymnasts, weightlifters, tennis players and others who play racquet sports, and swimmers, especially with the backstroke or butterfly stroke. The flexibility that allows an athlete to compete at a high level may be attributed to a generalized ligamentous laxity, which also predisposes the athlete to injury. Trauma may cause decompensation of a previously stable capsuloligamentous complex. A thorough history of the initial traumatic event, symptoms, and family history and a thorough examination of the injured shoulder, contralateral shoulder, and other joints are necessary.

Age also is important in predicting pathologic lesions and outcomes, with recurrence rates of more than 90% reported in patients younger than 20 years old compared with a recurrence rate of about 10% to 20% in patients older than 40 years old.

In most studies, the recurrence rate for adolescents treated with surgical stabilization was higher than that for patients in other age groups. These differences can be explained by the greater elasticity in adolescent ligaments that results in greater plastic deformation before failure of the system. This deformation must be considered in surgical treatment approaches.

Although recurrence of the dislocation is uncommon in patients 40 years old or older, associated rotator cuff tears are present in 30%, and such tears are present in more than 80% of patients older than 60 years. Fractures of the greater tuberosity also are more prevalent in patients older than 40 years old; some series report an incidence of 42%. In this age group, surgical treatment of rotator cuff tears or fractures of the greater tuberosity generally takes precedence over treatment of the capsular injury.

The mental set of the patient must be evaluated before treatment is started. Some patients with posterior instability learn to dislocate their shoulder through selective muscular contractions. Although voluntary dislocation does not indicate pathologic overlay, some of these patients have learned to use voluntary dislocation for secondary gain, and in these patients surgical treatment is doomed to failure.

In patients with primary neuromuscular disorders or syndromes and recurrent dislocation, conservative, nonoperative treatment should be the initial approach. If instability remains after appropriate medical treatment, surgery may be necessary in conjunction with continued nonoperative treatment. Patients with primary collagen disorders, Ehlers-Danlos syndrome, or Marfan syndrome should be treated with extensive supervised conservative treatment. If surgical intervention becomes necessary, the possibility of the abnormal tissue stretching out and allowing dislocation to recur should be stressed to the patient and family. When severe dysplastic or traumatic glenohumeral deformity is present, capsular and bony procedures may be necessary. Reformatted 3D CT images are beneficial in determining the need for osteotomy or bone grafting procedures in these patients.

Matsen's simplified classification system is useful for categorizing instability patterns: TUBS (traumatic, unidirectional Bankart surgery) and AMBRII (atraumatic, multidirectional, bilateral, rehabilitation, inferior capsular shift, and internal closure). Microtraumatic or developmental lesions fall between the extremes of macrotraumatic and atraumatic lesions and can overlap these extreme lesions (Fig. 3.18). Classification of 168 shoulders according to four systems used for describing shoulder instability revealed variations in the criteria that resulted in marked variations in the number of patients diagnosed with multidirectional instability.

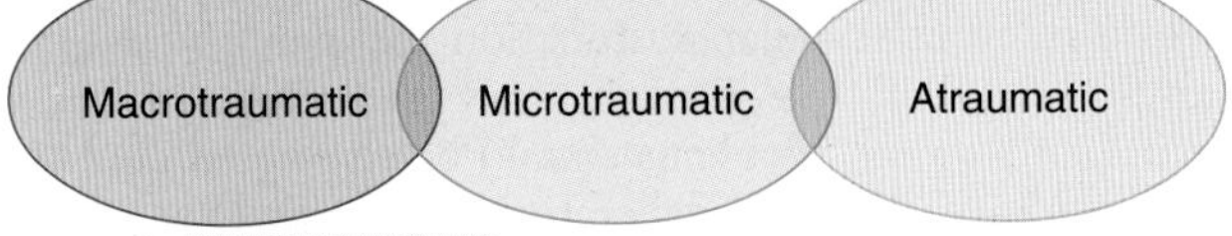

HISTORY

The history is important in recurrent instability of the shoulder joint. The amount of initial trauma, if any, should be determined. High-energy traumatic collision sports and motor vehicle accidents are associated with an increased risk of glenoid or humeral bone defects. Recurrence with minimal trauma in the midrange of motion often is associated with bony lesions, which must be treated. The position in which the dislocation or subluxation occurs should be elicited. In complete dislocations, the ease with which the shoulder is relocated is determined. Dislocations that occur during sleep or with the arm in an overhead position often are associated with a significant glenoid defect that requires surgical treatment.

Dislocations that are reduced by the patient often are subluxations or dislocations associated with generalized ligamentous laxity. The signs and symptoms of any nerve injury should be elicited. Most important, the physical limitations caused by this instability should be documented.

Recurrent subluxation of the shoulder is commonly overlooked by physicians because the symptoms are vague and there is no history of actual dislocation. The patient may complain of a sensation of the shoulder sliding in and out of place, or he or she may not be aware of any shoulder instability. The patient may complain of having a "dead arm" as a result of stretching of the axillary nerve or of secondary rotator cuff symptoms. It is important to differentiate primary from secondary rotator cuff impingement. Rotator cuff symptoms develop secondary to ligamentous dysfunction. Internal impingement of the undersurface of the posterior rotator cuff against the posterior glenoid and labrum is caused by anterior humeral subluxation with the shoulder externally rotated. This secondary impingement is more common than primary impingement in patients younger than 35 years old who are involved in upper extremity–dominant sports. Posterior shoulder instability may present as posterior pain or fatigue with repeated activity (e.g., blocking in football, swimming, bench press, rowing, and sports requiring overhead arm movement).

PHYSICAL EXAMINATION

The physical examination of a patient with instability begins by asking the patient which arm position creates the instability, what direction the shoulder subluxes, and if he or she can safely demonstrate the subluxation. Both shoulders should be thoroughly examined, with the normal shoulder used as a reference. The examination includes evaluation of the shoulders for atrophy or asymmetry, followed by palpation to determine the amount of tenderness present in the anterior or posterior capsule, the rotator cuff, and the acromioclavicular joint. Active and passive ranges of motion are evaluated with the patient upright and supine to record accurately the motion in all planes. The strengths of the deltoid, rotator cuff, and scapular stabilizers are evaluated, recorded, and graded from 0 to 5, with 5 being normal. Scapular winging or dysfunction should be noted during active range of motion and during strength examination. Winging may indicate scapular weakness and can be evaluated by having the patient do a press-up from the examination table or an incline type of push-up off the wall.

Stability is evaluated with the patient upright. A "shift-and-load" test is done by placing one hand along the edge of

FIGURE 3.18 Matsen's classification system.

Macrotraumatic   Microtraumatic   Atraumatic

the scapula to stabilize it and grasping the humeral head with the other hand and applying a slight compressive force. The amount of anterior and posterior translation of the humeral head in the glenoid is observed with the arm abducted 0 degrees. Easy subluxation of the shoulder indicates loss of the glenoid concavity, which must be surgically treated.

The sulcus test is done with the arm in 0 degrees and 45 degrees of abduction. This test is done by pulling distally on the extremity and observing for a sulcus or dimple between the humeral head and the acromion that does not reduce with 45 degrees of external rotation. The distance between the humeral head and acromion should be graded from 0 to 3 with the arm in 0 degrees and 45 degrees of abduction, with 1+ indicating subluxation of less than 1 cm, 2+ indicating 1 to 2 cm of subluxation, and 3+ indicating more than 2 cm of inferior subluxation that does not reduce with external rotation. Subluxation at 0 degrees of abduction is more indicative of laxity at the rotator interval, and subluxation at 45 degrees indicates laxity of the inferior glenohumeral ligament complex.

Anterior apprehension is evaluated with the shoulder in 90 degrees of abduction and the elbow in 90 degrees of flexion, with a slight external rotation force applied to the extremity as anterior stress is applied to the humerus. This generally produces an apprehension reaction in a patient who has anterior instability. Control of the proximal humerus should be maintained during any of the apprehension or stress tests to prevent dislocation during these procedures. Posterior instability can be evaluated with a Kim test or a posterior clunk test, in which the 90-degree abducted extremity is brought to a forward flexed, internally rotated position while posterior stress is applied to the elbow. The clunk is felt as the humeral head subluxes posteriorly, producing pain or a feeling of subluxation in an unstable shoulder.

The shoulder anterior drawer test should be performed with the patient supine and the extremity in various degrees of abduction and external rotation in the plane of the scapula. When examining the patient's right shoulder, the examiner's left hand is used to grasp the proximal humerus while the right hand is used to hold the elbow lightly. Anterior stress is applied to the proximal humerus using the left hand, and the amount of translation and the end point are evaluated. In performing this and other anterior or posterior instability tests, the amount of instability is graded from 0 to 3. Grade 1 means that the humeral head slips up to the rim of the glenoid, and grade 2 means that it slips over the labrum but then spontaneously relocates. Grade 3 indicates dislocation. A grade 3 instability should not be exhibited in an awake patient. Anterior stress is applied with the shoulder in various degrees of abduction and external rotation, and posterior stress is applied to evaluate for posterior instability with the arm in 90 degrees of abduction and various degrees of flexion. When examining the patient's right shoulder, posterior stress is applied with the examiner's right hand, starting at 0 degrees of forward flexion and internal rotation and proceeding to 110 degrees. The examiner's left hand stabilizes the scapula and palpates the posterior part of the glenohumeral joint with the palm. It also can be used as a buttress to ensure that posterior dislocation does not occur during this procedure. Apprehension is evaluated with anterior and posterior stress during these procedures.

The Jobe relocation test can be used for evaluating instability in athletes involved in sports requiring overhead motion (Fig. 3.19). This test is done with the patient supine and the

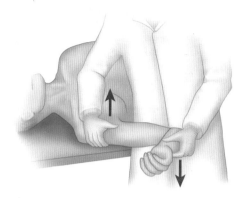
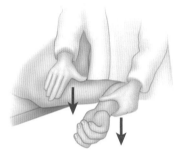

FIGURE 3.19   Jobe's relocation test (see text). A positive relocation test and a positive apprehension test are highly predictive of recurrent instability.

shoulder in 90 degrees of abduction and external rotation. Various degrees of abduction are evaluated while anterior stress is applied by the examiner's hand to the posterior part of the humerus. If this produces pain or apprehension, posteriorly directed force is applied to the humerus to relocate the humeral head in the glenohumeral joint while the shoulder is placed in abduction and external rotation. The posteriorly directed stress used to relocate the humerus is released. A feeling of apprehension or subluxation on the part of the patient indicates anterior instability.

Bony deformity of the glenoid or humerus is indicated by apprehension or instability at low ranges of motion (<90 degrees of abduction) and when inferior instability is prominent. Hyperlaxity is indicated by a positive sulcus test, a positive Gagey hyperabduction test, and the Beighton hyperlaxity scale (Table 3.4). The hyperabduction test is done by stabilizing the scapula with one hand placed superiorly while passively abducting the shoulder with the other hand. A side-to-side difference of more than 20 degrees is suggestive of inferior capsular laxity. External rotation of more than 85 degrees at 0 degrees of abduction is indicative of hyperlaxity, which may need to be corrected with rotator interval closure.

It is imperative to distinguish secondary rotator cuff impingement from primary impingement. The relocation and anterior apprehension tests are valuable in young athletes in sports requiring throwing or overhead motion. It also is imperative to rule out scapular dysfunction that can be corrected with physical therapy. Although rarely associated with shoulder instability, neck problems should be also ruled out, such as degenerative discs or degenerative arthritis that causes pain radiating into the posterior or lateral aspect of the shoulder.

TABLE 3.4

Beighton Hyperlaxity Score

CHARACTERISTIC	SCORING*
Passive dorsiflexion of the little finger beyond 90 degrees	1 point for each hand
Passive apposition of the thumb to the ipsilateral forearm	1 point for each hand
Active hyperextension of the elbow beyond 10 degrees	1 point for each elbow
Acute hyperextension of the knee beyond 10 degrees	1 point for each knee
Forward flexion of the trunk with the knees fully extended so that the palms of the hands rest flat on the floor	1 point

*A score of ≤4 points, on a 9-point scale, is diagnostic of hyperlaxity.

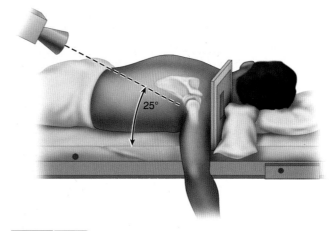

FIGURE 3.21 Radiographic technique for West Point view of shoulder to show glenoid labrum lesions. With patient prone and pillow beneath shoulder, cassette is placed superior to shoulder.

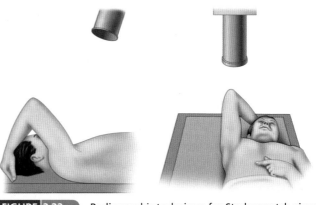

FIGURE 3.22 Radiographic technique for Stryker notch view of humerus.

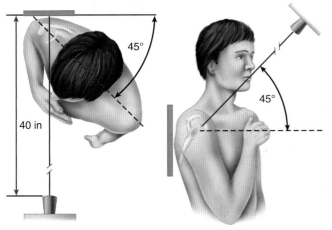

FIGURE 3.20 Garth et al. radiographic technique for apical oblique view of shoulder. With patient seated and injured shoulder adjacent to vertical cassette, chest is rotated to 45-degree oblique position. Beam is directed 45 degrees caudally, passing longitudinally through scapula, which rests at 45-degree angle on thorax while extremity is adducted. Origin of coracoid, midway between anterior and posterior margins of glenoid, aids in orientation on radiograph.

RADIOGRAPHIC EVALUATION

The diagnosis of an unstable shoulder often is made by history and physical examination, but an unstable shoulder can be documented by routine radiographs. The initial radiographic examination should include anteroposterior and axillary lateral views of the shoulder. If the initial radiographic evaluation is inconclusive, special views, gadolinium-enhanced MRI, or CT arthrography can be used to show posttraumatic changes not otherwise detected. The most common special views that can be obtained in the office are the anteroposterior view of the shoulder in internal rotation, the West Point or Rokous view, and the Stryker notch view. An anteroposterior radiograph of the shoulder in internal rotation often shows a Hill-Sachs lesion that may not be apparent on routine views. Garth et al. also described an apical oblique radiograph that frequently shows posterior humeral head defects that might not be seen on

routine films (Fig. 3.20). The West Point view is used to show calcification or small fractures at the anteroinferior glenoid rim. This is a modified, prone, axillary lateral view of the shoulder obtained with the shoulder abducted 90 degrees and the elbow bent with the arm hanging over the side of the table. The x-ray beam is directed 25 degrees medially and 25 degrees cephalad with the cassette placed above the shoulder perpendicular to the table (Fig. 3.21). The Stryker notch view is obtained with the patient supine and the elbow elevated over the head. The x-ray beam is directed 10 degrees cephalad (Fig. 3.22).

MRI or MRA is indicated for evaluating soft-tissue lesions associated with instability. MRI obtained within a few days of dislocation generally shows blood in the joint, which can aid in visualization and make MRA unnecessary. MRA is helpful in evaluating humeral avulsion glenohumeral ligament (HAGL) lesions, but occasionally it may show a tear but actually cover up the details of the exact tear site (Fig. 3.23). Evaluation of the glenoid track, as described by Yamamoto et al., evaluates Hill-Sachs lesions based on both the location and size of the humeral head defect and the amount of glenoid bone loss. It has been shown to be highly predictive in a clinical setting. Metzger et al. found that lesions falling outside the track engaged more than 85% of the time. The examination is measured on MRI (Fig. 3.24) and is essential

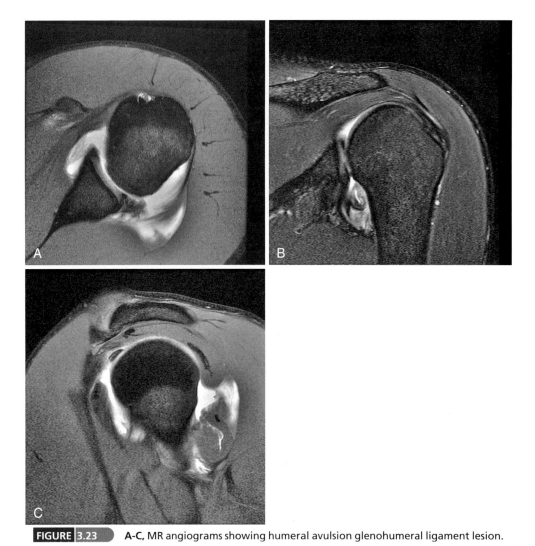

FIGURE 3.23 A-C, MR angiograms showing humeral avulsion glenohumeral ligament lesion.

in determining appropriate surgical intervention for on-track versus off-track lesions.

CT, particularly 3D CT, is the most sensitive test for detecting and measuring bone deficiency or retroversion of the glenoid or humerus for evaluation of recurrent instability. CT is indicated when there is blunting of the glenoid cortical outline or an obvious bone defect on plain radiographs. CT also is indicated for evaluating recurrences that occur with trivial trauma, low-angle instability, and failed surgical procedures (Fig. 3.25).

EXAMINATION USING ANESTHETIC AND ARTHROSCOPY

Examination with the patient under anesthesia may support the clinical diagnosis or sometimes show unsuspected planes of instability, especially in multidirectional instability patterns. For anterior instability, the arm is abducted. Anterior and posterior stress is applied with the scapula stabilized. Minimal anterior translation of the humeral head occurs unless there is instability. The most significant findings of instability are demonstrable at 40 degrees and 80 degrees of external rotation. Translation of two grades more than the opposite uninvolved side resulted in 93% sensitivity and 100% specificity for instability. For posterior instability, the arm is pushed posteriorly.

Normal shoulders may permit posterior displacement of 50% of the diameter of the glenoid without pathologic instability.

Arthroscopy can be combined with examination using anesthesia and is an excellent technique for confirming the presence of shoulder instabilities. The examiner should grade the instability in all planes as previously described, remembering that this examination under anesthesia is used to support the clinical history and examination with the patient awake. Arthroscopy should be performed to identify all intraarticular pathology so that treatment may be rendered accordingly. Arthroscopy portals and time should be limited to reduce extravasation into the soft tissues, which can make surgical exposure more difficult.

ANTERIOR INSTABILITY OF THE SHOULDER
■ SURGICAL TREATMENT

More than 150 operations and many modifications have been devised to treat traumatic recurrent anterior instability of the shoulder. There is no single best procedure. Factors that have been stressed as important in achieving a successful result are adequate exposure and accurate surgical technique. The pathologic condition should be defined, and a procedure should be done that corrects this condition most anatomically. Ideally, the procedure for recurrent instability

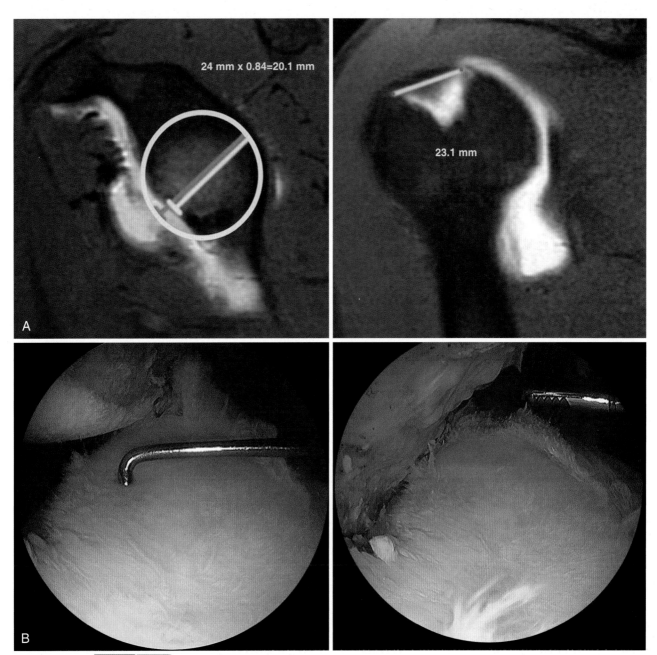

FIGURE 3.24   **A,** The glenoid track is calculated as 84% of the actual glenoid width measured on the sagittal oblique MR image. A best-fit circle is placed on the glenoid to calculate the expected width before bone loss; therefore, both percentage of bone loss and glenoid track can be determined. In this case, the actual glenoid width is 24 mm, with 4 mm of bone loss (17%). The glenoid track is 84% of 24 mm, or 20.1 mm. **B,** The distance from the rotator cuff footprint to the medial margin of the Hill-Sachs lesion is measured on the coronal MR image. In this case, it is 23.1 mm. Because the Hill-Sachs width to the footprint (23.1 mm) is greater than the glenoid track measurement (20.1 mm), it is considered outside the glenoid track and at high risk for engaging. (From Metzger PD, Barlow B, Leonardelli D, et al: Clinical application of the "glenoid track" concept for defining humeral head engagement in anterior shoulder instability. A preliminary report, *Orthop J Sports Med* 1:1, 2013.)

should include the following factors: (1) low recurrence rate, (2) low complication rate, (3) low reoperation rate, (4) does no harm (arthritis), (5) maintains motion, (6) is applicable in most cases, (7) allows observation of the joint, (8) corrects the pathologic condition, and (9) is not too difficult.

Operative procedures can be done open or arthroscopically with comparable results. When the appropriate procedure is accomplished to restore the anatomy, outcomes of Bankart repairs are affected by what Balg and Boileau described as the Instability Severity Index Score (ISIS; Table 3.5).

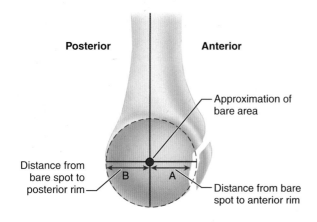

Posterior   Anterior

Approximation of bare area

Distance from bare spot to posterior rim

B   A

Distance from bare spot to anterior rim

$$\text{Percent bone loss} = \frac{(B - A)}{2 \times B} \times 100\%$$

FIGURE 3.25 Estimation of bone loss based on glenoid rim distances. En face view of glenoid is viewed on a CT scan. With use of intersection of longitudinal axis and widest anteroposterior diameter of glenoid, the bare spot is approximated on the glenoid fossa. A best-fit circle centered at the bare-spot approximation is drawn about the inferior two thirds of the glenoid *(red)*. Distances from the bare spot to anterior rim *(A)* and posterior rim *(B)* are measured. The percent bone loss is calculated according to the indicated equation. (From Provencher MT, Bhatia S, Ghodadra NS, et al: Recurrent shoulder instability: current concepts for evaluation and management of glenoid bone loss, *J Bone Joint Surg* 92A:133–151, 2010).

At present, our preferred surgical procedures are arthroscopic Bankart or capsular plication procedures as indicated. When an open procedure is desired, we prefer the Jobe capsulolabral reconstruction or Neer capsular shift for anterior instability and a glenoid-based shift for posterior instability. For glenoid bony defects that cannot be repaired, we reconstruct the anterior defects with a Latarjet procedure and use an autograft iliac crest extracapsular bone graft posteriorly. Moderately sized (20% to 30%) humeral head defects are treated with an arthroscopic remplissage procedure and Bankart repair, and larger defects (35% to 45%) are treated indirectly by increasing the glenoid arc using a Latarjet procedure or by allograft repair of the defect. In a contact or collision athlete any significant Hill-Sachs lesion is treated with a remplissage procedure, unless in a throwing athlete (Table 3.6).

BANKART OPERATION

In the original Bankart operation, the subscapularis and shoulder capsule are opened vertically. The lateral leaf of the capsule is reattached to the anterior glenoid rim. A medial leaf of the capsule is imbricated, and the subscapularis is approximated. The Bankart operation is indicated when the labrum and the capsule are separated from the glenoid rim or if the capsule is thin. The advantage of this procedure is that it corrects the labral defect and imbricates the capsule without requiring any metallic internal fixation devices. The main disadvantage of the original procedure is its technical difficulty.

TABLE 3.5

Instability Severity Index Score Based on a Preoperative Questionnaire, Clinical Examination, and Radiographs

PROGNOSTIC FACTORS	POINTS
AGE AT SURGERY (YEARS)	
<20	2
>20	0
DEGREE OF SPORT PARTICIPATION (PREOPERATIVE)	
Competitive	2
Recreational or none	0
TYPE OF SPORT (PREOPERATIVE)	
Contact or forced overhead	1
Other	0
SHOULDER HYPERLAXITY	
Shoulder hyperlaxity (anterior or inferior)	1
Normal laxity	0
HILL-SACHS LESION ON ANTEROPOSTERIOR RADIOGRAPH	
Visible in external rotation	2
Not visible in external rotation	0
GLENOID LOSS OF CONTOUR ON ANTEROPOSTERIOR RADIOGRAPHS	
Loss of contour	2
No lesion	0
***TOTAL* (POINTS)**	10

From Balg F, Boileau P: The instability severity index score: a simple preoperative score to select patients for arthroscopic or open shoulder stabilisation, *J Bone Joint Surg* 89B:1470–1477, 2007. Copyright British Editorial Society of Bone and Joint Surgery.

Since the original description of the Bankart procedure, modifications have allowed the procedure to be done with more ease and less surgical trauma. The procedure can be done through a subscapularis split; or in larger, more muscular individuals, the subscapularis split can be extended superiorly approximately 1 cm medial to the biceps tendon, releasing the subscapularis muscle in an L-shaped fashion. This L-type release provides excellent exposure of the rotator interval, and the inferior third of the subscapular muscle can be retracted inferiorly to expose the inferior capsule, while protecting the axillary nerve. The subscapularis split approach preserves neuromuscular function and minimizes the possibility of postoperative tendon detachment. We have had success using either the subscapularis split or the L-split, depending on the patient, and the modified Bankart procedure (Fig. 3.26). We have used a procedure similar to that described by Montgomery and Jobe for recurrent traumatic dislocations and recurrent microtraumatic subluxations with anterior and inferior instability. A 17-year follow-up of 127 patients with open Bankart repair found only two patients with recurrent instability, reminding us that his procedure produces results that are hard to duplicate by any other means. Keys to success of this procedure are (1) maximizing the healing potential by abrading the

TABLE 3.6

Our Preferred Open Surgical Treatment (90% to 95% Are Done Arthroscopically)	
Traumatic Bankart	Jobe capsulolabral reconstruction
Acute bony Bankart	Screw or anchor fixation
+Hyperlaxity	Rotator interval closure
HAGL	Suture anchor repair
MULTIDIRECTIONAL	**REPAIR BANKART/KIM LESIONS**
Anteroinferior prominent	Humeral side Neer capsular shift
Posterior prominent—glenoid side	Glenoid side shift
BONE LOSS—GLENOID	
Erosional bone loss >25%	Laterjet procedure
Erosional bone loss >40%	Eden-Hybinette procedure
BONE LOSS—HUMERAL HEAD	
20% + glenoid defect	Jobe capsular reconstruction + capsular shift + remplissage
25% (6 mm deep)	Remplissage
40%	Laterjet to increase glenoid rotational arc
BONE LOSS—ANTERIOR HUMERAL HEAD	
>30%	McLaughlin
Capsular deficiency	Achilles allograft capsular reinforcement

HAGL, Humeral avulsion glenohumeral ligament.

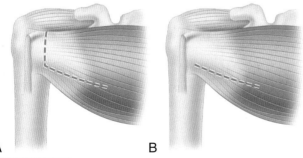

A   B

FIGURE 3.26 Division of subscapularis tendon. **A,** Lower fourth of subscapularis tendon is left intact to protect anterior humeral circumflex artery and axillary nerve. **B,** Subscapularis muscle is split horizontally and retracted superiorly and inferiorly to expose underlying capsule.

scapular neck, (2) restoring glenoid concavity, (3) securing anatomic capsular fixation at the edge of the glenoid articular surface, (4) re-creating physiologic capsular tension by superior and inferior capsular advancement and imbrication, and (5) performing supervised goal-oriented rehabilitation.

MODIFIED BANKART REPAIR

TECHNIQUE 3.5

(MONTGOMERY AND JOBE)

- Make an incision along the Langer lines, beginning 2 cm distal and lateral to the coracoid process and going inferiorly to the anterior axillary crease.
- Develop the deltopectoral interval, retracting the deltoid and cephalic vein laterally and the pectoralis major muscle medially. Leave the conjoined tendon intact, and retract it medially.
- Split the subscapularis tendon transversely in line with its fibers at the junction of the upper two thirds and lower one third of the tendon, and carefully dissect it from the underlying anterior capsule. Maintain the subscapularis tendon interval with a modified Gelpi retractor (Anspach, Inc., Lake Park, FL), and place a three-pronged retractor medially on the glenoid neck.
- Make a horizontal anterior capsulotomy in line with the split in the subscapularis tendon from the humeral insertion laterally to the anterior glenoid neck medially (Fig. 3.27A). Place stay sutures in the superior and inferior capsular flaps at the glenoid margin.
- Insert a narrow humeral head retractor, and retract the head laterally. Elevate the capsule on the anterior neck subperiosteally. Leave the labrum intact if it is still attached. Decorticate the anterior neck to bleeding bone with a rongeur.
- Drill holes near the glenoid rim at approximately the 3-, 4-, and 5:30-o'clock positions, keeping the drill bit parallel to the glenoid surface (Fig. 3.27B).
- Place suture anchors in each hole and check for security of the anchors (Fig. 3.27C). During this portion of the procedure, maintain the shoulder in approximately 90 degrees of abduction and 60 degrees of external rotation for throwing athletes. Maintain the shoulder in 60 degrees abduction and 30 to 45 degrees external rotation in nonthrowing athletes and other patients.
- Tie the inferior flap down in mattress fashion, shifting the capsule superiorly but not medially (Fig. 3.27D). The stay sutures help prevent medialization of the capsule. Shift the superior flap interiorly, overlapping and reinforcing the inferior flap (Fig. 3.27E).
- Loosely close the remaining gap in the capsule (Fig. 3.27F). The reconstruction has two layers of reinforced capsule outside the joint.

POSTOPERATIVE CARE Postoperative rehabilitation is carried out as described in Box 3.2.

Humeral avulsion of the glenohumeral ligament should always be evaluated with MRI or, better, an MRA. Anterior lesions are best treated open with a lower-third scapularis split and suture anchors placed in the anatomic footprint on the humerus. These lesions can be bipolar, involving detachment from the humerus and the glenoid, and should be carefully examined to produce a stable repair.

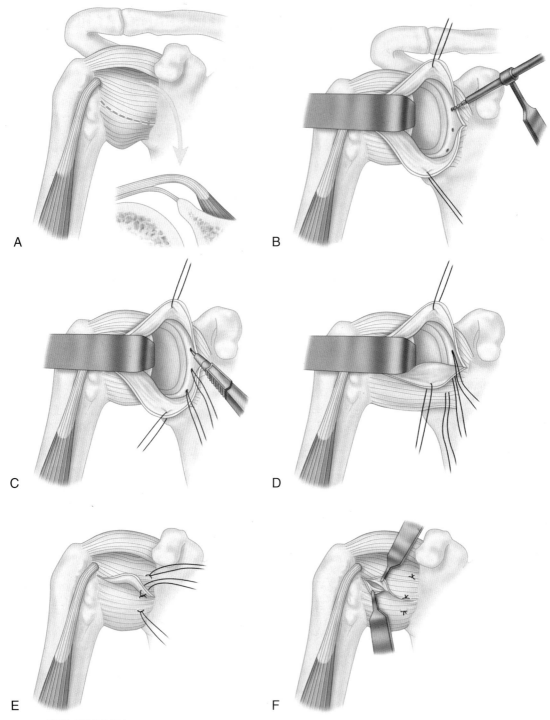

A

B

C

D

E

F

FIGURE 3.27 Montgomery and Jobe technique. **A,** Capsular incision made at center (3-o'clock position) of glenoid. Incision is extended medially over neck of glenoid. Stay suture is placed in capsule to mark glenoid attachment site. **B,** Suture anchor drill holes are started in scapular neck adjacent to glenoid articular surface and directed medially away from joint surface. For exposure of neck, sharp Hohmann retractor is placed along superior and inferior neck for capsular retraction *(not pictured).* **C,** Suture anchors are placed in each prepared drill hole. Sutures are pulled to set anchor. Each individual suture is pulled to ensure suture slides in anchor. **D,** Approximation of capsule to freshened neck. Two or three suture anchors are used to secure inferior capsule firmly to scapular neck. An Allis clamp is used by assistant to advance capsule superiorly against neck while sutures are placed. **E,** Superior and middle suture anchors are used to secure and advance superior flap in inferior direction. **F,** Final imbrication of capsule is done with interrupted nonabsorbable sutures. Extremity is maintained in 45 degrees abduction and 45 degrees external rotation during closure to prevent overconstraint. *Technical note:* Suture anchors should be at edge of glenoid articular surface and aimed medially 20 degrees. **SEE TECHNIQUE 3.5.**

Rehabilitation Program After Anterior Capsulolabral Reconstruction

Postoperative Period (0-3 Weeks)
Abduction pillow
Passive/active ROM: abduction (90 degrees), flexion (90 degrees), and external rotation (45 degrees); no extension
Isometric abduction, horizontal adduction, and external rotation
Elbow ROM
Ball squeeze
Ice

Phase I (3-6 Weeks)
Discontinue brace/pillow
Modalities as needed
Progressive passive and active ROM, protecting anterior capsule
Active internal rotation (full) and external rotation (neutral) using tubing and free weights
Prone extension (not posterior to trunk)
Shoulder shrugs and active abduction
Supraspinatus strengthening
Ice

Phase II (6 Weeks to 3 Months)
Continue ROM, gradually increasing external rotation (goal is full ROM by 2 months)
Continue strengthening exercises, with emphasis on rotator cuff and parascapular muscles
Add shoulder flexion and horizontal adduction exercises
Joint mobilization
Begin upper body ergometer for endurance at low resistance
Ice

Phase III (3-6 Months)
Continue capsular stretching and strengthening and ergometer
May include isokinetic strengthening and endurance exercises for internal and external rotation
Add push-ups (begin with wall push-up with body always posterior to elbows)
Start chin-ups at 4-5 months
Total body conditioning
Advance to throwing program or skill-specific training as tolerated
Ice

ROM, Range of motion.
From Montgomery WH, Jobe FW: Functional outcomes in athletes after modified anterior capsulolabral reconstruction, *Am J Sports Med* 22:352–358, 1994.

ANTERIOR STABILIZATION WITH ASSOCIATED GLENOID DEFICIENCY (LATERJET PROCEDURE)

In patients who have an inverted pear-shaped glenoid and an engaging Hill-Sachs lesion, we have found that the Laterjet procedure alone usually is adequate to treat this combined bone deficiency. The bone graft corrects the glenoid deficiency so that it can resist axial forces across an expanded glenoid diameter. The graft also lengthens the glenoid articular arc to prevent the Hill-Sachs lesion from engaging and is used when a large (35% to 45%) humeral head lesion is present (Fig. 3.28).

TECHNIQUE 3.6

(WALCH AND BOILEAU)
- With the patient secured in a beach-chair position and after induction of general endotracheal anesthesia, place a small pillow behind the scapula to position the glenoid surface perpendicular to the operative table. Sterilize and drape free the neck, chest, axilla, and entire arm.
- Make a 4 to 7-cm skin incision beginning under the tip of the coracoid process (Fig. 3.29A). Open the deltopectoral interval and retract the cephalic vein laterally with the deltoid. Place a self-retaining retractor into the deltopectoral interval and a Hohmann retractor on the top of the coracoid process.

HARVESTING AND PREPARATION OF THE BONE BLOCK
- Position the patient's arm in 90 degrees of abduction and external rotation, and section the coracoacromial ligament 1 cm from the coracoid.
- Adduct and internally rotate the arm to release the pectoralis minor insertion from the coracoid, and expose the base of the coracoid with a periosteal elevator to allow observation of the "knee" of the coracoid process. Use an osteotome or small angulated saw to osteotomize the coracoid process from medial to lateral at the junction of the horizontal-vertical parts (Fig. 3.29B).
- Bring the arm back into abduction and external rotation and release the coracohumeral ligament from the lateral part of the coracoid.
- Grasp the bone graft firmly with forceps and carefully release it from its deep attachments. Dissect the lateral part of the conjoined tendon, avoiding the medial aspect and potential damage to the musculocutaneous nerve.
- Evert the bone graft and decorticate its deep surface with a cutting rongeur or saw.
- With a 3.2-mm drill, drill two parallel holes in the deep surface of the bone graft.
- Measure the thickness of the bone graft with a caliper and place the graft under the pectoralis major for subsequent use; hold it in place with the self-retaining retractor, which keeps the deltopectoral interval open.

DIVISION OF THE SUBSCAPULARIS, CAPSULOTOMY, AND EXPOSURE
- With the upper limb in full external rotation, identify the inferior and superior margins of the subscapularis tendon. Use electrocautery and then Mayo scissors to divide the muscle at the superior two thirds or inferior one third junction in line with its fibers, carefully obtaining hemostasis at each step.
- Carefully carry division down to the white capsule, and then extend it medially by inserting a 4 × 4-inch sponge into the cleavage plane, thus exposing the subscapular fossa. Extend the division laterally as far as the lesser tuberosity. Place a Hohmann retractor in the subscapular fossa.

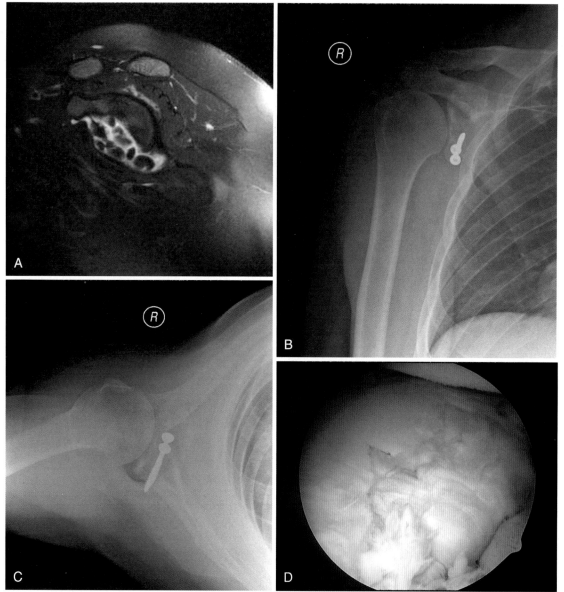

FIGURE 3.28   **A,** Preoperative sagittal MRI of shoulder with multiple loose bodies and loss of 35% of glenoid articular surface. Anteroposterior **(B)** and lateral **(C)** views after Laterjet procedure with parallel screw fixation. **D,** Arthroscopic view showing healed Laterjet procedure.

- Place the upper limb in neutral rotation to provide full exposure of the capsule, and make a 1.5-cm vertical capsulotomy at the level of the anteroinferior margin of the glenoid.
- Move the arm into full internal rotation to allow insertion of a humeral head retractor, which rests on the posterior margin of the glenoid.
- Retract the superior two thirds of the subscapularis superiorly with a Steinmann pin impacted at the superior part of the scapular neck; retract the inferior part inferiorly with a Hohmann retractor pushed under the neck of the scapula between the capsule and the subscapularis.
- With the anteroinferior rim of the scapula exposed, inspect the labrum, cartilage, and insertion site of the glenohumer-

al ligaments. Resect the medial capsular flap along with damaged portions of the labrum or fracture fragments.
- Use a scalpel to expose the anteroinferior margin of the glenoid and decorticate it with a curet or osteotome (Fig. 3.29C).

FIXATION OF THE BONE BLOCK

- Insert the bone block through the soft tissues and position it flush to the anteroinferior margin of the glenoid. Check the position of the bone block with the arm in internal rotation, taking care to avoid any lateral overhang; a slight medial position (no more than 1 to 2 mm) is acceptable. Never accept a lateral overhang of the coracoid in the joint; it can lead to rapid degenerative joint disease.

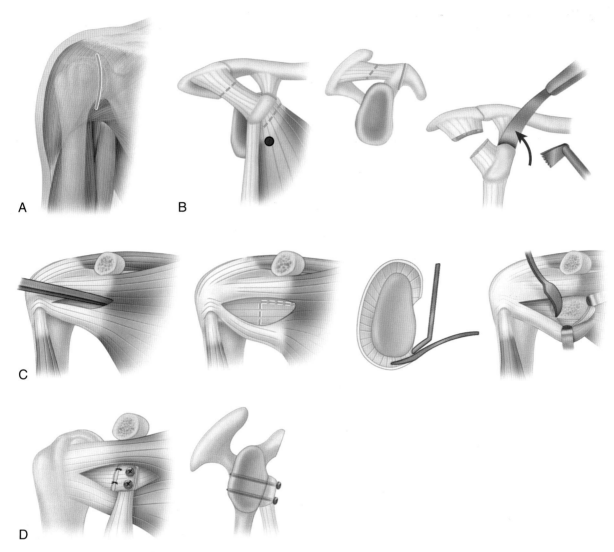

FIGURE 3.29 Laterjet-Bristow procedure (Walch and Boileau). **A,** Vertical incision under tip of coracoid process. **B,** Harvest of bone block corresponding to horizontal part of coracoid process, retaining conjoined coracobrachialis tendon and coracoacromial ligament. **C,** Division of subscapularis horizontally. Anteroinferior glenoid rim is decorticated. **D,** Bicortical fixation of bone block. Outer capsular flap is sutured to remainder of coracoacromial ligament. **SEE TECHNIQUE 3.6.**

■ Insert a 3.2-mm drill through the inferior hole in the bone graft and into the glenoid neck in an anteroposterior and superior direction. Check the orientation of the articular surface and direct the drill parallel to this plane. Temporarily reflect the bone block to allow measurement of the drilling depth with a depth gauge.

■ Place an AO malleolar screw into the posterior cortex to secure the bone block to the glenoid. Tighten this screw loosely to allow easy rotation and proper positioning of the superior part of the bone block. When positioning is correct, insert a second AO malleolar screw through the superior hole in the bone block and tighten both screws firmly (Fig. 3.29D). To avoid impingement with the humeral head, do not use washers with the screws.

CLOSURE

■ With the arm in external rotation, repair the remnant of the coracoacromial ligament to the lateral capsular flap with two interrupted absorbable sutures.

■ Remove the sponge placed earlier in the subscapular fossa, and move the arm through all ranges of motion to evaluate mobility.

■ Coat the cut surface of the coracoid with bone wax, place a suction drain, and close the superficial soft-tissue layers.

POSTOPERATIVE CARE Patients require immobilization in a sling or shoulder immobilizer for 2 weeks after surgery. Forward flexion is begun thereafter, and external rotation is begun at 6 weeks. Strengthening exercises are started 8 weeks after surgery.

RECONSTRUCTION OF ANTERIOR GLENOID USING ILIAC CREST BONE AUTOGRAFT

The Eden-Hybbinette procedure was originally described using an iliac crest autograft to reconstruct the anterior glenoid. Glenoid bone loss approaching 40% of the anterior glenoid or posterior bone loss of 25% with recurrent posterior dislocation should be reconstructed with an autogenous iliac crest bone graft, or, occasionally for posterior lesions, the medial aspect of the acromion can be used as a graft. Provencher et al. described using allograft from the lateral aspect of a distal tibia for reconstruction. At present, however, an iliac crest autograft is recommended because of its availability, greater healing potential, and less potential for resorption than an allograft.

TECHNIQUE 3.7

(WARNER ET AL.)
- Harvest a tricortical iliac crest autograft 2 cm wide and 3 cm long and contour it to make a smooth continuation of the glenoid arc.
- Drill two holes in the graft and use these to align the graft to form a smooth articular arc.
- Drill holes in the glenoid neck and mark them with electrocautery for ease in finding.
- Place sutures in the capsule and pass them around the screw shaft between the glenoid and graft sutures. Secure the graft extracapsularly.
- Appropriate graft position is vertical before closure of the lateral extent of the capsular incision.
- Decorticate the glenoid neck and secure the graft with two 4.0-mm cannulated bicortical screws.
- Anteriorly, place the graft intracapsularly, securing the capsule around the screwheads.
- Posteriorly, perform a medial-based plication.

POSTOPERATIVE CARE Postoperative care is as described for Technique 3.6.

■ UNSUCCESSFUL SURGICAL REPAIRS FOR ANTERIOR INSTABILITY

Failure of stabilization may occur because of failure to correct the pathology, failure to heal, or poor patient compliance. All potential causes of failure must be fully evaluated and should include a 3D CT evaluation for bony deficiency of the glenoid and humeral head and, on occasion, an arthrogram to identify the site of capsular failure. If failure of stabilization is determined to be caused by failure to heal, the procedure may be revised arthroscopically with the option of open repair if it is thought to be advantageous. Bony deficiency of the humeral head usually is corrected with an arthroscopic remplissage procedure. Deficiency of the glenoid more than 25% should be approached with an open Latarjet procedure (see Table 3.6). Loss of as little as 13.5% of the glenoid bone may give a sense of instability.

Recent studies have reported complication rates of up to 25% and return to previous level of sport of about 50% in patients with glenoid deformities treated with Latarjet procedures. Stability is increased with Latarjet procedures, but a meta-analysis showed arthroscopic soft-tissue procedures to have the lowest complication rates (1%) compared with arthroscopic Latarjet procedures (13.6%).

Reported complications of recurrent instability or loss of motion, neurovascular problems, infection, and postoperative degenerative changes can be reduced significantly with appropriate planning preoperatively, intraoperatively, and postoperatively. The patient's expectations and any secondary gains must be realized. Secure repair of the pathologic lesion is necessary to restore stability and preserve motion. Excessive loss of motion and injury to the glenohumeral joint from hardware have been indicated as causes of degenerative changes. Excessive loss of motion can be treated with an arthroscopic capsular release. If severe restriction of rotation (i.e., <15 degrees of external rotation) is present, an open coronal subscapularis lengthening should be considered.

The basic principles for approaching failed repairs are the same as for the primary procedure: (1) creating an optimal healing environment, (2) re-creating the glenoid concavity, (3) securing anatomic capsular fixation at the articular edge, (4) re-creating physiologic capsular tension, and (5) having supervised, goal-specific therapy. Procedures in which a bone block or a coracoid transfer is done can result in degenerative changes if malposition of the transfer causes impingement on the humeral head. The keys for successful surgical repair include appropriate patient selection, selection of the appropriate procedure to correct the pathologic lesion, a thorough understanding of the local anatomy, identification and protection of important neurovascular structures, use of a postoperative rehabilitation program consistent with the type of surgical correction done, and an understanding of the patient's goals.

MULTIDIRECTIONAL INSTABILITY OF THE SHOULDER

Neer and Foster introduced the term *multidirectional instability* in 1980. It describes glenohumeral subluxation or dislocation in multiple directions. The primary abnormality in multidirectional instability is a loose, redundant inferior pouch. It is important to distinguish multidirectional instability from routine unidirectional dislocation because the former problem is not correctable by standard repairs. Surgery in these patients is not indicated unless disability is frequent and significant, an adequate trial of conservative treatment emphasizing muscular and rotator cuff rehabilitative exercises has failed, and the patient is not a voluntary dislocator.

The principle of the procedure is to detach the capsule from the neck of the humerus and shift it to the opposite side of the calcar (inferior portion of the neck of the humerus), not only to obliterate the inferior pouch and capsular redundancy on the side of the surgical approach but also to reduce laxity on the opposite side. To reduce inferior laxity with the arm in 0 degrees of abduction, closure of the rotator interval is indicated. Internal closure also has been shown to decrease posterior translation. The approach can be anterior or posterior depending on the direction of greatest instability. When the findings include a 3+ sulcus sign and symptoms related to inferior instability, associated with anterior or posterior instability, an anterior capsular shift and closure of the rotator interval allow better correction of inferior laxity. If the finding is posterior instability with a 1+ to 2+ sulcus sign and only mild inferior symptoms, a posterior capsular procedure is indicated.

CAPSULAR SHIFT

TECHNIQUE 3.8

(NEER AND FOSTER)

- The patient is carefully examined and questioned preoperatively to determine the probable direction of greatest instability. After delivery of a general anesthetic, the instability of the shoulder is evaluated again. Anterior instability is tested with the arm in external rotation and extension at various levels of abduction. Inferior instability is tested with the arm in 0 degrees and 45 degrees of abduction. Posterior instability is tested with the arm in internal rotation at various levels of forward elevation. If this examination and the preoperative evaluation correlate with anteroinferior instability, use an anterior approach.

- Place the patient in a tilted position with the front and the back of the shoulder exposed. Drape the arm free. Attach an arm board to the side of the table.

- Make a 9-cm incision in the skin creases from the anterior border of the axilla to the coracoid process.

- Develop the deltopectoral interval medial to the cephalic vein, and retract the deltoid laterally. Divide the clavipectoral fascia, and retract the muscles attached to the coracoid process medially.

- With the arm in external rotation, divide the superficial half of the thickness of the subscapularis tendon transversely, 1 cm medial to the biceps groove (Fig. 3.30A). Leave the deep half of the subscapularis tendon attached to reinforce the anterior aspect of the capsule, and tag the superficial half of the tendon with stay sutures and retract it medially. It is important that this superficial portion of

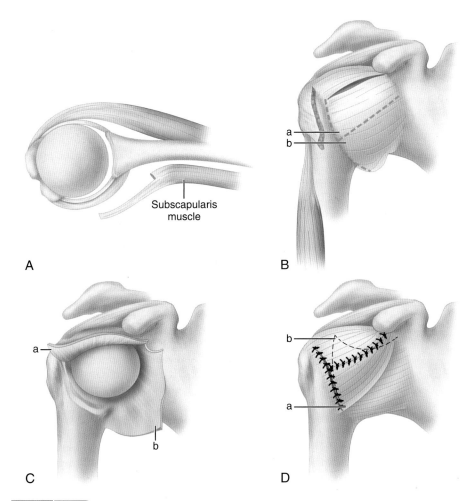

Subscapularis muscle

A

B

C

D

FIGURE 3.30 Neer technique of inferior capsular shift for shoulder instability. **A,** Reinforcement of capsular flaps; about half thickness of subscapularis tendon is left attached to reinforce capsule. **B,** Capsular incision. **C,** Preparation of flaps and slot. Arm is externally rotated as inferior flap is detached. **D,** Relocation of flaps with arm in slight flexion and 10 degrees of external rotation. Inferior flap *(b)* is relocated first and is pulled forward and upward. Superior flap *(a)* is brought down over inferior flap. **SEE TECHNIQUE 3.8.**

the subscapularis tendon be free so that the action of the subscapularis muscle is not tethered.

- Close the cleft between the middle and superior glenohumeral ligaments with nonabsorbable sutures.
- Make a T-shaped opening by incising between the middle and inferior glenohumeral ligaments (Fig. 3.30B).
- With a flat elevator to protect the axillary nerve and with the arm in external rotation, develop a capsular flap by detaching the reinforced part of the capsule containing the inferior glenohumeral ligament from the inferior aspect of the neck of the humerus around to the posterior aspect of the neck of the humerus (Fig. 3.30C).
- Inspect the interior of the joint, and remove any osteochondral bodies or tags of labrum.
- Test for posterior instability with and without forward traction on the inferior capsular flap to estimate the new location for the flap.
- Using curets and a small gouge, make a shallow slot in the bone at the anterior and inferior sulcus of the neck of the humerus (Fig. 3.30C). Suture the capsular flap to the stump of the subscapularis tendon and to the part of the capsule that remains on the humerus so that the capsular flap is held against the slot of raw bone. Suture anchors can be used to secure the capsule and generally are preferred.
- The tension on the capsular flap that is selected must eliminate the inferior pouch and reduce the posterior capsular redundancy (Fig. 3.30D). Suture the inferior flap first, drawing the superior flap down over it, and suture it so as to cause the middle glenohumeral ligament to reinforce the capsule anteriorly and to act as a sling against inferior subluxation.
- Hold the arm in slight flexion and about 10 degrees of external rotation on the arm board while the anterior portion of the capsule is reattached with nonabsorbable sutures. Bigliani et al. recommended repairing the capsule with the arm held in approximately 25 degrees of external rotation and 20 degrees of abduction. For throwers, they recommended relatively more abduction and external rotation to ensure full range of motion.
- Bring the subscapularis tendon over the reattached anterior portion, and reattach the tendon at its normal location.
- After closure of the deltopectoral interval with absorbable sutures and after closure of the skin with a skin stitch, maintain the arm at the side in neutral flexion-extension and in about 20 degrees of internal rotation by light plastic splints.

POSTOPERATIVE CARE Postoperatively, the extremity is placed in a commercially available shoulder immobilizer with the shoulder in 30 to 40 degrees of abduction and slight external rotation. Range-of-motion exercises for the elbow, wrist, and hand are started immediately, with Codman's exercises of the shoulder being added on the third postoperative day. External rotation to 10 degrees, forward elevation to 90 degrees, and isometric exercises are begun after 10 days. For 2 to 4 weeks, isometric strengthening is continued and external rotation is increased to 30 degrees and forward elevation to 140 degrees. At 4 to 6 weeks, resistive exercises are begun and external rotation is increased to 40 degrees and forward elevation to 160 degrees. At 6 weeks, external rotation is increased to

50 degrees and forward elevation to 180 degrees. At 3 months, external rotation can be progressed. In the dominant shoulder of throwers, external rotation should be progressed more quickly; however, progression that is too quick can lead to recurrent instability, especially in patients in late adolescence.

The internal and external rotators curb anterior and posterior displacement, and the supraspinatus and middle part of the deltoid curb inferior displacement. Complete recovery of the muscles probably is necessary to protect the repair because the capsule and ligaments normally function only as a checkrein. Lifting more than 9 kg and participating in sports are prohibited for 9 months and until muscle strength is normal on manual testing compared with the contralateral side. Ligament healing is more mature at 1 year, and patients are advised against swimming with the backstroke or butterfly stroke, heavy overhead use of the involved arm, and participation in contact sports during the first year after surgery.

■ CAPSULAR SHIFT WITH INCISION ADJACENT TO THE GLENOID

O'Brien, Warren, and Schwartz described a technique for a capsular shift procedure in which the T portion of the incision is made adjacent to the glenoid. This technique allows much easier repair of a detached glenoid labrum if this is present. If the instability is mainly an inferior instability with no glenoid labrum tear, however, and it is necessary to tighten well around to the posterior aspect of the humerus, we have found the technique of Neer to allow more posterior tightening. With the Neer technique, the posterior portion of the T can be extended farther as the humerus is externally rotated.

■ HILL-SACHS LESIONS

Large, engaging Hill-Sachs lesions involving 20% to 30% of the humeral head may be treated by disimpaction and bone grafting in the acute stage. Transfer of the infraspinatus tendon is useful in the chronic setting. Wolf et al. described an arthroscopic procedure to suture the infraspinatus tendon into the defect and reported good results. Larger defects of 30% to 40% may be treated indirectly with a Latarjet procedure, extending to the glenoid articulation; this prevents engagement of the Hill-Sachs defect. This is our preferred technique. The humeral head defect also can be approached directly and filled to prevent engagement. Small series of allograft reconstructions have shown satisfactory results, although some patients had to have the screws removed at a later date.

POSTERIOR INSTABILITY OF THE SHOULDER

Posterior shoulder dislocations and recurrent posterior instability of the shoulder account for only about 5% to 10% of all dislocations of the shoulder. Traumatic events that result in posterior dislocation often are associated with altered consciousness, such as occurs with seizures, electrical shock, and intoxication. Posterior dislocation also can be caused by a direct blow to the anterior shoulder or by a fall on a forward-flexed extremity.

Recurrent posterior subluxation, atraumatic or acquired as a result of repetitive microtrauma, is much more common than recurrence after a traumatic posterior dislocation. These instability patterns must be evaluated carefully and categorized as unidirectional, bidirectional, or multidirectional, and the direction of dislocations and symptomatic subluxations must be determined. Repetitive overuse and microtraumatic injuries that result in posterior instability include sports requiring overhead motion, such as pitching, tennis, and swimming (especially backstroke and breaststroke), weight lifting (especially bench press), and blocking by offensive linemen, all of which inflict repetitive trauma on the posterior capsule. Andrews and Phillips described recurrent posterior instability of the dominant shoulder in batters. This most commonly occurs with a check swing or pulling of an outside pitch, which alters the normal synchronous swing mechanics and increases the posteriorly directed shear forces on the shoulder.

Many patients with instability of microtraumatic or atraumatic origin learn to sublux their shoulder voluntarily with horizontal adduction and internal rotation; however, this does not mean there is a psychologic overlay. A patient who has a bland type of affect and who is able to sublux his shoulder with muscular contraction alone is more likely to have some psychologic overlay and secondary gain. With the shoulder in the abducted position, such patients selectively use internal rotators to sublux the shoulder posteriorly. These patients rarely, if ever, should be surgically treated.

In the past, glenoid version has been implicated in posterior instability; however, we believe that glenoid version contributes significantly to posterior instability only in patients with severe congenital dysplasia or traumatic disruption of the bony architecture. Fuchs, Jost, and Gerber stated that glenoid osteotomy is indicated when more than 10 degrees of retroversion is present. Because of high complication rates, osteotomies have fallen out of favor.

■ CONSERVATIVE TREATMENT

The initial treatment of posterior shoulder instability should be nonoperative. The regimen includes having the patient avoid provocative activities and educating the patient to avoid specific voluntary maneuvers that would cause the posterior subluxation. A strengthening exercise program aimed at the external rotators and posterior deltoid is carried out. Normal motion also should be obtained.

Most patients with posterior instability respond to an aggressive exercise program, especially patients with generalized ligamentous laxity and instability occurring as a result of repetitive microtrauma. In athletes who use overhead motion, observation and instruction by a knowledgeable coach can provide slight alterations in mechanics that may reduce the instability episodes.

Patients who have traumatic dislocations are less likely to be helped by an exercise program. Traumatic dislocations are most common in athletes who have repetitive posteriorly directed forces to the shoulder, such as football linemen, hockey players, and platform divers. If at least 4 to 6 months of an appropriate rehabilitation program has failed, if habitual dislocation has been ruled out, and if the patient is emotionally stable, surgery may be indicated if the pain and instability preclude adequate function of the involved shoulder.

■ SURGICAL TREATMENT

Through the years, various types of procedures have been proposed to correct posterior instability, including soft-tissue procedures such as the "reverse" Bankart and Putti-Platt procedures, muscle transfers and capsulorrhaphies, bone blocks, and glenoid osteotomies. The results of surgical treatment of posterior shoulder instability have been as varied as the techniques designed to correct it. In general, the best results with any procedure done to correct posterior instability are obtained in patients with recurrent traumatic posterior dislocation, not the more common posterior instability syndromes.

We do not recommend surgery on patients with this atraumatic type of posterior instability, unless they have frequent and significant disability and conservative treatment has failed. The dislocation must not be habitual, and the patient must be emotionally stable.

In any patient who has persistence of instability, a positive jerk test, and a positive shift in load test and any labral pathology (as indicated by the clunk test anterior or posterior), further workup is indicated. This includes T2-weighted axial MRI with contrast enhancement to evaluate for capsular deficiency and loss of chondral labral containment as described by Kim et al. and Antoniou and Harryman (Fig. 3.31). Both authors found chondrolabral cavity lesions in more than 80% of patients with erosion, cracking, or partial detachment posteriorly and inferiorly (i.e., the Kim lesion of the labrum). These deficiencies should be evaluated as noted with MRI, but, more importantly, arthroscopically at the time of stabilization. If an open technique is to be done, arthroscopic examination for these lesions is indicated in most instances and to

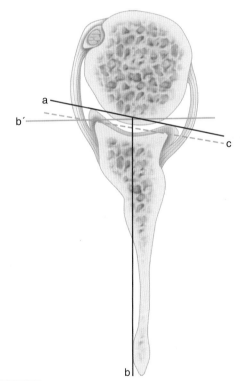

FIGURE 3.31 Measurement of version of chondrolabral and osseous portions of the glenoid. *a,* reference line representing plane of chondrolabral portion of glenoid; *b,* reference line representing plane of scapular body; *c,* reference line representing plane of osseous portion of glenoid. Angle between *a* and *b'* (perpendicular to *b*) represents version of chondrolabral portion of glenoid. Angle between *c* and *b'* represents version of osseous portion of glenoid (Kim et al.).

evaluate the rotator interval anteriorly. With a large rotator interval, a greater than 1 cm gap between the superior and middle glenohumeral ligaments at the edge of the glenoid, closure of the rotator interval should be done, particularly with external rotation of more 90 degrees at 0 degrees of abduction and a positive sulcus sign. If an open procedure is to be done posteriorly, this can be performed after completion of the arthroscopic examination and interval closure anteriorly. Also to be evaluated by MRI is severe glenoid retroversion, which is fairly unusual as previously described or, more commonly, loss of the bony glenoid rim. In the case of a fracture involving the rim, either arthroscopic or open fixation is indicated. For a larger fracture, an open procedure is indicated. For labral detachment producing pain but without true instability, the lesion is repaired in situ without capsular plication.

Treatment of posterior instability is approached the same as anterior instability by restoring the anatomy and tensioning the capsule appropriately. If surgery is required for a disabling posterior subluxation, or if posterior is the most significant plane in a multidirectional instability syndrome, the procedure that we have found most successful is the inferior capsular shift procedure through a posterior approach. We prefer either the capsular shift technique of Tibone or that of Neer and Foster for atraumatic multidirectional instability in a patient who is not an athlete who uses throwing or overhead motions. For an athlete with recurrent posterior subluxation who requires overhead movement, we prefer the muscle-splitting technique with medial shift as described by Tibone et al. The technique described by Hawkins and Janda is best reserved for a laborer or an athlete involved in contact sports, such as football or ice hockey, with recurrent posterior subluxation secondary to capsular deficiency. We have observed good to excellent results with this open procedure, but have had superior results with arthroscopic procedures unless severe bone deficiency must be treated.

NEER INFERIOR CAPSULAR SHIFT PROCEDURE THROUGH A POSTERIOR APPROACH

Neer and Foster described an inferior capsular shift procedure performed through a posterior approach. In this procedure, the posterior capsule is split longitudinally, and the capsular attachment along the humeral neck is released as far inferiorly and anteriorly as possible. The superior capsule is advanced inferiorly, and the inferior capsule is advanced superiorly. The infraspinatus is cut so that it is overlapped and shortened, adding further buttress to the posterior capsule. This procedure obliterates the axillary pouch and redundancy. It and other capsular shift procedures are indicated in posterior subluxation syndromes that are not true traumatic recurrent posterior dislocations.

TECHNIQUE 3.9

(NEER AND FOSTER)
- For the posterior approach, place the patient on the operating table in the lateral decubitus position with the

involved shoulder up. The patient is held in position with a beanbag and kidney rest.
- Make a 10-cm incision vertically over the posterior aspect of the acromion and the spine of the scapula (Fig. 3.32A).
- Undermine the subcutaneous tissue to expose the deltoid muscle. Split the deltoid muscle from an area on the spine of the scapula, beginning 2 to 3 cm medial to the posterolateral corner of the acromion and extending distally 5 to 6 cm (Fig. 3.32B). To protect the axillary nerve, the deltoid muscle should not be split distally beyond the teres minor. In a muscular individual, the deltoid muscle can be reflected from the spine of the scapula or the acromion.
- Expose the teres minor and infraspinatus muscles, and develop the interval between these muscles (Fig. 3.32C).
- Detach the infraspinatus obliquely so that the superficial piece of tendon can be used later to reinforce the posterior part of the capsule (Fig. 3.33).
- Make a T-shaped opening in the posterior pouch in the posterior part of the capsule (Fig. 3.34A).
- Form a superior capsular flap by detaching 1.5 cm of capsule above the initial longitudinal capsular incision.
- Use a flat elevator to protect the axillary nerve and, with the arm in progressive internal rotation, form the inferior capsular flap by detaching the capsule from the neck of the humerus around to the anterior portion of the calcar.

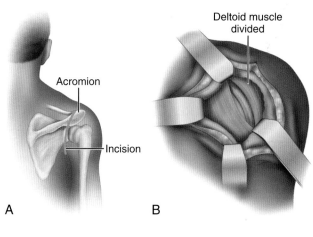

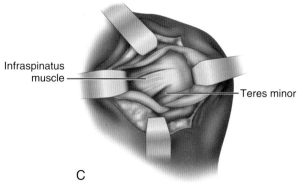

FIGURE 3.32 Neer and Foster posterior capsulorrhaphy for posterior shoulder subluxation. **A,** Saber cut skin incision just posterior to acromioclavicular joint toward posterior axillary fold. **B,** Deltoid muscle is split in line with fibers beginning 2–3 cm medial to posterolateral corner of acromion. **C,** Exposure of underlying infraspinatus and teres minor muscles. **SEE TECHNIQUE 3.9.**

- Elevate the teres minor from the capsule and leave it intact.
- Distract the joint (with the addition of muscle relaxants as necessary) so that the glenoid labrum can be inspected anteriorly. If the anterior portion of the glenoid labrum has been detached, make a second approach anteriorly through which the labrum is sutured to the bone of the glenoid (Bankart repair). If the anterior part of the labrum is intact, draw the posterior part of the capsule backward to eliminate the inferior pouch and to reduce anterior capsular laxity (Fig. 3.34B).
- With curets and a small gouge, make a shallow slot in the sulcus of the humeral neck so that the capsular flap is approximated to raw bone. Hold the arm in slight extension and moderate external rotation as the capsule is reattached (Fig. 3.34B).
- During tensioning of the flaps, Bigliani suggested holding the extremity in 5 to 10 degrees of external rotation, 10 to 15 degrees of abduction, and neutral flexion and extension. Reattach the superior flap first while drawing it downward to eliminate the posterior pouch. Next, draw the longer inferior flap over it, and turn back the excess part of the capsule for reinforcement posteriorly. Use the superficial portion of the infraspinatus to reinforce the posterior portion of the capsule further (Fig. 3.34C).
- Reattach the deep part of the infraspinatus superficially to preserve active external rotation, and carefully reattach the deltoid if it has been detached.
- Close the wound, and immobilize the arm at the side in neutral flexion-extension and 10 degrees of external rotation by means of a light plaster splint extending from the wrist to the middle part of the arm and around the waist, with the elbow bent 90 degrees. Rigid external immobilization is needed to ensure that 10 degrees of external rotation is maintained.

POSTOPERATIVE CARE The shoulder is immobilized with the arm at the side in slight abduction and neutral rotation for 6 weeks after surgery. A plastic brace maintains this position, supports the weight of the arm, and prevents inferior stress on the repair. Range-of-motion exercises with elevation in the scapular plane and external rotation and isometric exercises are begun 6 weeks after the surgery when the brace is removed. These exercises are progressed over the next 3 months to a full strengthening program. Elevation of more than 150 degrees and internal rotation exercises that might stress the repair are avoided for 3 months. Sports activities such as swimming and throwing are not allowed for 9 months to 1 year after surgery.

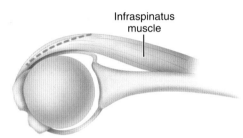

FIGURE 3.33 Neer and Foster inferior capsular shift through posterior approach. Detachment of infraspinatus tendon. **SEE TECHNIQUE 3.9.**

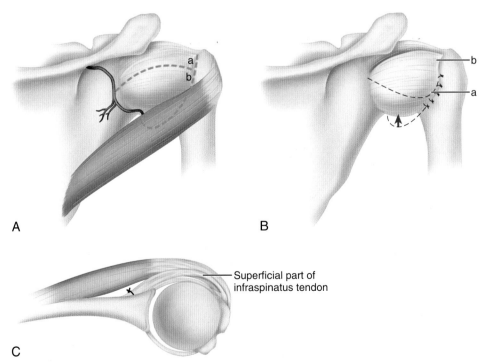

A

B

C

Superficial part of infraspinatus tendon

FIGURE 3.34 Neer and Foster inferior capsular shift through posterior approach. **A,** T-shaped incision to form superior flap *(a)* and inferior flap *(b)*. **B,** Relocation of flaps. **C,** Reinforcement of capsular flaps. Superficial part of infraspinatus tendon is brought down and sutured against raw bone on scapular neck; deep portion is sutured over this. **SEE TECHNIQUE 3.9.**

TIBONE AND BRADLEY TECHNIQUE

Tibone and Bradley recommended a variation on the posterior capsular shift procedure in which the interval between the infraspinatus and teres minor muscles is split to expose the posterior capsule. The capsule is shifted on the glenoid side to reduce the volume of the posterior capsule in a manner similar to that described by Neer and Foster and Bigliani et al. Shaffer et al. described an infraspinatus muscle–splitting incision in which the bipennate muscle is split between its two innervations, resulting in no long-term trauma to the muscle. They stated that this may allow better exposure of the middle portion of the posterior capsule and make the capsular shift easier. Whether the split of the bipennate infraspinatus or the split between the infraspinatus and the teres minor is used, damage to the posterior rotator cuff is reduced. The advantage of this approach is that imbrication of the posterior capsule produces a thicker posterior soft-tissue restraint. This is our preferred technique in athletes with a moderate amount of posterior instability.

TECHNIQUE 3.10

(TIBONE AND BRADLEY)

- Place the patient in the lateral decubitus position, and approach the shoulder as described in the technique for the Neer posterior capsular shift procedure.
- When the capsule has been sufficiently separated from the overlying muscles, make a transverse arthrotomy incision into the posterior capsule from a lateral to medial direction up to the labrum (Fig. 3.35A and B) and inspect the joint.
- Develop two capsular flaps by making a T-shaped incision into the capsule parallel to the glenoid cavity and just adjacent to the labrum. Tag these flaps with sutures to control them (Fig. 3.35C). The inferior capsular flap must be developed carefully because of the close proximity of the axillary nerve on the undersurface of the capsule. Usually the labrum is found intact.
- If the labrum is torn, reflect it so that holes can be made in the posterior glenoid cavity and sutures can be passed

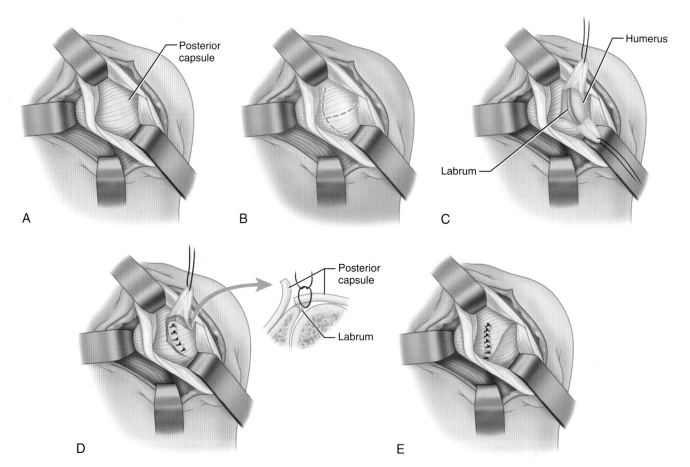

FIGURE 3.35 Tibone and Bradley posterior capsulorrhaphy for posterior shoulder subluxation. **A,** Development of interval between teres minor and infraspinatus muscle to expose capsule. **B,** Capsular incision from lateral to medial, up to glenoid labrum. **C,** Vertical capsular incision parallel to glenoid labrum. **D,** Medial and superior advancement of inferior capsular flap and attachment to labrum. *Inset,* Suture of flap to labrum. **E,** Suture of superior capsular flap over inferior flap. **SEE TECHNIQUE 3.10.**

directly through the bone as in a typical anterior Bankart repair. (Suture anchors can be used to secure the capsule to the neck adjacent to the glenoid articular cartilage.)

- When the labrum is intact, the sutures can be placed directly into the labrum.
- Advance the inferior capsular flap superiorly and medially, and attach it to the glenoid labrum with nonabsorbable sutures (Fig. 3.35D). This usually eliminates the posterior and any inferior instability.
- Suture the superior capsular flap over the inferior flap by advancing it inferiorly and medially.
- Close any remaining transverse gap in the capsule laterally with interrupted mattress sutures (Fig. 3.35E). The teres minor and infraspinatus muscles come together and usually do not need sutures.
- Close the wound in layers.

POSTOPERATIVE CARE The shoulder is placed in an abduction pillow in slight extension and neutral rotation to take stress off the repair. The pillow is removed at 3 weeks. Active and active-assisted range-of-motion exercises are started. At this time, emphasis is placed on elevating the arm in the scapular plane of the body and regaining internal and external rotation of the shoulder. At 6 weeks, forward flexion is allowed. At 12 weeks, weightlifting is started and progressed to increase strength and endurance. At 6 months, light throwing and noncontact sports can be resumed. At 1 year, a throwing athlete can return to competition.

CAPSULAR SHIFT RECONSTRUCTION WITH POSTERIOR GLENOID OSTEOTOMY

Posterior glenoplasty rarely is indicated, although it can be used if severe developmental or traumatic glenoid retroversion of more than 20 degrees is confirmed on CT reconstructed films. High recurrence rates of up to 53% have been reported with this procedure. Hawkins et al. reported a complication rate of 29%, including osteonecrosis of the glenoid and degenerative arthritis of the glenohumeral joint, after this procedure. Currently, a similar but simpler procedure using a glenoid osteotomy is preferred for severe glenoid dysplasia, whether traumatic or congenital. The same exposure can be used for bone graft reconstruction of a deficient posterior glenoid.

TECHNIQUE 3.11

(ROCKWOOD)
- Place the patient in the lateral decubitus position with the involved shoulder upward.
- Make a skin incision beginning 2.5 cm medial to the posterolateral corner of the acromion and extending downward 10 cm to the posterior axillary crease (Fig. 3.36A).
- Dissect and retract the subcutaneous tissues to expose the deltoid fibers.

- At a point 2.5 cm medial to the posterior corner of the acromion, split the deltoid distally 10 cm in line with its fibers (Fig. 3.36B). Retract the deltoid medially and laterally to expose the underlying infraspinatus and teres minor muscles.
- Reflect the teres minor tendon inferiorly down to the level of the inferior joint capsule, and divide the infraspinatus tendon. Reflect it medially and laterally, avoiding injury to the suprascapular nerve (Fig. 3.36C).
- Make a vertical incision in the posterior capsule to explore the joint. Make the incision midway between the humeral and glenoid attachments so that a double-breasted closure can be done (Fig. 3.36D). The teres minor muscle must be reflected sufficiently inferior so that the vertical cut in the capsule goes all the way down to the most inferior recess of the capsule.
- Pass a straight blunt instrument into the glenohumeral joint so that it lies on the anterior and posterior glenoid rims (Fig. 3.36E). Place an osteotome intracapsularly and direct it parallel to the blunt instrument. This is done to lessen the chance of the osteotomy cut entering the joint.
- The osteotomy site is not more than 0.6 cm medial to the articular surface of the glenoid. If the osteotomy site is more medial than this, injury to the suprascapular nerve is possible as it passes around the base of the spine of the scapula to supply the infraspinatus muscle. Each time the osteotome is advanced, pry open the osteotomy site; this helps create a lateral plastic deformation of the posterior glenoid.
- The osteotomy incision should not exit anteriorly, but should stop just at the anterior cortex of the scapula (Fig. 3.36F). The intact anterior cortex, periosteum, and soft tissue act as a hinge, which allows the graft to be secure in the osteotomy without the need for internal fixation.
- Take bone graft approximately 8 mm × 30 mm from the acromion. Use osteotomes to open up the osteotomy site, and place the bone graft into position (Fig. 3.36G).
- Place nonabsorbable sutures in the edge of the medial capsule.
- Hold the arm in neutral rotation, and suture the medial capsule laterally and superiorly under the lateral capsule (Fig. 3.36H). Suture the lateral capsule medially and superiorly over the medial capsule (Fig. 3.36I). Repair the infraspinatus tendon with the arm in neutral rotation. If the tendon is lax, double-breast it (Fig. 3.36J).
- Close the incision in layers.

POSTOPERATIVE CARE For the first 24 hours, the arm is maintained in neutral position and supported by skin traction. When the patient can comfortably stand, a modified shoulder immobilizer cast is applied by attaching a lightweight long arm cast to a belly band that sits around the abdomen and iliac crest. The arm is connected to this belly band through supports to maintain the arm in 10 to 15 degrees of abduction and neutral rotation. The cast is left in place for 6 to 8 weeks. After removal of the cast, the patient is allowed to use the arm for 4 to 6 weeks for activities of daily living. A rehabilitation program is begun, including pendulum exercises, isometric exercises, and stretching of the shoulder with the use of an overhead pulley. Afterward, resistive exercises are gradually increased.

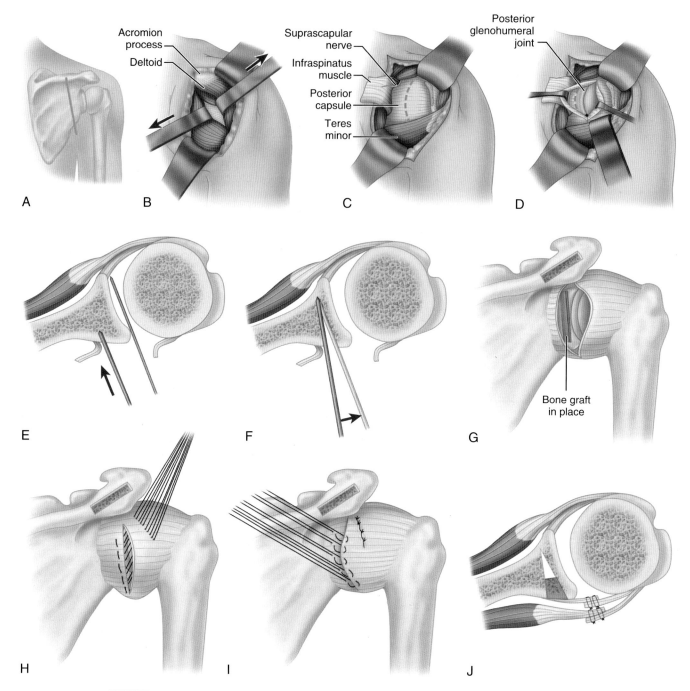

FIGURE 3.36 Rockwood technique of posterior shoulder reconstruction. **A,** Incision. **B,** Splitting of deltoid in line with its fibers. **C** and **D,** Capsular incision midway between humeral and glenoid attachments. **E,** Determination of angle of slope of glenoid. **F,** Glenoid osteotomy. **G,** Bone graft in place. **H,** Suture of medial capsule. **I,** Suture of lateral capsule. **J,** Suture of tendon to reduce laxity. **SEE TECHNIQUE 3.11.**

MCLAUGHLIN PROCEDURE

For recurrent posterior dislocation associated with a large anterior medial Hill-Sachs lesion, McLaughlin described transfer of the subscapularis tendon into the defect. Neer and Foster subsequently described transfer of the subscap-ularis with the lesser tuberosity into the defect and securing it with a bone screw. In a rare reverse Hill-Sachs lesion with involvement of 20% to 25% of the articular surface, trans-fer of the subscapularis with the tuberosity placed into the defect has been shown to produce satisfactory results in moderate-size defects; also, allografts in case reports involving larger lesions have provided satisfactory results.

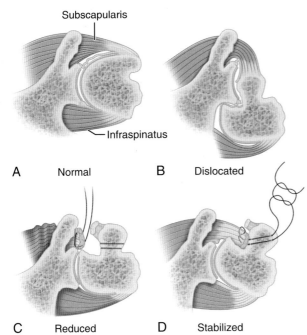

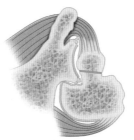

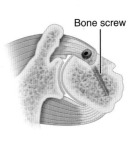

FIGURE 3.38 Neer and Foster modification of McLaughlin technique. Lesser tuberosity, with attached subscapularis tendon, is transferred into defect and fixed with bone screw. **SEE TECHNIQUE 3.12.**

FIGURE 3.37 McLaughlin technique for posterior dislocation of shoulder. **A,** Cross section of left shoulder viewed from above. **B,** Deformity in posterior dislocation with engagement of posterior glenoid rim in defect of anterior aspect of humeral head. **C,** Dislocation has been reduced, but instability remains; redislocation occurs with internal rotation, flexion, or adduction. Subscapularis has been divided. **D,** Stabilization by medial transposition of subscapularis insertion into defect. **SEE TECHNIQUE 3.12.**

BOX 3.3

Causes of Failure in Surgical Repair of Posterior Shoulder Instability

- Inadequate soft-tissue healing
- Ligamentous laxity
- Deficient capsule
- Deficient subscapularis
- Deficient glenoid
- Engaging Hill-Sachs lesion
- Overconstrained joint
- Nerve dysfunction

TECHNIQUE 3.12

(MCLAUGHLIN)

- Approach the shoulder anteriorly through the deltopectoral interval.
- Retract the conjoined tendon medially, exposing the subscapularis tendon. Divide the subscapularis tendon transversely as close to its insertion as possible.
- Alternatively, as described by Neer and Foster, osteotomize the lesser tuberosity with the insertion of the tendon. The added fragment of the lesser tuberosity helps fill the defect in the anteromedial humeral neck.
- Debride the surfaces of the defect in the anteromedial humeral neck.
- Reattach the subscapularis tendon to the humerus in the depths of the defect by mattress sutures passed through holes drilled in the bone (Fig. 3.37). Alternatively, as described by Neer and Foster, fix the lesser tuberosity together with the subscapularis tendon in the defect with a bone screw (Fig. 3.38).

POSTOPERATIVE CARE A shoulder immobilizer is applied. Pendulum exercises are started after the wound has healed, and gradual resumption of normal use is encouraged. The patient is protected from any forced external rotation forces for at least 3 months.

■ SURGICAL FAILURES

Causes of surgical failures are listed in Box 3.3. A thorough physical examination and 3D CT imaging are indicated to evaluate bony defects (see Fig. 3.17). Significant glenoid bone loss has been identified as a major factor in surgical failures, as have hyperlaxity and Hill-Sachs lesions. A Latarjet procedure, structural bone grafts, or remplissage procedures can be used as previously described for revision surgeries. Capsular deficiencies can be treated with a Latarjet procedure or soft-tissue allograft supplementation of the capsule with Achilles or posterior tibial tendon allografts. Subscapular deficiency is reconstructed with a pectoralis transfer. Finally, a careful search should be made to determine that a humeral avulsion of the glenohumeral ligament (HAGL lesion) is not present. Excessive loss of motion after arthroscopic procedures generally can be corrected by precision arthroscopic releases. Open procedures may be necessary when a previous open procedure was used.

ARTHROSCOPIC SURGERY

Arthroscopic repair of shoulder instability is an area of increasing interest and continued improvement. As experience increases with these techniques, the operative results have improved to be comparable to, and in some cases surpass, results obtained with more standard open techniques. Arthroscopic shoulder surgery is discussed in other chapter.

ELBOW

Acute dislocation of the elbow occurs relatively frequently, accounting for 28% of all injuries to the elbow. Elbow dislocation usually is a high-energy episode with severe soft-tissue injury, and residual loss of motion is common. Recurrent dislocation of the elbow is relatively rare, however, and usually is posterior. Persistence of posterolateral or medial instability is more common and, when symptomatic, should be surgically corrected in appropriate patients.

ANATOMY

The lateral ulnar collateral ligament of the elbow arises from the epicondyle and inserts on the annular ligament (Fig. 3.39). A separate band of the lateral ligamentous complex, the lateral ulnar collateral ligament, arises at the lateral epicondyle and blends with fibers of the annular ligament before inserting on the tubercle on the crest of the supinator of the ulna. This band has been described as the main lateral stabilizer, taut in flexion and extension, with disruption of this portion of the lateral complex resulting in posterolateral rotatory instability. The lateral collateral ligament contributes only 14% of the varus stability of the elbow with the joint in full extension and only 9% with the joint in 90 degrees of flexion. The remainder of the stability is contributed by the bony articular surfaces and the anterior capsule, with the bony surfaces supplying most of the stability.

The ulnar collateral ligament of the elbow is a well-developed ligament that can be described as three distinct portions (Fig. 3.40). In contrast to the lateral collateral ligament, the ulnar collateral ligament plays an important role in valgus stability. Valgus stability is divided equally among the ulnar collateral ligament, the anterior capsule, and the bony articulation with the elbow in full extension. At 90 degrees of flexion, the ulnar collateral ligament provides 55% of the stability

to valgus stress, with the anterior bundle being the primary stabilizer.

PATHOPHYSIOLOGY

Elbow instability may be congenital, traumatic, or attritional. The primary stabilizers of the elbow are the anterior band of the medial ulnar collateral ligament and the lateral collateral ligament complex, consisting of the lateral collateral ligament, annular ligament, and the lateral ulnar collateral ligament. Secondary stabilizers consist of the capsule, the ulnohumeral and radiocapitellar articulations, and the dynamic stabilizers, consisting of all muscle-tendon units that cross the elbow joint (i.e., biceps, brachialis, triceps, wrist flexors, and wrist extensors). Insufficiency of one or more of the stabilizers may result in a spectrum of instability from subtle valgus or posterolateral rotatory instability to recurrent dislocation.

In a long-term follow-up study of simple elbow dislocations, Anakwe et al. found that 60% of patients had residual stiffness with loss of extension and residual pain. Only 8% had functional instability. When fractures are associated with the dislocation, resulting in loss of bony stability being provided by the greater sigmoid notch of the ulna or the radiocapitellar joint, greater instability and disability can be anticipated.

O'Driscoll et al. described the typical injury pattern for traumatic elbow dislocation, with the individual falling on a slightly flexed extremity and a valgus internal rotation force of the humerus on the pronated fixed position of the forearm. Structures are disrupted on the lateral side, progressing medially as more force is applied (Fig. 3.41). When recurrence or persistence in instability results, the posterolateral structures are most commonly affected, but the medial structures also can be involved and cause significant instability. A coronoid fracture in association with disruption of the posterior band of the ulnar collateral ligament can result in symptomatic posteromedial instability. Thus close evaluation of both primary stabilizers is warranted. Isolated medial side disruptions from valgus stress can result from football tackling, gymnastics, or throwing a javelin.

Valgus instability from attritional disruption of the anterior bundle of the medial ulnar collateral ligament is by far the most common form of recurrent elbow instability. The anterior bundle is divided into two nonisometric bands: an anterior band, which is taut at 0 to 60 degrees, and a posterior

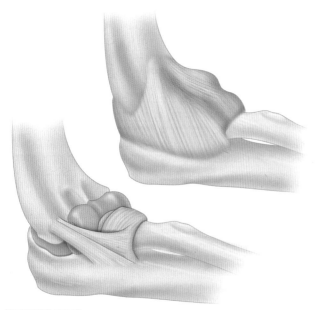

FIGURE 3.39   Lateral soft-tissue structures of elbow, including ulnar and radial part of lateral collateral ligament, annular ligament, and overlying capsule.

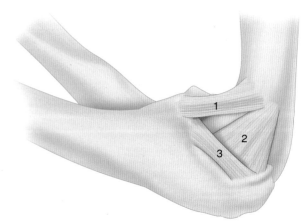

FIGURE 3.40   Medial elbow ligaments. *1,* Anterior oblique; *2,* posterior oblique; *3,* transverse oblique.

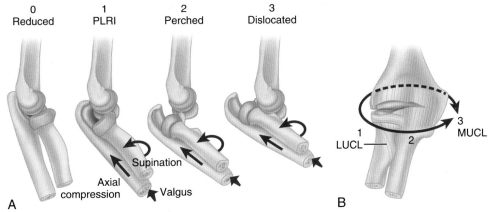

FIGURE 3.41 Injury pattern for traumatic elbow dislocation described by O'Driscoll et al. **A,** Three stages of elbow instability from subluxation to dislocation: stage 1, disruption of the ulnar part of the lateral collateral ligament; stage 2, disruption of the other lateral ligamentous structures and posterior capsule; stage 3A, partial disruption of the medial ulnar collateral ligament and posterior medial ulnar collateral ligament only; and stage 3B, complete disruption of the medial ulnar collateral ligament and posterior medial ulnar collateral ligament. **B,** Soft-tissue injury progresses in a circle from lateral to medial correlating with those shown in **A**. *LUCL,* lateral ulnar collateral ligament; *MUCL,* medial ulnar collateral ligament; *PLRI,* posterolateral rotatory instability

band, which is taut at 60 to 120 degrees. During the acceleration phase of throwing, up to 60 N of force is applied to the ligament, which is near its tensile failure point. Pitcher fatigue, poor mechanics, or repetition overuse can result in bundle fiber failure, partial tearing, and eventual complete disruption.

Failure of the primary stabilizer results in increased stress on secondary stabilizers, with resulting capsular contractures, chondromalacia, osteophytes, and loose bodies from compression of the radiocapitellar joint and shear forces to the posteromedial tip of the olecranon. Ulnar nerve symptoms may develop from traction, scarring, or osteophyte impingement.

PHYSICAL EXAMINATION

Examination of the elbow begins with a visual inspection for atrophy, swelling, or ecchymosis. The forearm circumference is measured 7 cm below the medial epicondyle to compare with the opposite extremity. Fluid can be detected in the soft spot posterolaterally. The flexor pronator mass, the ulnar collateral ligament, and the tip of the olecranon posteromedially are carefully palpated for the area of most tenderness. Tenderness and swelling 2 to 3 cm distal to the olecranon tip may indicate an olecranon stress fracture. Active and passive range of motion is recorded, and a valgus stress is applied to the elbow with the forearm in the supinated and the pronated positions and the elbow in about 30 degrees of flexion. The amount of medial opening, the firmness of the end point, and the production of medial pain should be noted when valgus is applied with the forearm pronated (Fig. 3.42).

The valgus extension overload test is done by maintaining a valgus stress on the elbow while the elbow is passively extended from 30 degrees down. Pain along the posteromedial aspect of the olecranon can be produced when subacute or chronic instability has resulted in posteromedial olecranon impingement. O'Driscoll described the active valgus extension overload test, which he thought was the most accurate test for ulnar collateral ligament competence. With the patient's shoulder abducted and externally rotated, a valgus stress is applied on the elbow as it is passively extended from 120 degrees down to 30 degrees and then flexed back in a rapid sequence.

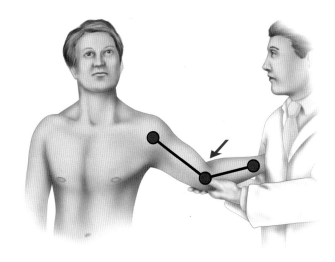

FIGURE 3.42 Test for elbow instability.

Generation of medial pain may indicate ligamentous incompetence. The milking maneuver is likewise performed by putting valgus stress on the elbow by pulling on the patient's thumb while stabilizing the arm and ranging the elbow between 30 and 120 degrees. Although valgus stress and compression are applied to the radiocapitellar joint, the forearm is pronated and supinated with the elbow in varying degrees of flexion to evaluate radiocapitellar crepitance or the production of pain, indicative of radiocapitellar chondromalacia.

The patient is placed prone, and the ulnar nerve is evaluated by the Tinel test. With the shoulder abducted to 90 degrees and the elbow flexed 90 degrees, the ulnar nerve is evaluated to see if it subluxes anteriorly from its groove with passive elbow motion or with manual stress on the nerve. Valgus stress again can be applied to the elbow when flexed greater than 30 degrees to detect medial instability.

Posterolateral instability can be evaluated by supinating the forearm and applying a valgus moment and axial force with the elbow flexed 20 to 30 degrees. A clunking sensation may indicate posterolateral laxity. The same test can be done with the extremity over the patient's head and the shoulder fully externally rotated. With the forearm fully supinated and valgus stress applied, the elbow is moved from a fully extended position to a flexed position. As the elbow is flexed near 40 degrees, a posterolateral prominence is produced by subluxation of the radial head; as the joint is flexed further, a dimple in the soft spot area appears and eventually disappears as the radius and ulna snap back into place on the humerus (Fig. 3.43). A variation of this examination, which reproduces functional posterolateral instability, is the table or seat press-up test, which is performed by having the patient push up with the forearm supinated while the examiner feels and observes for radial head instability. Wall or floor push-ups with the forearm in supination accomplish the same objective.

Diagnostic radiographs should include anteroposterior and lateral views and two 45-degree oblique views to evaluate the radiocapitellar joint and the trochlear joint. In patients with chronic medial symptoms, a Jones view of the elbow is indicated to determine if posteromedial osteophytes are present. In the presence of recent elbow subluxation or dislocation, the drop sign, widening of the ulnohumeral joint, may represent significant capsular disruption and persistent subluxation. A gravity

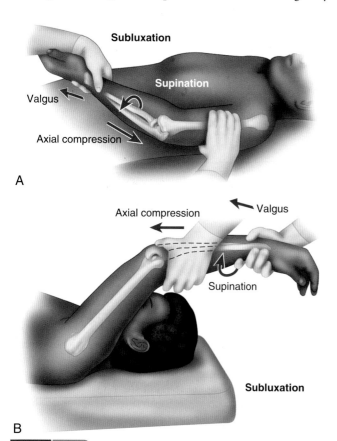

FIGURE 3.43   Test for posterolateral rotatory instability of elbow. **A,** With arm at side and forearm in supination, supination and valgus moments and axial forces are applied to elbow, which is flexed 20–30 degrees. Posterolateral subluxation is visibly and palpably reduced when elbow is flexed farther. **B,** Same procedure is done much more easily with patient's arm over his or her head. Full external rotation of shoulder provides counterforce for supination of forearm and leaves one of examiner's hands free to control valgus moments.

stress radiograph can be obtained with the patient supine, the shoulder abducted 90 degrees and externally rotated, the forearm supinated, and the elbow flexed 20 to 30 degrees. A lateral radiograph is obtained to show the opening of the medial side of the elbow to gravity stress. This is not a highly sensitive test, although a positive test does indicate a significant injury to the ulnar collateral ligament. Gadolinium-enhanced MR arthrograms or CT arthrograms are indicated to evaluate for complete or incomplete undersurface tears of the ulnar collateral ligament. Timmerman and Andrews described the *T sign* as a leak of contrast material around the humerus or ulna without extracapsular leakage. Currently the best test of ulnar collateral ligament instability is a gadolinium-enhanced MRI of the elbow to evaluate for extravasation of fluid (T sign) or degenerative changes in the ulnar collateral ligament. Edema of the soft tissues medial to the ulnar collateral ligament generally indicates ligamentous damage. Some centers use ultrasound to evaluate the ulnar collateral ligament in the relaxed and stressed positions. Nonetheless, MRI allows for better visualization.

NONOPERATIVE TREATMENT

Acute complete simple dislocations are categorized as stable or unstable after reduction. For stable elbows, early range of motion is indicated. For unstable elbows, an elbow splint is used to control range of motion, blocking extension at 45 degrees for 1 week, 30 degrees for the next week, and allowing full motion thereafter. If a contracture of more than 30 degrees is still present after 6 weeks, an extension splint can be used to improve motion. For incomplete injuries that involve disruption of the medial side of the elbow, the forearm is placed in supination. Lateral injuries are treated by placing the forearm in pronation with the elbow flexed 70 degrees for 1 to 2 weeks, followed by use of an elbow brace. Repair and primary reconstruction with strong tendon grafts of the lateral or medial side, or both, depending on the instability pattern, are indicated when instability persists or recurs.

ARTHROSCOPY

Arthroscopy of the elbow can be used to confirm the presence of medial instability or loose bodies and to remove posteromedial osteophytes. Medial instability may be associated with chondromalacia of the radiocapitellar joint, synovitis of the medial capsule, or the formation of posteromedial olecranon osteophytes. Andrews et al. described a valgus stress test done arthroscopically with the patient under general anesthesia. Using the anterolateral portal to view the medial compartment, valgus stress is applied to the elbow, which is flexed to 70 to 90 degrees, and the opening between the ulna and trochlea is measured. An opening of more than 1 to 2 mm indicates medial instability. With high-resolution MRA, most surgeons forgo arthroscopy unless specifically indicated. A more complete description of elbow arthroscopy is given in other chapter.

SURGICAL TREATMENT

Surgery generally is not indicated for simple elbow dislocations unless the dislocation recurs despite immobilization. In these instances, examination and MRI evaluation are used to delineate the soft tissues and bony anatomy to identify all damaged structures. Surgical intervention is directed toward the side of greatest instability, generally the lateral side, or in the case of global instability, both the lateral and medial sides may need to be treated. Repair of the capsule, primary ligamentous reconstruction, and reattachment of the tendon origins usually is necessary to obtain a stable joint. Significant fractures that result in joint instability must always be repaired.

The number of ulnar collateral ligament reconstructions has increased yearly for the past 2 decades. The procedure, first done in 1974 by Dr. Frank Jobe, has become a relatively common operation. Twenty-five percent of Major League Baseball pitchers and 15% of minor league pitchers have had ulnar collateral ligament reconstruction. The incidence of ulnar collateral ligament reconstruction in 15- to 19-year old players is 22 per 100,000 in the PearlDiver insurance database. With more primary procedures being done, more revisions also are performed. Athletes with primary reconstruction return to the same level of play 83% of the time, while those with revisions return 42% to 63% of time. After 21 months of rehabilitation, those with primary reconstructions generally return to play at about 13 months but continue to improve for an additional year; revisions tend to be associated with a decline in performance.

Ulnar collateral ligament tears have been associated with increased pitching velocity, innings, and pitches; a small repertoire of pitches; smaller stature; lack of rest within and between seasons; poor mechanics; and glenohumeral joint internal rotation deficit (GIRD). Revision failures are associated with increased workload. Results for the modified Jobe and docking techniques are similar. Ulnar nerve transfer results in neuropraxia in 12% of patients and some decrease in Conway (return-to-play) scores. Graft types have had comparable results for return-to-play, although symptomatic proximal graft heterotopic ossification occurs in about 0.6% of patients, and when the gracilis tendon is used, it occurs in 10% of patients. Ossification may require excision for persistent pain or loss of motion.

Suggested indications for ulnar collateral ligament reconstruction are an acute complete or high-grade partial rupture in a competitive throwing athlete who wishes to remain active and a partial tear with chronic pain or instability without improvement after at least 4 to 6 weeks of supervised conservative treatment. Conservative treatment consists of relative rest with forearm and shoulder strengthening exercises. Core strengthening and lower extremity and cardiovascular exercises are maintained. Medications and antiinflammatory agents are routinely prescribed. A short toss program is started at 4 to 6 weeks and progressed as the athlete tolerates. Recurrence of medial pain with throwing that prevents skillful progression of the athlete's monitored throwing program is indicative of ligamentous incompetence.

Jobe originally described the technique for reconstruction of the ulnar collateral ligament in 1986. Since that time, a number of modifications of the technique have been devised. In the original technique, the flexor mass was released from the epicondyle and open-ended tunnels were placed in the ulna and the medial humeral condyle (Fig. 3.44). A palmaris longus graft was used to reconstruct the ligament, and the ulnar nerve was transferred anteriorly under the flexor muscle mass. Jobe later modified the technique to involve splitting the common flexor mass to expose the ulnar collateral ligament tear, using a closed-ended tunnel in the medial epicondyle, and transferring the ulnar nerve only if heavy scar tissue is found around the nerve or if chronic changes are present in the ulnar nerve. Andrews et al. described dissection of the muscle belly of the flexor carpi ulnaris, retracting the muscle anteriorly to expose the ulnar collateral ligament. They did not detach the muscle from the epicondyle and used the

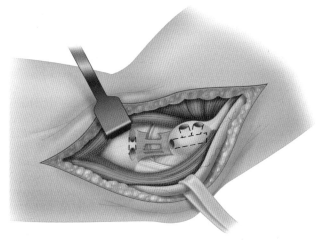

FIGURE 3.44 Jobe ulnar collateral ligament reconstruction. Medial aspect of right elbow before reconstruction showing remnant of ulnar collateral ligament and proper placement of bone tunnels in ulna and medial humeral condyle. Holes are drilled in ulna 5 mm from joint. Ulnar tunnel and closed-end tunnel in medial epicondyle are centered over bony attachments of ligament. Altchek et al. use same tunnel configuration, except anterior humeral tunnels are made with small drill bit for suture passage. **SEE TECHNIQUE 3.13.**

open-ended tunnels. The graft is sutured securely to the posterior epicondyle, and the soft-tissue graft is secured onto itself and the imbricated collateral ligament. The ulnar nerve is transferred anteriorly, where it is held by fascial slings. Cain et al. evaluated 743 athletes who had ulnar collateral ligament reconstruction with a minimum of 2 years' follow-up. Eighty-three percent returned to the same level or a higher level of competition at less than 1 year from surgical stabilization. In a statistical analysis of 147 Major League Baseball pitchers, Makhni et al. found that 67% were able to return to same competitive level as before their surgery. Overall, the group had a decline in performance comparable to age-matched controls. Reconstruction in immature athletes who progress to professional status has shown similar or slightly better results when compared with athletes who did not need surgery as an amateur.

Absence of the palmaris longus tendon occurs in 15% to 20% of individuals. When the palmaris longus tendon is present on one side only, it often has muscle extending distally, which usually is a short deficient tendon. One must be aware and prepared for the potential need of a hamstring graft, with the patient being informed of the possibility. Attritional tears with a bony ossicle in the ulnar collateral ligament also may be best treated with the larger hamstring graft.

A medial collateral ligament reconstruction done through a muscle-splitting approach and use of a single closed-end humeral tunnel was reported to allow 39 of 40 athletes to return to their previous level of competition. The benefits of this "docking procedure" include (1) reconstruction through a split in the muscle in a safe zone, (2) avoidance of obligatory nerve transfer, (3) placement of tendon grafts in bone tunnels, (4) reduction in number of humeral tunnels, and (5) simplification of graft tensioning (see Technique 3.15.) There has been interest in graft fixation with interference screws. Pullout studies have shown the use of a docking technique to be superior to use of screws. With the potential for bone resorption around absorbable screws, at present we do not advocate the use of the interference screw.

Repair of ligamentous avulsions in otherwise healthy ligaments has been reported by Savoie et al. and O'Brien et al. to have 93% good-to-excellent results and return-to-play at 6 months. Repair and backing up with an internal brace was shown by Dugas et al. to have good results for earlier to return to play. Biomechanical studies have shown the augmented repair to be as strong as traditional graft reconstruction at time-zero, with more resistance to gapping. Dugas et al. recommended the use of collagen-coated fiber tape to augment avulsions and partial tears in athletes without degenerative ligamentous changes. In early reports, 102 of 111 patients were able to return to play at the same or higher level by 6.7 months. In a small group of professional pitchers, the Kerlan-Jobe Orthopaedic Clinic (KJOC) overhead athlete scores averaged 88. There currently are no long-term results reported because the initial procedure using this technique was done in 2013.

ULNAR COLLATERAL LIGAMENT RECONSTRUCTION—MODIFIED JOBE TECHNIQUE

Important technical points to remember when performing this procedure are (1) calcification should be removed from the ligament (Fig. 3.45); (2) drill holes must correspond to ulnar collateral ligament attachment sites; (3) the graft should not rub on the epicondyle or ulna, and the ends of the graft should be buried in the tunnels; (4) a figure-of-eight configuration of the graft ensures strength and approximates ulnar collateral ligament biomechanics; and (5) meticulous handling of medial antebrachial cutaneous and ulnar nerves, their branches, and their vasculature is essential.

TECHNIQUE 3.13

- Apply a pneumatic tourniquet. Place the arm on an arm board with the elbow extended, and put a rolled towel beneath it. If appropriate, prepare the contralateral arm and ipsilateral leg for graft harvest.
- Make a 10-cm incision over the medial epicondyle.
- Protect the medial antebrachial cutaneous nerve, and incise the common flexor pronator mass at the posterior third to expose the ulnar collateral ligament.
- Split the muscle, but do not take it down, and incise the ulnar collateral ligament to evaluate the quality of the ligament and joint.
- Lightly retract the ulnar nerve until it is off the bone to allow for drilling of the holes. Do not transfer the nerve.
- Using a 3.2-mm bit at slow speed with a tissue protector, drill anterior and posterior holes in the proximal ulna. Leaving a 1-cm bone bridge, drill the tunnel at the level of the coronoid tubercle (see Fig. 3.44). In the medial epicondyle, drill a common anterior hole at the origin of the ulnar collateral ligament for 1 cm, using a 4-mm drill, and then, with a 3.2-mm drill bit, make divergent tunnels (lazy "Y") exiting anterior to the intermuscular septum 0.5 cm apart (see Fig. 3.44).
- Obtain a graft 15 cm long from the palmaris longus tendon, plantaris tendon, or Achilles tendon. Place a 1-0 nonabsorbable suture through each end of the graft, and thread it through the tunnels in a figure-of-eight fashion.
- Remove the rolled towel from beneath the elbow, and tension and suture the graft with the elbow in neutral (varus-valgus) and 45 degrees of flexion. Evaluate the range of motion. Suture the graft to the remnants of the ulnar collateral ligament.
- If ulnar nerve symptoms and heavy scar tissue are found, transposition of the ulnar nerve may be necessary. Elevate the flexor pronator musculature, leaving a ring of soft tissue on the medial epicondyle. Decompress the nerve proximally to the arcade of Struthers and distally to the end of the intermuscular septum, avoiding devascularization. Transfer the nerve anterior to the epicondyle, and reattach the flexor pronator mass to the epicondyle superficial to the transferred nerve.
- Release the tourniquet, and obtain hemostasis. Bathe the nerve with dexamethasone (Decadron) solution, and perform routine subcutaneous and skin closure. Apply a padded posterior splint with the elbow in 90 degrees of flexion and neutral rotation, leaving the wrist and hand free.

POSTOPERATIVE CARE The elbow is immobilized in the posterior splint for 7 to 10 days. Gentle hand grip exercises are begun as soon as the patient is comfortable. Active range-of-motion exercises for the elbow and shoulder are started at 10 days, and exercises to strengthen the muscles of the wrist and forearm are begun at 4 to 6 weeks. After 6 weeks, elbow strengthening exercises are

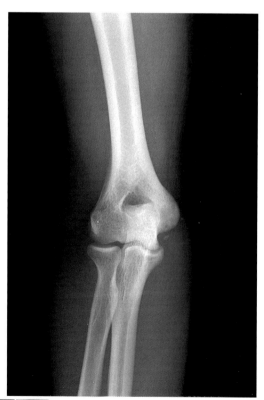

FIGURE 3.45   Anteroposterior radiograph showing calcification of deficient ulnar collateral ligament.

begun, but valgus stress on the elbow is avoided until 4 months postoperatively.

Athletes can begin a progressive, supervised throwing program. They continue with a progressive strengthening program for the forearm and shoulder and a general conditioning program. They are allowed to return to competitive pitching in approximately 1 year.

ULNAR COLLATERAL LIGAMENT RECONSTRUCTION—ANDREWS ET AL. TECHNIQUE

The goal of the procedure described by Andrews et al. is to reconstruct the anterior bundle of the ulnar collateral ligament. They recommend transposition of the ulnar nerve in all ulnar collateral ligament reconstructions because (1) the nerve must be mobilized to expose the ulnar collateral ligament through the interval used; (2) during drilling of the humeral tunnels the drill is aimed directly at the ulnar nerve if it is left in situ; and (3) athletes often have ulnar nerve symptoms and ulnar collateral ligament pathology. Preoperatively, the presence or absence of the palmaris longus tendon should be documented. Alternative sources of tendon graft include the contralateral palmaris longus tendon and gracilis tendon.

TECHNIQUE 3.14

PALMARIS LONGUS GRAFT HARVEST

- After induction of general anesthesia, apply a nonsterile tourniquet to the upper arm. Prepare and drape the arm and then exsanguinate it with an Esmarch bandage. Inflate the tourniquet to 250 mm Hg.
- Harvest the palmaris longus tendon first. Because of the close proximity of the other flexor tendons and the median nerve, great care must be taken when harvesting this tendon.
- Make three transverse incisions, each 7-10 mm long, directly over the palmaris tendon.
- Make the first incision at the wrist flexion crease, directly over the palmaris tendon. Use a no. 15 blade to incise the skin and blunt dissection to isolate the tendon, which is immediately subcutaneous.
- Place a small hemostat around the tendon and pull to place tension on the tendon. This shows the course of the tendon along the length of the forearm.
- Make a second incision 3 to 5 cm proximal and parallel to the first, directly over the tendon. After the skin is sharply incised, deliver the tendon out of the second incision with a blunt hemostat.
- Make the final incision parallel to the others at the site of the musculotendinous junction, near the junction of the proximal and middle thirds of the forearm. Deliver the tendon out of the wound with a hemostat and confirm that the correct structure has been identified in all three locations.
- Cut the tendon at the most distal incision and use a no. 0 absorbable suture to whip stitch the exposed end.

- Deliver the tendon out of the proximal incision and cut it free at the musculotendinous junction (Fig. 3.46A).
- On a back table, remove any remaining muscle from the proximal end of the tendon, and whip stitch the end of the tendon with a no. 0 absorbable suture. Protect the tendon with a moist sponge.
- Close the three incisions with subcutaneous no. 2-0 absorbable and subcuticular 3-0 nonabsorbable sutures.

ULNAR NERVE EXPOSURE AND PROTECTION
- Make an incision over the medial elbow directly over the medial epicondyle, extending approximately 3 cm proximal and 6 cm distal to the medial epicondyle.
- Use blunt dissection to identify and protect the medial antebrachial cutaneous nerve. This nerve is variable in size and location and often has multiple branches at this location. It most commonly is located in the distal third of the incision (Fig. 3.46B).
- Once this nerve is protected, elevate full-thickness flaps to expose the medial epicondyle, the flexor/pronator mass, and the cubital tunnel.
- Open the cubital tunnel with a no. 15 blade or tenotomy scissors and identify the ulnar nerve. Release the ulnar nerve and mobilize it from as far proximal into the posterior compartment as can be safely reached (Fig. 3.46C).
- Sharply split the fascia of the flexor carpi ulnaris and then bluntly spread the muscle fibers overlying the ulnar nerve.
- Identify and protect the first motor branch to the flexor carpi ulnaris.
- Place a vessel loop around the ulnar nerve for gentle retraction during the procedure.
- Divide the medial intermuscular septum of the upper arm at the most proximal aspect of the incision. Take down the remaining distal septum from the medial humerus, leaving it attached distally to the superior edge of the medial epicondyle. This strip of tissue will be used as a sling at the end of the procedure to hold the ulnar nerve in its anteriorly transposed position.
- Coagulate blood vessels at the posterosuperior edge of the medial epicondyle to prepare for drilling of the humeral tunnels.
- If posteromedial olecranon osteophytes are present, make a small incision in the joint capsule to expose the posteromedial olecranon tip. With the ulnar nerve protected, remove osteophytes with a rongeur, osteotome, or 4-mm burr. Close the capsule with interrupted no. 0 absorbable sutures.

JOINT EXPOSURE
- Expose the injured ulnar collateral ligament. The native ulnar collateral ligament inserts on the sublime tubercle of the ulnar, which lies deep and anterior to the ulnar nerve. Once it is mobilized, the posterior fibers can be easily seen.
- Elevate the flexor digitorum profundus muscle, which overlies the anterior fibers of the ulnar collateral ligament, off the ligament with a no. 15 or no. 69 blade and a small periosteal elevator (Fig. 3.46D). Begin this dissection distally and carry it proximally up the humeral origin on the medial epicondyle. Depending on the location, severity, and chronicity of the injury, a defect in the ligament may be visible at this point.

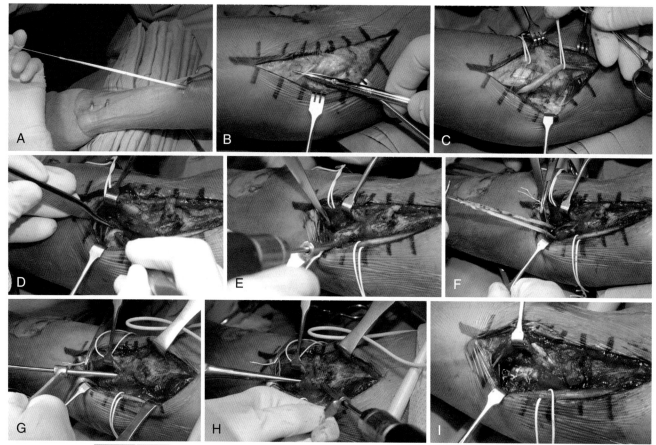

FIGURE 3.46 Andrews ulnar collateral ligament reconstruction. **A,** Harvest of palmaris graft. **B,** Medial antebrachial cutaneous nerve visible in distal third of exposure. **C,** Dissection of ulnar nerve from the cubital tunnel and mobilization with a vessel loop. **D,** Flexor digitorum profundus muscle belly elevated to expose the native ulnar collateral ligament, which is directly below the scalpel blade. **E,** Drilling of ulnar tunnels on either side of the sublime tubercle, perpendicular to the joint surface. **F,** Passage of graft through the ulnar tunnel. **G,** Drilling of the humeral tunnel from distal to proximal, starting at the native insertion of the ulnar collateral ligament onto the humerus. **H,** Placement of a curet in the first humeral tunnel while second tunnel is drilled. **I,** Graft sewn together between the humeral and ulnar tunnels to increase tension within the graft and re-create the course of the native ligament. (From Andrews JR, Jost PW, Cain EL: The ulnar collateral ligament procedure revisited: the procedure we use, *Sports Health* 4:438–441, 2012.) **SEE TECHNIQUE 3.14.**

- Split the remaining fibers of the injured ulnar collateral ligament longitudinally to expose the ulnohumeral articulation. Exposure of the joint surfaces provides a visual reference for proper ulnar tunnel position and allows inspection of partial undersurface ulnar collateral ligament tears.

TUNNEL PREPARATION AND GRAFT PASSAGE

- Use a 3.6-mm drill to make a hole at the posterior edge of the sublime tubercle, aiming anterior and parallel to the joint line (Fig. 3.46E).
- Place a hemostat in this hole and, with the same drill and starting at the anterior border of the sublime tubercle, make a second hole 1 cm distal to the joint line. When the drill is deep enough, it will hit the hemostat.
- Use angled curets to clean and connect the tunnels and to remove bone debris for easier graft passage. Wash away

any remaining bone debris in the soft tissues to prevent heterotopic ossification.
- Bend a Hewson suture passer to fit through the curved tunnel and use it to pass the palmaris graft through the ulnar tunnels, leaving equal length of tendon on each side (Fig. 3.46F).
- Begin the humeral tunnels by placing a 3.6-mm drill at the humeral origin of the UCL and aiming it proximal and lateral to exit the posterosuperior border of the medial epicondyle (Fig. 3.46G). Take care to exit as close as possible to the medial border of the humeral shaft to leave the largest bone bridge possible. Place a no. 0 curet in the tunnel.
- Drill a second hole, starting at the medial prominence of the medial epicondyle and aiming toward the humeral insertion of the UCL. This creates a Y-shaped tunnel config-

uration. The starting point of this second tunnel must be sufficiently distant from the exit point of the first tunnel to prevent fracturing of the bone bridge between them (Fig. 3.46H). The drill contacts the curet when it has reached the proper depth.

- Use straight and curved curets to clear bone debris from the tunnels.
- Pass a straight Hewson suture passer through one of the limbs of the Y-shaped humeral tunnel and use it to pass the suture on the end of the graft; place a clamp on the suture. Pass only the suture through the tunnel to allow adequate space for the Hewson suture passer to go through the tunnel a second time.
- Pass the suture passer through the second limb of the humeral tunnel and past the other end of the graft. Use the clamped suture to deliver the final limb of the graft through the remaining humeral tunnel.

GRAFT FIXATION

- With one assistant holding the elbow in 30 degrees of flexion and with a slight varus stress so that the articular surfaces of the ulnohumeral joint are in contact, and a second assistant holding tension on the two ends of the graft in an overlapping position on the posteromedial epicondyle, use no. 0 nonabsorbable, braided coated polyester to sew the two limbs to each other and to the underlying periosteum.
- Use three to five no. 0 nonabsorbable, braided coated polyester sutures to sew together the two limbs of the graft between the humeral and ulnar tunnels to increase tension within the graft and re-create the course of the native ulnar collateral ligament (Fig. 3.46I). Resect excess graft with a no. 15 blade.

ULNAR NERVE TRANSPOSITION

- Transfer the ulnar nerve anterior to the medial epicondyle and lay the sling of medial intermuscular septum over the nerve. Sew the end of the sling to the fascia of the flexor/pronator mass with no. 3-0 nonabsorbable, braided coated polyester sutures, taking care to leave the sling of septum very loose so that the ulnar nerve is not compressed under it and can move freely.

CLOSURE

- Close the flexor carpi ulnaris fascia and the fascia of the cubital tunnel with no. 0 absorbable suture.
- Release the tourniquet and obtain hemostasis with electrocautery.
- Irrigate the wound with normal saline and place a Hemovac drain in the dependent portion of the wound, exiting proximally.
- Close the wound with subcutaneous no. 2-0 absorbable and subcuticular no. 3-0 nonabsorbable suture, followed by Steri-Strips.
- Place sterile dressings and a posterior splint molded at 90 degrees of flexion.

POSTOPERATIVE CARE The splint is worn for 1 week; when it is removed, a functional brace set at 30 to 100 degrees is applied. Wrist gripping exercises are begun during the first week, and elbow isometric flexion and extension exercises are started during the second week. The brace is advanced from 15 to 110 degrees by week 3. Light isotonic exercises are started the fourth week, and full motion should be regained by 6 to 8 weeks. From 9 to 13 weeks, advanced strengthening exercises are begun, with eccentric elbow exercises and isometric and isotonic exercises. An interval throwing program is started during week 14, and return to competitive throwing is allowed in 22 to 26 weeks.

ULNAR COLLATERAL LIGAMENT RECONSTRUCTION

TECHNIQUE 3.15

(ALTCHEK ET AL.)

- If a reconstruction is planned, harvest the graft at this time. Usually the ipsilateral palmaris longus is harvested through a 5-mm to 1-cm incision placed in the distal wrist crease. Rather than make multiple incisions, use a tendon stripper specially made for this purpose.
- Place a no. 1 braided nonabsorbable suture using a curved needle in a Krackow fashion in one end of the tendon. After harvest, place the tendon on a moist sponge on the back table.
- To expose the medial collateral ligament, use a tourniquet to exsanguinate the arm.
- Make an incision from the distal third of the intermuscular septum across the medial epicondyle to a point 2 cm beyond the sublime tubercle of the ulna. While exposing the fascia of the flexor pronator, identify and preserve the antebrachial cutaneous branch of the median nerve, which frequently crosses the operative field.
- Incise the fascia of the flexor carpi ulnaris longitudinally, and split the underlying ligament (Fig. 3.47A).
- Place a deep, blunt, self-retaining retractor to maintain the exposure. Incise the anterior bundle of the medial collateral ligament longitudinally, exposing the joint. At this point, medial collateral ligament laxity can be confirmed by observing 2 mm or more separation of the joint surfaces with valgus stress (Fig. 3.47B).
- Expose the tunnel positions for the ulna. For the posterior tunnel, subperiosteally expose the posterior ulna at all times and meticulously protect the nerve. If the nerve subluxes anteriorly so that it cannot be protected, transpose it.
- Using a no. 3 burr, create tunnels anterior and posterior to the sublime tubercle so that a 2-cm bridge exists between them. Connect the tunnels using a small curved curet. Do not violate the bony bridge. Pass a looped no. 2-0 braided nonabsorbable suture using a curved needle.
- The humeral tunnel position is located in the anterior half of the medial epicondyle in the anterior position of the existing medial collateral ligament. Using a no. 4 burr, create a longitudinal tunnel up the axis of the

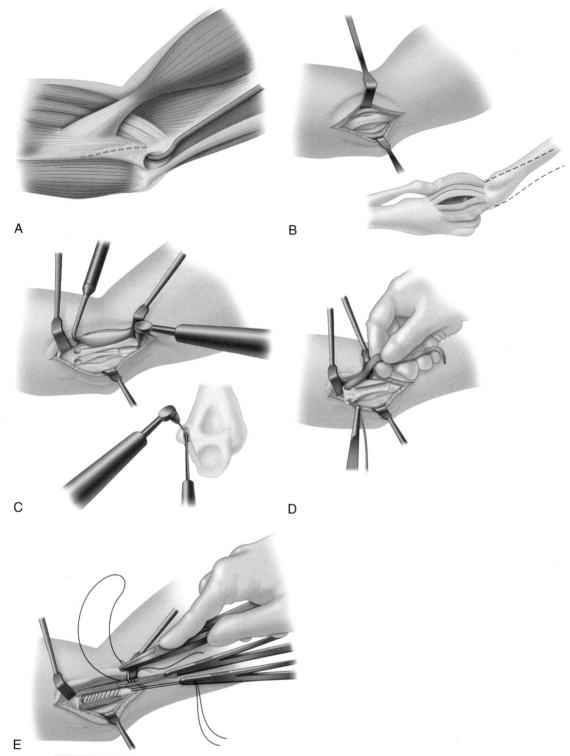

A

B

C

D

E

FIGURE 3.47   Altchek et al. medial collateral ligament reconstruction through muscle-splitting approach and using single closed-end humeral tunnel. **A,** Incision through flexor carpi ulnaris. **B,** Submuscular exposure of medial collateral ligament. **C,** Ulnar tunnel and single humeral tunnel and exit holes for two suture bundles. **D,** Graft passage through ulnar tunnel from anterior to posterior. **E,** Posterior limb of graft is docked in humeral tunnel. Elbow is reduced with varus stress; and after final tensioning of graft, Krackow stitch is placed in anterior limb of graft. **SEE TECHNIQUE 3.15.**

epicondyle to a depth of 15 mm. Expose the upper border of the epicondyle, just anterior to the intermuscular septum. Create two small tunnels separated by 5 mm to 1 cm with a dental drill with a small bit. This allows suture passage from the primary humeral tunnel (Fig. 3.47C). Use a suture passer from each of the two upper humeral tunnels to pass a looped suture for later graft passage.
- With the elbow reduced, repair the longitudinal incision in the medial collateral ligament with a 2-0 absorbable suture.
- Pass the graft through the ulnar tunnel from anterior to posterior (Fig. 3.47D). Pass the limb of the graft that has sutures already in place into the humeral tunnel exiting into one of the small superior humeral tunnels.
- With the first limb of the graft securely docked in the humerus, reduce the elbow with forearm supination and gentle varus stress. Maintain tension on the graft while flexing and extending the elbow to avoid potential creep within the graft.
- Measure the final length of the graft by placing the free limb of the graft adjacent to the humeral tunnel and visually estimating the length of the graft that can be tensioned within the humeral tunnel. Mark this point with dye, and place a no. 1 braided nonabsorbable suture in a Krackow fashion. Dock this end of the graft securely in the humeral tunnel with the sutures exiting the small superior humeral tunnel (Fig. 3.47E). The graft may be quadrupled and secured with one braided nonabsorbable suture in a Krackow fashion in the looped end, as well as in both tails. These are then folded over and secured on the docking position as described by Paletta et al.
- Perform final graft tensioning by moving the elbow through a full range of motion with varus stress placed on the elbow.
- When satisfied with graft tension, tie two sets of graft sutures over the bony bridge on the humeral condyle.
- Deflate the tourniquet, and copiously irrigate the wound.
- Approximate the flexor carpi ulnaris fascia, and perform subcutaneous and subcuticular closure.
- Place the elbow in a plaster splint at 60 degrees of flexion.

POSTOPERATIVE CARE The sutures are removed 1 week after surgery, and the elbow is placed in a hinged brace. Motion is allowed between 45 degrees of extension and 90 degrees of flexion. Over the next 3 weeks, motion is gradually advanced to full. A formal physical therapy program is begun at 6 weeks, and gradual strengthening of the forearm and shoulder is started. Care is taken to prevent a valgus load across the elbow during this phase of rehabilitation. At 12 weeks, the strengthening program is more vigorous, and bench-pressing with light-to-moderate weights is allowed. At 4 months, a throwing program is begun for throwing athletes.

For revision procedures or tunnel blow-out, a single ulnar tunnel with endobutton fixation can be used as a salvage procedure. A small interference screw can also be used, but generally poor bone quality makes this a less desirable fixation option.

ULNAR COLLATERAL LIGAMENT REPAIR WITH AN INTERNAL BRACE

TECHNIQUE 3.16

(DUGAS ET AL.)
- With the patient supine and the operative arm on a hand table, after anesthesia administration, examine the elbow with attention to any preoperative range of motion restrictions, particularly in extension.
- Make in incision from the posterior aspect of the medial epicondyle, extending distally.
- If ulnar nerve transposition is planned, extend the excision proximally and unroof and mobilize the ulnar nerve. Take care not to dissect the nerve proximally to prevent iatrogenic ulnar nerve instability.
- Elevate the flexor pronator mass off the ulnar collateral ligament and split the ulnar collateral ligament in line with its fibers.
- Visually examine the ligament for the location of the tear and the tissue quality. Midsubstance injuries, significant tissue degeneration, and/or tissue loss that prevents approximation of the ulnar collateral ligament to either the sublime tubercle or medial epicondyle are considered relative contraindications to repair.
- If repair is indicated, an InternalBrace (Arthrex) technique can be used.
- For most overhead throwing athletes, use 3.5-mm Swivel-Lock anchors (Arthrex). Larger anchors are available and can be used if required.
- Place the first anchor, loaded with collagen-dipped FiberTape and 0 FiberWire (Arthrex), in the location of the tear using a 2.7-mm drill and then tapping to the size of the anchor.
- Use a free needle to pass the FiberWire in a mattress fashion into the ulnar collateral ligament and tie this down to approximate the torn tissue to the ulnar collateral ligament footprint on the medial epicondyle or sublime tubercle.
- Close the remainder of the native ligament using 0 TiCron suture (Medtronic).
- Place the second anchor at the opposing attachment site with collagen-dipped FiberWire loosely tensioned. Allow enough slack on the brace to align the third thread on the anchor with a drill hole for the anchor.
- Dock the eyelet and advance the anchor to the aperture of the drill hole.
- Move the elbow through a range of motion to ensure adequate isometry and tension of the internal brace.
- To achieve isometry, choose a starting point for the medial epicondyle anchor in the center of the attachment point of the ulnar collateral ligament. Place the center of the sublime tubercle tunnel approximately 6 to 8 mm distal to the joint, slightly anterior on the ridge of the sublime tubercle. Drill the tunnel in a direction aimed slightly away from the articular surface of the ulna.
- Drill the medial epicondyle tunnel in a similar orientation to the tunnel created for ulnar collateral ligament reconstruction, proximally and slightly laterally toward the posterosuperior border of the medial epicondyle. This provides adequate tunnel length for anchor placement and avoids drilling into the cubital tunnel or olecranon fossa.

- If perfect isometry is not obtained, the brace may become taut at certain points during range of motion. If this occurs, remove the anchor and loosen the brace. If anisometry exists, laxity is preferred rather than overconstraint.
- Once the desired tension is achieved and the anchor is placed, suture the brace to the native ligament to prevent motion of the brace over the ligament and potential abrasion.
- Move the elbow through a range of motion to ensure full motion without overtensioning of the graft and to assess for instability of the ulnar nerve.

POSTOPERATIVE MANAGEMENT The patient is discharged home the same day. The splint is removed 5 to 7 days after surgery, and range-of-motion and strengthening exercises are begun in a protective hinged elbow brace. A supervised throwing program is initiated at 10 weeks, with the goal of returning to competition by 6 months after surgery.

LATERAL ULNAR COLLATERAL LIGAMENT RECONSTRUCTION FOR POSTEROLATERAL ROTATORY INSTABILITY

For posterolateral rotatory instability that persists because of disruption of the lateral ulnar collateral ligament and incompetence of the lateral capsular structures, Nestor, Morrey, and O'Driscoll described the use of a Kocher lateral incision for repair or reconstruction of the lateral side.

TECHNIQUE 3.17

(NESTOR, MORREY, AND O'DRISCOLL)
- Approach the elbow through a modified Kocher incision.
- By sharp dissection, carefully elevate the common extensor origin, including a portion of the extensor carpi radialis, to reveal the origin of the radial collateral ligament complex at the lateral epicondyle.
- Distally, reflect the anconeus muscle posteriorly and the extensor carpi ulnaris anteriorly. Reflect the extension of the origin of the anconeus to the lateral aspect of the triceps fascia sufficiently to expose the ligament adequately. Identify the supinator crest of the ulna.
- Typically, a lax ulnar band of the radial collateral ligament is observed and the abnormal portion of the ligament is proximal to the annular ligament. The pivot-shift maneuver reveals laxity of the anterior part of the capsule over the radial head and of the posterior part of the capsule at the posterior aspect of the radiohumeral joint. The subluxation of the joint clearly shows the stretched ulnar part of the collateral ligament.
- Enter the joint, and inspect for loose bodies and abrasion of the articular surfaces.
- Tighten the anterior and posterior aspects of the capsule with plication sutures, but do not tie these sutures

(Fig. 3.48A, *left*). If the radial collateral ligament complex appears intact but stretched or detached from its origin, imbricate and advance it with a Bunnell suture technique. Suture and plicate the ulnar and the radial parts of the radial collateral ligament complex. Advance the suture through holes placed in the bone at the humeral anatomic origin of the ligament (Fig. 3.48A, *right*).
- If the tissue of the collateral ligament is of poor quality, as is the usual case, reconstruct the ulnar part of the radial collateral ligament with an autogenous graft from the palmaris longus tendon.
- Pass the tendon through an osseous tunnel created by a small burr just posterior to the tubercle of the crest of the supinator. Make the entry holes about 7 mm apart to lessen the likelihood of rupture of the osseous tunnel roof. Thread the tendon through a humeral tunnel that emerges at the origin of the ligaments. Determine the location of the tunnel in the humerus by placing a temporary suture in the ulnar tunnel and holding the ends of the suture against the humerus with a hemostat while the elbow is moved. Reflect the tendon graft back onto itself, crossing the joint again, and attach it into its origin with 1-0 nonabsorbable sutures (Fig. 3.48B-E).
- If the tendon graft seems to be inadequate for the size of the arm or for the anticipated activity or stress, use an autogenous or allograft hamstring tendon to reinforce the reconstruction with the same sites of attachment to bone and crossing the joint twice.
- Tie all the sutures with the elbow flexed 30 degrees and with the forearm fully pronated.
- After completing the reconstruction, test the elbow for anterolateral rotatory instability. Allow the anconeus and triceps muscles to assume their normal positions, and close the interval between the anconeus and the extensor carpi ulnaris with absorbable sutures.
- Apply a splint with the forearm flexed 90 degrees and pronated.

　We prefer to use a closed-end tunnel and docking technique in the humerus comparable to that used with the ulnar collateral ligament. When the palmaris is deficient, we use a 3.2-mm thick portion of the gracilis tendon. One hamstring may be split for medial and lateral reconstructions in the case of global instability after dislocation. The humeral tunnel is drilled at the point on the epicondyle where the line drawn along the anterior humeral cortex intersects a line through the center of the radiocapitellar axis between the 3- and 4:30-o'clock position on the epicondyle (Fig. 3.49). Stability and isometry are less affected by the location of the ulnar tunnels. Placement of drill holes 4 mm posterior to the radial head at the crista supinatoris and at the proximal aspect of the lesser sigmoid notch provides reproducible landmarks.

POSTOPERATIVE CARE With the forearm in full pronation, the elbow is placed in 70 to 80 degrees of flexion and held in this position for 10 to 14 days. Protected movement is allowed in a hinged brace 2 to 6 weeks after surgery. After 6 weeks, the hinged brace can be removed for light activity. The brace is discontinued completely at the end of an additional 6 weeks, but patients are encouraged to protect the elbow from heavy activity. Full activity is

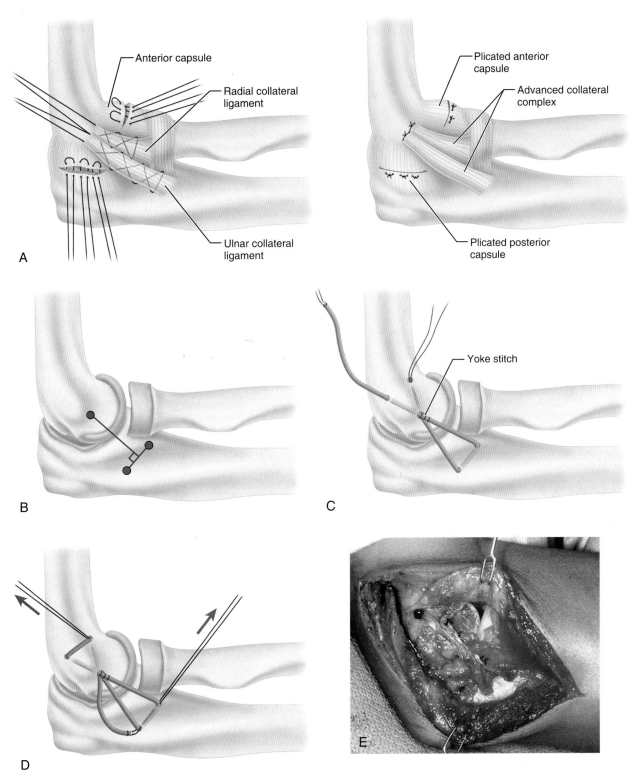

FIGURE 3.48 Technique of Nestor et al. **A,** Imbrication and advancement of ulnar band of radial collateral ligament and radial part of radial collateral ligament with Bunnell suture technique, accomplished by placing sutures through drill holes at anatomic origin of ligament in humerus. **B,** Ulnar tunnel placed in crista supinatoris tubercle and oriented to have optimal alignment with isometric point. **C,** Placement of graft into ulnar tunnel and creation of yoke stitch. **D,** Graft tensioning after introduction into humeral tunnels. **E,** Tunnel is made in humerus and expanded in posterosuperior direction to emerge posterior and superior to point of isometry. Second humeral tunnel exits posterior and inferior from common entry site. Palmaris longus tendon is drawn through ulnar and humeral tunnels and tied to itself after recrossing joint. **SEE TECHNIQUE 3.17.**

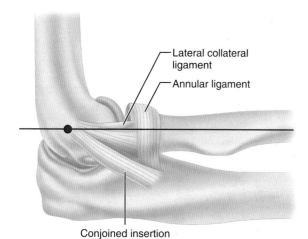

FIGURE 3.49 Lateral collateral and annular ligament complex of elbow. Lateral collateral ligament originates off humerus at axis point of ulnohumeral joint, which lies at intersection of anterior humeral line and radiocapitellar axis. Radial collateral ligament blends with annular ligament to insert in conjoined fashion onto proximal ulna. **SEE TECHNIQUE 3.17.**

allowed at 6 months, and participation in contact sports is allowed at 1 year. The patient is advised to protect the elbow from stresses during activities of daily living, such as lifting weights. We recommend that patients lift weights only in the plane of elbow flexion and extension, keeping the shoulder adducted and the elbow close to the body.

REFERENCES

PATELLA

Arendt EA, Askenberger M, Agel J, et al.: Risk of redislocation after primary patellar dislocation: a clinical prediction model based on magnetic resonance imaging variables, *Am J Sports Med* 46:3385, 2018.

Askenberger M, Janarv PM, Finnbogason T, et al.: Morphology and anatomic patellar instability risk factors in first-time traumatic lateral patellar dislocations. A prospective magnetic resonance imaging study in skeletally immature children, *Am J Sports Med* 45:50, 2016.

Azimi H, Anakwenze O: Medial patellofemoral ligament reconstruction using dual patella docking technique, *Arthrosc Tech* 6:e2093, 2017.

Bedi H, Marzo J: The biomechanics of medial patellofemoral ligament repair followed by lateral retinacular release, *Am J Sports Med* 38:1462, 2010.

Boddula MR, Adamson GJ, Pink MM: Medial reefing without lateral release for recurrent patellar instability: midterm and long-term outcomes, *Am J Sports Med* 42:216, 2014.

Bollier M, Fulkerson JP: The role of trochlear dysplasia in patellofemoral instability, *J Am Acad Orthop Surg* 19:8, 2011.

Camathias C, Speth BM, Rutz E, et al.: Solitary trochleoplasty for treatment of recurrent patellar dislocation, *JBJS Essent Surg Tech* 8:e11, 2018.

Camathias C, Studer K, Kiapour A, et al.: Trochleoplasty as a solitary treatment for recurrent patellar dislocation results in good clinical outcome in adolescents, *Am J Sports Med* 44:2855, 2016.

Camp CL, Krych AJ, Dahm DL, et al.: Medial patellofemoral ligament repair for recurrent patellar dislocation, *Am J Sports Med* 38:2248, 2010.

Camp CL, Stuart MJ, Krych AH, et al.: CT and MRI measurements of tibial tubercle—trochlear groove distances are not equivalent in patients with patellar instability, *Am J Sports Med* 41:1835, 2013.

Christensen TC, Sanders TL, Pareek A, et al.: Risk factors and time to recurrent ipsilateral and contralateral patellar dislocations, *Am J Sports Med* 45:2105, 2017.

Damasena I, Blythe M, Wysocki D, et al.: Medial patellofemoral ligament reconstruction combined with distal realignment for recurrent dislocations of the patella: 5-year results of a randomized controlled trial, *Am J Sports Med* 45:369, 2017.

DeJour D, Saggin P: The sulcus deepening trochleoplasty—the Lyon's procedure, *Int Orthop* 34:311, 2010.

Diduch DR, Kandil A, Burrus MT: Lateral patellar instability in the skeletally mature patient: evaluation and surgical management, *J Am Acad Orthop Surg* 26:429, 2018.

Hackl M, Müller LP, Wegmann K: The circumferential graft technique for treatment of chronic multidirectional ligamentous elbow instability, *JBJS Essent Surg Tech* 7:e6, 2017.

Hopper GP, Leach WJ, Rooney BP, et al.: Does degree of trochlear dysplasia and position of femoral tunnel influence outcomes after medial patellofemoral ligament reconstruction, *Am J Sports Med* 42:716, 2014.

Kita K, Tanaka Y, Toritsuka Y, et al.: Patellofemoral chondral status after medial patellofemoral ligament reconstruction using second-look arthroscopy in patients with recurrent patellar dislocation, *J Orthop Sci* 19:925, 2014.

Lewallen LW, McIntosh AL, Dahm DL: Predictors of recurrent instability after acute patellofemoral dislocation in pediatric and adolescent patients, *Am J Sports Med* 41:575, 2013.

Lippacher S, Dreyhaupt J, Williams SR, et al.: Reconstruction of the medial patellofemoral ligament: clinical outcomes and return to sports, *Am J Sports Med* 42:1661, 2014.

Ma LF, Wang F, Chen BC, et al.: Medial retinaculum plasty versus medial patellofemoral ligament reconstruction for recurrent patellar instability in adults: a randomized controlled trial, *Arthroscopy* 29:891, 2013.

Matic GT, Magnussen RA, Kolovich GP, Flanigan DC: Return to activity after medial patellofemoral ligament repair or reconstruction, *Arthroscopy* 30:1018, 2014.

Matsushita T, Kuroda R, Oka S, et al.: Clinical outcomes of medial patellofemoral ligament reconstruction in patients with an increased tibial tuberosity-trochlear groove distance, *Knee Surg Sports Traumatol Arthrosc* 22:2438, 2014.

Nelitz M, Dreyhaupt J, Reichel H, et al.: Anatomic reconstruction of the medial patellofemoral ligament in children and adolescents with open growth plates: surgical technique and clinical outcome, *Am J Sports Med* 41:58, 2013.

Nelitz M, Dreyhaupt J, Williams SRM: No growth disturbance after trochleoplasty for recurrent patellar dislocation in adolescents with open growth plates, *Am J Sports Med* 46:3209, 2018.

Ntagiopoulos PG, Byn P, Dejour D: Midterm results of comprehensive surgical reconstruction including sulcus-deepening trochleoplasty in recurrent patellar dislocations with high-grade trochlear dysplasia, *Am J Sports Med* 41:998, 2013.

Panni AS, Cerciello S, Maffulli N, et al.: Patellar shape can be a predisposing factor in patellar instability, *Knee Surg Sports Traumatol Arthrosc* 19:663, 2011.

Redfern J, Kamath G, Burks R: Anatomical confirmation of the use of radiographic landmarks in medial patellofemoral ligament reconstruction, *Am J Sports Med* 38:293, 2010.

Redler LH, Wright ML: Surgical management of patellofemoral instability in the skeletally immature patient, *J Am Acad Orthop Surg* 26:e405, 2018.

Sanchis-Alfonso V: Guidelines for medial patellofemoral ligament reconstruction in chronic lateral patellar instability, *J Am Acad Orthop Surg* 22:175, 2014.

Schneider DK, Grase B, Magnussen RA, et al.: Outcomes after isolated medial patellofemoral ligament reconstruction for the treatment of recurrent lateral patellar dislocations: a systematic review and meta-analysis, *Am J Sports Med* 44:2993, 2016.

Sherman SL, Erickson BJ, Cvetanovich GL, et al.: Tibial tuberosity osteotomy: indications, techniques, and outcomes, *Am J Sports Med* 42:2006, 2013.

Smith TO, Davies L, Toms AP, et al.: The reliability and validity of radiological assessment for patellar instability: a systematic review and meta-analysis, *Skeletal Radiol* 40:399, 2011.

Tensho K, Shimodaira H, Akaoka Y, et al.: Lateralization of the tibial tubercle in recurrent patellar dislocation. Verification using multiple methods to evaluate the tibial tubercle, *J Bone Joint Surg* 100:e58, 2018.

Tjoumakaris P, Forsythe B, Bradley JP: Patellofemoral instability in athletes: treatment via modified Fulkerson osteotomy and lateral release, *Am J Sports Med* 38:992, 2010.

Vavken P, Wimmer MD, Camathias C, et al.: Treating patella instability in skeletally immature patients, *Arthroscopy* 29:1410, 2013.

Weber AE, Nathani A, Dines JS, et al.: An algorithmic approach to the management of recurrent lateral patellar dislocation, *J Bone Joint Surg Am* 98:417, 2016.

HIP

Aly AS, Al-Kersh MA: Femoral and Dega osteotomies in the treatment of habitual hip dislocation in Down syndrome patients—is it efficient or not? *J Child Orthop* 12:227, 2018.

Aoki H, Nagao Y, Ishii S, et al.: Acetabular and proximal femoral alignment in patients with osteoarthritis of the dysplastic hip and its influence on the progression of disease, *J Bone Joint Surg* 92B:1703, 2010.

Blakey CM, Field MH, Singh PJ, et al.: Secondary capsular laxity of the hip, *Hip Int* 20:497, 2010.

Boykin RE, Anz AW, Bushnell BD, et al.: Hip instability, *J Am Acad Orthop Surg* 19:340, 2011.

Brunner A, Hamers AT, Fitze M, Herzog RE: The plain beta-angle measured on radiographs in the assessment to femoroacetabular impingement, *J Bone Joint Surg* 92B:1203, 2010.

Canham CD, Domb BG, Giordano BD: Atraumatic hip instability, *JBJS Rev* 4: pii: 01874474-201605000-00001, 2016.

Dumont GD: Hip instability: current concepts and treatment options, *Clin Sports Med* 35:435, 2016.

Field RE, Rajakulendran K: The labro-acetabular complex, *J Bone Joint Surg* 93A(Suppl 2):22, 2011.

Kalisvaart MM, Safran MR: Hip instability treated with arthroscopic capsular plication, *Knee Surg Sports Traumatol Arthroc* 25:24, 2017.

Maranho DA, Fuchs K, Kim YJ, et al.: Hip instability in patients with Down syndrome, *J Am Acad Orthop Surg* 26:455, 2018.

Mayer SW, Abdo JC, Hill MK, et al.: Femoroacetabular impingement is associated with sports-related posterior hip instability in adolescents: a matched-cohort study, *Am J Sports Med* 44:2299, 2016.

Novais EN, Heare TC, Hill MK, et al.: Surgical hip dislocation for the treatment of intra-articular injuries and hip instability following traumatic posterior dislocation in children and adolescents, *J Pediatr Orthop* 36:673, 2016.

Rhee PC, Woodcock JS, Clohisy JC, et al.: The Shenton line in the diagnosis of acetabular dysplasia in the skeletally mature patient, *J Bone Joint Surg* 93A:35, 2011.

Safran MR, Giordan G, Lindsey DP, et al.: Strains across the acetabular labrum during hip motion: a cadaveric model, *Am J Sports Med* 39(Suppl):92S, 2011.

Shu B, Safran MR: Hip instability: anatomic and clinical considerations of traumatic and atraumatic instability, *Clin Sports Med* 30:349, 2011.

STERNOCLAVICULAR/ACROMIOCLAVICULAR JOINT

Boström Windhamre HA, von Heideken JP, Une-Larsson VE, Ekelund AL: Surgical treatment of chronic acromioclavicular dislocations: a comparative study of Weaver-Dunn augmented with PDS-braid or hook plate, *J Shoulder Elbow Surg* 19:1040, 2010.

Fraschini G, Ciampi P, Scotti C, et al.: Surgical treatment of chronic acromioclavicular dislocation: comparison between two surgical procedures for anatomic reconstruction, *Injury* 41:1103, 2010.

Guan JJ, Wolf BR: Reconstruction for anterior sternoclavicular joint dislocation and instability, *J Shoulder Elbow Surg* 22:775, 2013.

Kawaguchi K, Tanaka S, Yoshitomi H, et al.: Double figure-of-eight reconstruction technique for chronic anterior sternoclavicular joint dislocation, *Knee Surg Sports Traumatol Arthrosc* 23:1559, 2015.

Lee SU, Park IJ, Kim YD, et al.: Stabilization for chronic sternoclavicular joint instability, *Knee Surg Sports Traumatol Arthrosc* 18:1795, 2010.

Martetschläger F, Warth RJ, Millett PJ: Instability and degenerative arthritis of the sternoclavicular joint: a current concepts review, *Am J Sports Med* 42:999, 2014.

Ting BL, Bae DS, Waters PM: Chronic posterior sternoclavicular joint fracture dislocations in children and young adults: results of surgical management, *J Pediatr Orthop* 34:542, 2014.

SHOULDER

Alkaduhimi H, van der Linde JA, Willigenburg NW, et al.: Redislocation risk after an arthroscopic Bankart procedure in collision athletes: a systematic review, *J Should Elbow Surg* 25:1549, 2016.

An VV, Sivakumar BS, Phan K, et al.: A systematic review and meta-analysis of clinical and patient-reported outcomes following two procedures for recurrent traumatic anterior instability of the shoulder: Latarjet procedure vs. Bankart repair, *J Shoulder Elbow Surg* 25:853, 2016.

Boone JL, Arciero RA: Management of failed instability surgery: how to get it right the next time, *Orthop Clin North Am* 41:367, 2010.

Boselli KJ, Cody EA, Bigliani LU: Open capsular shift: there still is a role, *Orthop Clin North Am* 41:427, 2010.

deBeer JF, Roberts C: Glenoid bone defects—open Latarjet with congruent arc modification, *Orthop Clin North Am* 41:407, 2010.

Elkousy H, Gartsman GM, Labriola J, et al.: Subscapularis function following the Latarjet coracoid transfer for recurrent anterior shoulder instability, *Orthopedics* 33:802, 2010.

Finestone A, Milgrom C, Radeva-Petrova DR, et al.: Immobilization in an external or internal rotation brace did not differ in preventing recurrent shoulder dislocation, *J Bone Joint Surg* 92A:1262, 2010.

Ghodadra N, Gupta A, Romeo AA, et al.: Normalization of glenohumeral articular contact pressures after Latarjet or iliac crest bone-grafting, *J Bone Joint Surg* 92A:1478, 2010.

Johnson SM, Robinson CM: Current concepts review. Shoulder instability in patients with joint hyperlaxity, *J Bone Joint Surg* 92A:1545, 2010.

Kaar SG, Fening SD, Jones MH, et al.: Effect of humeral head defect size on glenohumeral stability: a cadaveric study of simulated Hill-Sachs defects, *Am J Sports Med* 38:594, 2010.

Kao JT, Chang CL, Su WR, et al.: Incidence of recurrence after shoulder dislocation: a nationwide database study, *J Shoulder Elbow Surg* 27:1519, 2018.

Kim DS, Yoon YS, Yi CH: Prevalence comparison of accompanying lesions between primary and recurrent anterior dislocation in the shoulder, *Am J Sports Med* 38:2071, 2010.

Kirchhoff C, Imhoff AB: Posterosuperior and anterosuperior impingement of the shoulder in overhead athletes—evolving concepts, *Int Orthop* 34:1049, 2010.

Lafosse L, Boyle S: Arthroscopic Latarjet procedure, *J Shoulder Elbow Surg* 19:2, 2010.

Longo UG, Loppini M, Rizzello G, et al.: Remplissage, humeral osteochondral grafts, Weber osteotomy, and shoulder arthroplasty for the management of humeral bone defects in shoulder instability: systematic review and quantitative synthesis of the literature, *Arthroscopy* 30:1650, 2014.

Marshall T, Vega J, Siqueira M, et al.: Outcomes after arthroscopic Bankart repair: patients with first-time versus recurrent dislocations, *Am J Sports Med* 45:1776, 2017.

Meuffels DE, Schuit H, van Biezen FC, et al.: The posterior bone block procedure in posterior shoulder instability: a long-term follow-up study, *J Bone Joint Surg* 92B:651, 2010.

Milgrom FA, Radeva-Petrova DR, Barchilon RE, et al.: Immobilization in an external or internal rotation brace did no differ in preventing recurrent shoulder dislocation, *J Bone Joint Surg* 92A:1626, 2010.

Millett PJ, Fritz EM, Frangiamore SJ, et al.: Arthroscopic management of glenohumeral arthritis: a joint preservation approach, *J Am Acad Orthop Surg* 26:745, 2018.

Neviaser RJ, Benke MT, Neviaser AS: Mid-term to long-term outcome of the open Bankart repair for recurrent traumatic anterior dislocation of the shoulder, *J Shoulder Elbow Surg* 26:1943, 2017.

Nho SJ, Strauss EJ, Lenart BA, et al.: Long head of the biceps tendinopathy: diagnosis and management, *J Am Acad Orthop Surg* 18:645, 2010.

Ogawa K, Yoshida A, Matsumoto H, Takeda T: Outcome of the open Bankart procedure for shoulder instability and development of osteoarthritis: a 5- to 20-year follow-up study, *Am J Sports Med* 38:1549, 2010.

Owens BD, Campbell SE, Cameron KL: Risk factors for anterior glenohumeral instability, *Am J Sports Med* 42:2591, 2014.

Mather III RC, Orlando LA, Henderson RA, et al.: A predictive model of shoulder instability after a first-time anterior shoulder dislocation, *J Shoulder Elbow Surg* 20:259, 2011.

Metzger PD, Barlow B, Leonardelli D, et al.: Clinical application of the "glenoid track" concept for defining humeral head engagement in anterior shoulder instability. A preliminary report, *Orthop J Sports Med* 1, 2013.

Ponce BA, Rosenzweig SD, Thompson KJ, Tokish J: Sequential volume reduction with capsular plications: relationship between cumulative size of plications and volumetric reduction for multidirectional instability of the shoulder, *Am J Sports Med* 39:526, 2011.

Provencher MT, Bhatia S, Ghodadra NS, et al.: Recurrent shoulder instability: current concepts for evaluation and management of glenoid bone loss, *J Bone Joint Surg* 92A:133, 2010.

Provencher MT, LeClere LE, King S, et al.: Posterior instability of the shoulder: Diagnosis and management, *Am J Sports Med* 39:874, 2011.

Rokito AS, Birdzell MG, Cuomo F, et al.: Recovery of shoulder strength and proprioception after open surgery for recurrent anterior instability: a comparison of two surgical techniques, *J Shoulder Elbow Surg* 19:564, 2010.

Rouleau DM, Hebert-Davies J, Robinson CM: Acute traumatic posterior shoulder dislocation, *J Am Acad Orthop Surg* 22:145, 2014.

Streubel PN, Krych AJ, Simone JP, et al.: Anterior glenohumeral instability: a pathology-based surgical treatment strategy, *J Am Acad Orthop Surg* 22:283, 2014.

Torrance E, Clarke CJ, Monga P, et al.: Recurrence after arthroscopic labral repair for traumatic anterior instability in adolescent rugby and contact athletes, *Am J Sports Med* 46:2969, 2018.

Vezeridis PS, Ishmael CR, Jones KJ, et al.: Glenohumeral dislocation arthropathy: etiology, diagnosis, and management, *J Am Acad Orthop Surg* 2018, [Epub ahead of print].

Williams HLM, Evans JP, Fugness ND, et al.: It's not all about redislocation: review of complications after anterior shoulder stabilization surgery, *Am J Sports Med* 363546518810711, 2018. [Epub ahead of print].

Yang JS, Mazzocca AD, Cote MP, et al.: Recurrent anterior shoulder instability with combined bone loss: treatment and results with the modified Latarjet procedure, *Am J Sports Med* 44:922, 2016.

Young AA, Maia R, Berhouet J, Walch G: Open Latarjet procedure for management of bone loss in anterior instability of the glenohumeral joint, *J Shoulder Elbow Surg* 20:S61, 2011.

Zhu Y, Jiang C, Song G: Arthroscopic versus open Latarjet in the treatment of recurrent anterior shoulder dislocation with marked glenoid bone loss: a prospective comparative study, *Am J Sports Med* 45:1645, 2017.

ELBOW

Anakwe RE, Middleton SD, Jenkins PJ, et al.: Patient reported outcomes after simple dislocation of the elbow, *J Bone Joint Surg* 93A:1220, 2011.

Andrachuk JS, Scillia SJ, Aune KT, et al.: Symptomatic heterotopic ossification after ulnar collateral ligament reconstruction: clinical significance and treatment outcome, *Am J Sports Med* 44:1324, 2016.

Andrews JR, Jost PW, Cain EL: The ulnar collateral ligament procedure revisited: the procedure we use, *Sports Health* 4:438, 2012.

Arner JW, Chang ES, Bayer S, et al.: Direct comparison of modified Jobe and docking ulnar collateral ligament reconstruction at midterm follow-up, *Am J Sports Med* 47:144, 2019.

Bodendorfer BM, Looney AM, Lipkin SL, et al.: Biomechanical comparison of ulnar collateral ligament reconstruction with the docking technique versus repair with internal bracing, *Am J Sports Med* 46:3495, 2018.

Bruce JR, Andrews JR: Ulnar collateral ligament injuries in the throwing athlete, *J Am Acad Orthop Surg* 22:315, 2014.

Bruce JR, ElAttrache NS, Andrews JR: Revision ulnar collateral ligament reconstruction, *J Am Acad Orthop Surg* 26:377, 2018.

Bruce JR, Hess R, Joyner P, Andrews JR: How much valgus instability can be expected with ulnar collateral ligament (UCL) injuries? A review of 273 baseball players with UCL injuries, *J Shoulder Elbow Surg* 23:1521, 2014.

Byram IR, Khanna K, Gardner TR, et al.: Characterizing bone tunnel placement in medial ulnar collateral ligament reconstruction using patient-specific 3-dimensional computed tomography modeling, *Am J Sports Med* 41:894, 2013.

Cain Jr EL, Andrews JR, Dugas JR, et al.: Outcome of ulnar collateral ligament reconstruction of the elbow in 1281 athletes: results in 743 athletes with minimum 2-year follow-up, *Am J Sports Med* 38:2426, 2010.

Camp CL, Conte S, D'Angelo J, et al.: Epidemiology of ulnar collateral ligament reconstruction in Major and Minor League Baseball pitchers: comprehensive report of 1429 cases, *J Shoulder Elbow Surg* 27:871, 2018.

Camp CL, Conte S, D'Angelo J, et al.: Effect of predraft ulnar collateral ligament reconstruction on future performance in professional baseball: a matched cohort comparison, *Am J Sports Med* 46:1459, 2018.

Chalmers PN, Erickson B, Ball B, et al.: Fastball pitch velocity helps predict ulnar collateral ligament reconstruction in Major League Baseball pitchers, *Am J Sports Med* 44:2130, 2016.

Chang ES, Dodson CC, Ciccotti MG: Comparison of surgical techniques for ulnar collateral ligament reconstruction in overhead athletes, *J Am Acad Orthop Surg* 24:135, 2016.

Clain JB, Vitale MA, Ahmad CS, et al.: Ulnar nerve complications after ulnar collateral ligament reconstruction of the elbw: a systematic review, *Am J Sports Med* 363546518765139, 2018. [Epub ahead of print].

Cohen SB, Woods DP, Siegler S, et al.: Biomechanical comparison of graft fixation at 30° and 90° of elbow flexion for ulnar collateral ligament reconstruction by the docking technique, *J Shoulder Elbow Surg* 24:265, 2015.

Conte SA, Fleisig GS, Dines JS, et al.: Prevalence of ulnar collateral ligament surgery in professional baseball players, *Am J Sports Med* 43:1764, 2015.

Coughlin RP, Gohal C, Horner NS, et al.: Return to play and in-game performance statistics among pitchers after ulnar collateral ligament reconstruction of the elbow: a systematic review, *Am J Sports Med* 363546518798768, 2018. [Epub ahead of print].

Donohue KW, Mehlhoff TL: Chronic elbow dislocation: evaluation and management, *J Am Acad Orthop Surg* 24:413, 2016.

Dugas JR: Ulnar collateral ligament repair: an old idea with a new wrinkle, *Am J Orthop* 45:124, 2016.

Dugas JR, Looze CA, Capogna B, et al.: Ulnar collateral ligament repair with collagen-dipped FiberTape augmentation in overhead-throwing athletes, *Am J Sports Med* 47:1096, 2019.

Dugas JR, Walters BL, Beason DP, et al.: Biomechanical comparison of ulnar collateral ligament repair with internal bracing versus modified Jobe reconstruction, *Am J Sports Med* 44:735, 2016.

Erickson BJ, Chalmers PN, Bach Jr BR, et al.: Length of time between surgery and return to sport after ulnar collateral ligament reconstruction in Major League Baseball pitchers does not predict need for revision surgery, *J Shoulder Elbow Surg* 26:699, 2017.

Erickson BJ, Cvetanovich GL, Bach Jr BR, et al.: Should we limit innings pitched after ulnar collateral ligament reconstruction in Major League Baseball pitchers? *Am J Sports Med* 44:2210, 2016.

Erickson BJ, Nwachukwu BU, Rosas S, et al.: Trends in medial ulnar collateral ligament reconstruction in the United States: a retrospective review of a large private-payer database from 2007 to 2011, *Am J Sports Med* 43:1770, 2015.

Ford GM, Genuario J, Kinkartz J, et al.: Return-to-play outcomes in professional baseball players after medial ulnar collateral ligament injuries: comparison of operative versus nonoperative treatment based on magnetic resonance imaging findings, *Am J Sports Med* 44:723, 2016.

Frangiamore SJ, Bigart K, Nagle T, et al.: Biomechanical analysis of elbow medial ulnar collateral ligament tear location and its effect on rotational stability, *J Shoulder Elbow Surg* 27:2068, 2018.

Glogovac G, Grawe BM: Outcomes with a focus on return to play for revision ulnar collateral ligament surgery among elite-level baseball players: a systematic review, *Am J Sports Med* 363546518816960, 2018. [Epub ahead of print].

Gluck MJ, Beck CM, Golan EJ, et al.: Varus posteromedial rotatory instability: a biomechanical analysis of posterior bundle of the medial ulnar collateral ligament reconstruction, *J Shoulder Elbow Surg* 27:1317, 2018.

Goren D, Budoff JE, Hipp JA: Isometric placement of lateral ulnar collateral ligament reconstruction: a biomechanical study, *Am J Sports Med* 38:153, 2010.

Hagemeijer NC, Claessen FMAP, de Haan R, et al.: Graft site morbidity in elbow ligament reconstruction procedures: a systematic review, *Am J Sports Med* 45:3382, 2017.

Jones KJ, Dines JS, Rebolledo BJ, et al.: Operative management of ulnar collateral ligament insufficiency in adolescent athletes, *Am J Sports Med* 42:117, 2014.

Kadri OM, Okoroha KR, Patel RB, et al.: Nonoperative treatment of medial ulnar collateral ligament injuries in the throwing athlete: indications, evaluation, and management, *JBJS Rev* 7:e6, 2019.

Keller RA, Marshall NE, Guest JM, et al.: Major League Baseball pitch velocity and pitch type associated with risk of ulnar collateral ligament injury, *J Shoulder Elbow Surg* 25:671, 2016.

Keller RA, Mehran N, Marschall NE, et al.: Major League pitching workload after primary ulnar collateral ligament reconstruction and risk for revision surgery, *J Shoulder Elbow Surg* 26:288, 2017.

Kim HM, Andrews CR, Roush EP, et al.: Effect of ulnar tunnel location on elbow stability in double-strand lateral collateral ligament reconstruction, *J Shoulder Elbow Surg* 26:409, 2017.

Leasure J, Reynolds K, Thorne M, et al.: Biomechanical comparison of ulnar collateral ligament reconstruction with a modified docking technique with and without suture augmentation, *Am J Sports Med* 363546518820304, 2019. [Epub ahead of print].

Lee GH, Limpisvasti O, Park MC, et al.: Revision ulnar collateral ligament reconstruction using a suspension button fixation technique, *Am J Sports Med* 38:575, 2010.

Liu JN, Garcia GH, Conte S, et al.: Outcomes in revision Tommy John surgery in Major League Baseball pitchers, *J Shoulder Elbow Surg* 25:90, 2016.

Makhni EC, Randall RW, Morrow ZS, et al.: Performance, return to competition, and reinjury after Tommy John surgery in Major League Baseball pitchers, *Am J Sports Med* 42:1323, 2014.

Marshall NE, Keller R, Limpisvasti O, et al.: Major League Baseball pitching performance after Tommy John surgery and the effect of tear characteristics, technique, and graft type, *Am J Sports Med* 363546518817750, 2019. [Epub ahead of print].

Marshall NE, Keller R, Limpisvasti O, et al.: Pitching performance after ulnar collateral ligament reconstruction at a single institution in Major League Baseball pitchers, *Am J Sports Med* 46:3245, 2018.

Marshall NE, Keller RA, Lynch JR, et al.: Pitching performance and longevity after revision ulnar collateral ligament reconstruction in Major League Baseball pitchers, *Am J Sports Med* 43:1051, 2015.

Moore AR, Gleisig GS, Dugas JR: Ulnar collateral ligament repair, *Orthop Clin North Am* 50:383, 2019.

Murthi AM, Keener JD, Armstrong AD, Getz CL: The recurrent unstable elbow: diagnosis and treatment, *Instr Course Lect* 60:215, 2011.

Myeroff C, Brock JL, Huffman R: Ulnar collateral ligament reconstruction in athletes using a cortical button suspension technique, *J Shoulder Elbow Surg* 27:1366, 2018.

O'Brien DF, O'Hagan T, Stewart R, et al.: Outcomes for ulnar collateral ligament reconstruction: a retrospective review using the KJOC assessment score with two-year follow-up in an overhead throwing population, *J Shoulder Elbow Surg* 24:934, 2015.

Park JY, Seo BH, Hong KH, et al.: Prevalence and clinical outcomes of heterotopic ossification after ulnar collateral ligament reconstruction, *J Shoulder Elbow Surg* 27:427, 2018.

Peters SD, Bullock GS, Goode AP, et al.: The success of return to sport after ulnar collateral ligament injury in baseball: a systematic review and meta-analysis, *J Shoulder Elbow Surg* 27:561, 2018.

Ramsey ML, Getz CL, Parson BG: What's new in shoulder and elbow surgery, *J Bone Joint Surg* 92A:1047, 2010.

Rebolledo BJ, Dugas JR, Bedi A, et al.: Avoiding Tommy John surgery. What are the alternatives? *Am J Sports Med* 45:3143, 2017.

Reiman MP, Walker MD, Peters S, et al.: Risk factors for ulnar collateral ligament injury in professional and amateur baseball players: a systematic review with meta-analysis, *J Shoulder Elbow Surg* 28:186, 2019.

Rodriguez MJ, Kusnezov NA, Dunn JC, et al.: Functional outcomes following lateral ulnar collateral ligament reconstruction for symptomatic posterolateral rotatory instability of the elbow in an athletic population, *J Shoulder Elbow Surg* 27:112, 2018.

Savoie 3rd FH, Morgan C, Yaste J, et al.: Medial ulnar collateral ligament reconstruction using hamstring allograft in overhead throwing athletes, *J Bone Joint Surg* 95A:1062, 2013.

Trofa DP, Lombardi JM, Noticewala MS, et al.: Ulnar collateral ligament repair with suture augmentation, *Arthrosc Tech* 7:e53, 2018.

Whiteside D, Martini DN, Lepley AS, et al.: Predictors of ulnar collateral ligament reconstruction in Major League Baseball pitchers, *Am J Sports Med* 44:2202, 2016.

Watkins JN, McQueen P, Hutchinson MR: A systematic review of ulnar collateral ligament reconstruction techniques, *Am J Sports Med* 42:2510, 2014.

Williams PN, McGarry MH, Ihn H, et al.: The biomechanical evaluation of a novel 3-strand docking technique for ulnar collateral ligament reconstruction in the elbow, *J Shoulder Elbow Surg* 27:1672, 2018.

Wymore L, Chin P, Geary C, et al.: Performance and injury of characteristics of pitchers entering Major League Baseball draft after ulnar collateral ligament reconstruction, *Am J Sports Med* 44:3165, 2016.

Yamagami N, Yamamoto S, Aoki A, et al.: Outcomes of surgical treatment for osteochondritis dissecans of the elbow: evaluation by lesion location, *J Shoulder Elbow Surg* 27:2262, 2018.

The complete list of references is available online at ExpertConsult.com.

CHAPTER 4

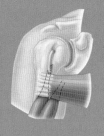

TRAUMATIC DISORDERS

Frederick M. Azar

COMPARTMENT SYNDROME

Compartment syndrome is an elevation of the interstitial pressure in a closed osteofascial compartment that results in microvascular compromise. Compartments with relatively noncompliant fascial or osseous structures most commonly are involved, especially the anterior and deep posterior compartments of the leg (Fig. 4.1) and the volar compartment of the forearm. Compartment syndrome can develop anywhere skeletal muscle is surrounded by substantial fascia, however, such as in the buttock, thigh, shoulder, hand, foot, arm, and lumbar paraspinous muscles.

Compartment syndromes can be classified as acute or chronic, depending on the cause of the increased pressure and the duration of symptoms. The most common causes of acute compartment syndrome are fractures, soft-tissue trauma, arterial injury, limb compression during altered consciousness, and burns. Other causes include intravenous fluid extravasation and anticoagulants. Acute exertional compartment syndromes have been reported in the foot in runners, basketball players, and other athletes. Chronic exertional compartment syndrome (CECS) is recurrence of increased pressure, most often in the anterior or deep posterior compartment of the leg. Exercise can increase muscle volume by 20%, causing an increase in pressure in a noncompliant compartment. Exertional compartment syndrome of the lower extremity is most common in long-distance runners and military recruits pushed past normal limits of functional tolerance. It also has been reported to occur elsewhere, including the forearms in weightlifters, rowers, welders, and others who place large demands on their upper extremities.

ANATOMY AND PATHOPHYSIOLOGY

The pathophysiology of compartment syndrome involves an insult to normal local tissue homeostasis that results in increased tissue pressure, decreased capillary blood flow, and local tissue necrosis caused by oxygen deprivation. Experimental evidence suggests that significant muscle necrosis can occur in patients with normal blood flow if intracompartmental pressure is increased to more than 30 mm Hg for longer than 8 hours. Higher pressures have been shown to cause greater compromise of neuromuscular viability in shorter periods of time.

Fascial hernias have been reported to have a definite association with the development of exertional compartment symptoms. Approximately 15% to 40% of patients treated for CECS have been found to have a fascial hernia, often despite a normal physical examination.

ACUTE COMPARTMENT SYNDROME
■ CLINICAL EVALUATION

Physical signs of acute compartment syndrome include tightness of the involved compartment, pain with passive motion of the muscles passing through the compartment, and weakness of the muscles. The most important sign is pain out of proportion to that expected with the injury. Hypesthesia or

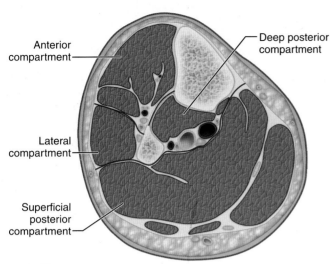

FIGURE 4.1 Four compartments of leg: transverse section through middle portion of left leg.

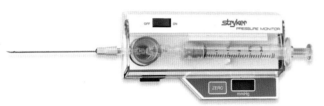

FIGURE 4.2 Stryker hand-held compartment pressure monitor. (Courtesy Stryker, Kalamazoo, MI.)

paresthesia should be evaluated by testing with pinprick, light touch, and two-point discrimination. The diagnosis of acute compartment syndrome may be delayed in patients with multiple injuries or altered consciousness and in children, in whom physical findings cannot be documented accurately. Because of the variability of clinical signs and symptoms of compartment syndrome, the sensitivity and positive predictive value of clinical findings are low; however, the specificity and negative predictive value are high. The absence of clinical findings associated with compartment syndrome is more useful for excluding the diagnosis than the presence of findings is for confirming the diagnosis.

If compartment syndrome is suspected and an adequate examination cannot be performed, pressure levels should be measured. Monitoring of compartment pressures also is helpful in patients with a fracture and altered neurologic function caused by vascular injuries, continuous epidural anesthesia, peripheral nerve injury, or tourniquet palsy.

A variety of invasive devices are available for measurement of compartment pressures, including a commercially available pressure monitor (Fig. 4.2), arterial line manometer, Whitesides three-way stopcock apparatus (Fig. 4.3A), and the wick monitor (Fig. 4.3B). Studies have shown, however, that pressure measurements are erroneous in as many as 30% to 35% of patients and should not be used as the primary determinant for or against fasciotomy. Noninvasive methods of evaluating compartment pressures include the use of ultrasonography to measure submicrometer displacement of the fascia wall caused by volume expansion of the muscle compartment, which is related to changes in intramuscular pressure. Although more study is necessary, in a model of compartment syndrome in the legs of healthy individuals, this technique had a diagnostic

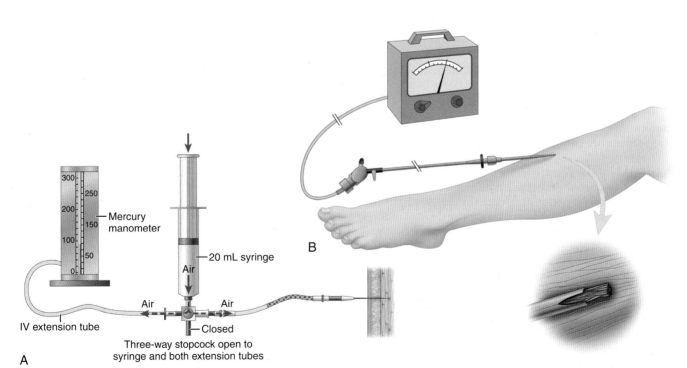

FIGURE 4.3 Technique of Whitesides et al. for determination of tissue pressure. **A,** Tissue pressure is measured by determining amount of pressure within closed system required to overcome pressure within closed compartment and inject minute amount of saline. **B,** Use of wick catheter for monitoring compartment pressures.

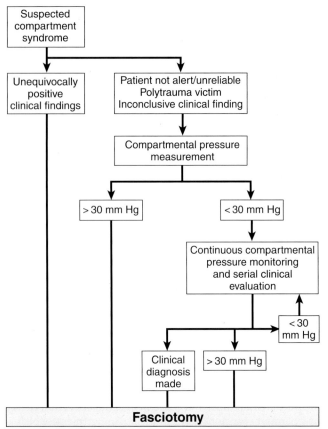

FIGURE 4.4 Algorithm for diagnosis and treatment of acute compartment syndrome of lower leg after tibial fracture. (From Bourne RB, Rorabeck CH: Compartment syndromes of the lower leg, *Clin Orthop Relat Res* 240:97, 1989.)

sensitivity of 77% and specificity of 93%. Infrared imaging also has been used in trauma patients to determine temperature differences between the proximal and distal skin surfaces to help make the diagnosis of compartment syndrome. Schmidt et al. determined that near-infrared spectroscopy data were not collected reliably, calling into question its utility for monitoring oxygenation in patients at risk for acute compartment syndrome. Currently, neither of these methods has been shown to be as accurate or easily available as the invasive methods.

■ TREATMENT

Significant controversy exists regarding appropriate compartmental pressures for performing fasciotomies. At our institution, if compartmental pressures are greater than 30 mm Hg in the presence of clinical findings, immediate fasciotomy is indicated. Equivocal readings require continuous monitoring and serial clinical examinations. In patients with major disruption of the arterial circulation or circumferential full-thickness burns, fasciotomy should be performed at the time of initial surgery. An algorithm for patients with tibial fractures has been developed to determine the roles of tissue pressure measurement and clinical findings (Fig. 4.4).

In isolated limb injuries, splitting of the cast and underlying padding can decrease compartment pressure by as much as 50% to 85%. Any circular constrictive bandages also should be released. Positioning of the limb is important; placing the limb at the level of the heart produces the highest arteriovenous gradient. On the other hand, elevation of the

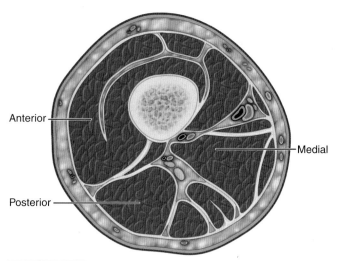

FIGURE 4.5 Three compartments of the thigh: anterior, medial, and posterior.

limb decreases arterial inflow without significantly increasing venous outflow, thus increasing local ischemia. If symptoms do not resolve within 30 to 60 minutes after appropriate treatment, pressure measurement should be repeated and, if results are equivocal, fasciotomy is indicated without delay. Although an exact timeframe has not been firmly established by evidence-based research in humans, fasciotomy after 12 hours has been associated with adverse outcomes.

■ ACUTE COMPARTMENT SYNDROME OF THIGH

Compartment syndrome of the thigh is much less frequent than that of the forearm or lower leg, but it is associated with a high level of morbidity. In one study of 23 patients with acute thigh compartment syndrome, four patients (17%) required amputations, whereas in another study of 18 patients more than half did not recover full thigh-muscle strength and had long-term functional deficits. Factors associated with an increased likelihood of functional deficits were high injury severity scores, ipsilateral femoral fracture, prolonged intervals to decompression, the presence of myonecrosis at the time of fasciotomy, and an age older than 30 years.

The most common causes of thigh compartment syndrome are blunt trauma (with or without fracture) and vascular injury; other cited causes of acute compartment syndrome of the thigh include polytrauma, arterial ischemia, burns, limb compression secondary to drug abuse, tourniquet use for lower leg surgery, use of military antishock trousers, muscle overuse, penetrating gunshot wounds, quadriceps tendon rupture and contusion or strain, other thigh muscle strains, and heterotopic ossification. Acute compartment syndrome of the thigh has been described mostly in case reports, and most often in young, active males participating in a contact sport (e.g., soccer, rugby). "Idiopathic" thigh compartment syndrome also has been described.

The myofascial compartments of the thigh have a considerably larger volume and potential capacity than those of the lower leg or forearm, accounting for the relative infrequency of thigh compartment syndrome. The thigh is divided into three distinct compartments (anterior, medial, and posterior) by intermuscular fascial extensions (Fig. 4.5); collectively, the compartments are encased by the fascia lata. Within the anterior compartment are the quadriceps muscle group and the

TABLE 4.1

Compartment-Specific Diagnostic Criteria of Acute Compartment Syndrome of the Thigh

	ANTERIOR COMPARTMENT	POSTERIOR COMPARTMENT	MEDIAL COMPARTMENT
Pain with passive stretch	Passive knee flexion with hip in extension	Passive knee extension with hip in flexion	Passive hip abduction with knee in extension
Motor deficit	Knee extension	Knee flexion, plantar flexion (sciatic tibial branch), dorsi-flexion, great toe extension (peroneal branch)	Hip adduction
Sensory deficit	Passive hip abduction with knee in extension	Hip adduction	Proximal-medial thigh (obturator nerve cutaneous branch)

Modified from Mithoefer K, Lhowe DW, Vrahas MS, et al: Functional outcome after acute compartment syndrome of the thigh, *J Bone Joint Surg* 88A:729, 2006.

sartorius muscle, the femoral nerve and its sensory branch, the saphenous nerve, and the femoral artery and vein. The medial compartment contains the adductor muscle group and its neurovascular supply, the profunda femoris and obturator arteries, and the obturator nerve. In the posterior compartment are the biceps femoris, semimembranosus and semitendinosus muscles, arterial branches of the profunda femoris, and the sciatic nerve. Most reported compartment syndromes of the thigh involve the anterior compartment because it is surrounded by the stiffest walls laterally and medially (fascia lata and iliotibial tract) and is the most vulnerable to trauma.

The diagnosis of acute compartment syndrome of the thigh is based on the criteria described earlier for acute compartment syndrome. The most common signs of thigh compartment syndrome are pain and increased thigh circumference compared with the opposite side. Weakness of the involved thigh muscles and sensory or motor deficits in the anatomic distribution of the nerves contained in specific compartments can help determine which compartments are involved (Table 4.1). Marmor et al., in a cadaver model of elevated muscle compartment pressures, used ultrasound to measure the width of the anterior compartment and the amount of pressure needed to flatten the bulging superficial compartment fascia, both of which showed strong correlation to compartment pressures, suggesting a clinical use for this modality in the future.

Although conservative management has been advocated for young patients with isolated anterior compartment syndrome of the thigh, most often immediate surgical decompression is indicated. A retrospective review of 29 patients with thigh compartment syndromes found that the frequency of complications correlated with the time to fasciotomy: delay of more than 12 hours was associated with a poor outcome in one study, and in another study patients who had decompression within 8 hours had significantly better outcomes than those with later surgery. High pressures in the thigh compartments have been found to cause long-term functional deficits even with shorter pressure durations, suggesting that the pressure level affects the time window until irreversible neuromuscular damage occurs. Some have suggested that fasciotomy should not be done when surgery is delayed for more than 12 hours because of the risk of infection in the ischemic muscle tissue, recommending that patients be treated medically (rapid fluid resuscitation) in an intensive care setting to manage rhabdomyolysis and avoid acute renal failure. When the condition of the involved muscles is unknown, a small incision has been recommended to allow access for testing of muscle viability before the extensive fasciotomy incision is made.

FASCIOTOMY FOR ACUTE COMPARTMENT SYNDROME OF THE THIGH

TECHNIQUE 4.1

(TARLOW ET AL.)
- Prepare and drape the thigh in a sterile fashion, exposing the limb from the iliac crest to the knee joint.
- Make a lateral incision beginning just distal to the inter-trochanteric line and extending to the lateral epicondyle (Fig. 4.6A).
- Use subcutaneous dissection to expose the iliotibial band and then make a straight incision in line with the skin incision through the iliotibial band (Fig. 4.6B).
- Carefully reflect the vastus lateralis off the lateral inter-muscular septum, making sure to coagulate all perforating vessels as they are encountered.
- Make a 1.5-cm incision in the lateral intermuscular septum and, using Metzenbaum scissors, extend it proximally and distally the length of the incision (Fig. 4.6C).
- After the anterior and posterior compartments have been released, measure the pressure of the medial compartment. If the pressure is elevated, make a separate medial incision to release the adductor compartment.
- Pack the wound open and apply a large, bulky dressing.
  See also Video 4.1.

POSTOPERATIVE CARE At 48 to 72 hours the patient is returned to the operating room for debridement of any necrotic material. Intravenous fluorescein and a Wood light can be helpful in evaluating muscle viability. If there is no evidence of muscle necrosis, the skin is loosely closed. Alternatively, a negative pressure wound device can be used. If closure is not accomplished, the debridement is repeated after another 48- to 72-hour interval, after which skin closure or skin grafting can be done.

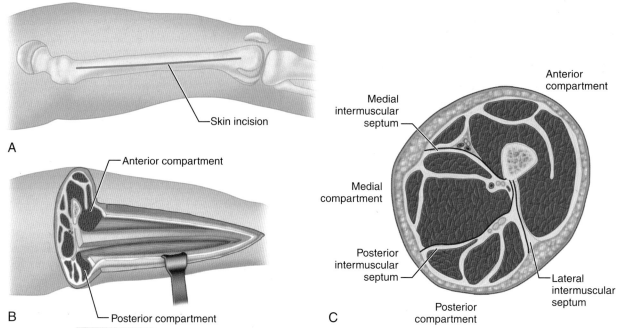

A

B

C

- Skin incision
- Anterior compartment
- Posterior compartment
- Anterior compartment
- Medial intermuscular septum
- Medial compartment
- Posterior intermuscular septum
- Posterior compartment
- Lateral intermuscular septum

FIGURE 4.6   Decompression of thigh compartments. **A,** Incision from intertrochanteric line to lateral epicondyle. **B,** Anterior compartment is opened by incising fascia lata, and vastus lateralis is retracted medially to expose lateral intermuscular septum, which is then incised to decompress posterior compartment. **C,** Drawing of thigh compartments and appropriate incisions. **SEE TECHNIQUE 4.1.**

■ ACUTE COMPARTMENT SYNDROME OF LOWER LEG

Most acute compartment syndromes of the lower leg (approximately 36%) are associated with tibial fractures; the second most common cause is blunt soft-tissue injury. During a 10-year period at a large trauma center, 288 (2.8%) of 10,315 patients with extremity trauma required fasciotomy for compartment syndrome. The need for fasciotomy varied widely according to mechanism of injury (<1% after motor vehicle accidents to almost 9% after gunshot wounds) and by type of injury (2% with closed fracture to 42% with combined vascular injury). Male sex and age younger than 55 years were among the independent predictors identified. An increasingly common risk factor for the development of compartment syndrome is the use of anticoagulation therapy in elderly trauma patients. As with all compartment syndromes, early diagnosis and treatment are essential to a good result. A review of the outcomes of fasciotomy found that 68% of patients treated within 12 hours of symptom onset had normal function, compared with only 8% in those treated more than 12 hours after symptom onset. Even with timely fasciotomy, many patients have long-term sequelae, including altered sensation, swelling, pain, functional deficits, and cosmetic concerns.

Two techniques for release of the compartments of the lower leg are commonly used: single-incision perifibular fasciotomy and double-incision fasciotomy. The single incision may be useful if the soft tissue of the limb is not extensively distorted. Because this is rarely true, the double-incision technique generally is safer and more effective. Neal et al., however, in a cadaver study determined that a single-incision four-compartment fasciotomy was as effective as fasciotomy with a double-incision technique. The role of selective compartment releases remains unclear. Thirty-eight patients with compartment syndromes in

association with tibial fractures were treated according to an algorithm in which standard anterior and lateral releases were done through a full-length lateral incision and then superficial and deep posterior compartment pressures were measured. If the difference between compartment pressure and preoperative diastolic blood pressure was greater than or equal to 30 mmHg, the posterior compartments were not released. Orthopaedic residents checked the patients every 2 hours on the floor and repeated compartment pressure measurements if symptomatology changed or the patient was obtunded. Although this management protocol seems safe and effective—only 8% of patients required posterior release and no patient without posterior release developed sequelae of a missed posterior compartment syndrome—the resources to follow patients closely and allow a rapid return to the operating room if needed may not be available to most practices. Release of all four compartments appears to be a safer approach for most patients.

SINGLE-INCISION FASCIOTOMY FOR LOWER LEG COMPARTMENT SYNDROME

TECHNIQUE 4.2

(DAVEY ET AL.)

- Make a single longitudinal, lateral incision in line with the fibula, extending from just distal to the head of the fibula to 3 to 4 cm proximal to the lateral malleolus (Fig. 4.7A).
- Undermine the skin anteriorly and avoid injuring the superficial peroneal nerve.

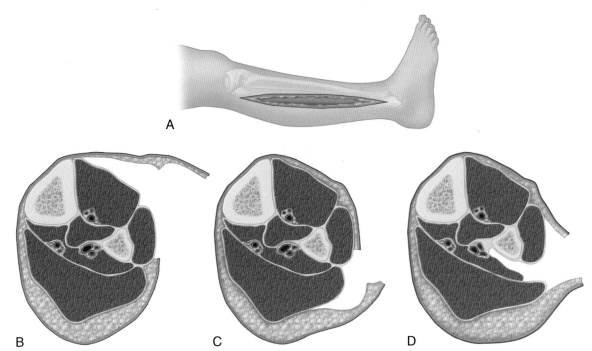

A

B   C   D

FIGURE 4.7 Technique of Davey et al. for decompression of leg compartments. **A,** Lateral skin incision from fibular neck to 3 to 4 cm proximal to lateral malleolus. **B,** Skin is undermined anteriorly, and fasciotomy of anterior and lateral compartments is performed. **C,** Skin is undermined posteriorly, and fasciotomy of superficial posterior compartment is performed. **D,** Interval between superficial posterior and lateral compartments is developed. Flexor hallucis longus muscle is dissected subperiosteally off fibula and retracted posteromedially. Fascial attachment of tibialis posterior muscle to fibula is incised to decompress muscle. **SEE TECHNIQUE 4.2.**

- Perform a longitudinal fasciotomy of the anterior and lateral compartments (Fig. 4.7B).
- Undermine the skin posteriorly and perform a fasciotomy of the superficial posterior compartment (Fig. 4.7C).
- Identify the interval between the superficial and lateral compartments distally and develop this interval proximally by detaching the soleus from the fibula.
- Subperiosteally dissect the flexor hallucis longus from the fibula.
- Retract the muscle and the peroneal vessels posteriorly.
- Identify the fascial attachment of the posterior tibial muscle to the fibula and incise this fascia longitudinally (Fig. 4.7D).
- Close only the skin over a suction drain or a negative pressure wound device.

DOUBLE-INCISION FASCIOTOMY FOR LOWER LEG COMPARTMENT SYNDROME

TECHNIQUE 4.3

(MUBARAK AND HARGENS)

- Make a 20- to 25-cm incision in the anterior compartment, centered halfway between the fibular shaft and the crest of the tibia (Fig. 4.8A). Use subcutaneous dissection for wide exposure of the fascial compartments.

- Make a transverse incision to expose the lateral intermuscular septum and identify the superficial peroneal nerve just posterior to the septum.
- Using Metzenbaum scissors, release the anterior compartment proximally and distally in line with the anterior tibial muscle.
- Perform a fasciotomy of the lateral compartment proximally and distally in line with the fibular shaft.
- Make a second longitudinal incision 2 cm posterior to the posterior margin of the tibia (Fig. 4.8B). Use wide subcutaneous dissection to allow identification of the fascial planes.
- Retract the saphenous vein and nerve anteriorly.
- Make a transverse incision to identify the septum between the deep and superficial posterior compartments. Release the fascia over the gastrocnemius-soleus complex for the length of the compartment.
- Make another fascial incision over the flexor digitorum longus muscle and release the entire deep posterior compartment. As dissection is carried proximally, if the soleus bridge extends more than halfway down the tibia, release this extended origin.
- After release of the posterior compartment, identify the deep posterior muscle compartment. If increased tension is evident in this compartment, release it over the extent of the muscle belly (Fig. 4.8C).
- Pack the wound open and apply a posterior plaster splint with the foot plantigrade.
- Management of fasciotomy wounds has included primary closure, healing by secondary intention, or split-thickness skin grafting to cover defects, which is necessary in

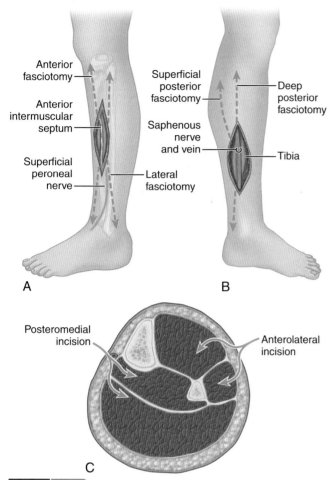

FIGURE 4.8   Method of Mubarak and Hargens for decompression of anterior and lateral compartments of leg. **A,** Anterolateral incision. **B,** Posteromedial incision. **C,** Decompression of all four compartments of leg. **SEE TECHNIQUE 4.3.**

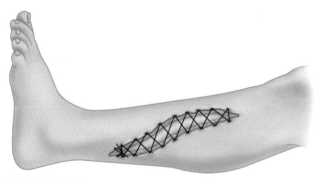

FIGURE 4.9   Delayed primary closure after fasciotomy with vessel loop shoelace technique. **SEE TECHNIQUE 4.3.**

approximately 50% of patients. An alternative is a delayed primary closure, which can be accomplished using the vessel loop shoelace technique (Fig. 4.9) or commercial closure devices. Vacuum-assisted wound closure can be used to reduce postoperative edema, which may improve wound closure with or without negative pressure therapy (Fig. 4.10).

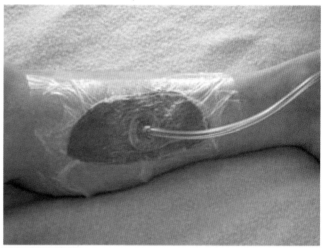

FIGURE 4.10   Fasciotomy wound with vacuum-assisted closure system in place. (From Saziye K, Mustafa C, Ilker U, Afksendyios K: Comparison of vacuum-assisted closure device and conservative treatment for fasciotomy wound healing in ischemia-reperfusion syndrome: preliminary results, *Int Wound J* 8:229, 2011.) **SEE TECHNIQUE 4.3.**

POSTOPERATIVE CARE At 48 to 72 hours, the patient is returned to the operating room for debridement of any necrotic material. Intravenous fluorescein and a Wood light can be helpful in evaluating muscle viability. If there is no evidence of muscle necrosis, the skin is loosely closed. If closure is not accomplished, the debridement is repeated after another 48- to 72-hour interval, after which skin closure or skin grafting can be done.

CHRONIC EXERTIONAL COMPARTMENT SYNDROME

Chronic exertional compartment syndrome (CECS) is defined as reversible ischemia secondary to a noncompliant osteofascial compartment that is unresponsive to the expansion of muscle volume that occurs with exercise. Factors believed to contribute to an increase in an intracompartmental pressure during exercise include increased volume of the skeletal muscle with exertion due to blood flow and edema (muscle volume can increase up to 20% of its resting size during exercise), dynamic contraction factors due to the gait cycle (rear-foot landing, overpronation), and muscle hypertrophy as a response of exercise. Anabolic steroid and creatine use also increases muscle volume.

CECS is most common in young adult recreational runners, elite athletes, and military recruits. The anterior and lateral compartments are most often affected, and symptoms are bilateral in about 75% of patients. Studies have indicated that a 2-year delay in diagnosis is typical for CECS.

■ CLINICAL EVALUATION

The importance of an accurate history cannot be overemphasized in the evaluation of patients with lower extremity pain. In many patients the diagnosis is delayed for months or even years. In their series of 42 patients, Winkes et al. reported a median time of 28 months from first symptom to diagnosis. A typical patient with CECS is a competitive runner, 20 to

Differential Diagnosis of Chronic Exertional Compartment Syndrome

- Medial tibial stress syndrome (shin splints)
- Stress fracture
- Tenosynovitis
- Periostitis
- Deep venous thrombosis
- Nerve entrapment syndrome
- Lumbosacral radiculopathy
- Neurogenic claudication
- Popliteal artery entrapment syndrome
- Vascular claudication
- Infection
- Myopathy
- Tumor

30 years old, who describes exercise-induced pain and a feeling of tightness that begins after 20 to 30 minutes of running. The pain usually resolves within 15 to 30 minutes of cessation of exercise. Paresthesias of the nerves running through the involved compartment often are reported. Physical examination may reveal tenderness over the musculature of the involved compartment, and muscle herniation through defects in fascia may be palpated. Patients should be examined after completing the exercise that reproduces symptoms. Other possible causes of the patient's symptoms also should be considered (Box 4.1).

If history and physical examination are not diagnostic, other studies can be instituted to arrive at a diagnosis. Periostitis is easily seen on bone scan, with diffuse uptake often covering one third of the bone. Stress fractures show a more localized, intense uptake of the radioactive isotope, although 90% of stress fractures can be diagnosed with plain radiographs. Stress reactions, precursors of stress fractures, can best be detected by MRI on short T1 inversion recovery sequence or a fat-suppressed T2-weighted fast spin-echo sequence. Entrapment of the peroneal nerve can be determined by provocative tests in which pressure over the point at which the superficial peroneal nerve emerges from the deep fascia produces pain during active, resisted dorsiflexion and eversion of the ankle. The Tinel sign also may be positive in the same area.

As with acute compartment syndrome, some controversy exists as to values for diagnosis of CECS. The most commonly accepted values are the presence of one or more of the following criteria: (1) preexercise, resting pressure of 15 mm Hg or more; (2) pressure of 30 mm Hg or more 1 minute after exercise; and (3) pressure of 20 mm Hg or more 5 minutes after exercise. One study found that the level of pain was significantly higher in patients with CECS than in controls at all phases of exercise. The authors noted that a pressure of 105 mm Hg immediately after 5 minutes of sustained walking at 4 miles per hour with a 5% incline and the patient wearing a 15-kg backpack had better diagnostic accuracy than the Pedowitz criteria above. Other authors have suggested use of postexercise MRI, near-infrared spectroscopy, triple-phase bone scan, methoxyisobutyl isonitrile (MIBI) perfusion imaging, and thallous chloride scintigraphy.

TREATMENT
NONOPERATIVE TREATMENT
Conservative measures include relative rest (limiting activity to a level that avoids all but minimal symptoms), antiinflammatory medications, manual therapy, stretching and strengthening of the involved muscles, and orthotics. Forefoot running (forefoot strike) also has been reported to improve pain and lower intracompartmental pressure with sustained results of up to 1 year, avoiding surgical intervention. Return to work or sports has been reported in 65% to 75% of patients with nonoperative treatment; however, Maksymiak et al. found that operatively treated patients were more satisfied, reported better recovery to former performance levels, and had better functional outcomes than those treated nonoperatively. If symptoms persist, if pressures are extremely elevated, or if the athlete desires to continue activity at the same level, fasciotomy of the involved compartments is indicated.

OPERATIVE TREATMENT
Failure after fasciotomy may be related to the compartments released. Anterior compartment fasciotomy has a success rate of 80% to 90%, whereas release of the deep posterior compartment has a lower rate of 50% to 70% as does a combined anterior and lateral release. Younger patient age (<23 years) also has been shown to be a factor in improved subjective function and satisfaction after fasciotomy. Most patients, however, are able to return to running without significant symptoms within 3 months of surgery. Winkes et al. reported that fasciotomy was beneficial in 71% of patients with CECS in the lower leg, with all symptoms improved at short-term and long-term follow-up. Several studies have indicated that patients who do not have all four compartments released have worse outcomes than those who have four-compartment release. Maher et al. reported that 91% of patients with four-compartment releases returned to sport at their desired level, compared to only 67% of those who did not have four-compartment release. In their literature review, Vajapey and Miller concluded that limited-incision fasciotomy remains the most effective treatment for CECS. Open fasciotomy remains the predominant surgical technique, although its comparative efficacy relative to newer endoscopic or other minimally invasive techniques is still being determined.

Subcutaneous and endoscopic techniques have been described for fasciotomy. Although increased complication rates and recurrence of symptoms have been reported with these techniques, a "double mini-incision" technique produced good results in 18 athletes; 14 had release of the anterior compartment only, and four had release of the anterior and lateral compartments. At 2-year follow-up, all 18 had resumed their sports activities; two had a transient sensation of weakness that resolved within 3 months. Endoscopic compartment release was reported to be successful in nine patients (14 legs), eight of whom were able to resume preoperative activities; the only reported complications were two postoperative hematomas that resolved. With anterior and posterior compartment release, extensive undermining and careful identification and retraction of the superficial peroneal nerve during anterior release and of the saphenous nerve and vein during posterior release are necessary. We believe the double-incision technique to be better for release of the posterior structures.

Fasciotomy may not be successful, resulting in recurrence of symptoms. Partial fasciectomy has been advocated by some authors, especially in patients with recurrence after fasciotomy. Other complications include numbness, bruising, skin infection, weakness, and vascular compromise.

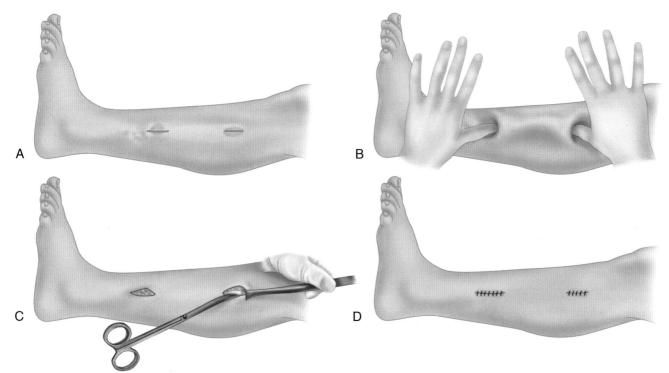

FIGURE 4.11 Mouhsine et al. double mini-incision fasciotomy for chronic anterior compartment syndrome. **A,** Two vertical 2-cm skin incisions. **B,** Development of subcutaneous flap with blunt dissection. **C,** Skin retraction to allow fasciotomy under direct vision. **D,** After wound closure. **SEE TECHNIQUE 4.4.**

DOUBLE MINI-INCISION FASCIOTOMY FOR CHRONIC ANTERIOR COMPARTMENT SYNDROME

TECHNIQUE 4.4

(MOUHSINE ET AL.)
- Without the use of a tourniquet, make two vertical 2-cm skin incisions over the anterior compartment 15 cm apart (Fig. 4.11A).
- Identify the fascia and carefully develop a subcutaneous flap with blunt dissection of the bridge of skin and subcutaneous tissue (Fig. 4.11B). Use retractors to mobilize this flap to allow a clear view of the deep fascia.
- Identify the anterior intermuscular septum and the superficial peroneal nerve through the distal incision (10 to 12 cm proximal to the lateral malleolus). Retract the skin anteriorly and posteriorly to allow anterior and/or lateral fasciotomy under direct vision (Fig. 4.11C). If needed, use a gloved finger to complete the release.
- Close the two incisions with 3.0 monofilament and sterile adhesive strips (Fig. 4.11D) and apply a firm bandage from midfoot to the knee.

POSTOPERATIVE CARE The limb is elevated for 24 to 48 hours and ice is applied. Then supervised active range-of-motion exercises and progressive weight bearing are begun. Most patients need to use crutches for up to 10 days. Sports activities are gradually resumed at 3 to 4 weeks after surgery.

SINGLE-INCISION FASCIOTOMY FOR CHRONIC ANTERIOR AND LATERAL COMPARTMENT SYNDROME

TECHNIQUE 4.5

(FRONEK ET AL.)
- Make a 5-cm longitudinal incision halfway between the fibula and the tibial crest in the midportion of the leg (Fig. 4.12A) or over the fascial defect if a muscular hernia is present at the exit of the superficial peroneal nerve (Fig. 4.12B,C).
- Identify the nerve and the intermuscular septum and pass a fasciotome into the anterior compartment in line with the anterior tibial muscle (Fig. 4.12D).
- In the lateral compartment, run the fasciotome posterior to the superficial peroneal nerve in line with the fibular shaft (Fig. 4.12E).
- Do not repair muscular hernias.
- Close the skin in the usual fashion and apply a sterile dressing.

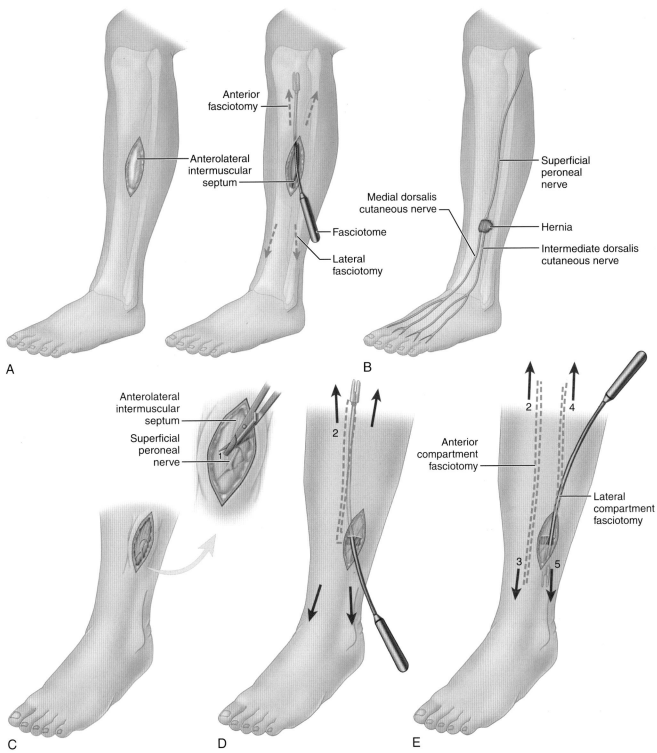

FIGURE 4.12 Fronek et al. single-incision fasciotomy. **A,** Incision between tibial crest and fibular shaft, over anterolateral intermuscular septum, when no fascial hernia exists. **B,** In presence of fascial hernia, incision is directly over fascial defect. **C,** Defect is enlarged across intermuscular septum (1). **D** and **E,** Complete longitudinal release of anterior compartment (2 and 3) and lateral compartment (4 and 5). **SEE TECHNIQUE 4.5.**

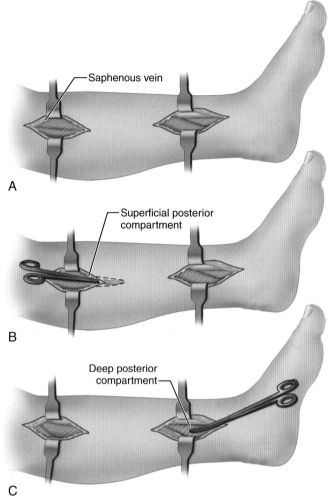

FIGURE 4.13 Rorabek two-incision release of chronic deep posterior compartment syndrome. **A,** Two vertical incisions; saphenous vein is identified and retracted anteriorly. **B,** Superficial compartment is entered and released. **C,** Deep fascia is incised, and deep posterior compartment is released. **SEE TECHNIQUE 4.6.**

DOUBLE-INCISION FASCIOTOMY FOR CHRONIC POSTERIOR COMPARTMENT SYNDROME

TECHNIQUE 4.6

(RORABECK)

- Make two incisions in the leg 1 cm behind the posteromedial border of the tibia (Fig. 4.13A). Identify the saphenous vein in the proximal incision and retract it anteriorly along with the nerve.
- Enter and release the superficial compartment (Fig. 4.13B).
- Incise the deep fascia (Fig. 4.13C).
- Expose the deep compartment, including the flexor digitorum longus and posterior tibial muscles, by detaching the soleal bridge.

- Identify the neurovascular bundle and posterior tibial tendon and incise proximally and distally the fascia overlying the tendon. The posterior tibial tendon is the key to posterior compartment decompression, and it usually is constricted proximally between the two origins of the flexor hallucis longus; enlarge the opening between these two structures to check for constriction.
- Release the tourniquet and obtain meticulous hemostasis.
- Close the wound over a suction drain to minimize the risk of hematoma formation.

POSTOPERATIVE CARE Early range-of-motion exercises are encouraged, and weight bearing to tolerance on crutches is allowed the day after surgery. Crutches are discarded when walking is possible without difficulty. Light jogging is allowed at 2 to 3 weeks if swelling and tenderness are absent.

Risk Factors for Achilles Tendon Rupture

Intrinsic: Anatomic Predisposition, Inability of Body's Biomechanics to Naturally Absorb Force
- Subtalar hyperpronation
- Excessive rearfoot/forefoot varus/valgus
- Increased femoral anteversion
- Limb-length discrepancy
- Muscle weakness/imbalance
- High body mass index
- Aging

Extrinsic: Errors in Training Technique, Environmental Factors
- Excessive running duration and intensity
- Unfamiliar running surface
- Drugs: fluoroquinolone antibiotics, corticosteroids

RUPTURE OF MUSCLES AND TENDONS
RUPTURE OF ACHILLES TENDON

Injuries of the Achilles tendon are relatively common in middle-aged athletes, and the frequency of these injuries is increasing (from 2/100,000 in 1986 to 2.5/100,000 in 2016) as more people remain active in recreational sports for longer times. Tendinitis, tendinosis, and peritendinitis accounted for 11% of lower extremity complaints at a large runners' clinic, and Achilles tendon ruptures have been estimated to be the third most frequent tendon rupture. Some studies have suggested that Achilles tendinopathy is present in 24% of competitive athletes and in up to 50% of competitive runners. Tendon ruptures are estimated to occur in approximately 8% of competitive athletes. The peak age for Achilles tendon rupture in both men and women is between 30 and 40 years of age. Several intrinsic and extrinsic risk factors for Achilles tendon rupture have been identified (Box 4.2). A survey of 154 patients with acute tendon ruptures found that at 4-year follow-up 6% had sustained a rupture on the contralateral side; according to the authors' calculations, patients with an acute Achilles tendon rupture have a nearly 200-fold increased risk of a contralateral tendon rupture. Patients who have an Achilles tendon rupture in their 30s have a significantly increased risk for contralateral tendon rupture.

Most commonly, the mechanisms of Achilles tendon rupture are pushing off with the weight-bearing forefoot while extending the knee, sudden unexpected dorsiflexion of the ankle, and violent dorsiflexion of the plantar flexed foot, as in a fall from a height. Disruption also can occur from a direct blow to the contracted tendon or from a laceration.

◼ ANATOMY AND PATHOPHYSIOLOGY

Achilles tendon rupture has been related to a relatively hypovascular area of the tendon, shown by angiography to be 2 to 6 cm above the tendon insertion into the calcaneus. The major blood supply of the tendon is through its mesotendon, with the richest supply through the anterior mesentery. With increasing age, this anterior mesenteric supply becomes reduced. Age-dependent changes in collagen crosslinking result in

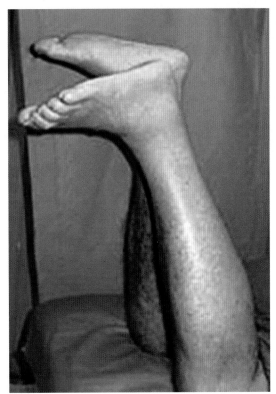

FIGURE 4.14   Matles test for Achilles tendon rupture. If the foot falls into neutral or slight dorsiflexion with this maneuver, the Achilles tendon is likely ruptured.

increased stiffness and loss of viscoelasticity, predisposing to injury. Repetitive microtrauma to this area may make it impossible for the reparative process to keep pace, and a degenerative attrition may be responsible for many Achilles tendon ruptures. Another theory concerning the cause of Achilles tendon rupture is the failure of inhibiting mechanisms at the musculotendinous unit as a result of fatigue, with resultant eccentric overload. The cause of Achilles tendon rupture probably is a combination of a relatively hypovascular area and repetitive microtrauma that causes an inflammatory reparative process that is unable to keep up with the stresses because of decreased vascularity. A mechanical overload completes the rupture.

◼ CLINICAL EVALUATION

The diagnosis of Achilles tendon rupture is reliably made by a palpable tendon defect, the inability to do a toe raise on the affected side, and a positive Thompson "squeeze test," which is performed by squeezing the calf muscle just distal to its maximal girth while the patient is prone to bring about plantar flexion of the ankle joint. The test is positive for complete rupture when there is no plantar flexion of the ankle. Another test that may be beneficial is that described by Matles. The patient is placed prone with the lower legs extending off the bed and is asked to actively flex the knees to 90 degrees. Active flexion of the knee should cause the gastrocnemius to shorten, causing plantar flexion of the foot. If the foot falls into neutral or slight dorsiflexion, the Achilles tendon is likely ruptured (Fig. 4.14). In the needle test described by O'Brien, a 25-gauge needle is placed percutaneously in the midline of the proximal tendon. Motion of the proximal tendon indicating continuity is detected by observing the needle when the foot is put through passive range of motion.

AAOS Recommendations: Achilles Tendon Ruptures

Strength of Recommendation: Consensus

- The physical examination should include two or more of the following tests to establish the diagnosis of acute Achilles tendon rupture:
  - Clinical Thompson test (Simmonds squeeze test)
  - Decreased ankle plantar flexion strength
  - Presence of a palpable gap (defect, loss of contour)
  - Increased passive ankle dorsiflexion with gentle manipulation
- Operative treatment should be approached more cautiously in patients with diabetes, neuropathy, immunocompromised states, age older than 65, tobacco use, sedentary lifestyle, obesity (body mass index > 30), peripheral vascular disease, or local/systemic dermatologic disorders.

Strength of Recommendation: Moderate

- Early (≤2 weeks) postoperative protected weight bearing (including limiting dorsiflexion) for patients with acute Achilles tendon rupture who have been treated operatively
- Use of a protective device that allows mobilization by 2 to 4 weeks postoperatively

Strength of Recommendation: Weak

- Nonoperative treatment as an option for patients with acute Achilles tendon rupture
- Open, limited open, and percutaneous techniques as options for treating patients with acute Achilles tendon rupture
- In patients who participate in sports, option of returning to sports within 3 to 6 months after operative treatment for acute Achilles tendon rupture

Strength of Recommendation: Inconclusive

- Routine use of magnetic resonance imaging, ultrasound, and radiography to confirm the diagnosis of acute Achilles tendon rupture
- Use of immediate functional bracing as nonoperative treatment for patients with acute Achilles tendon rupture
- Preoperative immobilization or restricted weight bearing before surgical treatment of acute Achilles tendon rupture
- Use of allograft, autograft, xenograft, synthetic tissue, or biologic adjuncts in acute Achilles tendon ruptures that are treated operatively
- Use of antithrombotic treatment for patients with acute Achilles tendon ruptures
- Postoperative physiotherapy for patients with acute Achilles tendon rupture

Modified from Chido CP, Glazebrook M, Bluman EM, et al: American Academy of Orthopaedic Surgeons clinical practice guideline on treatment of Achilles tendon rupture, *J Bone Joint Surg* 92A:2466, 2010.

■ TREATMENT

The decision to treat acute Achilles tendon ruptures conservatively or operatively is somewhat controversial, with evidence to support either form of treatment. Despite the multitude of articles in the medical literature about Achilles tendon rupture, there is still no consensus as to the best treatment and few high-level studies to support various recommendations. The American Academy of Orthopaedic Surgeons' recommendations (Box 4.3) are primarily consensus or based on weak or inconclusive evidence. Important considerations include return to sport and to activities of daily living (pain, range of motion, strength), rerupture rate, and risks associated with surgery.

Current nonoperative treatment of Achilles tendon ruptures involves functional bracing and an aggressive rehabilitation protocol that allows early motion (Table 4.2). Suggested ultrasound-based criteria for choosing nonoperative treatment include (1) gap of less than 5 mm with maximal plantar flexion, (2) gap of less than 10 mm with the foot in neutral position, and (3) more than 75% tendon apposition with the foot in 20 degrees of plantar flexion.

Historically, operative treatment has been shown to have a significantly lower rerupture rate than nonoperative treatment but to be associated with a higher complication rate. More recent comparisons, however, show less difference in rerupture rates, rates of other complications, and functional outcomes, perhaps because improved operative techniques have decreased the frequency of postoperative complications and the use of functional bracing and aggressive rehabilitation has improved rerupture rates and function after nonoperative treatment. A systematic review and meta-analysis involving 762 patients found no significant differences between conservative and operative treatment in terms of deep venous thrombosis (DVT), return to sport, ankle range of motion, or physical activity scale; however, the rate of rerupture was significantly lower in the operative group than in the nonoperative group. Overall the risk of rerupture is low and differences between treatment groups are small.

Regardless of treatment, 30% to 50% of patients are reported to have functional impairments, including pain, reduced strength, and decreased range of motion, at 1 to 5 years after injury. A study of 31 National Football League (NFL) players who had an acute Achilles tendon rupture found that only 21 (64%) returned to play at an average of 11 months after injury, and all 21 had significant decreases in the number of games played and in their power ratings compared with the three seasons preceding the injury. Despite the persistence of functional deficits and lower activity levels, in most patient populations the patient-reported outcomes are relatively high, suggesting that patients learn to adjust to any impairments.

Contraindications to operative repair of Achilles tendon ruptures include arterial insufficiency, poor skin and soft-tissue quality, poorly controlled medical comorbidities (e.g., diabetes), and an inability to comply with postoperative rehabilitation protocols. Advanced age alone is not a contraindication to operative repair; good results have been reported with both open and percutaneous repair techniques in older patients. Although obesity has been cited as a risk factor for poorer outcomes after a number of orthopaedic procedures, current studies have found that both obese and non-obese patients can achieve good outcomes with Achilles tendon repair. Hillam et al. compared outcomes in obese and non-obese patients and found that obesity had an increased association with wound dehiscence but was not significantly associated with any other complication.

TABLE 4.2

Protocol for Nonoperative Treatment of Achilles Tendon Rupture and Rehabilitation After Operative Repair

0-2 weeks	Posterior slab/splint; non–weight bearing with crutches (immediately postoperative or after injury)
2-4 weeks	Aircast walking boot with 2-cm heel lift* Protected weight bearing with crutches. Active plantar flexion and dorsiflexion to neutral, inversion/eversion below neutral, modalities to control swelling Incision mobilization modalities[†] (e.g., friction, ultrasound, stretching) Knee/hip exercises with no ankle involvement (e.g., leg lifts from sitting, prone, or side-lying position) Non–weight-bearing fitness/cardiovascular exercises (e.g., bicycling with one leg, deep-water running) Hydrotherapy (within motion and weight-bearing limitations)
4-6 weeks	Weight bearing as tolerated* Continue activities as above
6-8 weeks	Remove heel lift from boot Weight bearing as tolerated *Dorsiflexion stretching, slowly graduated resistance exercises (open and closed kinetic chain, functional activities) Proprioceptive and gait training Modalities, including ice, heat, and ultrasound as indicated Incision mobilization [†]Fitness/cardiovascular exercises, including weight bearing as tolerated (e.g., bicycling, elliptical machine, walking and/or running on treadmill, StairMaster) Hydrotherapy
8-12 weeks	Wean off boot Return to crutches and/or cane as necessary and gradually wean off Continue to progress range of motion, strength, proprioception
>12 weeks	Continue to progress range of motion, strength, proprioception Retrain strength, power, endurance Increase dynamic weight-bearing exercise, include plyometric training Sport-specific training

*Patients are required to wear the boot while sleeping; may be removed for bathing and dressing but weight-bearing restrictions must be observed.
[†]If deemed necessary by the physical therapist (scar tight or not moving well).
Modified from Willits K, Amendola A, Bryant D, et al: Operative versus nonoperative treatment of acute Achilles tendon ruptures: a multicenter randomized trial using accelerated functional rehabilitation, *J Bone Joint Surg* 92A:2767, 2010.

◼ ACUTE RUPTURE

A variety of techniques and modifications have been described for repair of acute Achilles tendon ruptures, including open repair, with or without augmentation (tendon transfer, local fascial turndown, allograft), and percutaneous or minimally invasive repair, with or without intraoperative ultrasound or endoscopy. In addition, numerous suture materials and configurations have been used for repair, including single and double Bunnell, Kessler, and Krackow (locking-loop) techniques and various modifications of these. Although proponents have suggested benefits for varied modifications, none has been firmly proved to be superior. A cadaver study found no difference in strength between Krackow, Bunnell, and Kessler sutures when all were done with a double-suture technique. One long-term follow-up study (12 years) reported that fibrin glue produced functional results equal to those obtained with sutures, with fewer complications.

Repairs of acute Achilles tendon ruptures have been augmented with "turn-down" flap of fascia, the plantaris and peroneus brevis tendons, and biologic or synthetic scaffolds. Two large studies found no benefit of turn-down flaps over simple end-to-end repair, noting that the augmentation required a longer incision and a longer operating time. Extracellular matrix xenografts have been reported to decrease gapping and increase load to failure immediately after surgery in cadaver models of Achilles rupture, as well as in animal studies; however, these benefits have not been clinically proven.

Another "biologic" treatment approach involves the use of platelet-rich plasma (PRP) injected into the area of tendon rupture to theoretically recruit platelet growth factors to promote rapid tendon healing. Animal studies have shown that local application of PRP stimulates tendon repair, and cell culture studies have shown that PRP can stimulate processes associated with tendon healing. A clinical study on the use of PRP in open repair of acute Achilles tendon injuries reported faster recovery of motion and quicker return to sports with PRP; however, others reached the opposite conclusion, reporting no effect on function and suggesting that PRP may actually have a negative effect on tendon healing. Until preparation and delivery methods, as well as patient selection, are more standardized, it is difficult to determine the effect of PRP on tendon healing. Animal studies using mesenchymal stem cells for tendon healing also have shown promise.

▌ OPEN REPAIR TECHNIQUES FOR ACHILLES TENDON RUPTURE

Open repair of acute Achilles tendon ruptures remains the "gold standard" of operative treatment, especially for athletic individuals, because of the historically low rate of reruptures,

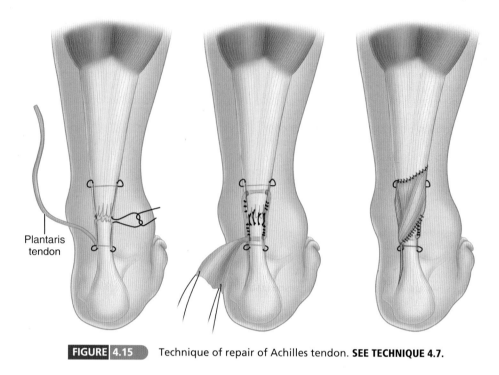

Plantaris
tendon

FIGURE 4.15 Technique of repair of Achilles tendon. **SEE TECHNIQUE 4.7.**

high rate of return to sports, and decreased complication rate with newer techniques. Of 62 professional athletes with acute Achilles tendon ruptures repaired operatively, 31% were unable to return to play. Athletes who did return played in fewer games, had less playing time, and performed at a lower level than their preinjury status. However, these functional deficits were seen at only 1 year after surgery compared to matched controls, suggesting that those who return to play can expect to perform at a level similar to that of uninjured controls 2 years after surgery. Advocates of open repair argue that Achilles tendon injuries often result in complex obliquely oriented tears that cannot be adequately apposed and repaired with percutaneous or minimally invasive techniques.

Complications of open Achilles tendon surgery have been well documented, with major complications reported in up to 10% of patients. The most frequently reported complications include wound infection, rerupture, and sural nerve injury. Traditionally, Achilles tendon repair has been done with the patient prone, which itself is associated with a number of complication risks. Marcel et al. described an alternative technique in which the surgery is done through a posterome-dial incision with the patient supine. They suggest that supine positioning can avoid risks associated with prone positioning and markedly reduce operating room time without increasing complications. None of their 45 patients in whom supine positioning was used had infections, sural nerve injuries, or reruptures.

Delayed time to surgery has been cited as a prognostic factor in outcomes after open repair of acute Achilles tendon ruptures. Svedman et al., in a study of 228 patients with acute Achilles tendon rupture who were treated with uniform anes-thetic and surgical techniques within 10 days of injury, found that those who had surgery within 48 hours of injury had better outcomes and fewer adverse events than those treated after 72 hours.

OPEN REPAIR OF ACUTE ACHILLES TENDON RUPTURE

TECHNIQUE 4.7   *Figure 4.15*

- With the patient prone, make a posteromedial longitudi-nal incision 8 to 10 cm long; make it about 1 cm medial to the tendon, and end it just proximal to where the shoe counter strikes the heel. The skin incision should be off center to prevent later irritation by shoes directly over the tendon in the midline.
- Carry the incision sharply through the skin, subcutaneous tissues, and tendon sheath.
- Reflect the tendon sheath with the subcutaneous tissue, minimizing subcutaneous dissection.
- Approximate the ruptured ends of the tendon with No. 5 nonabsorbable tension suture, using a modified Kessler stitch through the stump 2.5 cm from the rupture. Plantar flex the foot 0 to 5 degrees, flex the knee 15 degrees, and approxi-mate the ends of the tendon by tying the tension suture.
- Use a tendon stripper and harvest the plantaris tendon, releasing it proximally. Lay it aside in a moist sponge.
- Place the frayed ends of the tendon in as nearly normal position as possible and repair the rupture with multiple 2-0 absorbable sutures anteriorly and posteriorly.
- Place the previously harvested plantaris tendon in a fascial needle and pass it circumferentially, first through the pos-terior and then through the anterior part of the tendon 2 cm from the rupture.
- Use multiple 2-0 absorbable sutures to tack the plantaris tendon to the Achilles tendon. The distal tendon usually is long enough to be fanned out and tacked over the repair, as described by Lynn (see Technique 4.10).

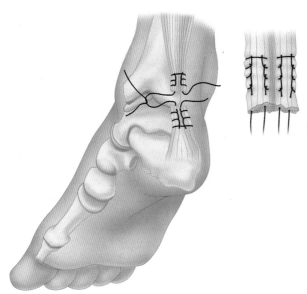

FIGURE 4.16   Krackow suture technique for Achilles tendon rupture. **SEE TECHNIQUE 4.8.**

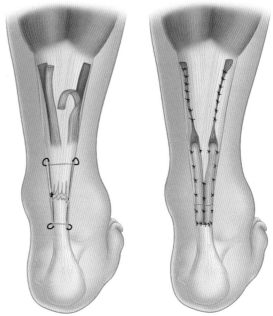

FIGURE 4.17   Lindholm technique for repairing ruptures of Achilles tendon. **SEE TECHNIQUE 4.9.**

- Close the fascial sheath and subcutaneous tissues with 2-0 absorbable sutures.
- Close the skin and apply a sterile dressing.
- Apply a short leg cast with the foot in gravity equinus.

OPEN REPAIR OF ACHILLES TENDON RUPTURE—KRACKOW ET AL.

TECHNIQUE 4.8

- With the patient prone, make a posteromedial incision approximately 10 cm long about 1 cm medial to the tendon and ending proximal to where the shoe counter strikes the heel.
- Sharply dissect through the skin, subcutaneous tissues, and tendon sheath. Reflect the tendon sheath with the subcutaneous tissue to minimize subcutaneous dissection.
- Approximate the ruptured ends of the tendon with a 2-0 nonabsorbable suture (Fig. 4.16).
- Check the repair for stability after the sutures are tied.
- Close the peritenon and subcutaneous tissues with 4-0 absorbable sutures.
- Close the skin and apply a sterile dressing and a posterior splint or short leg cast with the foot in gravity equinus.

OPEN REPAIR OF ACHILLES TENDON RUPTURE—LINDHOLM

TECHNIQUE 4.9

- With the patient prone, make a posterior curvilinear incision extending from the midcalf to the calcaneus.
- Incise the deep fascia in the midline and expose the tendon rupture.
- Debride the ragged ends of the tendon and appose them with a box type of mattress suture of heavy nonabsorbable suture material or wire; also use fine interrupted sutures (Fig. 4.17).
- Fashion two flaps from the proximal tendon and gastrocnemius aponeurosis, each approximately 1 cm wide and 7 to 8 cm long. Leave these flaps attached at a point 3 cm proximal to the site of rupture.
- Twist each flap 180 degrees on itself so that its smooth external surface lies next to the subcutaneous tissue as it is turned distally over the rupture.
- Suture each flap to the distal stump of the tendon and to one another so that they cover the site of rupture completely.
- Close the wound, being careful to approximate the tendon sheath over the site of repair.

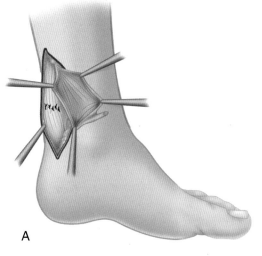

A

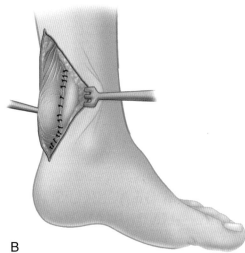

B

FIGURE 4.18   Lynn technique for repairing fresh rupture of Achilles tendon. **A,** Ruptured Achilles tendon has been sutured, and plantaris tendon has been divided distally and is being fanned out to form membrane. **B,** Fanned-out plantaris tendon has been placed over repair of Achilles tendon and sutured in place. **SEE TECHNIQUES 4.10 AND 4.16.**

REPAIR OF ACUTE ACHILLES TENDON RUPTURE USING PLANTARIS TENDON

Lynn described a method of repairing ruptures of the Achilles tendon in which the plantaris tendon is fanned out to make a membrane 2.5 cm or wider for reinforcing the repair. The method is useful for injuries less than 10 days old; later the plantaris tendon becomes incorporated in the scar tissue and cannot be identified easily.

TECHNIQUE 4.10

(LYNN)
- Make an incision 12.5 to 17.5 cm long parallel to the medial border of the Achilles tendon.

- Open the tendon sheath in the midline and, with the foot held in 20 degrees of plantar flexion and without excising the irregular edges, sew the ends of the Achilles tendon together with 2-0 absorbable sutures.
- If the plantaris tendon is intact (Fig. 4.18A), divide its insertion on the calcaneus; then, using forceps and beginning distally, fan out the tendon to form a membrane.
- Place this membrane over the repair of the Achilles tendon and suture it in place with interrupted sutures (Fig. 4.18B). When possible, cover the Achilles tendon for 2.5 cm both proximal and distal to the repair.
- If the plantaris tendon also is ruptured, dissect it free from the Achilles tendon for several centimeters and divide it proximally, using a tendon stripper.
- Then pull the tendon distally into the incision, fan it out as a free graft, and cover the repair as already described.
- Close the sheath of the Achilles tendon as far distally as possible without tension and close the wound.

POSTOPERATIVE CARE   Postoperative care is the same as that used after treatment of acute rupture of the Achilles tendon (see Technique 4.11).

DYNAMIC LOOP SUTURE TECHNIQUE FOR ACUTE ACHILLES TENDON RUPTURE

TECHNIQUE 4.11

(TEUFFER)
- Expose the Achilles tendon and the tuberosity of the calcaneus through a posterolateral longitudinal incision.
- Identify and retract the sural nerve in the proximal part of the wound.
- Detach the peroneus brevis tendon from its insertion through a small incision at the base of the fifth metatarsal.
- Excise the aponeurotic septum, separating the lateral and posterior compartments, and deliver the freed peroneus brevis into the first incision.
- Dissect the tuberosity of the calcaneus and drill a hole large enough for passage of the tendon through the transverse diameter of the bone.
- Pass the peroneus brevis tendon through this hole and back proximally beside the Achilles tendon, reinforcing the site of rupture, and suture it to the peroneus brevis itself, producing a dynamic loop (Fig. 4.19).

Turco and Spinella described a modification in which the peroneus brevis is passed through a midcoronal slit in the distal stump of the Achilles tendon. The graft is sutured medially and laterally to the stump and proximally to the tendon with multiple interrupted sutures to prevent splitting of the distal tendon stump (Fig. 4.20). This modification can be beneficial if a long distal stump is present.

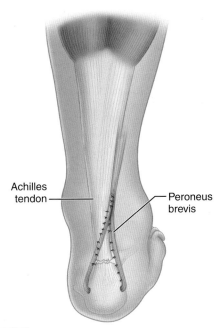

FIGURE 4.19 Dynamic loop suture of peroneus brevis to itself when end-to-end suture is not possible. **SEE TECHNIQUE 4.11.**

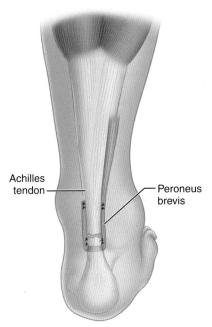

FIGURE 4.20 Turco and Spinella modification. Peroneus brevis is passed through midcoronal slit in distal stump of Achilles tendon and sutured to stump and to tendon. **SEE TECHNIQUE 4.11.**

POSTOPERATIVE CARE The cast is removed at 2 weeks, the wound is inspected, and the staples or sutures are removed unless subcuticular sutures were used for wound closure. Occasionally, another week is required for proper wound healing before sutures are removed. Another short leg cast with the foot in gravity equinus is worn for an additional 2 weeks. At 4 weeks, the cast is changed again and the foot is gradually brought to the plantigrade position over the next 2 weeks. Walking is gradually resumed with partial weight bearing on crutches during a 2-week period. At 6 to 8 weeks, a short leg walking cast is applied with the foot in the plantigrade position and full weight bearing is allowed. Alternatively, a removable brace allowing only plantar flexion can be used as early as 4 to 6 weeks after surgery. Gentle active range-of-motion exercises for 20 minutes twice a day are begun. Isometric ankle exercises along with a knee-strengthening and hip-strengthening program can be instituted. Toe raises, progressive resistance exercises, and proprioceptive exercises, in combination with a general strengthening program, constitute the third stage of rehabilitation. In reliable, well-supervised patients with good tissue repair, this program can be accelerated, with earlier use of dorsiflexion-stop orthoses and active range-of-motion exercises. Return to full unrestricted activity usually requires at least 6 months and often more.

MINIMALLY INVASIVE AND PERCUTANEOUS REPAIR OF ACUTE ACHILLES TENDON RUPTURE

A number of techniques have been developed to allow repair through smaller incisions to speed recovery and minimize complications, especially infection and sural nerve damage. Because of the risk of sural nerve injuries with "blind" suturing of the tendon, some of these techniques use multiple incisions (e.g., three-incision technique), endoscopy, or specially designed devices.

Comparisons of open repairs with minimally invasive or percutaneous techniques have shown functional results comparable to those obtained with open repair, with fewer complications, no apparent increased risk of rerupture, and better cosmetic results. A recent systematic review involving 182 patients found a significantly decreased risk of postoperative complications, especially wound infection, in acute Achilles tendon ruptures treated with minimally invasive surgery compared with open surgery. In their systematic review and meta-analysis of 2060 patients treated with six commonly used surgery and rehabilitation protocols, Wu et al. determined that minimally invasive surgery with accelerated rehabilitation had the lowest risk of DVT, deep infection, and rerupture. Cited disadvantages of minimally invasive techniques include risk of sural nerve injury, failure to appose tendon ends or malalignment of tendon ends, and a lower strength of the repair. In a study of 211 patients with minimally invasive repairs, sural nerve injury occurred in 41 (19%) and reruptures in 17 (8%).

Keller et al. described a mini-open Achilles tendon rupture technique that does not open the paratenon and avoids the sural nerve. In their 100 patients with this procedure, there were no infections, wound dehiscence, scar adherence, or sural nerve damage; 98% of patients were satisfied with their results, and 80 returned to their previous sport activity at the same or higher level. The technique requires the use of custom-made suture retrievers. In a later description of the technique, Wagner and Wagner listed important tips for performing the procedure: (1) operate within 10 days of the rupture to avoid scar formation at the rupture site; (2) plan the procedure according to the level of the rupture to ensure that the suture passers are long enough to span the rupture site from the proximal incision up to the calcaneus; (3) ensure that the bone anchors are placed in the middle of the total height of the calcaneus, avoiding the enthesis, and align the anchors

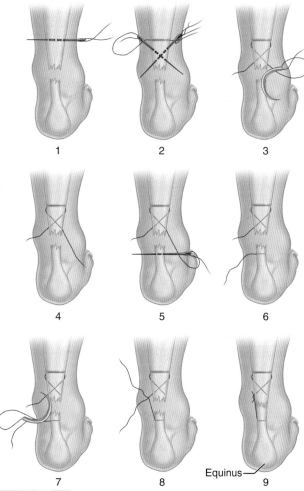

1 2 3

4 5 6

7 8 Equinus 9

FIGURE 4.21 Ma and Griffith technique for percutaneous repair of acute rupture of Achilles tendon. **SEE TECHNIQUE 4.12.**

to be perpendicular to the axis of the calcaneus; (4) follow the proximal suturing technique to obtain the best resistance of the repair; and (5) taking care to not overtighten consecutive sutures, restore the appropriate level of physiologic equinus. A percutaneous technique using a device (percutaneous Achilles repair system, PARS, Arthrex) has been developed to improve recovery and reduce postoperative complications. Hsu et al. compared the PARS technique in 101 patients to open repair in 169 patients and found that the percutaneous group had shorter surgical times and more patients who returned to baseline physical activities by 5 months compared to the open repair group. The overall postoperative complication rate was 5% in the percutaneous group and 11% in the open group. As noted by Lichti et al., the PARS technique requires that the surgeon be familiar with the instrumentation and suture management must be meticulous to avoid entanglement of the sutures.

TECHNIQUE 4.12

(MA AND GRIFFITH)

- In the operating room with the patient under local, regional, or general anesthesia, and with the extremity prepared as for open surgery, palpate the tendon defect

and make small stab wounds on each side of the Achilles tendon 2.5 cm proximal to the rupture defect.
- Use a small hemostat to free the underlying tendon sheath from the subcutaneous tissue; pass a No. 0 or a No. 1 nonabsorbable suture threaded on a straight needle from the lateral stab wound through the body of the tendon and exit in the medial stab wound (Fig. 4.21, *step 1*).
- With a straight needle on each end of the inserted suture, crisscross the needles within the body of the tendon and puncture the skin just distal to the site of tendon rupture; enlarge the sites of needle puncture with a scalpel (Fig. 4.21, *step 2*) and pull the suture completely through the stab wounds; snug the suture within the proximal portion of the ruptured tendon.
- With the lateral suture now threaded on a curved cutting needle, pass the suture back through the last stab wound to exit at about the midportion of the distal stump of the ruptured tendon on the lateral side (Fig. 4.21, *step 3*). Enlarge the hole with a scalpel before pulling the suture through.
- Use a hemostat to free the subcutaneous tissue from the underlying tendon sheath (Fig. 4.21, *step 4*).
- Using a straight needle, pass the lateral suture through the body of the distal stump of the tendon; enlarge the puncture wound in the skin as before (Fig. 4.21, *steps 5 and 6*).
- Using a curved cutting needle, pass the suture from this distalmost stab wound on the medial side and exit at the middle stab wound on the medial side of the ruptured tendon (Fig. 4.21, *step 7*).
- With the ankle maintained in equinus position, apply tension to the suture in a crisscross manner and bring the tendon ends together; tie the suture in this position and, with a small hemostat, bury the knot in the depths of the wound (Fig. 4.21, *steps 8 and 9*).
- Suturing the skin is unnecessary. Apply a sterile dressing to the stab wounds, and apply a short leg cast in gravity equinus position.

POSTOPERATIVE CARE The short leg cast is worn with non–weight bearing for 4 weeks, at which time a weight-bearing, low-heeled, short leg equinus cast is applied. At 8 weeks, the cast is removed and a therapy program of toe-heel raising and gastrocnemius-soleus exercises is begun. The patient gradually restores the foot to a neutral position during a 4-week period. Then the patient begins heel cord stretching exercises for an additional 4 weeks.

PERCUTANEOUS ACHILLES TENDON REPAIR

TECHNIQUE 4.13

(HSU, BERLET, ANDERSON)

- Position the patient prone and apply a thigh tourniquet. Place the feet slightly hanging off the end of the bed with a bump beneath the operative side ankle to adjust

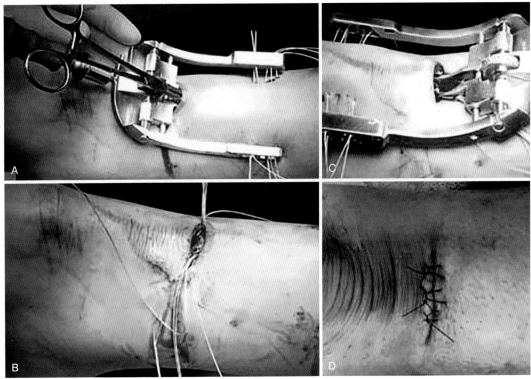

FIGURE 4.22 **A,** Proximal jig insertion. **B,** Passage of sutures creating locking sutures in either side of the tendon. **C,** Distal jig insertion. **D,** Completed repair. (From Hsu AR, Jones CP, Cohen BE: Clinical outcomes and complications of percutaneous Achilles repair system versus open technique for acute Achilles tendon ruptures, *Foot Ankle Int* 36:1279, 2015.) **SEE TECHNIQUE 4.13.**

plantar flexion and Achilles tension and avoid interference with the contralateral leg. The operative leg should be in neutral rotation to allow subsequent central positioning of the PARS jig.

■ After preparation and draping, exsanguinate the extremity and inflate the tourniquet.

■ Palpate the defect in the Achilles tendon and make a 2-cm transverse or vertical incision just proximal to the defect in the center of the tendon. Placing the incision just proximal to the rupture site ensures proper visualization and control of the proximal Achilles tendon stump, which can be retracted proximally into the calf. The distal stump can be brought into the incision by plantar flexing the ankle. A transverse incision follows the natural skin creases in the back of the ankle and allows for percutaneous jig insertion with minimal paratenon disruption. A vertical incision can be used and extended in cases of tendinosis, calcifications, or delayed presentation, but it requires increased paratenon and soft-tissue disruption.

■ Incise the skin and soft tissues using a "no-touch" technique without pickups. Carefully carry dissection down to the paratenon and sharply incise it. Preservation of the paratenon helps minimize disruption to the vascular supply of the tendon and allows repair at the end of the procedure.

■ The sural nerve is not typically seen in the operative field, but if it is, dissect it out and retract it out of the way with a vessel loop.

■ Use an index finger or Freer elevator within the wound to confirm that the center of the rupture has been located.

■ Insert an Allis clamp into the wound, secure the proximal tendon stump, and pull it through the wound 1 to 2 cm. Run a Freer elevator along the dorsal aspect of the proximal tendon to release potential adhesions that may limit distal excursion. Avoid dissection along the ventral aspect of the tendon to preserve native tendon blood supply.

PROXIMAL JIG INSERTION

■ Insert the proximal jig into the wound with the inner prongs in the narrowest position possible while gently placing traction on the proximal tendon stump with a clamp (Fig. 4.22A).

■ Use the center turn wheel to widen the inner prongs so that they slide along the sides of the tendon in the paratenon. Proper jig placement should allow the jig to slide along the tendon with minimal resistance.

■ Palpate the proximal tendon under the skin to check that the tendon is centered within the prongs of the jig. The most common error is to insert the jig too deep, which causes subsequent needles and sutures to miss the tendon and pull through.

■ Once it is properly located, keep the jig centered and stabilized so that it does not veer medially or laterally.

■ During suture passing, first use all the needles (1.6 mm) with Nitinol loops that are not loaded with suture.

■ Insert the first two needles into their respective numbered holes through the tendon and then through the opposite side of the jig. Check each needle to make sure it does not pass outside the jig. The placement of two needles within the jig and tendon at all times during suture passing helps stabilize the jig and avoids adjacent suture piercing with the subsequent needle.

- Pass a #2 FiberWire suture or SutureTape suture through the jig with the needle suture passer, making them of equal length on both sides. SutureTape has a broader, flatter surface to increase contact surface area between the suture and tendon and reduce any suture cutting through frayed tendon.

- The colors of the sutures are not as important as the order in which they are placed. An assistant can write down the colors and order of the sutures passed, as needed. The two central sutures—#3 and #4—have one looped end and one end with a tail. They are passed in an oblique, crossing pattern. These sutures create locking sutures on either side of the tendon (Fig. 4.22B). Holes #6 and #7 can be used if a second locking suture is needed.

JIG REMOVAL, SUTURE MANAGEMENT

- After all sutures are passed, use the turn wheel to narrow the inner prongs while applying controlled tension to the jig to remove it. Remove all sutures from both sides of the tendon from the wound. Before the jig is completely removed, use a hemostat through each loop of sutures to guide them out of the wound. Test both pairs of sutures by pulling them distally to ensure that adequate proximal fixation has been obtained.

- If any or all of the sutures pull out of the tendon, this indicates that the tendon was not centered in the jig or the jig was placed too deep or not proximal enough along the tendon during suture passing. If this occurs, remove the sutures and repeat the previous steps paying attention to tendon positioning within the jig.

- Do not extend the incision longitudinally on either end of a transverse incision as this may lead to wound healing complications.

- Once proximal fixation is achieved, neatly spread apart the sutures on each side of the tendon in the following order from proximal to distal: first suture, second suture, looped, green striped suture (third), tail of the green striped suture (fourth), and fifth suture. Loop the second suture on both sides around the two green striped sutures and back proximally through the looped end of the green striped suture.

- Pull the green striped suture tail through the tendon onto the opposite side to create a locking suture on both sides of the tendon. In the end, there are two nonlocking sutures and one locking suture on either side of the tendon. Pull each pair of sutures individually distally to confirm fixation and remove creep from the sutures. Place a hemostat on each group of three sutures to keep these out of the way during distal tendon preparation.

- For distal tendon preparation using this technique, repeat the above steps. Secure the distal tendon stump with an Allis clamp and deliver it out of the wound while inserting the jig (Fig. 4.22C). Insert the jig as distal as possible to the Achilles insertion to ensure that all sutures are passed through the tendon. Suture passing, jig removal, and creation of locking sutures follow the previously outlined steps. Test and pull on each pair of sutures to ensure that adequate distal tendon fixation was achieved.

- Place and hold the ankle in maximal plantar flexion during suture tying for a secure repair. We have never found the Achilles tendon repair to be too tight when using the percutaneous technique. The tendon will always gradually stretch out during weight bearing and physical therapy.

- When tying nonlocking sutures, have an assistant hold tension on the opposite side as the suture will continue to slide through the tendon with increasing force applied to the suture during knot tying. During tying, pull out any remaining slack from the sutures before securing them with five or six knots. After each suture is tied, cut it above the knot and away from the other sutures to avoid tangling.

- After the sutures are tied, the ankle should be plantar flexed with improved resting tension. After wound irrigation, ensure the suture knots are tucked ventrally into the wound and do not protrude into the subcutaneous tissue. Sharply debride residual strands of tendon and tuck them within the wound for adequate paratenon closure (Fig. 4.22D). Use absorbable sutures to close the paratenon and subcutaneous tissues and nylon sutures for skin closure.

■ CHRONIC RUPTURE

The definition of a "chronic" rupture has ranged from those diagnosed and treated more than 48 hours after injury to those diagnosed and treated up to 2 months after injury. There appears to be some consensus that a rupture diagnosed 4 to 6 weeks after injury should be considered a chronic rupture and that these are more difficult to treat than acute injuries. At about 1 week after rupture of the Achilles tendon, any space between the tendon ends fills with scar tissue. If left untreated, the tendon heals elongated, leaving the patient unable to push off on the affected side. Running, jumping, and activities such as ascending or descending stairs are severely compromised. Calf atrophy usually is present, the Achilles tendon often loses its normal contour, and a visible tendon defect may be present. MRI can be helpful to estimate the gap between the ruptured ends of the tendon (Fig. 4.23). Chronic ruptures appear as an area of low-intensity signal on T1-weighted images and alteration in T2-weighted signal.

If posterior heel pain, swelling, or functional impairment is disabling, delayed repair or reconstruction is indicated. In most active adults, repair is preferable but often is not possible. For ruptures more than 3 months old, treatment depends on the patient's physiologic age, activity level, and amount of functional impairment. A number of techniques have been described for reconstruction of a neglected Achilles tendon rupture (Box 4.4). If the tendon defect is less than 3 cm after debridement and the injury is less than 3 months old, direct repair often is possible. If, however, the tendon gap is more than 3 cm (more common), additional techniques must be used, such as local tissue transfer, tissue augmentation, synthetics, and allografts.

V-Y quadricepsplasty (see Technique 4.18) and gastrocnemius-soleus fascia turn-down graft (see Technique 4.17) techniques can be used for augmentation, and local tendon transfers (flexor hallucis longus, flexor digitorum longus, peroneus brevis and longus, plantaris) can be used to bridge larger defects (Table 4.3). Minimally invasive and endoscopically assisted techniques have been described for tendon transfers, but there are few reports of the long-term outcomes of these procedures. Maffulli et al. described a "less-invasive" technique

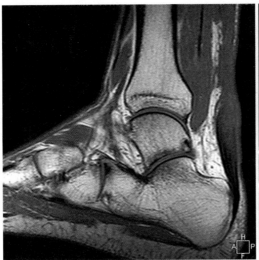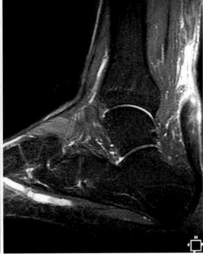

FIGURE 4.23   MRI appearance of chronic Achilles tendon rupture.

BOX 4.4

Techniques for Reconstruction of Chronic Achilles Tendon Ruptures

- Primary repair (uncommon)
- Augmentation
    - Free fascia tendon graft
        Fascia lata
        Donor tendons (semitendinosus, peroneal, gracilis, patellar tendon)
    - Fascia advancement
        V-Y quadriceps plasty
        Gastrocnemius-soleus fascia turn-down graft
    - Local tendon transfer
        Flexor hallucis longus
        Flexor digitorum longus
        Peroneus brevis
        Peroneus longus
        Plantaris
        Posterior tibial
- Synthetic or allograft augmentation
    - Polyglycol threads
    - Marlex mesh
    - Dacron vascular graft
    - Carbon fiber
    - Allograft tendon

Modified from Coughlin MJ, Schon LC: Disorders of tendons. In Coughlin MJ, Mann RA, Saltzman CL, editors: *Surgery of the foot and ankle*, ed 8, Philadelphia, 2007, Elsevier.

---

for transfer of the peroneus brevis through two paramidline incisions and recommended this technique for tendon gaps of less than 6 cm. In a later report, he and his colleagues compared outcomes of three less invasive tendon transfer procedures: free ipsilateral semitendinosus graft (gaps of more than 6 cm), ipsilateral peroneus brevis transfer (smaller gaps), and ipsilateral flexor hallucis longus transfer. All three techniques produced significant functional improvement, and return to sports was possible in most patients; no clear advantage of one technique over the others was demonstrated.

TRANSFER OF THE PERONEUS BREVIS TENDON FOR NEGLECTED ACHILLES TENDON RUPTURES

TECHNIQUE 4.14

(MAFFULLI ET AL.)

- Make a 5-cm longitudinal incision 2 cm proximal and just medial to the palpable end of the proximal stump.
- Make a second longitudinal incision, 3 cm long, 2 cm distal, and just lateral to the lateral margin of the distal stump (Fig. 4.24A). Take care to avoid sural nerve injury by making this incision as close as possible to the anterior aspect of the lateral border of the Achilles tendon (posterior to the sural nerve).
- Make a 2-cm longitudinal incision at the base of the fifth metatarsal.
- Mobilize the distal Achilles tendon stump, freeing it of all peritendinous adhesions, particularly on its lateral aspect. Resect the ruptured tendon end back to healthy tendon and place a locking suture (No. 1 Vicryl) along the free tendon edge to prevent separation of the bundles.
- Mobilize the proximal tendon stump through the proximal incision, divide any adhesions, and release the soft tissues anterior to the soleus and gastrocnemius muscle to allow maximal excursion and minimize the gap between the tendon stumps.
- Plantar flex the ankle and measure the gap between the two tendon ends. If less than 6 cm, the peroneus brevis tendon can be used to bridge the gap.
- Identify the peroneus brevis tendon through the incision on the lateral border of the foot. Expose the tendon and place a locking suture in the tendon end before releasing it from the metatarsal base.
- Through the distal incision over the Achilles tendon, incise the deep fascia overlying the peroneal muscle compartment and identify the peroneus brevis tendon at the base

TABLE 4.3

Comparison of Tendons for Tendon Transfer in Treatment of Chronic Achilles Tendon Rupture

TENDON	STRENGTH RELATIVE TO GSC	ADVANTAGES	CONCERNS
Peroneus brevis	18 times weaker	In phase with GSC during normal gait Shared role as plantar flexor of ankle Relatively close proximity to Achilles tendon but in separate muscle compartment	Loss of eversion strength Lateral-to-medial pull after transfer to calcaneus, which does not reproduce inversion normally created by Achilles tendon Sural nerve damage during harvest
Flexor digitorum longus	27 times weaker	In phase with GSC during normal gait Shared role as plantar flexor of ankle Relatively close proximity to Achilles tendon	Weakened flexion of toes Lesser toe deformities Nerve or artery injury during harvest
Flexor hallucis longus	13 times weaker	In phase with GSC during normal gait Shared role as plantar flexor of ankle Closest proximity to Achilles tendon	Loss of push-off strength during gait Clawed hallux deformity Transfer metatarsalgia Nerve or artery injury during harvest

GSC, Gastrocnemius-soleus.

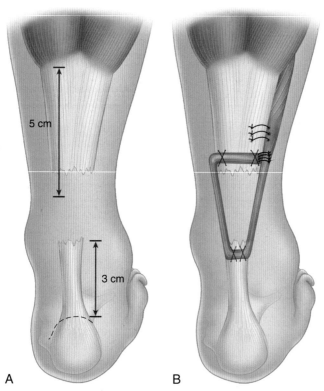

A   B

FIGURE 4.24 Peroneus brevis transfer for chronic Achilles tendon rupture. **A,** Longitudinal incisions.**B,** Completed transfer. **SEE TECHNIQUE 4.14.**

of the incision. Withdraw the peroneus brevis tendon through the distal incision; tendinous strands between the two peroneal tendons distally may require strong force to withdraw the tendon.

- Mobilize the muscular portion of the peroneus brevis proximally to increase its excursion.
- Make a longitudinal tenotomy parallel to the tendon fibers in both tendon stumps.
- Use a clamp to develop the plane, from lateral to medial, in the distal Achilles tendon stump, and pass the peroneus brevis graft through the tenotomy.

- With the ankle in maximal plantar flexion, suture the peroneus brevis to both sides of the distal stump.
- Pass the peroneus brevis tendon beneath the intact skin bridge into the proximal incision, then from medial to lateral through the transverse tenotomy in the proximal stump, and secure it with sutures.
- Suture the peroneus brevis tendon back onto itself on the lateral side of the proximal incision (Fig. 4.24B).
- Close the incisions in standard fashion and apply a previously prepared removable fiberglass cast support with the foot in maximal equinus.

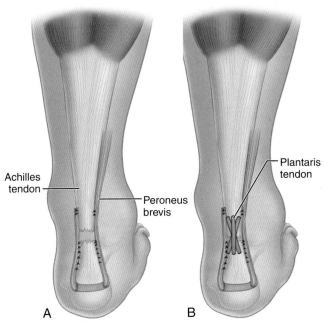

- Achilles tendon
- Peroneus brevis
- Plantaris tendon

A   B

FIGURE 4.25 Technique for chronic rupture of Achilles tendon. **A,** Exposure of Achilles tendon and tuberosity through posterolateral incision. Peroneus brevis is passed through hole drilled in tuberosity and sutured to Achilles tendon. **B,** Plantaris tendon is passed through ruptured ends of tendon. **SEE TECHNIQUE 4.16.**

POSTOPERATIVE CARE Weight bearing to tolerance on the metatarsal heads is allowed with the use of elbow crutches. Active flexion and extension of the hallux and lesser toes are encouraged, as are isometric exercises of the calf muscles and toes. At 2 weeks, the back shell of the cast is removed and physical therapy focusing on proprioception, plantar flexion, inversion, and eversion is begun with the front shell in place to prevent ankle dorsiflexion. Full weight bearing is allowed with the front shell of the cast in place, but this rarely is possible because of balance difficulties, and most patients still require the assistance of a single elbow crutch. The front shell of the cast is removed at 6 weeks and physical therapy is continued. Patients normally regain a plantigrade ankle over the next 2 to 3 weeks.

DIRECT REPAIR OF NEGLECTED ACHILLES TENDON RUPTURES

TECHNIQUE 4.15

- Make a curvilinear, posteromedial incision, extending proximally as far as necessary for mobilization of the tendon.
- Free the gastrocnemius and soleus muscles individually in the proximal leg with combinations of sharp and blunt dissection to provide additional mobilization.

- Resect most of the scar tissue and proceed with repair as described for acute ruptures, using tension sutures and reinforcement with the plantaris tendon.
- Keep the knee flexed and the foot in equinus during the repair to relieve tension.

POSTOPERATIVE CARE Postoperative care is as described for after repair of an acute rupture of the Achilles tendon (see Technique 4.11).

REPAIR OF NEGLECTED ACHILLES TENDON RUPTURES USING PERONEUS BREVIS AND PLANTARIS TENDONS

Repair of significant tendon defects in active patients may be best accomplished using a modification of local tendon transfer described by White and Kraynick and Teuffer.

TECHNIQUE 4.16

(WHITE AND KRAYNICK; TEUFFER, MODIFIED)

- Expose the Achilles tendon and the tuberosity of the calcaneus through a posterolateral incision; identify and retract the sural nerve in the proximal part of the wound.
- Through a small second incision, detach the peroneus brevis from the base of the fifth metatarsal.
- Incise the lateral septum and draw the peroneus brevis tendon through the first incision.
- Make an incision through the sheath of the Achilles tendon to expose the ruptured ends.
- Resect the scarred tissue and dissect proximally to free the gastrocnemius-soleus.
- Identify the plantaris tendon and release it with a tendon stripper.
- Take the peroneus brevis tendon from lateral to medial through a hole drilled in the calcaneal tuberosity and suture it to the Achilles tendon with multiple interrupted nonabsorbable sutures to form a dynamic loop (Fig. 4.25A).
- Place the harvested plantaris tendon on a fascial needle and pass it in a figure-of-eight manner from posterior to anterior through the ruptured ends of the tendon (Fig. 4.25B).
- Leave enough of the tendon to be fanned over the distal part of the tendon and tack it over the repair for a smoother closure of the tendon graft (see Fig. 4.18).
- Close the tendon sheath and subcutaneous tissues with nonabsorbable sutures.
- Close the skin and apply a sterile dressing and a short leg cast in gravity equinus.

POSTOPERATIVE CARE Postoperative care is the same as described after repair of an acute rupture of the Achilles tendon (see Technique 4.11).

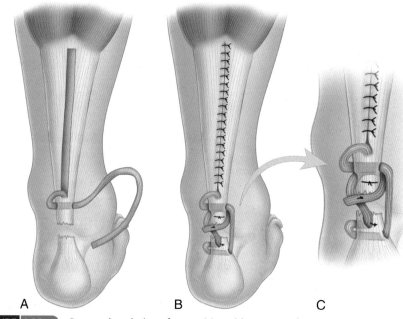

A   B   C

FIGURE **4.26**   Bosworth technique for repairing old ruptures of Achilles tendon. **SEE TECHNIQUE 4.17.**

REPAIR OF NEGLECTED ACHILLES TENDON RUPTURES USING GASTROCNEMIUS-SOLEUS TURN-DOWN GRAFT

TECHNIQUE 4.17

(BOSWORTH)
- Make a posterior longitudinal midline incision, extending from the calcaneus to the proximal one third of the calf.
- Expose the ruptured tendon and, using sharp dissection, excise the scar tissue from between the ends.
- Free from the median raphe of the gastrocnemius muscle a strip of tendon 1.5 cm wide and 17.5 to 22.5 cm long and leave it attached just proximal to the site of rupture.
- Turn the strip distally, pass it transversely through the proximal tendon (Fig. 4.26A), and anchor it there with absorbable suture.
- Pass the strip distally and then transversely through the distal end of the tendon; pass it again through this end from anterior to posterior.
- While holding the knee at 90 degrees and the ankle in plantar flexion, draw the fascial strip tight and anchor it with chromic catgut sutures.
- Bring the strip proximally and pass it transversely through the proximal end of the tendon; carry it distally and suture it on itself (Fig. 4.26B,C).
- Close the wound and apply a long leg cast, holding the knee in flexion and the foot in plantar flexion.

POSTOPERATIVE CARE Postoperative care is as described for after repair of an acute rupture of the Achilles tendon (see Technique 4.11).

V-Y REPAIR OF NEGLECTED ACHILLES TENDON RUPTURES

Abraham and Pankovich described a V-Y tendinous flap for repair of chronic ruptures of the Achilles tendon. V-Y advancement may be required if more than 80% of the tendon width is involved. It also is useful when 1 to 3 cm of tendon must be resected.

TECHNIQUE 4.18

(ABRAHAM AND PANKOVICH)
- With the patient prone and under tourniquet control, make a lazy "S" incision from the lateral aspect of the Achilles tendon insertion to the midpart of the calf (Fig. 4.27A).
- Identify and retract the sural nerve.
- Incise the deep fascia in line with the skin incision.
- Resect the scar tissue from the tendon ends.
- Measure the length of the tendon defect with the knee in 30 degrees of flexion and the ankle in 20 degrees of plantar flexion.
- Make an inverted-V incision through the aponeurosis with the apex over its central part. Make the arms of the incision at least one and a half times longer than the tendon defect to allow approximation in a Y configuration (Fig. 4.27B).
- Pull the flap distally and approximate the ends of the ruptured tendon with interrupted nonabsorbable sutures.
- Close the proximal part of the incision in a Y configuration (Fig. 4.27C).
- Suture the peritenon with interrupted nonabsorbable sutures.
- Close the deep fascia and subcutaneous tissue in a routine manner and apply a long leg cast with the knee in 30 degrees of flexion and the ankle in 20 degrees of plantar flexion.

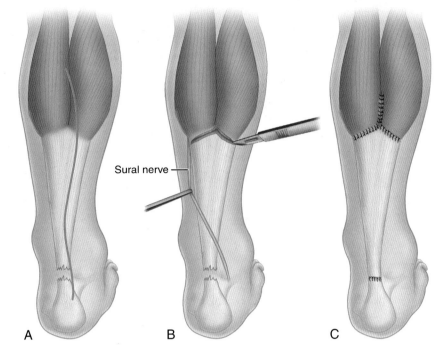

A   B   C

Sural nerve

FIGURE 4.27 V-Y repair of neglected rupture of Achilles tendon. **A,** Incision. **B,** Design of V flap. **C,** Y repair and end-to-end anastomosis. **SEE TECHNIQUE 4.18.**

POSTOPERATIVE CARE At 6 to 8 weeks, the long leg cast is removed, a short leg cast is applied and worn for 1 month, and weight bearing is allowed. After cast removal, a 3- to 5-cm heel lift is used for 1 month and progressive stretching exercises are begun immediately.

REPAIR OF NEGLECTED ACHILLES TENDON RUPTURES USING FLEXOR HALLUCIS LONGUS TENDON TRANSFER

TECHNIQUE 4.19

(WAPNER ET AL.)

- Place the patient supine and apply a tourniquet.
- Make a longitudinal incision on the medial border of the foot just above the abductor muscle, extending from the head of the first metatarsal to the navicular (Fig. 4.28A).
- Carry the dissection sharply through the subcutaneous tissue to the fascia of the abductor.
- Reflect the abductor with the flexor hallucis brevis plantarward.
- Identify the flexor hallucis longus and the flexor digitorum longus tendons and divide the flexor hallucis longus as far distally as possible, allowing an adequate distal stump for repair to the flexor digitorum longus.

- Place a tag suture into the divided proximal end of the flexor hallucis longus.
- Suture the distal end of the flexor hallucis longus into the flexor digitorum longus with the toes in neutral position.
- Make a posteromedial incision about 1 cm medial to the Achilles tendon from its musculotendinous junction proximally to approximately 2.5 cm below its calcaneal insertion (Fig. 4.28A).
- Carry the incision sharply through the skin, subcutaneous tissues, and tendon sheath, minimizing subcutaneous dissection. Inspect the substance of the tendon.
- Carry the dissection deep to the paratenon, creating full-thickness flaps to avoid skin slough.
- Incise the deep fascia longitudinally over the posterior compartment and expose the flexor hallucis longus. Retract the flexor hallucis tendon from the midfoot into the posterior wound.
- Drill a transverse hole just distal to the insertion of the Achilles tendon halfway from medial to lateral (Fig. 4.28B).
- Drill a second hole vertically just deep to the insertion of the Achilles tendon to join the first drill hole. Enlarge the tunnel with a large towel clip.
- Pull the tag suture through the tunnel from proximal to distal using a suture passer.
- Pass the flexor hallucis longus tendon through the tunnel and weave from distal to proximal through the Achilles tendon using a tendon weaver until the full length of the harvested tendon is used (Fig. 4.28C).
- Secure the weave with multiple 1-0 Dacron sutures.
- If desired, the repair can be supplemented using the plantaris tendon or a central slip of the Achilles tendon as previously described.
- Close the paratenon using absorbable suture. Close the subcutaneous tissues and skin of both incisions.

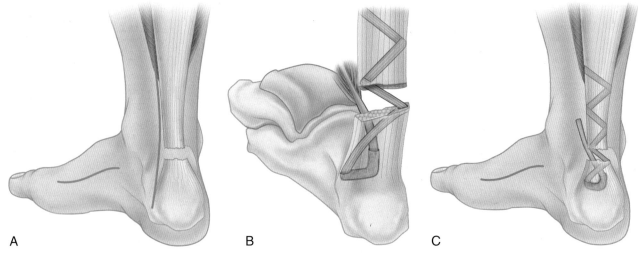

A   B   C

FIGURE 4.28 Repair of chronic Achilles tendon rupture with flexor hallucis longus. **A,** Two incisions are made. Medial midline incision on midfoot is used to harvest flexor tendon. Posteromedial incision anterior to Achilles tendon is used to expose tendon. **B,** Hole is drilled just deep to Achilles tendon insertion and is directed plantarward. Second drill hole is made from medial to lateral to intersect first drill hole midway through posterior body of calcaneus. **C,** Flexor hallucis longus is woven through remaining portion of Achilles tendon for secure fixation and supplementation of tendon. **SEE TECHNIQUE 4.19.**

■ Apply sterile bandages and place the leg in a posterior plaster, non–weight-bearing cast in 15 degrees of plantar flexion.

POSTOPERATIVE CARE The cast is changed at 4 weeks to a short leg walking cast or a removable cast brace with the ankle in neutral; the cast brace is worn for an additional 4 weeks. A rehabilitation program is begun with strengthening and range-of-motion exercises at 8 weeks. The removable brace remains in place until grade 4 to 5 strength and 10 degrees of dorsiflexion are obtained. Athletic activity is restricted for 6 months.

■ COMPLICATIONS

Wong et al. and Kocher et al. classified complications after open repair of Achilles tendon ruptures as minor, moderate, or major (Box 4.5). The most common complication appears to be rerupture. Reported rerupture rates after operative treatment are approximately 3%, with higher rates reported after nonoperative treatment. MRI is helpful to delineate the length of the tendon defect, evaluate the morphology of the tendon ends, and identify any pathologic processes. Sural nerve damage has been reported in 3% to 40% of percutaneous repairs and 0% to 20% of open repairs. Wound healing problems can occur after operative treatment of Achilles tendon ruptures, ranging from adhesions to deep infection associated with wound breakdown and tendon necrosis. Patients with deep infection typically are older, have received corticosteroid medication more often, sustained the tendon injury during everyday activities, and had a longer delay before treatment. Major wound breakdown, skin loss, and tendon necrosis may require complex reconstructive procedures, including local pedicle flaps and free flaps.

RUPTURE OF GASTROCNEMIUS MUSCLE

Musculotendinous rupture of the gastrocnemius muscle usually occurs at the insertion of the medial head into the soleus aponeurosis. It is most common in middle-aged, male athletes during eccentric overload with the knee extended and the ankle dorsiflexed, as may occur in tennis or jogging. This condition, although rarely confused with rupture of the Achilles tendon, may be confused with rupture of the plantaris tendon, or more important, with thrombophlebitis. Patients may be mistakenly treated for thrombophlebitis with anticoagulants, which can cause other complications, as well as an increase in bleeding in the torn gastrocnemius muscle. Patients may report hearing an audible pop or a feeling of being struck in the back of the leg when the injury occurred. Swelling and bruising in the leg may extend to the foot and ankle. A defect in the medial gastrocnemius muscle may be visible or palpable. If the diagnosis is uncertain, MRI shows the area of disruption better than CT or ultrasonography. Only conservative management is required to treat ruptures of the gastrocnemius muscle. Initial management includes relative rest, ice, compression, elevation (RICE) and early weight bearing as tolerated. Ankle or foot bracing that holds the ankle in a position of slight plantarflexion may be helpful, and some studies have shown an increased rate of healing with the use of bracing. Physical therapy progresses until the patient is pain free and has full, symmetric range of motion and strength; sport-specific exercises can then be initiated. Depending on the severity of the rupture, return to play may require from 1 to 12 weeks of rehabilitation.

TENDINOSIS OF EXTENSOR MECHANISM OF KNEE (JUMPER'S KNEE)

Tendinosis of the extensor mechanism ("jumper's knee") is most common in elite athletes in jumping sports but can affect athletes in other sports. The prevalence of jumper's knee has been estimated to range from 40% to 50% in high-level volleyball players and from 35% to 40% in elite basketball players.

Classification of Complications After Open Repair of Achilles Tendon Rupture

Classification of Wong et al.

Minor
- Wound
  - Superficial infection
  - Wound hematoma
  - Delayed wound healing
  - Adhesion of scar
  - Suture granuloma
  - Skin necrosis
- General
  - Pain
  - Disturbances in sensibility
  - Suture rupture

Major
- Wound
  - Deep infection
  - Chronic fistula
- General
  - Deep venous thrombosis
  - Tendon lengthening
  - Death

Classification of Kocher et al.

Major
- Death
- Pulmonary embolism
- Deep venous thrombosis
- Pneumonia
- Skin slough
- Sinus formation
- Fistula
- Tendon lengthening
- Second operation

Moderate
- Delayed healing
- Granuloma
- Medical infection
- Nerve injury

Minor
- Adhesion

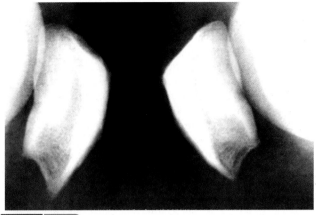

FIGURE 4.29   Elongation of lower pole of patella in tennis player with long history of patellar tendinitis. (From Roels J, Martins M, Mulior JC, Burssens A: Patellar tendinitis [jumper's knee], *Am J Sports Med* 6:362, 1978.)

Classification of Jumper's Knee According to Symptoms

STAGE	SYMPTOMS
0	No pain
1	Pain only after intense sports activity; no undue functional impairment
2	Pain at the beginning and after sports activity; still able to perform at a satisfactory level
3	Pain during sports activity; increasing difficulty in performing at a satisfactory level
4	Pain during sports activity; unable to participate in sport at a satisfactory level
5	Pain during daily activity; unable to participate in sport at any level

Modified from Ferretti A, Conteduca F, Camerucci E, et al: Patellar tendinosis: a follow-up study of surgical treatment, *J Bone Joint Surg* 84A:2179, 2002.

Tendinosis of the extensor mechanism ("jumper's knee") usually occurs at the tendo-osseous junction at the inferior pole of the patella and is caused by repetitive traction or overload injury during sports. Prolonged, repetitive microtrauma causes focal mucoid degeneration, fraying, and microtearing of the collagen fibrils. Occasionally, a single episode of eccentric overload or a direct blow to the tendon may cause onset of symptoms. Physical examination usually reveals tenderness at the inferior pole of the patella and often associated abnormalities of patellar tracking, chondromalacia, Osgood-Schlatter disease, or mechanical malalignment of the leg. The tenderness usually is worse with extension than with flexion. Anteroposterior, lateral, and tangential views of the patella may show radiolucency of the involved pole early in the process. With prolonged symptoms, the involved pole may become elongated (Fig. 4.29). Periosteal reaction of the anterior patellar surface ("tooth sign") and tendon calcification may be evident, and in long-standing disease stress fracture or disruption of the extensor mechanism may occur.

Blazina et al. described three stages of jumper's knee based on symptoms: phase 1, pain only after activity; phase 2, pain during and after activity but no significant functional impairment; and phase 3, pain during and after activities with progressive difficulty in satisfactory performance. Phase 4, end-stage disease with stress fracture through the patella or disruption of the extensor mechanism, was later added. Ferretti et al. classified jumper's knee symptoms into six stages (Table 4.4) based on the system of Blazina et al. MRI demonstrated medial focal thickening in almost all 11 knees, and all demonstrated a focus of abnormal signal intensity in the proximal third of the patellar tendon. MRI findings correlated with intraoperative findings of degenerative pathologic changes consistent with angiofibroblastic tendinosis. The medial thickening was thought to represent the greater stresses across the medial portion of the extensor mechanism. Advances in ultrasonography have provided more options for diagnosis and conservative treatment of patellar tendinitis.

Patients with symptoms of phase 1 or 2 usually respond well to conservative treatment with activity modification, rest, and antiinflammatory medication. Jumping and eccentric exercises are discouraged, although some now recommend eccentric exercise for treatment of jumper's knee. Functional, pain-free physical therapy is begun after symptoms resolve, with a gradual return to activity. Cortisone injections should not be used because they may increase the risk of tendon rupture. The same nonoperative protocol, with a longer rest period, can be tried initially in patients with symptoms of phase 3 involvement, but operative treatment is indicated if symptoms persist. Patients with "end-stage" or phase 4 symptoms generally require operative treatment. Several studies have indicated that delays in operative treatment result in worse outcomes, whereas others have found no such correlation. As early as 2 weeks but more commonly at 4 to 8 weeks after patellar tendon rupture, muscle retraction of up to 5 cm may be present, necessitating quadriceps lengthening, tendon or muscle transfer, or a combination of these techniques. For end-stage disruption of the extensor mechanism (phase four), repair is as described for acute rupture of the quadriceps (see Technique 4.26) or patellar (see Techniques 4.21 or 4.22) tendon.

▓ CHRONIC PATELLAR TENDINOSIS

Suggested alternatives to open patellar tenotomy of chronic jumper's knee include eccentric exercise, sclerosing injections targeting the area of neovessels and nerves on the dorsal side of the patellar tendon, injections of PRP, arthroscopic shaving of the same area, and extracorporeal shockwave therapy. Studies of the effectiveness of eccentric training have had conflicting results, with one randomized controlled study reporting results comparable to surgery and another reporting no effect of a 12-week eccentric training program. A systematic review and meta-analysis of 2530 patients found that eccentric exercise therapies obtained the best results at short-term, but multiple injections of PRP obtained the best results at long-term follow-up. A randomized controlled trial comparing ultrasound-guided injection of autologous skin-derived tendon-like cells and injection of autologous plasma alone found faster response and greater improvements in pain and function with cell therapy. Satisfactory results were obtained in 74% of 83 knees treated with extracorporeal shockwave therapy, with athletes returning to participation in their sport in an average of 6 weeks. Two studies, however, compared extracorporeal shockwave therapy with PRP injection and found that PRP had significantly better results at 6 and 12 months. Mesenchymal stem cells also may have therapeutic utility in the future.

TENOTOMY AND REPAIR FOR CHRONIC PATELLAR TENDINOSIS

TECHNIQUE 4.20

- Incise the tendon sheath longitudinally and identify and excise the area of degeneration using longitudinal incisions in the tendon.

- The inferior pole of the patella can be curetted or drilled to incite a healing response.
- Suture the defect in the tendon with side-to-side interrupted 2-0 Vicryl sutures.
- Close the peritenon with interrupted absorbable sutures and close the skin and subcutaneous tissue in routine fashion.
- Apply a knee immobilizer.

POSTOPERATIVE CARE The knee immobilizer is worn for 3 to 4 weeks, and crutches are used for partial weight bearing. Stage 1 of rehabilitation should emphasize range of motion and isometric strengthening. Closed-chain kinetics are started in stage 2 when swelling and tenderness have resolved. Stage 3 should consist of activity-specific exercises, avoiding eccentric overload. Return to full activities can be allowed when 85% to 90% of strength and full range of motion are achieved.

▓ STRESS FRACTURE THROUGH THE PATELLA

The same repetitive loading that can cause patellar tendinosis or even patellar tendon rupture can result in a stress fracture of the patella, usually in a young athlete. Initially a stress reaction may produce low-grade symptoms, which if recognized and treated with activity restriction may resolve. If activities are continued, a stress fracture may develop. The most common site of stress fracture is at the junction of the middle and distal thirds of the patella where the fibers of the distal quadriceps and proximal patellar tendons merge and insert.

FIXATION OF PATELLAR STRESS FRACTURE

TECHNIQUE 4.21

- For stress fracture through the inferior pole of the patella (Fig. 4.30), make a longitudinal midline or curvilinear transverse incision to expose the fracture.
- If the fracture is several weeks old, freshen the fracture surface and insert parallel, vertical 4.0 cancellous screws through the inferior pole. If needed, this can be augmented with nonabsorbable sutures passed circumferentially through the screw holes.
- As an optional step, use an oscillating saw to take a slot graft 10 mm wide × 15 mm long and slide it distally across the fracture site.
- Close the wound in routine fashion and apply a cylinder cast.

POSTOPERATIVE CARE The cast is worn for 6 weeks, after which active range-of-motion and strengthening exercises are begun. Return to full activity usually is possible at 10 to 16 weeks.

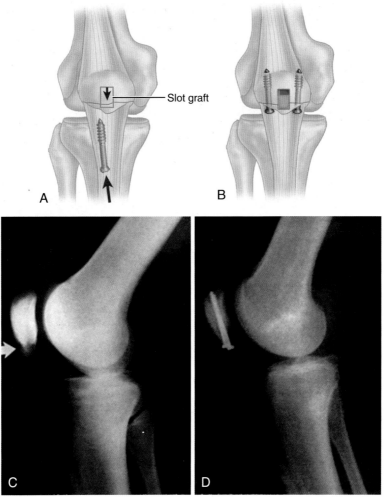

A

B

C

D

FIGURE 4.30 Stress fracture of inferior pole of patella. Fracture is secured with parallel screws; corticocancellous slot graft is placed distally across fracture. **SEE TECHNIQUE 4.21.**

RUPTURE OF EXTENSOR MECHANISM OF KNEE

Disruption of the extensor mechanism of the knee most commonly is caused by fracture of the patella. Disruption of the quadriceps mechanism and disruption of the patellar tendon are the next most common causes. The mechanism of injury usually is an eccentric overload to the extensor mechanism with the foot planted and the knee partially flexed. Patellar tendon rupture or avulsion is more common in patients younger than 40 years old, especially athletes. Quadriceps rupture is more common in older patients and in patients with systemic disease or degenerative changes. Systemic diseases, such as lupus erythematosus, diabetes, gout, hyperparathyroidism, uremia, and obesity, have been associated with disruption of the quadriceps mechanism. A relationship between prior steroid injection, as well as use of corticosteroids or fluoroquinolone antibiotics, and tendon rupture has been documented.

■ ANATOMY AND PATHOPHYSIOLOGY

Many studies have indicated that degenerative tendinopathy is present before tendon rupture; however, a more recent histologic analysis of 22 ruptured quadriceps tendons found degenerative changes in only 64%, with the frequency of degenerative changes increasing with age. Numerous authors have documented a history of pain before rupture. Occasionally, as may be the case in an athlete, no history of pain is reported. This is consistent with a subclinical process. Degenerative spurring ("tooth sign"), as seen on a tangential view of the patella, may indicate significant changes in the quadriceps mechanism (Fig. 4.31).

■ CLINICAL EVALUATION

Diagnosis of a disrupted extensor mechanism can be difficult, and often diagnosis is delayed, especially in patients with large lower extremities. Extensor mechanism disruption should be suspected in middle-aged or elderly patients with swelling, pain, and dysfunction of the knee, especially if a history of jumping, squatting, or stumbling is reported. An audible pop may be heard. Physical examination usually reveals a palpable gap in the quadriceps tendon, and the patella can be displaced inferiorly. Swelling and ecchymosis may be present. Straight-leg raising reveals a significant extension lag. This may be less evident with an intact extensor mechanism. Disruption of the patellar tendon causes similar findings, in addition to a superiorly displaced patella. A lateral radiograph may reveal a

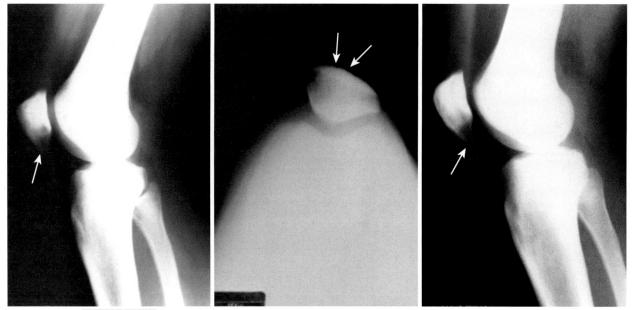

FIGURE 4.31   Degenerative spurring (tooth sign) on tangential view of patella indicates significant changes in quadriceps mechanism.

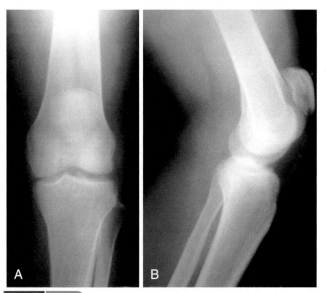

FIGURE 4.32   Anteroposterior **(A)** and lateral **(B)** radiographs of patellar tendon rupture.

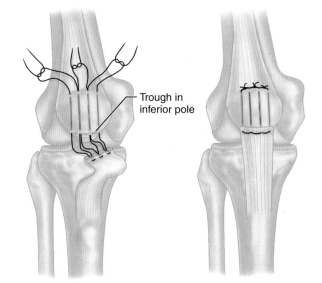

Trough in inferior pole

FIGURE 4.33   Technique of repair of fresh rupture of patellar tendon. **SEE TECHNIQUE 4.22.**

superiorly displaced patella, especially if the knee is flexed. If the diagnosis is in doubt, ultrasound or MRI can be helpful.

■ TREATMENT OF ACUTE RUPTURE OF PATELLAR TENDON

Rupture of the patellar tendon usually occurs at the inferior pole of the patella; the patella is a part of the proximal segment of the tendon and may be retracted 3 to 5 cm proximal to its normal position by contracture of the quadriceps muscle (Fig. 4.32). Fresh ruptures should be repaired if skin conditions are optimal. It is important to pay close attention to the position of the patella in the sagittal plane to prevent excessive baja or alta. Tensioning of the suture to allow 90 to 100 degrees of passive flexion has been recommended.

SUTURE REPAIR OF PATELLAR TENDON RUPTURE

TECHNIQUE 4.22   *Figure 4.33*

- With the patient supine and a tourniquet around the upper thigh, make a longitudinal incision centered over the defect.
- With careful subcutaneous dissection, expose the area of the rupture. Identify the infrapatellar branch of the saphenous nerve and retract it during the procedure; the patient

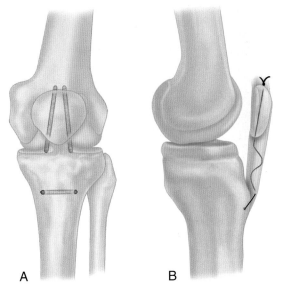

FIGURE 4.34 Mersilene loop tendon repair. **A,** Route of burr channels. **B,** Suturing of ruptured tendon. **SEE TECHNIQUE 4.22.**

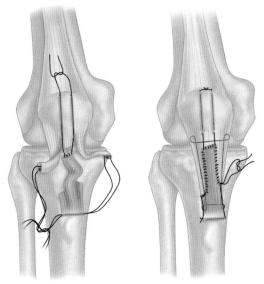

FIGURE 4.35 Technique of repair of fresh rupture of patellar tendon. Interlocking sutures are secured through parallel vertical holes drilled in patella and transverse hole drilled in tibial tuberosity. **SEE TECHNIQUE 4.22.**

- should be informed before surgery that there will likely be a permanent anesthetic area lateral to the incision.
- Use sharp dissection to open the peritenon longitudinally in the midline proximally and distally from the defect.
- Carefully realign the tear, which is most commonly at the tendon-bone junction, replacing the tendon in its anatomic position to allow normal patellar tracking.
- With a rongeur, make a small horizontal trough at the inferior pole of the patella, place three horizontal No. 5 nonabsorbable mattress sutures through the patellar tendon stump and bring the tendon through holes drilled in the patella, drawing the tendon securely to the inferior pole of the patella. This can be accomplished with a suture passer or Beath pin.
- Flex the knee to 45 degrees and place a hemostat parallel to the roof of the intercondylar notch to ensure that patella baja has not been produced. The inferior pole of the patella should be at or just slightly above the hemostat.
- Bury the nonabsorbable suture knots superior to the patella deep to the quadriceps tendon and hold them there during closing of the two vertical windows in the quadriceps with No. 0 absorbable sutures.
- The tendon should be repaired adjacent to the articular surface and not to the anterior surface of the patella. Failure to do this causes tilting of the patella and an increase in patellofemoral forces.
- Identify the full extent of the retinacular tear and repair it with No. 0 absorbable sutures or No. 2 nonabsorbable sutures.
- If the patellar tendon is extensively frayed, two running interlocking No. 5 nonabsorbable sutures can be used to secure the tendon, as described subsequently. Use a suture retriever or Beath pin to thread the suture strands through 3-mm drill tunnels, one horizontally into the tibial tubercle and two vertically into the patella (Fig. 4.34). If secure fixation cannot be obtained with this method, augment the repair with the semitendinosus or gracilis tendon.

- Ruptures through the substance of the tendon can be repaired with running interlocking sutures placed in the proximally and distally based bundles and secured through parallel vertical holes drilled in the patella and a transverse hole drilled in the tibial tuberosity (Fig. 4.35). Repair the individual bundles side-to-side after appropriate tendon length is determined.
- If needed after completion of the repair, place a circumferential tension suture of No. 5 nonabsorbable box wire.

POSTOPERATIVE CARE A cylinder cast with the knee in extension or a hinged brace locked in extension is applied, and weight bearing to tolerance is allowed. Straight-leg raising exercises are begun at 3 weeks. At 6 weeks, the cast is removed and a controlled motion brace with a range of motion 0 to 45 degrees is fitted. Motion is increased 10 to 15 degrees each week. Crutches are used for ambulation in the brace until sufficient strength and motion have been regained. If a tension wire was used for protection, it can be removed electively at 10 to 12 weeks under local anesthesia.

SUTURE ANCHOR REPAIR OF PATELLAR TENDON RUPTURE

TECHNIQUE 4.23

(DEBERARDINO AND OWENS)
- Through a midline longitudinal incision over the patellar tendon, incise the peritenon longitudinally and dissect it away from the underlying tendon.

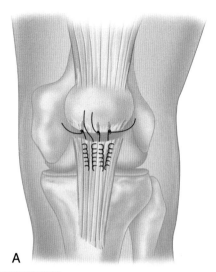 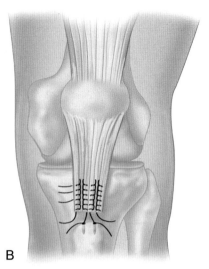

A   B

FIGURE 4.36 Repair of patellar tendon avulsion with suture anchors (see text). **A,** For proximal avulsions, three suture anchors are placed in anatomic tendon footprint. **B,** For distal avulsions, suture anchors are placed in the tibial tubercle. **SEE TECHNIQUE 4.23.**

- Debride or resect any grossly pathologic tendon tissue.
- For ruptures in the midsubstance of the tendon, expose the full length of the tendon and place two Krackow locking stitches in each tendon stump with No. 2 or No. 5 nonabsorbable suture. Repair the retinaculum with absorbable sutures. With the knee fully extended, tie the four proximal core sutures to the distal ones.
- For proximal avulsion of the tendon from the patella, expose the inferior patellar pole and place three suture anchors equidistant along the anatomic tendon footprint. Pull the suture through the anchor eyelet to produce long and short suture arms. Pass the long suture arm down and back of the tendon stump in a locking Krackow fashion, and use the short arm to reduce the tendon to the patella (Fig. 4.36A). Tie each suture repair securely.
- For distal avulsion of the tendon, the same procedure is used but the suture anchors are placed in the tibial tubercle and the tendon is repaired to the tubercle (Fig. 4.36B).
- Flex the knee to check for gap formation. Close the peritenon with absorbable sutures.

POSTOPERATIVE CARE Weight bearing is allowed with the knee braced in full extension. The stability of the tendon repair determines the amount of early flexion allowed with active-assisted range of motion. Motion is progressed as tolerated, with the goal of 90 degrees of flexion by 4 to 6 weeks and full motion by 10 to 12 weeks. Isometric quadriceps contractions can be done immediately after surgery, progressing to straight-leg raises at 6 weeks. Full return to activities is not allowed for 6 months.

▉ TREATMENT OF CHRONIC RUPTURE OF PATELLAR TENDON

When a rupture of the patellar tendon is more than 6 weeks old, the patella is retracted proximally and may require extensive surgical release to draw it distally to the appropriate level.

Although preoperative traction through a Kirschner wire placed transversely in the patella has been recommended, we now believe better results can be obtained with proximal release of scar tissue and a modified Thompson quadricepsplasty (see chapter 1), if necessary. Before surgery, lateral radiographs of the uninvolved extremity should be obtained with the knee flexed to 45 degrees to evaluate patellar height; these are compared with radiographs of the involved knee during surgery to determine the appropriate tendon length.

Various methods of reconstruction of the patellar tendon have been described. If sufficient patellar tendon is left for repair, augmentation with the semitendinosus or gracilis tendon may be indicated. If the rupture is several months old, an allograft can be used, and an Achilles tendon allograft has been used with some success in this situation.

ACHILLES TENDON ALLOGRAFT FOR CHRONIC PATELLAR TENDON RUPTURE

TECHNIQUE 4.24

- Make a longitudinal incision beginning 3 to 4 cm above the superior pole of the patella and extending just distal to the tibial tuberosity.
- With sharp subcutaneous dissection, expose the extensor mechanism medially and laterally through the plane of the prepatellar bursa. Medially protect the infrapatellar branch of the saphenous nerve if possible.
- Make a sharp longitudinal incision through the tendon sheath and scar tissue in the midportion of the patellar tendon and expose the remains of the tendon. If sufficient tissue is present to add structural strength to the

repair, freshen the ends of the tendon to be used later as described for hamstring augmentation.

- Perform a lateral retinacular release and use blunt and sharp dissection to free the medial and lateral gutters in the suprapatellar pouch.
- If further mobilization is necessary, use a periosteal elevator to dissect the vastus intermedius muscle proximally off the femur. Rarely, a medial release may be required to complete the quadricepsplasty as described by Thompson, but this should be avoided, if possible, to decrease the likelihood of avascular changes in the patella. The lateral incision allows inspection of the intraarticular structures and the patellofemoral articulation.
- If an allograft is necessary, we have had good results using the Achilles tendon, as well as the tibialis and hamstring tendons. Place the allograft over the tibial tuberosity about 4 cm distal to the joint line to estimate the proper length of the trough to be made in this area.
- Use an oscillating saw to make the trough 2.5 to 3.0 cm long, 1.5 to 2.0 cm wide, and 1.5 cm deep.
- Contour the corticocancellous bone attached to the Achilles tendon to fit flush in the trough (Fig. 4.37A). After ensuring proper alignment, secure it in this position with two staggered 4-mm cancellous screws using a lag screw technique or two 6.5-mm partially threaded cancellous screws.
- Identify the attachment of the patellar tendon in the central area of the inferior pole of the patella and place a Kirschner wire through this area, exiting superiorly 3 mm posterior to the central part of the quadriceps tendon.
- Pass an 8- or 9-mm reamer over the Kirschner wire and use a rasp to contour the tunnel edges.
- Fashion the Achilles tendon graft into three branches, the central third consisting of the thick half to two thirds of the tendon. This central branch should be 8 to 9 mm in diameter and should be freed distally far enough to allow

the graft to be pulled up to the inferior pole of the patella without hindering the two lateral branches.

- Place a whipstitch of No. 2 nonabsorbable suture in the central branch and pass it from inferior to superior through the tunnel, exiting through a slit in the quadriceps tendon just superior to the patellar insertion (Fig. 4.37B). A ligament passer may be helpful.
- Tack the tendon in place with multiple interrupted nonabsorbable sutures through the graft in the soft tissue of the inferior pole of the patella and at the edges of the quadriceps tendon just superior to the superior pole of the patella (Fig. 4.37C).
- The appropriate graft length is determined by ensuring the knee flexes to 90 degrees, evaluating Insall's index, and measuring the alignment of the inferior pole of the patella and ensuring that it is parallel to the roof of the intercondylar notch with the knee at 45 degrees. With the knee extended, there should be about 1.5 cm of slack in the patellar tendon. Obtain a lateral radiograph to confirm correct patellar height compared with the uninvolved extremity.
- When the appropriate patellar level has been determined, use multiple interrupted sutures to tack the patellar tendon stump to the graft, which was passed through the midline slit in the patellar stump.
- Close the lateral release with the knee flexed 30 degrees and carefully check patellar tracking and the quadriceps angle.
- Tack the medial and lateral branches of the graft to the medial and lateral retinaculum using No. 0 nonabsorbable sutures.
- Close the tendon sheath with interrupted 2-0 absorbable sutures, close the subcutaneous tissue with 2-0 absorbable sutures, and close the skin in the usual fashion.
- Alternatively, place suture anchors in the distal pole of the patella and the anterior cortex of the patella and use

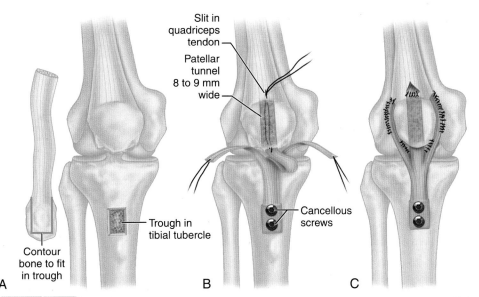

Slit in quadriceps tendon
Patellar tunnel 8 to 9 mm wide
Trough in tibial tubercle
Contour bone to fit in trough
Cancellous screws

A   B   C

FIGURE **4.37** Technique of reconstruction of chronic rupture of patellar tendon using Achilles tendon allograft. **A,** Slot measuring 3.0 cm long, 2.0 cm wide, and 1.5 cm deep is cut in tuberosity; graft is contoured to fit. **B,** Central arm of graft is placed through 9 mm longitudinal tunnel and then through vertical slit in quadriceps tendon. Tunnel is placed centrally to avoid penetration of articular cartilage. **C,** Graft is secured with multiple sutures. **SEE TECHNIQUE 4.24.**

these to secure the allograft tendon to the patella. Drape the allograft tendon over the quadriceps tendon and muscle fascia and secure it with nonabsorbable sutures.

- If augmentation of the repair is necessary, use No. 5 nonabsorbable suture placed in a box-stitch fashion through holes drilled in the patella and tibial tubercle. Steel wire or cerclage cables also can be used.
- Apply a cylinder cast or knee immobilizer locked in extension.

POSTOPERATIVE CARE At 10 to 14 days, the cast is removed for wound evaluation and removal of sutures or staples if needed. A cylinder cast or locked brace is worn for 4 to 6 weeks. Active and passive range-of-motion exercises are begun at 4 to 6 weeks. Weight bearing to tolerance with crutches is allowed until sufficient motion and strength allow unassisted ambulation. A progressive strengthening and range-of-motion exercise program is essential to regain function. The timing of rehabilitation can be adjusted depending on the intraoperative findings.

HAMSTRING (SEMITENDINOSUS AND GRACILIS) AUTOGRAFT AUGMENTATION FOR CHRONIC PATELLAR TENDON RUPTURE

We have in the past advocated the use of autogenous hamstring tendon grafts in a two-stage procedure in which the quadriceps mechanism is freed and traction is applied through the patella with a Kirschner wire as the first stage.

The second stage is reconstruction of the patellar tendon with the semitendinosus tendon. We now believe a one-stage procedure is preferable and that use of both the gracilis and semitendinosus is necessary for augmentation. The semitendinosus is a suitable graft because it is strong native tissue, does not require an additional surgery for removal, and allows immediate postoperative mobilization; harvesting the hamstrings has been shown to cause little functional deficit. A biomechanical study showed that augmentation of the patellar tendon repair decreased gap formation at the repair site after cyclic loading.

TECHNIQUE 4.25

(ECKER, LOTKE, AND GLAZER)

- Make an incision beginning just proximal and lateral to the patella, extending distally, crossing the midline of the limb inferior to the patella, and ending along the medial flare of the tibia. Expose the patella, quadriceps tendon, and tibial tuberosity.
- Place a Steinmann pin transversely through the midportion of the patella for distal traction (Fig. 4.38A).
- Remove all scar tissue from the remnants of the patellar tendon.
- Now flex the knee and expose the insertions of the gracilis and semitendinosus tendons into the pes anserinus.
- Use a tendon stripper to release the tendons from their proximal musculotendinous junctions and bring the tendons into the primary incision.
- Pass the semitendinosus tendon through an oblique hole drilled in the tibial tuberosity and through one of two transverse holes drilled through the distal part of the patella.
- Then pass the gracilis tendon through the other hole in the patella (Fig. 4.38B).

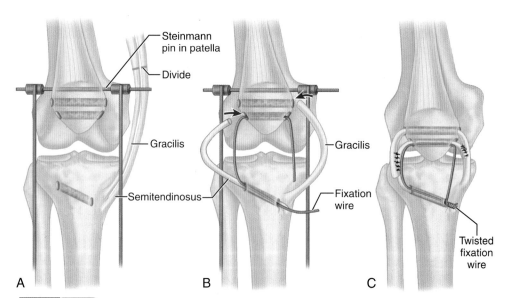

FIGURE 4.38 Technique for one-stage delayed reconstruction of patellar tendon. **A,** Steinmann pin through transverse hole in patella is used for distal traction. **B,** Proximally divided semitendinosus and gracilis tendons are placed through holes and fixation wire is inserted. **C,** With patella in normal position, fixation wire is secured and gracilis and semitendinosus tendons are sutured to each other. **SEE TECHNIQUE 4.25.**

- Pass a wire through the patella and the tibial tuberosity and tighten it to maintain a distance between the patella and the tibial tuberosity equal to the length of the patella.
- Suture the semitendinosus and gracilis tendons under tension (Fig. 4.38C).
- Remove the transverse traction pin, close the wound, and apply a cylinder cast.

POSTOPERATIVE CARE At 2 weeks, the cast is removed for wound evaluation and a new cylinder cast or locked brace is applied. At 6 weeks, vigorous straight-leg raising with weights and active flexion exercises are instituted.

HAMSTRING AUTOGRAFT AUGMENTATION FOR CHRONIC PATELLAR TENDON RUPTURE

TECHNIQUE 4.26

(MANDELBAUM ET AL.)
- Make a midline approach to the patellar tendon. Make a medial arthrotomy for inspection of the joint and lysis of adhesions as necessary.
- Make a Z-lengthening incision in the quadriceps tendon and a Z-shortening incision through the patellar tendon, using careful dissection to preserve the vascular pedicle in the proximal and the distal flaps (Fig. 4.39A).
- Place sutures in the tendon (Fig. 4.39B) and obtain an anteroposterior radiograph; compare it with the preoperative film of the uninvolved extremity to determine appropriate patellar height.
- When a satisfactory position is obtained, place multiple absorbable sutures in the quadriceps and patellar tendons to secure the repair.
- Expose the distal insertion of the pes anserinus and with a tendon stripper harvest the semitendinosus and gracilis tendons (Fig. 4.39C).
- Suture the tendons together with multiple interrupted absorbable sutures.
- Pass the tendons through a transverse hole in the midportion of the patella and through a transverse hole in the tibial tuberosity in a figure-of-eight fashion.
- Use running interlocking sutures, as described by Krackow, Thomas, and Jones, to suture the tendon to itself (Fig. 4.39D).
- Tack the tendons to the underlying patellar tendon (Fig. 4.39E) and close the wound in the usual fashion.

POSTOPERATIVE CARE Postoperative care is the same as after reconstruction of a neglected rupture of the patellar tendon (see Technique 4.23).

RUPTURE OF TENDON OF QUADRICEPS FEMORIS MUSCLE
ACUTE RUPTURE

Acute ruptures of the quadriceps tendon generally result from eccentric contraction of the extensor mechanism against a sudden load of body weight with the foot planted and the knee flexed. The quadriceps tendon usually ruptures transversely at the osteotendinous junction in older patients and at the midtendon or musculotendinous area in younger patients. A cadaver study identified a hypovascular zone in the quadriceps tendon 1 to 2 cm from the superior pole of the patella, corresponding to the site of spontaneous ruptures reported in the literature. The rupture often extends through the vastus intermedius tendon, slightly proximal to the rupture of the rectus femoris tendon. Incomplete ruptures usually can be treated nonoperatively, depending on the extent of the tear and the patient's occupation or sports activity, with immobilization of the knee in full extension for 6 weeks, followed by protected range-of-motion and strengthening exercises. When good quadriceps muscle control is regained, and the patient can perform a straight-leg raise without discomfort, the immobilizer is progressively discontinued.

For complete ruptures, operative repair should be done as soon as possible. Delays in operative repair can complicate the repair process and lead to unsatisfactory results. Without its distal tendinous insertion intact, the quadriceps apparatus begins to retract in the first few days after injury. After days or weeks, retraction can make apposition of the torn tendon ends difficult and can increase tension on the suture line.

Although various techniques have been described for repair of quadriceps tendon ruptures, none has been proved to be the most reliable and effective. Most techniques involve repair of the tendon with sutures passed through holes drilled in the patella, although suture anchors have been used instead. If a local flap technique is to be used for reinforcement, the tendon proximal to the rupture should be evaluated carefully to avoid formation of an additional weakened area. The repair can be protected by a circumferential wire or strong nonabsorbable sutures or by a Bunnell pull-out wire through the medial and lateral retinaculum. PRP injection may aid in the reparative process, although more studies are needed.

REPAIR OF ACUTE RUPTURE OF THE TENDON OF THE QUADRICEPS FEMORIS MUSCLE

TECHNIQUE 4.27   *Figure 4.40*

- Make a midline longitudinal incision 15 to 20 cm long to expose the rupture.
- Irrigate the hematoma and freshen the tendon ends.
- If sufficient tendon is left distally, make an end-to-end repair using multiple No. 2 or No. 5 nonabsorbable mattress sutures through the tendon and No. 0 absorbable sutures to repair the retinaculum. Carefully align the tendon and evaluate patellar tracking and position. Use a circumferential wire or suture for protection of the repair.

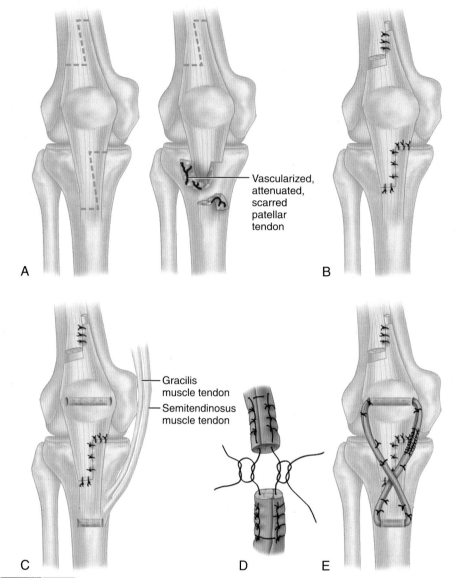

Vascularized, attenuated, scarred patellar tendon

Gracilis muscle tendon

Semitendinosus muscle tendon

A   B

C   D   E

FIGURE 4.39   Technique of reconstruction of neglected ruptures of patellar tendon. **A,** Z-shortening of patellar tendon and Z-lengthening of quadriceps tendon. **B,** Tack sutures are placed in tendons. **C,** Semitendinosus and gracilis tendons are harvested with tendon stripper and sutured together. **D,** Tendons are passed through transverse hole in patella and sutured together with Krackow technique. **E,** Tendons are tacked to underlying patellar tendon. **SEE TECHNIQUE 4.26.**

- In ruptures at the osteotendinous junction, an 8- to 10-mm stump of vastus intermedius often is left attached to the patella. Place No. 0 nonabsorbable sutures through the stump and lay them aside for later use.
- With a rongeur, make a small trough in the superior pole of the patella.
- Drill three longitudinal holes about 1 cm apart centered over the anticipated area of attachment of the quadriceps tendon.
- Pass a No. 5 nonabsorbable suture proximally through the quadriceps tendon, using a running interlocking suture, for a distance of about 2.5 cm, until normal-appearing tendon is reached. Pass the suture distally in a similar manner, ending just lateral to the midline of the ruptured tendon.

- Pass similar sutures along the medial side of the tendon and distally as previously described.
- Pass the suture distally with a suture retriever or Beath pin, place a single throw in the suture, and secure it with a hemostat.
- Move the knee through a range of motion to check patellar tracking and position.
- If placement is satisfactory, bring the sutures in the vastus intermedius stump anteriorly and secure them through the quadriceps tendon while maintaining anatomic position.
- Tie the sutures distally, drawing the tendon into the bony trough.
- Repair the retinaculum with interrupted absorbable sutures and close the skin and subcutaneous tissue in a rou-

tine manner. Apply a cylinder cast or locked brace with the knee in extension.

POSTOPERATIVE CARE The cylinder cast or locked brace is worn for 6 weeks. Weight bearing with crutches is allowed at 3 weeks. Cast removal and a dial-locked brace is fitted, allowing a range of knee motion from 0 to 60 degrees; the range is increased 10 to 15 degrees each week. An aggressive strengthening program is essential for good functional recovery.

■ CHRONIC RUPTURE

When a rupture of the quadriceps tendon is not treated for months or years, its repair is difficult. A defect of 2.5 to 5.0 cm

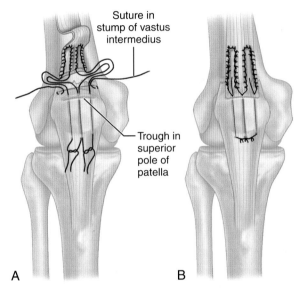

Suture in stump of vastus intermedius

Trough in superior pole of patella

A   B

FIGURE 4.40 Technique for repair of fresh rupture of quadriceps femoris muscle. **A,** Two parallel interlocking sutures are placed in quadriceps tendon. Small trough is made in anterior aspect of superior pole of patella. Horizontal mattress sutures are placed in vastus intermedius stump. **B,** Sutures in vastus intermedius are pulled anteriorly through rectus and are tied while tendon is held in anatomic position, using sutures placed distally through drill holes; sutures are then tied distally. **SEE TECHNIQUE 4.27.**

or more may be present between the ends of the tendon and must be repaired with fascia lata. If the ends can be apposed, the repair is done as described for fresh rupture of the tendon of the quadriceps femoris muscle.

If shortening makes apposing the ends of the tendon impossible, tendon lengthening can be helpful. An inverted V is cut through the full thickness of the proximal segment of the quadriceps tendon, with the inferior ends of the V ending 1.5 to 2.0 cm proximal to the rupture (Fig. 4.41). The triangular flap thus fashioned is split into an anterior part of one third of its thickness and a posterior part of two thirds. The tendon ends are apposed with interrupted sutures, and the anterior part of the flap is turned distally and is sutured. The open upper part of the V is closed with interrupted sutures. Pull-out wire sutures can be used to protect the repair but typically are not necessary.

■ COMPLICATIONS

Loss of motion, especially flexion, is a common complication after rupture of the quadriceps tendon. Extensor mechanism weakness, manifested by quadriceps atrophy and extensor lag, may occur, although this can be corrected with time and proper rehabilitation. Infection and wound problems may occur with subcutaneous placement of nonabsorbable sutures or wires and with an incision directly over the tibial tubercle. Occasionally, these sutures or wires require removal, especially when wire breakage has occurred. Patella alta or baja can be avoided by paying close attention to the position of the patella within the sagittal plane during surgery. Malalignment can lead to degenerative changes at the patellofemoral joint by increasing joint reactive forces. Rerupture that requires repeat repair also is a potential complication.

RUPTURE OF ADDUCTOR LONGUS MUSCLE

Rupture of the adductor longus muscle is characterized by the sudden or gradual appearance of swelling on the medial aspect of the upper third of the thigh with an inconsistent history of trauma. Soccer, ice hockey, and football players seem prone to this condition, and the mechanism of injury may be a combination of wide abduction of the thighs with flexion of one hip and internal rotation of the other. The palpable mass becomes more prominent during contraction of the adductor longus muscle. In 19 NFL players with adductor ruptures, nearly half (9) reported prior abdominal or groin pain.

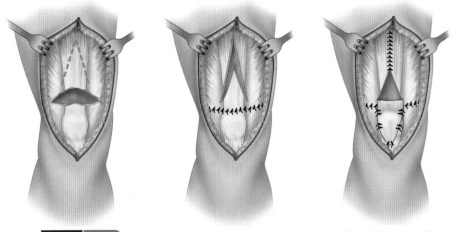

FIGURE 4.41 Codivilla tendon lengthening and repair of quadriceps tendon.

We have found repair of adductor longus ruptures difficult when they occur at the musculotendinous junction. Conservative therapy consisting of ice, thigh compression using a thigh sleeve, and relative rest using crutches if necessary generally is successful. When the acute inflammatory response has subsided, stretching and strengthening exercises are begun for rehabilitation of the hip and thigh musculature, concentrating on the adductors. Minimal functional deficit can be expected with this treatment. Nonoperative treatment was reported to result in a significantly faster return to play (6 weeks) in 14 NFL players compared with operative repair in five players (12 weeks).

RUPTURE OF GLUTEUS MEDIUS AND MINIMUS TENDONS

Often misdiagnosed as greater trochanteric pain syndrome or trochanteric bursitis, avulsion or rupture of the gluteus medius or minimus tendons ("rotator cuff of the hip") can cause prolonged lateral hip pain. The cause of tendinosis and rupture of these tendons is uncertain but may be related to local mechanical trauma or predisposing systemic conditions. The incidence of gluteal ruptures is unknown, but gluteal medius or minimus tears have been reported in 4% to 20% of patients undergoing total hip replacement and in approximately 25% of patients with femoral neck fractures. Most reported gluteus medius ruptures have been in women older than age 50 years. The two most reliable signs of a gluteus medius rupture are a Trendelenburg gait and pain on resisted hip abduction, both of which are reported to have a more than 70% specificity and sensitivity. In patients with chronic tears, plain radiographs usually are unremarkable but may show sclerosis, an irregular border, or osteophytes at the anterior edge of the greater trochanter. MRI (91% accuracy) and ultrasound can be used for confirmation of the diagnosis.

If diagnosed early, gluteus tendon ruptures can be treated conservatively by unloading the involved hip with crutches or a cane, NSAIDs, and physical therapy once acute symptoms subside. If symptoms persist, operative treatment may involve conjoined tendon debridement, transosseous fixation, and possibly augmentation with a soft-tissue graft. Transosseous fixation can be obtained with suture fixation through drill holes or suture anchors in the greater trochanteric footprint of the tendons. Open repair has been reported to successfully relieve pain in 90% to 95% of patients. Techniques for endoscopic repair of the gluteus tendon also have been described.

HAMSTRING TENDON INJURIES

Although hamstring tendon injuries are among the most common musculoskeletal injuries in athletes, there is little information in the literature concerning their diagnosis, treatment, and outcomes. Proximal hamstring avulsions can cause considerable morbidity. A variety of forms of damage exist, including inflammation, degeneration, partial tearing, complete tearing, and a combination of these pathologies. Injuries can range from mild strains of the muscles or myotendinous junction to complete avulsions from the ischial tuberosity with tendon retraction. Complete proximal rupture of the hamstring tendons represents the most severe and uncommon form of hamstring injuries with a prevalence of 9%. A complete rupture is defined as the tearing of all three tendons (biceps femoris, semitendinosus, and semimembranosus) from the ischial tuberosity.

The clinical diagnosis can be made when several physical examination findings are present, including absence of palpable tension in the distal part of the hamstrings with the patient prone and the knee flexed to 90 degrees (positive bowstring sign) (Fig. 4.42). Ecchymosis of the posterior aspect of the thigh, a palpable defect of the proximal part of the hamstrings, and weakness in prone knee flexion are also indicative of a proximal avulsion. The diagnosis of a three-tendon avulsion can be confirmed with noncontrast MRI, with use of a combination of fat-suppressed inversion recovery and proton density–weighted fast-spin-echo sequences in multiple orthogonal planes (Fig. 4.43).

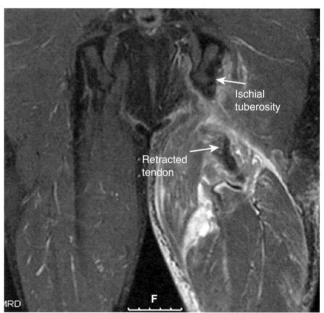

FIGURE 4.43   Fat-suppressed inversion-recovery MRI in the coronal plane, showing retracted tear of proximal hamstrings with surrounding edema. (From Birmingham P, Muller M, Wickiewicz T, et al: Functional outcome after repair of proximal hamstring avulsions, *J Bone Joint Surg Am* 93:1819, 2011.)

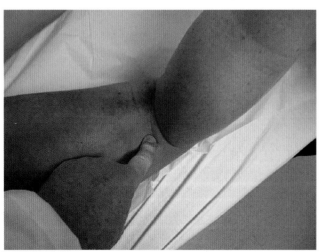

FIGURE 4.42   Positive bowstring sign: absence of palpable hamstring tendons distally. (From Birmingham P, Muller M, Wickiewicz T, et al: Functional outcome after repair of proximal hamstring avulsions, *J Bone Joint Surg Am* 93:1819, 2011.)

Benazzo et al. and Lempainen et al. detailed specific tendon involvement seen on MRI: 33% of patients had semitendinosus and biceps tendon involvement, and 48% had semimembranosus and three-tendon involvement. Of those with single-tendon involvement, 8% had only semimembranosus involvement, 11% had only biceps femoris involvement, and 1.5% had only semitendinosus involvement. The central or paramuscular tendons of the hamstrings may be the site of chronic and recurrent hamstring injuries. These central tendon tears are mainly located 10 to 20 cm distally from the origin of the hamstrings, and they often are difficult to diagnose because they can mimic a simple muscle strain injury. The central tendons of the hamstrings run from the ischial tuberosity to different insertion sites medially (the semimembranosus and semitendinosus muscles) and laterally (the biceps femoris muscle) around the knee joint. Studies have mainly reported the benefits of surgical treatment of proximal and distal ruptures of the hamstring tendon. Information on central hamstring tendon injuries and the outcome of operative treatment is limited.

TREATMENT
▥ NONOPERATIVE TREATMENT

In the treatment of chronic proximal hamstring tendinosis and partial tearing of the proximal hamstring origin, a trial of conservative measures is typically completed before surgical intervention. Nonoperative treatment has been recommended for single-tendon tears with or without retraction, although more recent studies have associated nonoperative treatment of hamstring (as low as 71%), and less patient satisfaction when compared with those treated surgically. Consequently, both acute and chronic repairs of complete and partial proximal hamstring ruptures have become more popular in recent years. Nonoperative treatment often results in sciatica, posterior thigh pain, and muscle weakness, leaving patients with poor function and more extensive rehabilitation.

Zissen et al. showed fair results with ultrasound-guided injection of corticosteroid in 38 patients, 29 of whom reported immediate relief of symptoms. Half experienced improvement of symptoms for at least 1 month, and a third reported prolonged resolution of symptoms. No complications were identified.

▥ OPERATIVE TREATMENT

Operative treatment of proximal hamstring tears has been suggested for osseous avulsions with 2 cm or more displacement, for partial tears for which nonoperative treatment is unsuccessful, and for complete three-tendon tears with or without displacement. The literature supports consideration of operative treatment primarily for competitive athletes, but a case-by-case decision is recommended.

Operative repair has variable outcomes. Multiple studies have demonstrated improved strength and endurance, with a low risk of reruptures. Functionally, 76% to 100% of patients eventually return to sports, 55% to 100% return to their preinjury activity level, and 88% to 100% of patients are satisfied with surgical outcomes. In their systematic review, Startzman et al. determined that of 266 patients involved, 99% returned to strenuous activities and sports after surgery.

Multiple series have shown that surgically repaired proximal hamstring avulsions yield better functional results and patient-reported outcome scores and a higher rate of return to preinjury activities than patients treated nonoperatively. Bodendorfer et al. found that satisfaction was much higher among patients treated operatively (93%) compared to those treated nonoperatively (53%), with higher strength in the surgical group compared with the contralateral extremity. In their series of 58 patients with hamstring repairs, Bowman et al. reported an overall satisfaction rate of 94%. At a mean of 7 months, 88% of patients were able to return to their usual sports or recreational activities, with 72% returning at the same level. Birmingham et al. reported that 21 of 23 patients returned to activity at an average of 95% of their preinjury activity level at an average of 9.8 months after repair of proximal hamstring tendon ruptures.

Some studies have suggested that delayed repair is associated with poorer results and reduced hamstring strength and endurance, while other studies showed no difference. Sarimo et al. reported that 29 of their 41 patients had good or excellent results, while 12 patients had moderate or poor results. The good or excellent group had an average delay of 2.4 months from the time of injury to the time of surgery, while the moderate or poor group had an average delay of 11.7 months, and the difference was significant. Rust et al., in their series of 72 patients who had either direct tendon repair with suture anchors or Achilles allograft tendon reconstruction, found that acute repair was superior to surgery for chronic tears with regard to return to sports. Neither Birmingham et al. nor Klingele and Sallay, however, found a difference in postoperative isokinetic testing between acute (repair less than 4 weeks after injury) and chronic (repair more than 4 weeks after injury) repairs. In their systematic review involving 387 participants, van der Made et al. found no to minimal difference in outcome between acute and delayed repair in terms of return to sports, patient satisfaction, hamstring strength, or pain.

REPAIR OF PROXIMAL HAMSTRING AVULSION

TECHNIQUE 4.28

(BIRMINGHAM ET AL.)

- With the patient prone, make a longitudinal incision at the edge of the gluteus maximus muscle. A longitudinal incision minimizes excessive traction on the gluteus maximus muscle and the inferior gluteal nerve and allows adequate mobilization of displaced soft-tissue tears.
- Retract the gluteus muscle proximally; identify the fascia distal to the transverse gluteus maximus fibers and open it, taking care to protect the posterior femoral cutaneous nerve and the inferior cluneal nerve.
- Identify the tendons and avulsion site. There usually is a large hematoma present in acute injuries.
- Place traction sutures in the tendon and debride the tuberosity avulsion site.
- The sciatic nerve lies lateral and anterior on the surface of the semimembranosus and semitendinosus. The sciatic nerve dissection is more difficult to perform after 4 weeks have passed since the occurrence of the injury, as scar

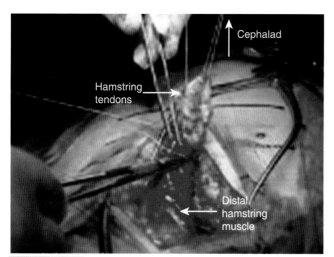

FIGURE 4.44 Mobilized proximal hamstring tendons with Krackow stitches in place and exiting proximally. (From Birmingham P, Muller M, Wickiewicz T, et al: Functional outcome after repair of proximal hamstring avulsions, *J Bone Joint Surg Am* 93:1819, 2011.) **SEE TECHNIQUE 4.28.**

tissue can begin to encase the nerve, making it difficult to mobilize the nerve safely; thus the dissection is best performed by someone experienced in nerve dissection.

- With use of two Orthocord sutures (DePuy Mitek, Raynham, MA), place two sets of Krackow stitches in the tendon, exiting proximally (Fig. 4.44).
- Debride the tuberosity to bone and place two UltraFix RC anchors (ConMed Linvatec, Utica, NY) in the tuberosity approximately 1 inch (2.54 cm) apart.
- Repair the tendons back to the lateral aspect of the ischial tuberosity.
- If the semimembranosus tendon is distinguishable, place it more lateral than the semitendinosus and the biceps femoris tendons in their anatomic locations.
- Pull one limb of the Krackow suture through the anchor, pulling the tendon to bone, and tie it in place. Use a minimum of two anchors to recreate a tendon footprint on the tuberosity, which creates more surface area for tendon-to-bone healing. This can usually be done with minimal knee flexion if done early (<4 weeks after injury). If the repair is performed later than that, knee flexion may be required to approximate the tendon to the ischial tuberosity.

POSTOPERATIVE MANAGEMENT The patient is placed in a custom pelvic-thigh-hip spica orthosis that is fitted preoperatively and allows the hip to be maintained in extension and the knee left free. The patient may bear full weight with the aid of crutches while wearing the brace. The brace is used for 6 weeks to protect the repair, after which a rehabilitation program is started with progressive hip motion and a strengthening program. Running is restricted for a minimum of 12 weeks because it takes this amount of time to reestablish hip motion, muscle strength, and endurance. There is some evidence in the literature to suggest that tendon-to-bone healing is not biomechanically mature until 12 weeks.

OPEN REPAIR OF PROXIMAL HAMSTRING AVULSION

TECHNIQUE 4.29

(BOWMAN ET AL.)
- With the patient prone, make an 8-cm horizontal incision in the gluteal crease. Carry out cautious subcutaneous dissection to identify and protect the posterior femoral cutaneous nerve.
- Identify the inferior gluteus maximus musculature and retract it superiorly and laterally.
- Identify the sciatic nerve, neurolyse it, and protect it throughout the procedure.
- Identify the hamstring sheath and incise it longitudinally to expose the invested hamstring tendons.
- Define the ischial tuberosity, perform bursectomy, and roughen the bone with a Cobb elevator and a rongeur.
- Place a double-loaded 2.3-mm Iconix (Stryker) or 4.5-mm PEEK Corkscrew (Arthrex) suture anchor in the oblique lateral facet of the ischial tuberosity.
- Insert a modified Krackow suture in the proximal hamstring tendons and use a tension-slide technique to bring the tendon down to the bone.
- Evaluate the adequacy of the repair and insert a second or third anchor as needed.
- Place the suture ends through a 4.75-mm SwiveLock (Arthrex) and set them proximally to complete double-row repair.

ENDOSCOPIC REPAIR OF PROXIMAL HAMSTRING AVULSION

TECHNIQUE 4.30

(BOWMAN ET AL.)
- With the patient prone, make a 4-cm incision in the gluteal crease, and place a 30-degree arthroscope into the space between the gluteus maximus and the ischial tuberosity.
- Through an accessory portal, use a shaver to perform ischial bursectomy.
- Identify the sciatic nerve, neurolyse it, and protect it.
- Identify the torn proximal hamstring tendons and debride them.
- Once the ischial tuberosity is clearly defined, use a 4-mm bur to prepare the bone.
- Place one or two suture anchors under direct visualization (Fig. 4.45A).
- Use a suture-passing device to place the sutures through the proximal hamstring tendons in a mattress fashion and

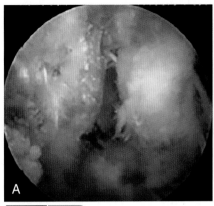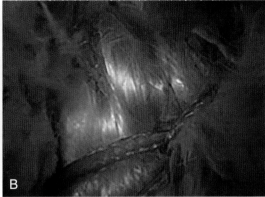

FIGURE 4.45 **A,** Suture anchor placement in the anatomic footprint on the ischium with sutures passed through the tendon. **B,** Final repair construct after reduction. (From Bowman EN, Marshall NE, Gehardt MB, et al: Predictors of clinical outcomes after proximal hamstring repair, *Orthop J Sports Med* 7: 2325967118823712, 2019.) **SEE TECHNIQUE 4.30.**

use a tension-slide technique to bring the tendons down to bone and tie an arthroscopic knot.

■ Place a lateral-row SwiveLock anchor as described in the open technique (Fig. 4.45B).

POSTOPERATIVE MANAGEMENT After both open and endoscopic procedures, patients are initially restricted to partial weight bearing with crutches for 6 weeks, followed by unrestricted weight bearing, stretching, and closed chain exercises for the next 6 weeks. No limitation is placed on range of motion. At 3 months, unrestricted strengthening is permitted, with gradual resumption of running, followed by sports or usual activities as strength improves.

■ COMPLICATIONS

The primary complication after hamstring repair is continued pain, weakness, or difficulty in returning to running or sports. Rerupture rates in the literature are typically low (<1% to 2%). In 23 patients with repairs described by Birmingham et al., there were no wound complications, infections, or reruptures; 14 reported some loss of sensation along the incision, and 14 reported cosmetic defects in the area of the incision. Four patients with chronic repairs had postoperative sciatica. Bowman et al. reported that patients with endoscopic repairs had outcomes similar to those after open repair in terms of satisfaction, pain, complication rates, and patient-reported functional outcomes.

RUPTURE OF BICEPS BRACHII TENDONS
■ PROXIMAL BICEPS TENDON RUPTURE

More than half of all ruptures involving the biceps brachii muscle occur through the tendon of its long head. The rupture usually is more or less transverse and is located either within the shoulder joint or within the proximal part of the intertubercular groove. Most of the remaining ruptures occur at the musculotendinous junction or at the attachment to the glenoid. A few ruptures occur through the tendon of the short head, the muscle proper, or the distal tendon of the biceps muscle. The injury is most common in individuals 40 to 60

years of age and often is due to impingement or chronic microtrauma on the tendon, but it may occur in younger individuals during heavy weightlifting or other sports activities (e.g., football, rugby, soccer, snowboarding) or in a traumatic fall.

Acute rupture of the proximal biceps tendon is associated with an up to 30% decrease in elbow flexion power, and the power of shoulder abduction with the arm in external rotation is about 17% less that of the opposite side. With an acute injury, ecchymosis and a lump may be noted on the lateral side of the arm from retraction of the tendon. With ruptures seen late, however, usually no appreciable weakness is noted in either flexion of the elbow or abduction of the shoulder. One difficulty in the diagnosis of rupture of the proximal biceps tendon is determining if the rupture is associated with concomitant rotator cuff tears or instability. The presentation of a patient with a proximal biceps tendon rupture is similar to that of a patient with a rotator cuff tear, and the standard tests for rotator cuff injury (see chapter 2) may be needed to define the injury. Two recent studies found proximal biceps tendon ruptures to be highly correlated with rotator cuff pathology (85% and 93%), indicating the necessity of a high index of suspicion concerning concomitant anterosuperior rotator cuff pathology in patients with acute proximal biceps ruptures and the need for early evaluation with advanced imaging.

Ruptures of the proximal biceps tendon traditionally have been treated nonoperatively because they rarely cause significant functional impairment. We prefer operative repair of acute proximal biceps tendon rupture in young, active patients who are unwilling to accept the deformity or slight weakness of supination. Occasionally, repair is indicated in a middle-aged patient whose profession, such as carpentry, requires full supination strength if the patient believes the time out of work is outweighed by the slight increase in supination power gained by operation.

Chronic biceps tendinitis or biceps tendon rupture is associated with impingement syndrome. In patients with a history of impingement symptoms and an acute rupture, arthrography or MRI is used for evaluation of rotator cuff pathology. Treatment is directed toward the impingement syndrome and repair of the rotator cuff defect. In an active patient younger than 40 years old with a rupture of less than 1 year's duration, tenodesis should be performed at the time of acromioplasty, resection of the coracoacromial ligament, and repair of the rotator cuff tendon. Tenotomy may be appropriate in older, less active patients who do not object to the supination weakness and cosmetic deformity. It is a technically simpler procedure, with a short rehabilitation time and requires no postoperative immobilization.

Techniques for tenodesis vary from open techniques to a mini-open subpectoral approach to all-arthroscopic techniques. Fixation can be done with suture anchors, interference screws, or bone tunnels.

REPAIR OF PROXIMAL BICEPS TENDON RUPTURE

TECHNIQUE 4.31

- Make an anterior incision and expose the deltopectoral groove and the tendon of the long head of the biceps by opening the intertubercular groove and dividing the transverse humeral ligament.
- Remove the infraglenoid portion of the tendon, and if the tendon was previously intact (as in biceps tendinitis), place a marking suture in it so that proper length can be retained.
- Make an inferior axillary approach, centered on the inferior border of the pectoralis major tendon.
- Identify the biceps and coracobrachialis and incise the overlying fascia longitudinally.
- Place a Hohmann retractor under the pectoralis major and retract the muscle proximally and laterally; deliver the long head of the biceps into the incision.
- At the location of the intended tenodesis, add 25 mm to the length of the biceps tendon and excise the remaining tendon.
- Fix the tendon to the bone with sutures through drill holes, suture anchors, or interference screws.

POSTOPERATIVE CARE Postoperatively, the arm is rested in a sling for several days. The patient is encouraged to resume activities as tolerated. Participation in sports should be delayed for at least 12 weeks.

SUBPECTORAL BICEPS TENODESIS

TECHNIQUE 4.32

(MAZZOCA ET AL.)
- With the patient in the beach chair position, perform a standard diagnostic arthroscopic examination.
- Identify the rotator interval between the supraspinatus and subscapularis tendons and make a standard anterior portal from inside-out or outside-in.

- With a probe in the anterior portal, pull the biceps tendon into the glenohumeral joint to evaluate its mobility and any structural lesions. Because pathologic processes of the biceps tendon are most often in the intertubercular groove portion, it is critical that this part be drawn into the joint.
- Evaluate the coracohumeral ligament and supraspinatus and subscapular tendons for any pathologic process.
- With an arthroscopic cutting instrument or thermal ablator through the anterior portal, tenotomize the biceps tendon at its base. A shaver can be used to debride the proximal portion for a stable base.
- With the arm abducted and internally rotated, palpate the inferior border of the pectoralis major tendon; on the medial aspect of the arm, make an incision 1 cm superior to this inferior border and continue it to 3 cm below the inferior border (Fig. 4.46A).
- Inject the incision site with a local anesthetic plus epinephrine for subcutaneous hemostasis and perioperative analgesia.
- Dissect through the subcuticular tissue, using electrocautery to control bleeding, and clear the overlying fatty tissue until the fascia overlying the pectoralis major, coracobrachialis, and biceps is identified. If these anatomic landmarks are not seen, the dissection may be too lateral; if the cephalic vein is seen in the deltopectoral groove, the dissection is too proximal and too lateral.
- Once the inferior border of the pectoralis major has been identified, incise the fascia over the coracobrachialis and biceps in a proximal to distal direction. It is important to see the horizontal fibers of the pectoralis muscle and dissect below this level.
- Use blunt finger dissection under the inferior edge of the pectoralis muscle, palpating up the anteromedial humerus, to identify the longitudinal, fusiform structure of the biceps tendon.
- Place a pointed Hohmann retractor into the pectoralis major tendon and on the proximal humerus to retract the muscle proximally and laterally (Fig. 4.46B).
- Position a blunt Chandler retractor on the medial aspect of the humerus and gently retract the coracobrachialis and short head of the biceps tendon. Avoid vigorous medial retraction to prevent injury to the musculocutaneous nerve.
- Once the biceps tendon is identified, place a right-angle clamp deep to it and pull the tendon into the wound (Fig. 4.46C).
- One centimeter proximal to the pectoralis major tendon, reflect the periosteum in a rectangle roughly 2 × 1 cm.
- To ensure appropriate tensioning of the biceps tendon, resect the proximal portion to leave 20 to 25 mm of tendon proximal to the musculotendinous portion of the biceps.
- Using a Krackow or whip stitch, weave a No. 2 nonabsorbable suture into the proximal 15 mm of the tendon (Fig. 4.46D). Secure enough of the tendon to ensure adequate interference fixation within bone and to position the musculotendinous portion of the biceps muscle beneath the inferior border of the pectoralis major tendon. This is critical for proper tensioning of the muscle-tendon unit as well as for cosmesis.
- Use a guidewire and an 8-mm reamer to make a 15-mm deep bone tunnel at the junction of the middle and distal

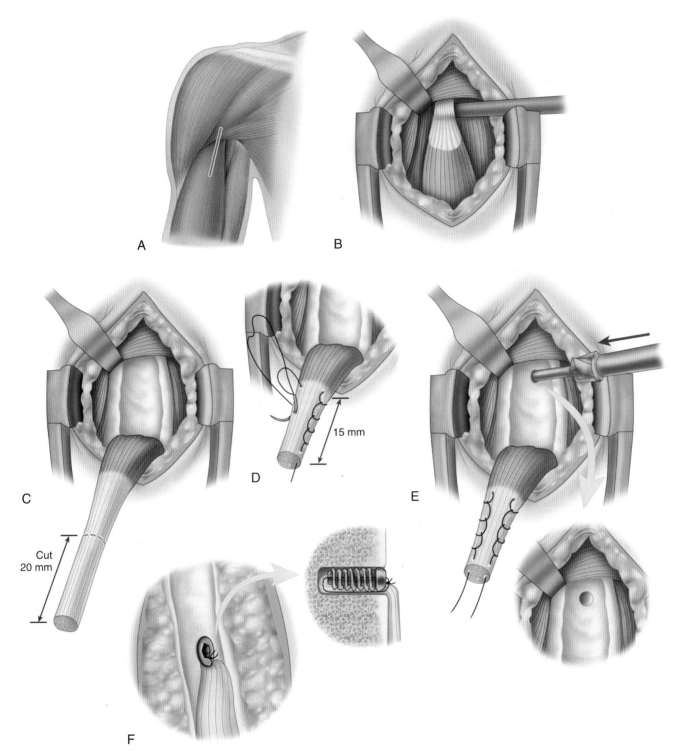

FIGURE 4.46   Subpectoral biceps tenodesis (see text). **A,** Skin incision. **B,** Retraction of pectoralis muscle. **C,** Biceps tendon pulled into wound. **D,** Krackow sutures woven into proximal tendon. **E,** Guidewire placed in bicipital groove for reaming. **F,** Placement of interference screw. (Redrawn from Mazzocca AD, Rios CG, Romeo AA, Arciero RA: Subpectoral biceps tenodesis with interference screw fixation, *Arthroscopy* 21:896, 2005.) **SEE TECHNIQUE 4.32.**

thirds of the intertubercular groove between the lesser and greater tuberosities (Fig. 4.46E).

- Clear all debris from the field with irrigation.
- Thread one limb of the suture through a biotenodesis screwdriver and screw (8 × 12 mm) and wrap the end of the suture into the screw cleat.
- Place the tenodesis screwdriver into the bone tunnel and advance the screw over the tendon; when the screw is flush with the bone tunnel, remove the screwdriver.
- Tie the limb of the suture next to the tendon and screw to the limb of the suture through the screw to provide both an interference fit and suture anchor stability (Fig. 4.46F).
- When the fixation is completed, the musculotendinous junction should rest in its exact anatomic location underneath the inferior border of the pectoralis major tendon.
- Complete the procedure with standard wound closure.

POSTOPERATIVE CARE A sling is worn during sleep for the first 4 weeks and is used only while awake if the patient is having difficulty keeping the elbow flexed passively or if he or she is going into public areas. The sling is discontinued completely after 4 weeks. Activity typically is dictated by procedures done in conjunction with the biceps tenodesis. If biceps tenodesis alone is done, strengthening activities should be restricted until 6 weeks after surgery; many patients are able to resume activity as tolerated at 2 weeks, but they should be informed of the risks.

Arthroscopic biceps tenodesis is described in other chapter.

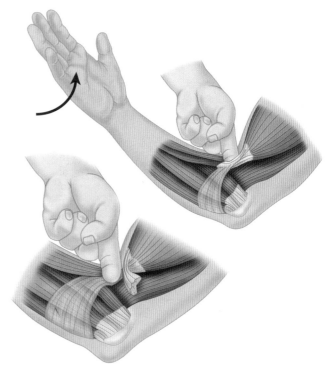

FIGURE 4.47   Hook test for distal biceps avulsion. With elbow actively flexed and supinated, examiner should be able to "hook" index finger under cordlike structure in antecubital fossa if biceps tendon is intact.

▉ DISTAL BICEPS TENDON RUPTURE

Distal rupture of the biceps tendon typically occurs in middle-aged men during heavy lifting with the elbow flexed 90 degrees, or when the biceps muscle contracts against unexpected resistance. A pop may be heard, which usually is followed by pain, swelling, and ecchymosis in the antecubital fossa. Superior migration of the muscle is evident, as is a palpable defect. Initially, there is weakness with flexion and supination.

The biceps squeeze test, similar to the Thompson test for Achilles tendon rupture, can be used for diagnosis of complete distal biceps rupture. The test is done with the patient seated and the elbow flexed 60 to 80 degrees. This amount of flexion minimizes tension on the brachialis and helps isolate the biceps to forearm supination. The forearm is slightly pronated to place tension on the biceps brachii tendon. The examiner stands on the same side as the extremity being tested. The biceps brachii is squeezed firmly with both hands, one hand at the distal myotendinous junction and the other around the muscle belly. As the biceps is squeezed, the muscle belly is drawn away from the underlying humerus, eliciting an anterior bow of the muscle. Lack of forearm supination with this maneuver is considered a positive text, indicating rupture of the biceps brachii tendon or muscle belly. The reported positive predictive value of this test is 95%, with a sensitivity of 100%. The hook test can be used for the diagnosis of complete biceps tendon avulsions: with the elbow actively flexed and supinated, the examiner should be able to "hook" an index finger under a cordlike structure in the antecubital fossa if the tendon is intact (Fig. 4.47). This test was reported to have 100% sensitivity and specificity; however, the examiner must be sure to hook the lateral edge of the

biceps tendon, not the medial edge, because the lacertus fibrosus might be mistaken for an intact biceps tendon.

Median nerve compression in the proximal forearm may result from a partial rupture. Although complete ruptures often are dramatic in appearance and relatively easy to diagnose, partial or incomplete ruptures are not and often exhibit features similar to that of complete disruption, including pain and weakness of elbow flexion and forearm supination, differing only in that the biceps tendon is still palpable.

MRI can be helpful in distinguishing complete from partial ruptures, as well as in defining tendinosis, tenosynovitis, hematoma, and brachialis contusion. A flexed abducted supinated (FABS) position (90 degrees of elbow flexion, 180 degrees of shoulder abduction, and forearm supination) has been recommended to obtain a true longitudinal view of the tendon. Ultrasound is a potentially faster and less expensive imaging method, but it is very user dependent. In a comparison of MRI to ultrasound for the diagnosis of complete distal biceps tendon ruptures, Lynch et al. found that accuracy rates were 86% with MRI and 45% with ultrasound. Sensitivity and specificity of MRI were 76% and 50%, respectively, while those of ultrasound were 62% and 20%.

Opinions differ as to the proper method and site for reattaching this tendon. Most authors agree that theoretically it should be reattached at its normal position on the radial tuberosity to restore the power of supination of the biceps muscle. When the elbow is extended, the biceps muscle is twice as powerful as the supinator muscle in supinating the forearm, and this power is even greater when the elbow is flexed. Surgical treatment of distal biceps tendon ruptures can be accomplished through a single-incision or two-incision technique. The two-incision technique of Boyd and Anderson restores the power of supination to the biceps but avoids the dangers of deep dissection in the antecubital fossa.

Occasionally, a distal biceps injury is not initially recognized and may present after a delay. Higher complication rates have been reported with delayed repair because of tendon retraction, muscle atrophy, and scar formation, and early repair has been reported to produce better functional and patient-reported outcomes than delayed repair or reconstruction. More recent reports, however, indicate that, despite a higher rate of initial complications, delayed reconstruction (more than 21 days) results in functional outcomes similar to those of acute repair. Frank et al. described delayed reconstruction with a semitendinosus autograft in 19 patients and determined that strength, range of motion, and complication rates were similar to those of acute repair, although functional outcome scores were not as good.

An endoscopic procedure has been described, but we have no experience with this technique.

There has been some concern about heterotopic ossification formation or radioulnar synostosis using the Boyd and Anderson approach; however, in our patients treated with this technique we have not found this to be a problem. We believe that using an osteotome instead of a drill to make the trapdoor prevents the disbursement of bone particles into the interosseous space, which might lead to ectopic ossification. We have modified the technique by substituting the trapdoor with a trough. We also recommend minimal disruption of the interosseous membrane when passing the tendon from the anterior incision to the posterolateral incision. In addition, a small transverse incision is made instead of the anterior curvilinear incision.

A "mini-open" two-incision technique has been described using a small (≤2 mm) transverse incision in the flexion crease of the antecubital fossa and a 3-cm posterolateral incision for transosseous fixation. In a report of 784 repairs of distal biceps tendons, the double-incision technique had higher rates of posterior interosseous nerve palsy, heterotopic bone formation, and reoperations. A more recent retrospective analysis of 970 distal biceps repairs using a single- or two-incision technique found that the use of a two-incision technique increased the risk of radioulnar synostosis and neuritis or numbness compared to a single-incision technique. Most studies, however, report similar outcomes with single- and double-incision techniques.

We use both single- and double-incision techniques but do not recommend immediate mobilization as described by

Barrett et al. They reported good results with this protocol; only two (3.4%) of 58 patients developed heterotopic ossification and only one required reoperation for a radioulnar synostosis. Good results also have been reported with single-incision techniques using suture anchors, interference screws, buttons, and tenodesis screws. Reported advantages of the single-incision techniques include limited exposure of the radial tuberosity, better cosmetic result, and decreased risk of heterotopic ossification. Disadvantages include increased costs (expensive hardware), possibility of less secure fixation, and no bony trough for tendon revascularization. In general, nerve injuries are more frequent with single-incision techniques, and heterotopic ossification is more common after two-incision techniques.

Biomechanical studies comparing fixation methods have had conflicting conclusions; some have shown button fixation to have significantly higher pull-out strength than suture anchors or bone tunnel fixation, whereas others have found transosseous sutures to be stronger than suture anchors. A biomechanical comparison of all-suture anchors to titanium suture anchors found that the two performed similarly, with similar load and mechanism of failure, while a comparison of cortical button fixation to suture anchor fixation did not find that one method was superior to the other. Interference screw fixation was found to pose a higher risk of anatomic failure of the tenodesis than suture anchor fixation, although functional outcomes were not different.

TWO-INCISION TECHNIQUE FOR REPAIR OF THE DISTAL BICEPS TENDON

TECHNIQUE 4.33

(BOYD AND ANDERSON)
- Make a 2-cm transverse anterior incision and a longer, 6- to 8-cm posterolateral incision over the radial aspect of the ulnar border (Fig. 4.48A).
- Open the deep fascia and identify the biceps tendon with palpation.

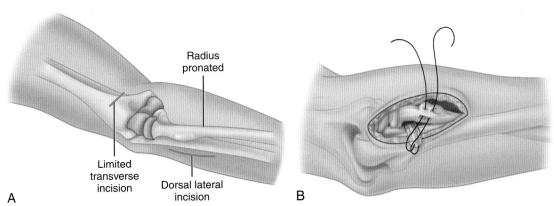

FIGURE 4.48   Two-incision technique for repair of distal biceps tendon. **A,** Incisions. **B,** Biceps tendon passed through "trapdoor" in tuberosity. **SEE TECHNIQUE 4.33.**

- Locate the original tunnel through the interosseous membrane.
- Place Krakow locking stitches in the tendon end. It is important to keep each locking throw in close proximity to the previous throw to avoid kinking the tendon and forming a bunched end to the tendon that would prohibit the tendon from seating into the groove or "trapdoor" created in the radial tuberosity.
- With a long curved hemostat, deliver the tendon from the anterior incision to the posterolateral incision. Avoid making multiple passes through the membrane to minimize the risk of heterotopic ossification and subsequent synostosis.
- Deepen the posterolateral incision, identify the anconeus, and sharply dissect it off the bone. Pronate the arm to protect the posterior interosseous nerve.
- Use a small ¼-inch curved osteotome to make a trough or "trapdoor" in the tuberosity.
- Drill two holes in the dorsal aspect of the trough, leaving a 10-mm bone bridge between them (Fig. 4.48B).
- Pass the sutures tied to the tendon, and with them the tendon, through the interosseous membrane.
- Use a suture passer to pass the first suture through the trough and out of the drill hole.
- Pass the second suture with the suture passer through the trough and out of the drill hole.
- Pulling carefully on the sutures in the tendon, guide it into the trough in the bone.
- Tie the sutures securely over the bone and cut off the ends of the sutures.
- Close the anterior incision with the elbow flexed about 60 degrees.
- Release the tourniquet and close the posterolateral incision.

POSTOPERATIVE CARE With the elbow flexed to 110 degrees and the forearm in moderate supination, a posterior plaster splint is applied. At 2 weeks, the splint and the sutures are removed. A hinged brace is applied and worn for 4 weeks. Passive flexion is allowed, as is active extension, progressing 15 to 20 degrees per week. Supination/pronation range-of-motion exercises are added at 4 to 6 weeks. At 6 to 8 weeks, full range of motion should be possible, but return to full activities should be delayed for 12 to 16 weeks.

SINGLE-INCISION TECHNIQUE FOR REPAIR OF THE DISTAL BICEPS TENDON

TECHNIQUE 4.34

- Make a 3- to 4-cm anterior longitudinal incision (Henry approach, see other chapter). Superficial antecubital veins may require ligation. Identify and preserve the lateral antebrachial cutaneous nerve.

- Identify the proximal torn biceps tendon and place it in a moist sponge.
- Ligate the radial recurrent vessels.
- Deep knee retractors allow excellent exposure of the radial tuberosity. Debride the remnant of the tuberosity free of remaining tendon and elevate the periosteum over the bone with a curet.
- Fix the tendon to the radial tuberosity with sutures through bone tunnels, suture anchors, button, or tenodesis or interference screws.
- Once the tendon is approximated, move the forearm through a full range of pronation and supination to ensure that the tendon tracks smoothly.

POSTOPERATIVE CARE The elbow is immobilized at 90 degrees for 2 weeks, at which time the sutures are removed. A hinged elbow brace is applied with extension stopped at 80 degrees. Full passive flexion is allowed with passive pronation and supination to 90 degrees. At 6 weeks, progressive extension in the brace is allowed at a rate of 20 degrees per week. At 8 weeks, active flexion is begun and strengthening is started at 12 weeks. Full, unrestricted use is allowed at 16 weeks.

RUPTURE OF PECTORALIS MAJOR MUSCLE

Rupture of the pectoralis major muscle most commonly is caused by forced abduction, external rotation, and extension of the shoulder against resistance. Once considered a rare injury, pectoralis major rupture has become more common over the past 2 decades, especially in athletes participating in sports such as weightlifting. Although the bench press is the most frequently cited cause of pectoralis major rupture, these injuries also have been reported in other sports, including rugby, snow and water skiing, football, wrestling, and hockey. Traumatic ruptures occur almost exclusively in men between the ages of 20 and 40 years. Swelling, ecchymosis, and later muscular deformity are evident at the site of the rupture, usually at the musculotendinous insertion into the humerus. Weakness in shoulder adduction and internal rotation is present. A more specific sign of pectoralis major rupture, both acute and chronic, is a loss or thinning of the anterior axillary fold on the side of the injury. A defect in the axillary fold often is accentuated by abduction or contracted adduction of the affected arm. The defect is palpable when compared with the opposite flexed pectoralis tendon. MRI and ultrasound are effective in determining the location and extent of ruptures of the pectoralis major.

Direct surgical repair usually is indicated for fresh, traumatic ruptures in young adults, especially if full muscle power is required or if the patient objects to the clinical deformity. Pectoralis tendon repair generally results in a high rate of return to sport (90%) and work (95%), pain relief, and improved cosmetic appearance. The tendon usually is avulsed from bone, and repair usually is done by tying nonabsorbable sutures through drill holes, with or without suture anchors, in the same manner as a rotator cuff repair (Fig. 4.49). Repair also can be accomplished with direct tendon-to-tendon suture using multiple nonabsorbable mattress sutures. In a biomechanical cadaver study, repair with a running, locked configuration appeared to improve performance by preventing suture pullout. Delayed repair, if warranted by symptoms, may be successful if the muscle ends have not significantly retracted. If testing of resistance

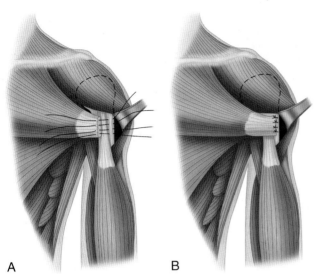

FIGURE 4.49 Repair of pectoralis major with bone trough technique. **A,** Sutures passed through bone trough in tendon footprint. **B,** Tying of sutures pulls ruptured tendon into bone trough. (Redrawn from Petilon J, Carr DR, Sekiya JK, Unger DV: Pectoralis major muscle injuries: evaluation and management, *J Am Acad Orthop Surg* 13:59, 2005.)

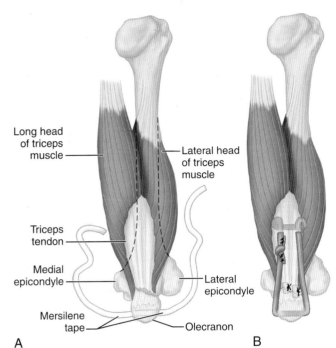

FIGURE 4.50 Repair of triceps tendon avulsion or rupture. **A,** Mersilene strip is passed through hole in olecranon. **B,** Strip is threaded through large needle and loop is made through tendon; needle is then passed transversely through tendon and another loop is fashioned.

to shoulder adduction and internal rotation indicates some remaining tendon function, delayed repair may be successful. If circumferential mobilization of the tendon does not restore sufficient tendon length to allow reattachment, an allograft, either Achilles or hamstring tendon, can be used to provide length and allow repair directly to the humerus. A shoulder immobilizer should be worn for 6 weeks after surgery. Pendulum exercises are started within the first or second week, and progressive resistance exercises are begun at about 3 months. Unrestricted activity usually is allowed at about 4 months after surgery.

RUPTURE OR AVULSION OF TRICEPS TENDON

Rupture of the triceps tendon is relatively uncommon. It usually occurs as an avulsion of the tendon and a small piece of bone from the olecranon tip. Triceps tendon rupture also is associated with steroid injections for olecranon bursitis, and an association with anabolic steroid use has been suggested.

Patients present with pain and swelling over the posterior aspect of the elbow. Physical examination reveals tenderness to palpation, swelling, and ecchymosis. A palpable defect may be present proximal to the olecranon. Although an inability to actively extend against resistance is a sign of complete rupture, not all complete ruptures cause this deficit. Sagittal MRI is helpful for determining the integrity of the triceps tendon. Partial ruptures are characterized by a small fluid-filled defect within the distal tendon that appears as a bright area on T2-weighted images. Complete ruptures are characterized by a large fluid-filled gap between the distal end of the triceps tendon and the olecranon process.

Nonoperative treatment of triceps tendon ruptures generally is reserved for elderly patients with low activity demands. Most ruptures at the olecranon insertion should be repaired with No. 2 or No. 5 nonabsorbable sutures passed through holes drilled in the olecranon (Fig. 4.50). A tension suture of No. 5

nonabsorbable suture can be used to relieve stress on the repair. Suture anchors also can be used, and this is the method we use most often. Mirzayan et al. found that repair with transosseous tunnels had a significantly higher rerupture rate, higher reoperation rate, and longer release from medical care than repair with anchor fixation. Yeh et al. described an "anatomic triceps tendon footprint repair" using suture anchors to create a suture bridge and restore a wider area of tendon-bone contact. An endoscopic technique has been reported but we have no experience with this.

For ruptures at the myotendinous junction, a V-Y triceps tendon advancement technique has been described, in which autologous plantaris tendon is interwoven with the remaining proximal and distal triceps tissue to augment the strength of the repair.

Multiple procedures have been described for treatment of chronic ruptures, including use of anconeus or Achilles rotation flaps, plantaris or hamstring tendon augmentation, and ligament augmentation devices.

DOUBLE-ROW REPAIR OF THE DISTAL TRICEPS TENDON

TECHNIQUE 4.35

(AZAR)
- Position the anesthetized patient supine with a sterile roll for the elbow.

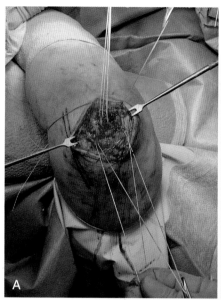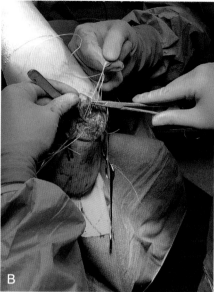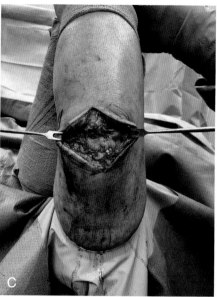

FIGURE 4.51 Double-row triceps repair. **A,** FiberWire suture through the tendon using a Krackow stitch technique. **B,** Parallel transosseous tunnels drilled in the olecranon. **C,** Completed repair. **SEE TECHNIQUE 4.35.**

- Make a straight posterior midline incision approximately 6 to 8 cm centered over the olecranon tip.
- Mobilize the subcutaneous tissues to expose the triceps tendon tear.
- Debride the edges of the ruptured triceps tendon and curet the olecranon footprint of the tear to bleeding bone.
- Place a #2 FiberWire suture (Arthrex, Naples, FL) through the tendon using a Krackow stitch technique.
- Drill parallel transosseous tunnels in the olecranon approximately 2 cm and approximately 4 cm in length using a 2.0-mm drill bit.
- For the double row, place two or three suture anchors just proximal to the tendon insertion site into the olecranon for augmentation of the reattachment (Fig. 4.51A).
- Pass the sutures of the bone anchors through the tendon in a horizontal mattress pattern and leave them untied.
- Pass the FiberWire sutures into the transosseous tunnel and advance them through the olecranon with a Hewson suture passer.
- With the elbow in full extension, reattach the tendon to the olecranon footprint (Fig. 4.51B).
- Tie the transosseous sutures first, followed by the bone anchor sutures (Fig. 4.51C).
- Evaluate the stability of the reattachment by moving the elbow through its total range of motion. Irrigate the wound and close in layers.

POSTOPERATIVE MANAGEMENT The arm is immobilized in a long arm posterior splint in 20 degrees of extension for 2 weeks, followed by a supervised assisted range of motion rehabilitation program, including progressive elbow flexion, full passive extension, and passive/active-assisted forearm rotation exercises with the elbow in extension for the next 4 weeks. At 6 weeks, active extension of the elbow is initiated, followed by strengthening exercises at 10 to 12 weeks. Unrestricted activity is allowed at 4 months.

DISPLACEMENT OF TENDONS
PERONEAL TENDONS

Subluxation and dislocation of the peroneal tendons are uncommon and often overlooked causes of lateral ankle pain. Because the acute injury may mimic lateral ankle sprain and may occur at the same time as lateral ankle ligament injury, diagnosis can be difficult. In one study, only 60% of peroneal tendon disorders were accurately diagnosed at the first clinical evaluation. These injuries are most frequent in young athletic individuals participating in such sports as skiing, soccer, basketball, rugby, ice skating, tennis, football, and gymnastics; chronic subluxation has been reported without any history of a specific traumatic event.

The superior peroneal retinaculum is a primary restraint to instability of the peroneal tendons at the fibular malleolus. It extends approximately 3.5 cm proximally from the tip of the lateral malleolus and attaches posterolaterally onto the calcaneus and the deep investing fascia adjacent to the Achilles tendon. The peroneal tendons may be displaced within the tendon sheaths but are more commonly displaced outside the sheaths and the tendon groove. The peroneal musculature contracts and overpowers the soft tissue. The tendons dislocate anteriorly from behind the distal fibula. Powerful contraction of the peroneals with the foot dorsiflexed may cause failure of the superior peroneal retinaculum, leading to subluxation or dislocation of the tendons. An inversion injury with the foot in plantar flexion also can stretch or avulse this structure.

Anatomic factors that may predispose to recurrent dislocation include incompetence of the superior retinaculum, a shallow sulcus, or a convex posterior surface of the distal fibula. Congenital deformities such as congenital vertical talus and talipes planovalgus also have been reported to contribute to peroneal tendon dislocation.

■ CLASSIFICATION

Peroneal tendon injuries have been classified primarily by location. In one classification system (Shawen and Anderson), zone I

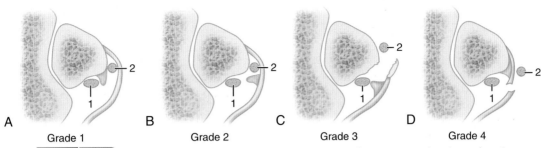

FIGURE 4.52 Classification of peroneal subluxation (see text): *1*, peroneus brevis tendon; *2*, peroneus longus tendon. (See text.) (Redrawn from Raikin SM, Elias I, Nazarian LN: Intrasheath subluxation of the peroneal tendon, *J Bone Joint Surg* 90A:992, 2008.)

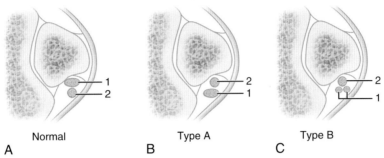

FIGURE 4.53 Two types of tendon intrasheath subluxation: *1*, peroneus brevis tendon; *2*, peroneus longus tendon. **A,** Normal location of tendons. **B,** Type A subluxation in which tendons snap over each other and switch their relative position. **C,** Type B subluxation in which peroneus longus tendon subluxes through a longitudinal split tear within the peroneus brevis tendon. (Redrawn from Raikin SM, Elias I, Nazarian LN: Intrasheath subluxation of the peroneal tendon, *J Bone Joint Surg* 90A:992, 2008.)

BOX 4.6

Differential Diagnosis of Peroneal Tendon Subluxation/Dislocation

- Lateral ligament ankle sprain
- Achilles tendon rupture
- Fracture: malleolus, fifth metatarsal, cuboid
- Stress fracture: calcaneus
- Sinus tarsi syndrome
- Calcaneocuboid syndrome
- Peroneal tendinopathy
- Degenerative joint disease
- Tarsal coalition
- Osteochondral lesion of the talus
- Loose bodies in the ankle or subtalar joint
- Sural neuritis
- Radiculopathy
- Malignant or benign neoplasm
- Accessory muscle or bone

---

injuries involve the fibular groove and usually the peroneus brevis tendon; zone II injuries are located in the cuboid tunnel and primarily involve the peroneus longus tendon. In Oden's modification of the classification of Eckert and Davis (Fig. 4.52), injuries are divided into four grades. In grade 1 lesions, the most common pattern (>50%), the superior peroneal retinaculum is elevated off the fibula with the peroneal tendons coming to lie between the bone and the periosteum. In grade 2 lesions the fibrocartilaginous ridge behind the lateral insertion of the superior peroneal retinaculum is avulsed along with the retinaculum and the tendons are displaced beneath the ridge. Grade 3 lesions involve an avulsion of a small cortical osseous fragment from the fibular insertion of the superior peroneal retinaculum with the tendons dislocating beneath the fibular fragment. Grade 4 lesions, the least common type, involve a complete avulsion or rupture of the superior peroneal retinaculum with the tendons lying external and superficial to the retinaculum. More recently, Raikin et al. proposed intrasheath subluxation within the peroneal groove beneath an otherwise intact superior peroneal retinaculum as a subgroup of peroneal subluxation. Two types of these intrasheath subluxations were described: type A, in which there is no peroneal tendon tear and the tendons momentarily switch their relative positions (the peroneus longus tendon lies deep to the peroneus brevis tendon), and type B, in which the peroneus longus subluxes through a longitudinal tear in the peroneus brevis tendon (Fig. 4.53).

■ CLINICAL AND RADIOGRAPHIC EVALUATION

The diagnosis can be confirmed by popping and clicking of the lateral ankle, especially while ascending stairs, and by provocative testing in which the foot is placed in dorsiflexion, eversion, and external rotation while resisting an inversion–plantar flexion force applied by the examiner. Dislocation of the tendon can be detected with circumduction of the foot while the examiner palpates the anterior tip of the peroneal groove. Patients with intrasheath subluxations may not have reproducible clinical signs. The differential diagnosis should include degenerative, traumatic, and congenital causes of lateral ankle pain (Box 4.6), especially lateral ankle ligament sprain (Table 4.5).

TABLE 4.5

Differentiating Peroneal Tendon Subluxation From Lateral Ankle Ligament Sprain

SIGN/SYMPTOM	PERONEAL TENDON SUBLUXATION	LATERAL ANKLE LIGAMENT SPRAIN
Tenderness	Proximal to tip of fibula	Distal to tip of fibula
Swelling	Posterolateral	Anteroinferior
History	Snapping	Giving way
Worse on uneven ground	Possible	Probable
Worse with circumduction	Yes	No
Worse on flexion-inversion	No	Yes

Radiographs usually are negative; with a grade 3 injury, a "fleck" of bone may be seen off the posterior distal fibula. MRI can be used to identify injury to the superior peroneal retinaculum, the peroneal tendons, and supporting soft tissues, as well as identify anomalous structures such as the peroneus quartus or a low-lying peroneal brevis muscle belly. Kinematic MRI of the ankle moving from dorsiflexion to plantar flexion has been suggested to be superior to static imaging because the pathologic process is position dependent. Ultrasonography also has been reported to be effective for dynamically evaluating peroneal tendon subluxation.

■ TREATMENT

Treatment depends on whether the injury is acute or chronic, the bone and soft-tissue anatomy, any associated clinical findings, and the age and activity level of the patient. Nonoperative treatment rarely is successful, and operative treatment is preferred, especially in young, athletic patients. Acute repair of the superior peroneal retinaculum is recommended. Symptomatic chronic or recurrent tendon dislocation should be treated surgically unless contraindicated. Operative procedures are of five general types: periosteal attachment, groove deepening, tenoplasty, bone block procedures, and rerouting procedures, such as incision of the calcaneofibular ligament and placement of the peroneal tendons deep to the ligament. We generally prefer a soft-tissue reconstruction using the deep fascia or periosteum in combination with groove deepening. If the fascia is insufficient, a posterior bone-block procedure can give excellent results. Use of a lateral band from the Achilles tendon is another alternative, although some of our patients have had persistent symptoms of Achilles tendinitis after this procedure. Other procedures described for treatment of peroneal tendon subluxation include use of half of the peroneus brevis tendon for repair of the superior peroneal retinaculum, transposition of the peroneal tendon under the calcaneofibular ligament, and various techniques of superior peroneal retinaculum reconstruction and deepening of the posterior fibular groove. An endoscopic technique for repair of the superior peroneal retinaculum also has been described. Bone-block procedures involve osteotomies of the fibula designed to produce a bony lip at the distal fibula to help prevent subluxation; although these procedures can have high rates of success, they also have high rates of complications because of

the internal fixation used. An endoscopic technique has been reported, but we have no experience with it.

REPAIR OF THE SUPERIOR PERONEAL RETINACULUM

TECHNIQUE 4.36

- Make a longitudinal incision over the posterior aspect of the distal third of the fibula and extend it over the lateral border of the foot to the cuboid.
- At the lateral malleolus superficially, elevate the posterior skin flap, and from the deep fascia, form an ample flap with its base attached to the tip of the lateral malleolus.
- Retract anteriorly the sheaths and tendons of the peroneal muscles.
- With an osteotome, make a groove in the posterior aspect of the lateral malleolus and place the peroneal tendons in it.
- Bring the fascial flap over the tendons and suture it to the remains of the retinacula or to the periosteum or soft tissue on the lateral side of the calcaneus to hold the tendons in their normal position.

POSTOPERATIVE CARE With a splint or cast, the foot is immobilized in slight eversion and at an angle of 90 degrees to the leg for 4 weeks, with protected weight bearing. At 2 to 4 weeks, full weight bearing is allowed in a cast or removable brace.

FIBULAR GROOVE DEEPENING WITH TISSUE TRANSFER (PERIOSTEAL FLAP) FOR RECURRENT PERONEAL TENDON DISLOCATION

TECHNIQUE 4.37

(ZOELLNER AND CLANCY)
- Make a 7-cm J-shaped curvilinear incision posterior to the lateral malleolus along the course of the peroneal tendons.
- Free the tendons from their sheath and retract them anteriorly over the malleolus.
- Raise a cortical osteoperiosteal flap measuring 3 × 1 cm along the posteromedial aspect of the distal fibula and lateral malleolus, leaving the posteromedial border intact to act as a hinge (Fig. 4.54A).
- Swing the flap posteriorly and remove cancellous bone from the posterior aspect of the fibula to deepen the groove 6 to 9 mm (Fig. 4.54B).

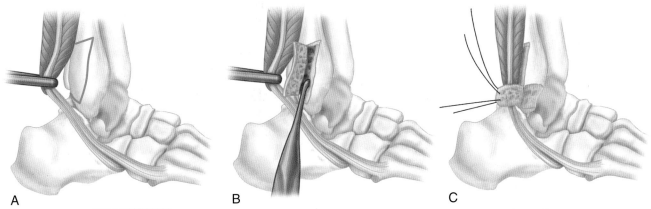

FIGURE 4.54 Technique for recurrent dislocation of peroneal tendon. **A,** With tendons retracted, cortical osteoperiosteal flap is raised along posterolateral aspect of distal fibula, leaving posteromedial border intact as hinge. **B,** Flap is hinged posteriorly, and cancellous bone is removed from posterior aspect of fibula to deepen groove. **C,** Periosteal flap is swung posteriorly over tendons in groove. **SEE TECHNIQUE 4.37.**

- Then tamp the flap back into position, creating a groove 3 to 4 cm long. The floor of the groove should provide a smooth gliding surface for the peroneal tendons.
- Replace the tendons in the groove and move the ankle through a full range of motion. The tendons should remain well seated and show no tendency to subluxate or dislocate.
- If the superior peroneal retinaculum is strong enough to use for repair, plicate it over the tendon. If the retinaculum is tenuous, as is often the case, raise an additional periosteal flap (1 cm²) from the lateral surface of the malleolus, leaving it hinged on its posterolateral side. Reflect this flap posteriorly and suture it to the medial part of the peroneal retinaculum (Fig. 4.54C).
- Close the wounds in the usual manner and apply a short-leg cast.

POSTOPERATIVE CARE At 3 weeks the initial cast is changed to a hinged short leg cast that allows dorsiflexion and plantar flexion exercises; this cast is worn for 3 more weeks. Strenuous athletic activities are not allowed until a full range of motion and normal strength are attained.

INDIRECT (IMPACTION) FIBULAR GROOVE DEEPENING FOR PERONEAL TENDON DISLOCATION

TECHNIQUE 4.38

(SHAWEN AND ANDERSON)
- Make a 6- to 8-cm longitudinal incision curved anteriorly over the tip of the fibula along the posterior edge of the fibula.

- Develop full-thickness skin flaps to avoid skin necrosis.
- Incise the distal 4 to 5 cm of the superior peroneal retinaculum from the fibula, leaving a 3-mm cuff of tissue to assist with soft-tissue repair.
- Elevate the remainder of the cuff on the fibula off the bone to expose the lateral cortex; roughen the cortex to bleeding bone.
- Excise any low-lying peroneus brevis muscle and supernumerary muscles of the lateral leg compartment (e.g., peroneus quartus) and remove any fibrinous tissue within the fibular groove.
- Expose the distal tip of the fibula and sequentially ream the distal fibula through a small entry site at the fibular tip. As an alternative, place an intramedullary guide pin from distal to proximal into the fibula, attempting to follow the posterior cortex, and sequentially ream over the guide pin to an appropriate size (usually 7 to 8 mm).
- Use a bone tamp and mallet to impact the posterior cortex. Be sure to impact the distal tip of the fibula inward to avoid a sharp edge that would impinge on the peroneal tendon.
- After groove deepening and all necessary tendon repairs are completed, repair the superior peroneal retinaculum, excising any redundant tissue. Advance the remaining superior peroneal retinaculum to the previously prepared cortical bed and secure it either through drill holes or with suture anchors.
- Suture the cuff of tissue left on the fibula in a "pants-over-vest" fashion over the repair, close the skin and subcutaneous tissue in standard fashion, and apply a cast with the leg and ankle in a neutral position.

POSTOPERATIVE CARE The patient remains non–weight bearing for 2 weeks, at which time the cast and sutures or staples are removed and a short leg walking cast is applied. The patient is allowed to bear weight as tolerated. At 6 weeks, the cast is removed and an Aircast (Summit, NJ) or a similar supportive device is applied to avoid ankle inversion. Active range of motion exercises are begun. At 8 to 10 weeks, aggressive peroneal strengthening is initiated. Full return to activities usually is possible between 4 and 6 months after surgery.

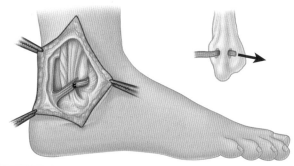

FIGURE 4.55 Jones technique for displacement of peroneal tendons. Check ligament formed by flap of Achilles tendon is inserted through hole drilled in lateral malleolus. **SEE TECHNIQUE 4.39.**

ACHILLES TENDON AUGMENTATION OF SUPERIOR PERONEAL RETINACULUM REPAIR

TECHNIQUE 4.39

(JONES)
- Make a longitudinal incision 5 cm long posterior to the lateral malleolus.
- Without disturbing their sheaths, replace the peroneal tendons in their normal position behind the malleolus.
- Expose the Achilles tendon and dissect from its lateral border a flap 5 cm long × 0.6 cm wide and leave it attached to the calcaneus (Fig. 4.55).
- Next expose the lateral malleolus and drill a hole through it in an anteroposterior direction.
- Draw the free end of the flap from the calcaneus through the hole and suture it to itself and to the periosteum.

POSTOPERATIVE CARE Postoperative care is the same as that after Technique 4.32.

■ COMPLICATIONS

Complications of operative treatment of peroneal tendon subluxation include sural and superficial nerve injury; this risk can be minimized by careful surgical technique. Peroneal tendon adhesions can develop and limit motion; early (4 weeks) range-of-motion exercises can help avoid this complication. Overtightening of the peroneal tendon sheath can cause stenosing flexor tenosynovitis. Undertightening or inadequate groove depth can lead to persistent instability. Satisfactory tendon excursion with ankle and hindfoot range of motion should be documented after superior peroneal retinaculum repair.

BICEPS BRACHII TENDON

The precise prevalence of isolated biceps dislocation, also referred to as the *bicipital syndrome,* is unknown. Some authors believe it to be more common than anterior shoulder

BOX 4.7

Arthroscopic Classification of Biceps Tendon Instability

Direction of instability
- Anterior
- Posterior
- Anteroposterior

Extent of instability
- None
- Subluxation
- Dislocation

Lesion grade
- 0 (normal)
- I (minor lesion)
- II (major lesion)

Rotator cuff tear/lesion
- A (intact)
- B (partial thickness)
- C (full thickness)

From Lafosse L, Reiland Y, Baier GP, et al: Anterior and posterior instability of the long head of the biceps tendon in rotator cuff tears: a new classification based on arthroscopic observations, *Arthroscopy* 23:73, 2007.

subluxation and often misdiagnosed, whereas others believe it to be extremely rare. Most often the biceps syndrome is associated with a large tear of the rotator cuff or a fracture of the lesser tuberosity, resulting in incompetence of the bicipital groove–transverse humeral ligament complex with resulting medial displacement of the tendon. One study of 200 patients with rotator cuff tears identified biceps tendon instability in 45%; 80% of those were subluxations. Posterior instability was most common (53%), followed by anteroposterior (27%) and anterior (20%). Subluxations were anterior or posterior, whereas dislocations were only anterior. Based on their arthroscopic examination of these patients, the authors developed an arthroscopic classification of biceps tendon instability according to the direction and extent of instability in relation to the bicipital groove (subluxation or dislocation) (Box 4.7).

■ CLINICAL EVALUATION

The diagnosis is based on the history of anterior shoulder pain and popping with stress of the biceps tendon. Provocative testing, such as the Yergason test and palpation over the bicipital groove with the shoulder abducted to 90 degrees and internally and externally rotated against moderate resistance, can help in making the diagnosis. The O'Brien and Speed tests are not reliable for detecting biceps brachii instability. A bicipital groove radiograph may show a shallow groove, a medial wall angle of less than 45 degrees, osteophyte formation, or a healed fracture of the lesser tuberosity. MRI or arthrography is useful to confirm the diagnosis. A rotator cuff tear often is identified, and medial displacement of the tendon may be visible on the external rotation bicipital groove view.

■ TREATMENT

Surgery is indicated for a persistently symptomatic shoulder. Based on the arthroscopic classification of biceps instability, biceps tenodesis was recommended for all anterior dislocations if not reliably reducible.

Tenodesis of the biceps tendon to the humerus can be performed, along with excision of the proximal intraarticular tendon through the rotator cuff interval and repair of cuff pathology as indicated. For acute injury involving fracture of the lesser tuberosity, fixation of the tuberosity and repair of the transverse humeral ligament should be done. Chronic symptoms from fracture of the medial aspect of the intertubercular groove should be treated with tenodesis, followed by excision of the intraarticular tendon through a small incision in the rotator interval.

TREATMENT OF BICEPS BRACHII TENDON DISPLACEMENT

TECHNIQUE 4.40

- In the rare instance when no pathologic condition exists in the rotator cuff, use an anterior approach through the deltopectoral interval. Identify the long head of the biceps tendon, and make an incision through the transverse humeral ligament, extending down through the proximal third of the pectoralis major tendon. Rarely, the biceps tendon can be placed back in the groove and the transverse humeral ligament can be repaired using interrupted sutures. More commonly, tenodesis should be performed.
- If a pathologic process of the rotator cuff is present with the subluxing biceps tendon, use an anterosuperior approach, beginning the incision just lateral to the acromioclavicular joint and extending it distally in line with the deltoid fibers.
- With wide subcutaneous dissection, expose the deltoid at its insertion.
- Split the deltoid, beginning just lateral to the acromioclavicular joint and continuing 5 cm distally in the deltoid raphe. Do not excise the acromial branch of the thoracoacromial artery in the proximal dissection.
- Carefully dissect the deltoid from the anterior acromion using electrocautery, perform an acromioplasty, and excise the coracoacromial ligament.
- Flex the shoulder, identify the long head of the biceps tendon, and tenodese it to the humerus with interference or tenodesis screws or suture anchors.
- Excise the intraarticular portion of the tendon and repair the rotator cuff.
- Close the wound in the usual manner.
- Alternatively, release the proximal biceps tendon attachment arthroscopically, and then perform a tenodesis procedure. A subpectoral technique (see Technique 4.28) also can be used.

POSTOPERATIVE CARE A shoulder immobilizer is worn for 2 weeks. A sling is used for an additional 2 weeks, and then active use and exercises are begun. If the rotator cuff was repaired, rehabilitation depends on the size of the tear.

Arthroscopic biceps tenodesis and release are described in other chapter.

REFERENCES

COMPARTMENT SYNDROME

Aweid O, Del Buono A, Malliaras P, et al.: Systematic review and recommendations for intracompartmental pressure monitoring in diagnosing chronic exertional compartment syndrome of the leg, *Clin J Sport Med* 22:356, 2012.

Bariteau JT, Beutel BG, Kamal R, et al.: The use of near-infrared spectrometry for the diagnosis of lower-extremity compartment syndrome, *Orthopedics* 34:178, 2011.

Brewer RB, Gregory AJ: Chronic lower leg pain in athletes: a guide for the differential diagnosis, evaluation, and treatment, *Sports Health* 4:121, 2012.

Campano D, Robaina JA, Kusnezov N, et al.: Surgical management for chronic exertional syndrome of the leg: a systematic review of the literature, *Arthroscopy* 32:1478, 2016.

Challa ST, Hargens AR, Uzosike A, et al.: Muscle microvascular blood flow, oxygenation, pH, and perfusion pressure decrease in simulated acute compartment syndrome, *J Bone Joint Surg Am* 99:1453, 2017.

Davis DE, Raikin S, Garras DN, et al.: Characteristic of patients with chronic exertional compartment syndrome, *Foot Ankle Int* 34:1349, 2013.

de Bruijn JA, van Zantvoort APM, van Klaveren D, et al.: Factors predicting lower leg chronic exertional compartment syndrome in a large population, *Int J Sports Med* 39:58, 2018.

de Bruijn JA, van Zanvoort APM, Winkes MB, et al.: Lower leg chronic exertional compartment syndrome in patients 50 years of age and older, *Orthop J Sports Med* 6: 2325967118757179, 2018.

Diebal A, Gregory R, Alitz C, Gerber JP: Forefoot running improves pain and disability associated with chronic exertional compartment syndrome, *Am J Sports Med* 40:1060, 2012.

Dunn JC: Waterman BR: chronic exertional compartment syndrome of the leg in the military, *Clin Sports Med* 33:693, 2014.

Farber A, Tan TW, Hamburg NM, et al.: Early fasciotomy in patients with extremity vascular injury is associated with decreased risk of adverse limb outcomes: a review of the National Trauma Data Bank, *Injury* 43:1486, 2012.

Flynn JM, Bashyal RK, Yeger-McKeever M, et al.: Acute traumatic compartment syndrome of the leg in children: diagnosis and outcome, *J Bone Joint Surg* 93A:937, 2011.

Fouasson-Chailloux A, Menu P, Dauty M: Evaluation of strength recovery after traumatic acute compartment syndrome of the thigh: a case study, *Ortop Traumatol Rehabil* 19:379, 2017.

Frink M, Hildebrand F, Krettek C, et al.: Compartment syndrome of the lower leg and foot, *Clin Orthop Relat Res* 468:940, 2010.

Gallo RA, Plakke M, Silvis ML: Common leg injuries of long-distance runners: anatomical and biomechanical approach, *Sports Health* 4:485, 2012.

Gill CS, Halstead ME, Matava MJ: Chronic exertional compartment syndrome of the leg in athletes: evaluation and management, *Phys Sportsmed* 38:126, 2010.

Gorczyca JT, Roberts CS, Pugh KJ, Ring D: Review of treatment and diagnosis of acute compartment syndrome of the calf: current evidence and best practices, *Instr Course Lect* 60:35, 2011.

Govaert GA, van Helden S: Ty-raps in trauma: a novel technique of extremity fasciotomy wounds, *J Trauma* 69:972, 2010.

Helmhout PH, Diebal AR, van der Kaaden L, et al.: The effectiveness of a 6-week intervention program aimed at modifying running style in patients with chronic exertional compartment syndrome: results from a series of case studies, *Orthop J Sports Med* 3: 2325967115575691, 2015.

Herring MJ, Donohoe E, Marmor MT: A novel non-invasive method for the detection of elevated intra-compartmental pressures of the leg, *J Vis Exp* 147, 2019, https://doi.org/10.3791/59887.

How MI, Lee PK, Wei TS, et al.: Delayed presentation of compartment syndrome of the thigh secondary to quadriceps trauma and vascular injury in a soccer player, *Int J Surg Case Rep* 11:56, 2015.

Irion V, Magnussen RA, Miller TL, Kaeding CC: Return to activity following fasciotomy for chronic exertional compartment syndrome, *Eur J Orthop Surg Traumatol* 24:1223, 2014.

Kanlic EM, Pinski SE, Verwiebe EG, et al.: Acute morbidity and complications of thigh compartment syndrome: a report of 26 cases, *Patient Saf Surg* 4:13, 2010.

Khan SK, Thati S, Gozzard C: Spontaneous thigh compartment syndrome, *West J Emerg Med* 12:134, 2011.

Knight JR, Daniels M, Roberson W: Endoscopic compartment release for chronic exertional compartment syndrome, *Arthrosc Tech* 2:e187, 2013.

Koepplinger ME, Ellis LA, Davis KR: Complicated thigh compartment syndrome, *Curr Orthop Prac* 22:116, 2011.

Maher JM, Brook EM, Chiodo C, et al.: Patient-reported outcomes following fasciotomy for chronic exertional compartment syndrome, *Foot Ankle Spec* 11:471, 2018.

Maksymiak R, Ritchie E, Zimmermann W, et al.: Historic cohort: outcome of chronic exertional compartment syndrome-suspected patients, *BMJ Mil Health*, 2020 Feb 3, [Epub ahead of print].

Marmor M, Charlu J, Knox R, et al.: Use of standard musculoskeletal ultrasound to determine the need for fasciotomy in an elevated muscle compartment pressure cadaver leg model, *Injury* 50:627, 2019.

Masquelet AC: Acute compartment syndrome of the leg: pressure measurement and fasciotomy, *Orthop Traumatol Surg Res* 96:913, 2010.

Mauser N, Gissel H, Henderson C, et al.: Acute lower-leg compartment syndrome, *Orthopedics* 36:619, 2013.

McQueen MM, Duckworth AD, Aitken SA, Court-Brown CM: The estimated sensitivity and specificity of compartment pressure monitoring for acute compartment syndrome, *J Bone Joint Surg* 95A:673, 2013.

Nathan S, Roberts CS, Deliberato D: Lumbar paraspinal compartment syndrome, *Int Orthop* 36:1221, 2012.

Neal M, Henebry A, Mamczak CN, et al.: The efficacy of a single-incision versus two-incision four-compartment fasciotomy of the leg: a cadaveric model, *J Orthop Trauma* 30:e164, 2016.

Ojike NI, Roberts CS, Giannoudis PV: Compartment syndrome of the thigh: a systematic review, *Injury* 41:133, 2010.

Packer JD, Day MS, Nguyen JT, et al.: Functional outcomes and patient satisfaction after fasciotomy for chronic exertional compartment syndrome, *Am J Sports Med* 41:430, 2013.

Pandya NK, Ganley TJ: Single-incision endoscopically-assisted compartment releases for exertional compartment syndrome in pediatric patients, *Curr Orthop Prac* 21:213, 2010.

Park S, Lee HS, Seo SG: Selective fasciotomy for chronic exertional compartment syndrome detected with exercise magnetic resonance imaging, *Orthopedics* 40:e1099, 2017.

Pasic N, Bryant D, Willits K, et al.: Assessing outcomes in individuals undergoing fasciotomy for chronic exertional compartment syndrome of the leg, *Arthroscopy* 31:707, 2015.

Rajasekaran S, Beavis C, Aly AR, Leswick D: The utility of ultrasound in detecting anterior compartment thickness changes in chronic exertional compartment syndrome: a pilot study, *Clin J Sport Med* 23:305, 2013.

Rajasekaran S, Hall MM: Nonoperative management of chronic exertional compartment syndrome: a systematic review, *Curr Sports Med Rep* 15:191, 2016.

Reisman WM, Shuleer MS, Kinsey TL, et al.: Relationship between near infrared spectroscopy and intracompartmental pressures, *J Emerg Med* 44:292, 2013.

Rennerfelt K, Zhang Q, Karlsson J, et al.: Changes in muscle oxygen saturation have low sensitivity in diagnosing chronic anterior compartment syndrome of the leg, *J Bone Joint Surg Am* 98:56, 2016.

Ringler MD, Litwiller DV, Felmlee JP, et al.: MRI accurately detects chronic exertional compartment syndrome: a validation study, *Skeletal Radiol* 42(3):385, 2013.

Roberts CS, Gorczyca JT, Ring D, Pugh KJ: Diagnosis and treatment of less common compartment syndromes of the upper and lower extremities: current evidence and best practices, *Instr Course Lect* 60:43, 2011.

Roscoe D, Roberts AJ, Hulse D: Intramuscular compartment pressure measurement in chronic exertional compartment syndrome: new and improved diagnostic criteria, *Am J Sports Med* 43:392, 2015.

Schmidt AH, Bosse MJ, Obremskey WT, et al.: Continuous near-infrared spectroscopy demonstrates limitations in monitoring the development of acute compartment syndrome in patients with leg injuries, *J Bone Joint Surg Am* 100:1645, 2018.

Scully WF, Benavides JM: Surgical tips for performing open fasciotomies for chronic exertional compartment syndrome of the leg, *Foot Ankle Int* 40:859, 2019.

Shagdan B, Menon M, Sanders D, et al.: Current thinking about acute compartment syndrome of the lower extremity, *Can J Surg* 53:329, 2010.

Shuler MS, Reisman WM, Kinsey TL, et al.: Correlation between muscle oxygenation and compartment pressures in acute compartment syndrome of the leg, *J Bone Joint Surg* 92A:863, 2010.

Smith RD, Rust-March H, Kluzek S: Acute compartment syndrome of the thigh in a rugby player, *BMJ Case Rep*, 2015: pii: bcr2015210856, 2015.

Sugimoto D, Brilliant AN, d'Hemecourt DA, et al.: Running mechanics of females with bilateral compartment syndrome, *J Phys Ther Sci* 30:1056, 2018.

Tam JPH, Gibson AGF, Murray JRD, et al.: Fasciotomy for chronic exertional compartment syndrome of the leg: clinical outcome in a large retrospective cohort, *Eur J Orthop Surg Traumatol* 29:479, 2019.

Thein R, Tilbor I, Rom E, et al.: Return to sports after chronic anterior exertional compartment syndrome of the leg: conservative treatment versus surgery, *J Orthop Surg* 27:2309499019835651, 2019.

Tiidus PM: Is intramuscular pressure a valid diagnostic criterion for chronic exertional compartment syndrome? *Clin J Sport Med* 24:87, 2014.

Tornetta P 3rd, Puskas B, Wang K: Compartment syndrome of the leg associated with fracture: an algorithm to avoid releasing the posterior compartments, presented at Orthopaedic Trauma Association, October 16, 2008. Available online at http://hwbf.org/ota/am/ota08/otapa/OTA0802 15.htm. Accessed May, 2011.

Tucker AK: Chronic exertional compartment syndrome of the leg, *Curr Rev Musculoskelet Med* 3:32, 2010.

Vajapey S, Miller TL: Evaluation, diagnosis, and treatment of chronic exertional compartment syndrome: a review of current literature, 45:391, 2017.

van Zantvoort AP, de Bruijn JA, Winkes MB, et al.: Isolated chronic exertional compartment syndrome of the lateral lower leg: a case series, *Orthop J Sports Med* 3: 2325967115617728, 2015.

van Zantvoort APM, de Bruijn JA, Hundscheid HPH, et al.: Fasciotomy for lateral lower-leg chronic exertional compartment syndrome, *Int J Sports Med* 39:1081, 2018.

Wall CJ, Lynch J, Harris IA, et al.: Clinical practice guidelines for the management of acute limb compartment syndrome following trauma, *ANZ J Surg* 80:151, 2010.

Waterman BR, Laughlin M, Kilcoyne K, et al.: Surgical treatment of chronic exertional compartment syndrome of the leg: failure rates and postoperative disability in an active patient population, *J Bone Joint Surg* 95A:592, 2013.

Waterman BR, Liu J, Newcomb R, et al.: Risk factors for chronic exertional compartment syndrome in a physically active military population, *Am J Sports Med* 41:2545, 2013.

Whitney A, O'Toole RV, Hui E, et al.: Do one-time intracompartmental pressure measurements have a high false-positive rate in diagnosing compartment syndrome? *J Trauma Acute Care Surg* 76:479, 2014.

Wilder RP, Magrum E: Exertional compartment syndrome, *Clin Sports Med* 29:429, 2010.

Winkes MB, van Zantvoort AP, de Bruijn JA, et al.: Fasciotomy for deep posterior compartment syndrome in the lower leg: a prospective study, *Am J Sports Med* 44:1309, 2016.

Wittstein J, Moorman 3rd CT, Levin LS: Endoscopic compartment release for chronic exertional compartment syndrome: surgical technique and results, *Am J Sports Med* 38:1661, 2010.

Zimmermann WO, Hutchinson MR, Van den Berg R, et al.: Conservative treatment of anterior chronic exertional compartment syndrome in the military, with a mid-term follow-up, *BMJ Open Sport Exer Med* 5:e000531, 2019, Rupture of Muscles and Tendons.

RUPTURE OF ACHILLES TENDON

Ahmad J, Jones K: The effect of obesity on surgical treatment of Achilles tendon ruptures, *J Am Acad Orthop Surg* 25:773, 2017.

Alhaug OK, Berdal G, Husebye EE, et al.: Flexor hallucis longus tendon transfer for chronic Achilles tendon rupture. A retrospective study, *Foot Ankle Surg* 25:630, 2019.

Amendola A: Outcomes of open surgery versus nonoperative management of acute Achilles tendon rupture, *Clin J Sport Med* 24:90, 2014.

Aufwerber S, Heijne A, Edman G, et al.: Early mobilization does not reduce the risk of deep venous thrombosis after Achilles tendon rupture: a randomized controlled trial, *Knee Surg Sports Traumatol Arthrosc* 28:312, 2020.

Barfod KW, Bencke J, Lauridsen HB, et al.: Nonoperative dynamic treatment of acute Achilles tendon rupture: the influence of early weight-bearing on clinical outcome: a blinded, randomized controlled trial, *J Bone Joint Surg* 96A:1497, 2014.

Barfod KW, Hansen MS, Hölmich P, et al.: Efficacy of early controlled motion of the ankle compared with immobilization in non-operative treatment of patients with an acute Achilles tendon rupture: an assessor-blinded, randomised controlled trial, *Br J Sports Med*, 2019 Oct 9, [Epub ahead of print].

Bisaccia M, Rinonapoli G, Meccariello L, et al.: Validity and reliability of mini-invasive surgery assisted by ultrasound in Achilles tendon rupture, *Acta Inform Med* 27:40, 2019.

Brumann M, Baumbach SF, Mutschler W, Polzer H: Accelerated rehabilitation following Achilles tendon repair after acute rupture—development of an evidence-based treatment protocol, *Injury* 45:1782, 2014.

Bullock MJ, DeCarbo WT, Hofbauer MH, et al.: Repair of chronic Achilles ruptures has a high incidence of venous thromboembolism, *Foot Ankle Spec* 10:415, 2017.

Chegini Kord M, Ebrahimpour A, Sadighi M, et al.: Minimally invasive repair of acute Achilles tendon rupture using gift box technique, *Arch Bone Jt Surg* 7:429, 2019.

Chen L, Liu JP, Tang KL, et al.: Tendon derived stem cells promote platelet-rich plasma healing in collagenase-induced rage Achilles tendinopathy, *Cell Physiol Biochem* 34:2143, 2014.

Chiodo CP, Glazebrook M, Bluman EM, et al.: American Academy of Orthopaedic Surgeons clinical practice guideline on treatment of Achilles tendon rupture, *J Bone Joint Surg* 92A:2466, 2010.

Claessen FM, de Vos RJ, Reijman M, Meuffels DE: Predictors of primary Achilles tendon ruptures, *Sports Med* 44:1241, 2014.

Clanton TO, Haytmanek CT, Williams BT, et al.: A biomechanical comparison of an open repair and 3 minimally invasive percutaneous Achilles tendon repair techniques during a simulated, progressive rehabilitation protocol, *Am J Sports Med* 43:1957, 2015.

Cretnik A, Kosir R, Kosanovic M: Incidence and outcome of operatively treated Achilles tendon rupture in the elderly, *Foot Ankle Int* 31:14, 2010.

de Jonge S, de Vos RJ, Weir A, et al.: One-year follow-up of platelet-rich plasma treatment in chronic Achilles tendinopathy: a double-blind randomized placebo-controlled trial, *Am J Sports Med* 39:1623, 2011.

Deng S, Sun Z, Zhang C, et al.: Surgical treatment versus conservative management for acute Achilles tendon rupture: a systematic review and meta-analysis of randomized controlled trials, *J Foot Ankle Surg* 56:1236, 2017.

de Vos RJ, Weir A, Tol JL, et al.: No effects of PRP on ultrasonographic tendon structure and neovascularisation in chronic midportion Achilles tendinopathy, *Br J Sports Med* 45:387, 2011.

El-Akkawi AI, Joanroy R, Barfod KW, et al.: Effect of early versus late weight-bearing in conservatively treated acute Achilles tendon rupture: a meta-analysis, *J Foot Ankle Surg* 57:346, 2018.

Filardo G, Presti ML, Kon E, Maracci M: Nonoperative biological treatment approach for partial Achilles tendon lesion, *Orthopedics* 33:120, 2010.

Frantz TL, Everhart JS, Jamieson M, et al.: Patient-reported outcomes of Achilles tendon repair using the modified gift-box technique with nonabsorbable suture loop: a consecutive case series, *J Foot Ankle Surg* 58:696, 2019.

Giannetti S, Patricola AA, Stacati A, Santucci A: Intraoperative ultrasound assistance for percutaneous repair of the acute Achilles tendon rupture, *Orthopedics* 37:820, 2014.

Glazebrook M, Rubinger D: Functional rehabilitation for nonsurgical treatment of acute Achilles tendon rupture, *Foot Ankle Clin* 24:387, 2019.

Grassi A, Amendola A, Samuelsson K, et al.: Minimally invasive versus open repair for acute Achilles tendon rupture: meta-analysis showing reduced complications with similar outcomes, after minimally invasive surgery, *J Bone Joint Surg Am* 100:1969, 2018.

Grassi A, Rossi G, D'Hooghe P, et al.: Eighty-two percent of male professional football (soccer) players return to play at the previous level two seasons after Achilles tendon rupture treated with surgical repair, *Br J Sports Med*, 2019 Jul 30, [Epub ahead of print].

Grieco PW, Frumberg DB, Weinberg M, et al.: Biomechaical evaluation of varying the number of loops in a physiological model of Achilles tendon rupture, *Foot Ankle Int* 36:444, 2015.

Henriquez H, Munoz R, Carcuro G, et al.: Is percutaneous repair better than open repair in acute Achilles tendon rupture? *Clin Orthop Relat Res* 470:998, 2012.

Hillam JS, Mohile N, Smyth N, et al.: The effect of obesity on Achilles rupture repair, *Foot Ankle Spec* 12:503, 2019.

Holm C, Kjaer M, Eliasson P: Achilles tendon rupture – treatment and complications: a systematic review, *Scand J Med Sci Sports* 25:e1, 2015.

Hsu AR, Jones CP, Cohen BE, et al.: Clinical outcomes and complications of percutaneous Achilles repair system versus open technique for acute Achilles tendon rupture, *Foot Ankle Int* 36:1279, 2015.

Kaniki N, Willits K, Mohtadi NG, et al.: A retrospective comparative study with historical control to determine the effectiveness of platelet-rich plasma as part of nonoperative treatment of acute Achilles tendon rupture, *Arthroscopy* 30:1139, 2014.

Keene DJ, Alsousou J, Harrison P, et al.: Platelet rich plasma injection for acute Achilles tendon rupture: PATH-2 randomized, placebo controlled, superiority trial, *MJ* 367:16132, 2019.

Khalid MA, Weiss WM, Iloanya M, et al.: Dual purpose use of flexor hallucis longus tendon for management of chronic Achilles tendon ruptures, *Foot Ankle Spec* 12:345, 2019.

Khan RJ, Carey Smith RL: Surgical interventions for treating acute Achilles tendon ruptures, *Cochrane Database Syst Rev* CD003674, 2010.

Kou J: AAOS clinical practice guideline: acute Achilles tendon rupture, *J Am Acad Orthop Surg* 18:511, 2010.

Lantto I, Heikkinen J, Flinkkila T, et al.: A prospective randomized trial comparing surgical and nonsurgical treatments of acute Achilles tendon ruptures, *Am J Sports Med* 44:2406, 2016.

Lemme NJ, Li NY, DeFroda SF, et al.: Epidemiology of Achilles tendon ruptures in the United States: athletic and nonathletic injuries from 2012 to 2016, *Orthop J Sports Med* 6:2325967118808238, 2018.

Lemme NJ, Li NY, Kleiner JE, et al.: Epidemiology and video analysis of Achilles tendon ruptures in the National basketball association, *Am J Sports Med* 47:2360, 2019.

Lu J, Liang X, Ma Q: Early functional rehabilitation for acute Achilles tendon ruptures: an update meta-analysis of randomized controlled trials, *J Foot Ankle Surg* 58:938, 2019.

Maffulli N, Longo U, Maffulli GD, et al.: Achilles tendon ruptures in elite athletes, *Foot Ankle Int* 32:9, 2011.

Maffulli N, Longo U, Ronga M, et al.: Favorable outcome of percutaneous repair of Achilles tendon ruptures in the elderly, *Clin Orthop Relat Res* 468:1039, 2010.

Maffulli N, Oliva F, Maffulli GD, et al.: Surgical management of chronic Achilles tendon ruptures using less invasive techniques, *Foot Ankle Surg* 24:164, 2018.

Maffulli N, Spiezia F, Longo UG, Denaro V: Less-invasive reconstruction of chronic Achilles tendon ruptures using a peroneus brevis tendon transfer, *Am J Sports Med* 38:2304, 2010.

Magnussen RA, Glisson RR, Moorman 3rd CT: Augmentation of Achilles tendon repair with exracellular matrix xenograft: a biomechanical analysis, *Am J Sports Med* 39:1522, 2011.

Manent A, Lopez L, Coromina H, et al.: Acute Achilles tendon ruptures: efficacy of conservative and surgical (percutaneous, open) treatment: a randomized, controlled, clinical trial, *Foot Ankle Surg* 58:1229, 2019.

Marcel Jr JJ, Sage K, Guyton GP: Complications of supine surgical Achilles tendon repair, *Foot Ankle Int* 39:720, 2018.

Metz R, van der Heijden GJ, Verleisdonk EJ, et al.: Effect of complications after minimally invasive surgical repair of acute Achilles tendon ruptures: report on 211 cases, *Am J Sports Med* 39:820, 2011.

Nilsson-Helander K, Silbernagel KG, Thomeé R, et al.: Acute Achilles tendon rupture: a randomized, controlled study comparing surgical and non-surgical treatments using validated outcome measures, *Am J Sports Med* 38:2186, 2010.

Ochen Y, Beksw RB, van Heijl M, et al.: Operative treatment versus non-operative treatment of Achilles tendon ruptures: systematic review and meta-analysis, *BMJ* 364:k5120, 2019.

Olsson N, Nilsson-Helander K, Karlsson J, et al.: Major functional deficits persist 2 years after acute Achilles tendon rupture, *Knee Surg Sports Traumatol Arthrosc* 19:1385, 2011.

Olsson N, Petzold M, Brorsson A, et al.: Predictors of clinical outcome after acute Achilles tendon ruptures, *Am J Sports Med* 42(6):1448, 2014.

Olsson N, Silbernagle KG, Eriksson BI, et al.: Stable surgical repair with accelerated rehabilitation versus nonsurgical treatment for acute Achilles tendon ruptures: a randomized controlled study, *Am J Sports Med* 41:2867, 2013.

Park YH, Kim TJ, Choi GW, et al.: Age is a risk factor for contralateral tendon rupture in patients with acute Achilles tendon rupture, *Knee Surg Sports Traumatol Arthrosc*, 2019.

Park YH, Kim TJ, Choi GW, et al.: Achilles tendinosis does not always precede Achilles tendon rupture, *Knee Surg Sports Traumatol Arthrosc* 27:3297, 2019.

Park YH, Lim JW, Choi GW, et al.: Quantitative magnetic resonance imaging analysis of the common site of acute Achilles tendon rupture: 5 to 8 cm above the distal end of the calcaneal insertion, *Am J Sports Med* 47:2374, 2019.

Pedersen MH, Wahlsten LR, Grønborg H, et al.: Symptomatic venous thromboembolism after Achilles tendon rupture: a nationwide Danish cohort study of 28,546 patients with Achilles tendon rupture, *Am J Sports Med* 47:3229, 2019.

Persson R, Jick S: Clinical implications of the association between fluoroquinolones and tendon rupture: the magnitude of the effect with and without corticosteroids, *Br J Clin Pharmacol* 85:949, 2019.

Porter DA, Barnes AF, Rund AM, et al.: Acute Achilles tendon repair: strength outcomes after an acute bout of exercise in recreational athletes, *Foot Ankle Int* 35:123, 2014.

Reda Y, Farouk A, Abdelmonem I, et al.: Surgical versus non-surgical treatment for acute Achilles tendon rupture. A systematic review of literature and meta-analysis, *Foot Ankle Surg*, 2019 Apr 4, [Epub ahead of print].

Rouvillain JL, Navarre T, Labrada-Blanco O, et al.: Percutaneous suture of acute Achilles tendon rupture: a study of 60 cases, *Acta Orthop Belg* 76:237, 2010.

Schepull T, Kvist J, Norrman H, et al.: Autologous platelets have no effect on the healing of human Achilles tendon ruptures: a randomized single-blind study, *Am J Sports Med* 39:38, 2011.

Schipper ON, Anderson RB, Cohen BE: Outcomes after primary repair of insertional ruptures of the Achilles tendon, *Foot Ankle Int* 39:664, 2018.

Soroceanu A, Sidhwa F, Aarabi S, et al.: Surgical versus nonsurgical treatment of acute Achilles tendon rupture: a meta-analysis of randomized trials, *J Bone Joint Surg* 94A:2136, 2012.

Stavenuiter XJR, Lubberts B, Prince 3rd RM, et al.: Postoperative complications following repair of acute Achilles tendon rupture, *Foot Ankle Int* 40:679, 2019.

Svedman S, Juthberg R, Edman G, et al.: Reduced time to surgery improves patient-reported outcome after Achilles tendon rupture, *Am J Sports Med* 46:2929, 2018.

Taylor DW, Petrera M, Hendry M, Theodoropoulos JS: A systematic review of the use of platelet-rich plasma in sports medicine as a new treatment for tendon and ligament injuries, *Clin J Sports Med* 21:344, 2011.

Tejwani NC, Lee J, Weatherall J, Sherman O: Acute Achilles tendon ruptures: a comparison of minimally invasive and open approach repairs followed by early rehabilitation, *Am J Orthop (Belle Mead NJ)* 43:E221, 2014.

Trofa DP, Miller JC, Jang ES, et al.: Professional athletes' return to play and performance after operative repair of an Achilles tendon rupture, *Am J Sports Med* 45:2864, 2017.

Van der Eng DM, Schepers T, Goslings JC, Schep NW: Rerupture rate after early weightbearing in operative versus conservative treatment of Achilles tendon rupture: a meta-analysis, *J Foot Ankle Surg* 52:622, 2013.

Vieira MH, Oliveira RJ, Eca LP, et al.: Therapeutic potential of mesenchymal stem cells to treat Achilles tendon injuries, *Genet Mol Res* 13:10434, 2014.

Wagner P, Wagner E, López M, et al.: Proximal and distal failure site analysis in percutaneous Achilles tendon rupture repair, *Foot Ankle Int* 40:1424, 2019.

Wegrzyn J, Luciani JF, Philippot R, et al.: Chronic Achilles tendon rupture reconstruction using a modified flexor hallucis longus transfer, *Int Orthop* 34:1187, 2010.

Westin O, Svedman S, Senorski EH, et al.: Older age predicts worse function 1 year after an acute Achilles tendon rupture: a prognostic multicenter study on 391 patients, *Orthop J Sports Med* :2325967118813904, 2018.

Wilkins R, Bisson LJ: Operative versus nonoperative management of acute Achilles tendon ruptures: a quantitative systematic review of randomized controlled trials, *Am J Sports Med* 40:2154, 2012.

Willits K, Amendola A, Bryant D, et al.: Operative versus nonoperative treatment of acute Achilles tendon ruptures: a multicenter randomized trial using accelerated functional rehabilitation, *J Bone Joint Surg* 92A:2767, 2010.

Wu Y, Mu Y, Yin L, et al.: Complications in the management of acute Achilles tendon rupture: a systematic review and network meta-analysis of 2060 patients, *Am J Sports Med* 47:2251, 2019.

RUPTURE OF PATELLAR TENDON

Andriolo L, Altamura SA, Reale D, et al.: Nonsurgical treatments of patellar tendinopathy: multiple injections of platelet-rich plasma area suitable option: a systematic review and meta-analysis, *Am J Sports Med* 47:1001, 2019.

Bahr MA, Bahr R: Jump frequency may contribute to risk of jumper's knee: a study of interindividual and sex differences in a total of 11,943 jumps video recorded during training and matches in young elite volleyball players, *Br J Sports Med* 48:1322, 2014.

Bright JM, Fields KB, Draper R: Ultrasound diagnosis of calf injuries, *Sports Health* 9:352, 2017.

Brockmeyer M, Diehl N, Schmitt C, et al.: Results of surgical treatment of chronic patellar tendinosis (jumper's knee): a systematic review of the literature, *Arthroscopy* 31:2424, 2015.

Charousset C, Zaoui A, Bellaiche L, Bouyer B: Are multiple platelet-rich plasma injections useful for treatment of chronic patellar tendinopathy in athletes? A prospective study, *Am J Sports Med* 42:906, 2014.

Clarke AW, Alyas F, Morris T, et al.: Skin-derived tenocyte-like cells for the treatment of patellar tendinopathy, *Am J Sports Med* 39:614, 2011.

Dan M, Phillips A, Johnston RV, et al.: Surgery for patellar tendinopathy (jumper's knee), *Cochrane Database Syst Rev* 9:CD013034, 2019.

DeBerardino TM, Owens BD: Repair of acute and chronic patellar tendon tears. In Miller MD, Weisel S, editors: *Operative techniques in sports medicine surgery*, Philadelphia, 2011, Lippincott Williams and Wilkins.

Filardo G, Kon E, Della Villa S, et al.: Use of platelet-rich plasma for the treatment of refractory jumper's knee, *Int Orthop* 34:909, 2010.

Hutchison MK, Houck J, Cuddeford T, et al.: Prevalence of patellar tendinopathy and patellar tendon abnormality in male collegiate basketball players: a cross-sectional study, *J Athl Train* 54:953, 2019.

Kaux JF, Croisier JL, Bruyere O, et al.: One injection of platelet-rich plasma associated to a submaximal eccentric protocol to treat chronic jumper's knee, *J Sports Med Phys Fitness* 55:953, 2015.

Kaux JF, Forthomme, Mh N, et al.: Description of a standardized rehabilitation program based on submaximal eccentric following a platelet-rich plasma infiltration for jumper's knee, *Muscles Ligaments Tendons J* 4(1):85, 2014, eCollection 2014.

Krushinski EM, Parks BG, Hinton RY: Gap formation in transpatellar patellar tendon repair: pretensioning Krackow sutures versus standard repair in a cadaver model, *Am J Sports Med* 38:171, 2010.

Labib SA, Wilczynski MC, Sweitzer BA: Two-layer repair of a chronic patellar tendon rupture: a novel technique and literature review, *Am J Orthop (Belle Mead NJ)* 39:277, 2010.

Massoud EI: Repair of fresh patellar tendon rupture: tension regulation at the suture line, *Int Orthop* 34:1153, 2010.

Morton S, Williams S, Valle X, et al.: Patellar tendinopathy and potential risk factors: an international database of cases and controls, *Clin J Sport Med* 27:468, 2017.

Nguene-Nyemb AG, Huten D, Ropars M: Chronic patellar tendon rupture reconstruction with a semitendinosus autograft, *Orthop Traumatol Surg Res* 97:447, 2011.

Nguyen MT, Hsu WK: Performance-based outcomes following patellar tendon repair in professional athletes, *Phys Sportsmed*, 2019 July 16, [Epub ahead of print].

Schwartz A, Watson JN, Hutchinson MR: Patellar tendinopathy, *Sports Health* 7:415, 2015.

Smith J, Sellon JL: Comparing PRP injections with ESWT for athletes with chronic patellar tendinopathy, *Clin J Sport Med* 24:88, 2014.

Van der Worp H, de Poel HJ, Diercks RL, et al.: Jumper's knee or lander's knee? A systematic review of the relation between jump biomechanics and patellar tendinopathy, *Int J Sports Med* 35:714, 2014.

Vetrano M, Castorina A, Vulpiani MC, et al.: Platelet-rich plasma versus focused shock waves in the treatment of jumper's knee in athletes, *Am J Sports Med* 41:795, 2013.

Valianatos P, Papadakou E, Erginoussakis D, et al.: Treatment of chronic patellar tendon rupture with hamstrings tendon autografts, *J Knee Surg*, 2019 May 8, [Epub ahead of print].

Willberg L, Sunding K, Forssblad M, et al.: Sclerosing polidocanol injections or arthroscopic shaving to treat patellar tendinopathy/jumper's knee? A randomised controlled study, *Br J Sports Med* 45:411, 2011.

Yen CY, Tsai YJ, Hsiao CK, et al.: Biomechanical evaluation of patellar tendon repair using Krackow suture technique, *Biomed Eng Online* 18:64, 2019.

RUPTURE OF TENDON OF QUADRICEPS FEMORIS MUSCLE/EXTENSOR MECHANISM OF KNEE

Garner MR, Gausden E, Berkes MB, et al.: Extensor mechanism injuries of the knee: demographic characteristics and comorbidities from a review of 726 patient records, *J Bone Joint Surg Am* 97:1592, 2015.

Govindu R, Ammar H, George V: Bilateral quadriceps tendon rupture, *J Clin Rheumatol* 25:e63, 2019.

Hak DJ, Sanchez A, Trobisch P: Quadriceps tendon injuries, *Orthopedics* 33:40, 2010.

Negrin LL, Nemecek E, Hajdu S: Extensor mechanism ruptures of the knee: differences in demographic data and long-term outcome after surgical treatment, *Injury* 46:1957, 2015.

RUPTURE OF GLUTEUS MEDIUS/MINIMUS TENDONS

Domb BG, Nasser RM, Botser IB: Partial-thickness tears of the gluteus medius: rationale and technique for trans-tendinous endoscopic repair, *Arthroscopy* 26:1697, 2010.

Ebert JR, Bucher TA, Ball SV, et al.: A review of surgical repair methods and patient outcomes for gluteal tendon tears, *Hip Int* 25:15, 2015.

El-Husseiny M, Patel S, Rayan F, Haddad F: Gluteus medius tears: an under-diagnosed pathology, *Br J Hosp Med (Lond)* 72:12, 2011.

Grimaldi A, Mellor R, Hodges P, et al.: Gluteal tendinopathy: a review of mechanisms, assessment and management, *Sports Med* 45:1107, 2015.

RUPTURES OF THE HAMSTRING

Belk JW, Kraeutler MJ, Mei-Dan O, et al.: Return to sport after proximal hamstring tendon repair: a systematic review, *Orthop J Sports Med* : 2325967119853218, 2019.

Birmingham P, Muller M, Wickiewicz T, et al.: Functional outcome after repair of proximal hamstring avulsions, *J Bone Joint Surg Am* 93:1819, 2011.

Blakeney WG, Zilko SR, Edmonston SJ, et al.: A prospective evaluation of proximal hamstring tendon avulsions: improved functional outcomes following surgical repair, *Knee Surg Sports Traumatol Arthrosc* 25:1943, 2017.

Bodendorfer BM, Curley AJ, Kotler JA, et al.: Outcomes after operative and nonoperative treatment of proximal hamstring avulsions: a systematic review and meta-analysis, *Am J Sports Med* 46:2798, 2018.

Bowman EN, Marshall NE, Gerhardt MB, et al.: Predictors of clinical outcomes after proximal hamstring repair, *Orthop J Sports Med* 2325967118823712, 2019.

Cohen SB, Rangavajjula A, Vyas D, et al.: Functional results and outcomes after repair of proximal hamstring avulsions, *Am J Sports Med* 40:2092, 2012.

Domb BG, Linder D, Sharp KG, et al.: Endoscopic repair of proximal hamstring avulsion, *Arthrosc Tech* 2:e35, 2013.

Guanche CA: Hamstring injuries, *J Hip Preserv Surg* 2:122, 2015.

Harris JD, Griesser MJ, Best TM, et al.: Treatment of proximal hamstring ruptures - a systematic review, *Int J Sports Med* 32:490, 2011.

Hofmann KJ, Paggi A, Connors D, et al.: Complete avulsion of the proximal hamstring insertion: functional outcomes after nonsurgical treatment, *J Bone Joint Surg Am* 96:1022, 2014.

Lempainen L, Banke IJ, Johansson K, et al.: Clinical principles in the management of hamstring injuries, *Knee Surg Sports Traumatol Arthrosc* 23:2449, 2015.

Lempinen L, Kosola J, Pruna R, et al.: Central tendon injuries of hamstring muscles: case series of operative treatment, *Orthop J Sports Med* 6:2325967118755992, 2018.

Otto A, DiCosmo AM, Baldino JB, et al.: Biomechanical evaluation of proximal hamstring repair: all-suture anchor versus titanium suture anchor, *Orthop J Sports Med* 23245967119892925, 2020.

Rust DA, Giveans MR, Stone RM, et al.: Functional outcomes and return to sports after acute repair, chronic repair, and allograft reconstruction for proximal hamstring ruptures, *Am J Sports Med* 42:1377, 2014.

Sandmann GH, Hahn D, Amereller M, et al.: Mid-term functional outcome and return to sports after proximal hamstring tendon repair, *Int J Sports Med* 37(7):570, 2016.

Startzman AN, Fowler O, Carreira D: Proximal hamstring tendinosis and partial ruptures, *Orthopedics* 40:e574, 2017, t al.:.

van der Made AD, Reurink G, Gouttebarge V, et al.: Outcome after surgical repair of proximal hamstring avulsions: a systematic review, *Am J Sports Med* 43:2841, 2015.

RUPTURE OF BICEPS BRACHII

Bain GI, Durrant AW: Sports-related injuries of the biceps and triceps, *Clin Sports Med* 29:555, 2010.

Banerjee M, Shafizadeh S, Bouillon B, et al.: High complication rate following distal biceps refixation with cortical button, *Arch Orthop Trauma Surg* 133:1361, 2013.

Barlow JD, McNeilan R, Speeckaert A, et al.: Use of a bicortical button to safely repair the distal biceps in a two-incision approach: a cadaveric analysis, *J Hand Surg Am* 42:570, 2017.

Barret H, Winter M, Gastaud O, et al.: Double incision repair technique with immediate mobilization for acute distal biceps tendon ruptures provides good results after 2 years in active patients, *Orthop Traumatol Surg Res* 105:323, 2019.

Beks RB, Claessen FM, Oh LS, et al.: Factors associated with adverse events after distal biceps tendon repair or reconstruction, *J Shoulder Elbow Surg* 25:1229, 2016.

Caekebeke P, Corten J, Duerinckx J: Distal biceps tendon repair: comparison of clinical and radiological outcome between bioabsorbable and nonabsorbable screws, *J Shoulder Elbow Surg* 25:349, 2016.

Cain RA, Nydick JA, Stein MI, et al.: Complications following distal biceps repair, *J Hand Surg [Am]* 37:2112, 2012.

Carroll MJ, DaCambra MP, Hildebrand KA: Neurologic complications of distal biceps tendon repair with 1-incision endobutton fixation, *Am J Orthop (Belle Mead NJ)* 43:3159, 2014.

Cohen SB, Buckley PS, Neuman B, et al.: A functional analysis of distal biceps tendon repair: single-incision Endobutton technique vs. two-incision modified Boyd-Anderson technique, *Phys Sportsmed* 44:59, 2016.

Cusick MC, Cottrell BJ, Cain RA, Mighell MA: Low incidence of tendon rerupture after distal biceps repair by cortical button and inteference screw, *J Shoulder Elbow Surg* 23:1532, 2014.

Dunphy TR, Hudson J, Batech M, et al.: Surgical treatment of distal biceps tendon ruptures: an analysis of complications in 784 surgical repairs, *Am J Sports Med* 45:3020, 2017.

Erickson BJ, Basques BA, Griffin JW, et al.: The effect of concomitant biceps tenodesis on reoperation rates after rotator cuff repair: a review of a large private-payer database from 2007 to 2014, *Arthroscopy* 33:1301, 2017.

Ford SE, Andersen JS, Macknet DM, et al.: Major complications after distal biceps tendon repairs: retrospective cohort analysis of 970 cases, *J Shoulder Elbow Surg* 27:1898, 2018.

Frank T, Seltser A, Grewal R, et al.: Management of chronic distal biceps tendon ruptures: primary repair vs semitendinosus autograft reconstruction, *J Shoulder Elbow Surg* 28:1104, 2019.

Frazier MS, Boardman MJ, Westland M, Imbriglia JE: Surgical treatment of partial distal biceps tendon ruptures, *J Hand Surg* 35A:1111, 2010.

Geaney LE, Brennerman DJ, Cole MP, et al.: Outcomes and practical information for patients choosing nonoperative treatment for distal biceps rupture, *Orthopedics* 33:391, 2010.

Grewal R, Athwal GS, MacDermid JC, et al.: Single versus double-incision technique for the repair of acute distal biceps tendon ruptures: a randomized clinical trial, *J Bone Joint Surg Am* 94:1166, 2012.

Hinchey JW, Aronowitz JG, Sanchez-Sotelo J, Morrey BF: Re-reruprute rate of primarily repaired distal biceps tendon injuries, *J Shoulder Elbow Surg* 23:850, 2014.

Kodde IF, Baerveldt RC, Mulder PG, et al.: Refixation techniques and approaches for distal biceps tendon ruptures: a systematic review of clinical studies, *J Shoulder Elbow Surg* 25:e29, 2016.

Lynch J, Yu CC, Chen C, et al.: Magnetic resonance imaging versus ultrasound in diagnosis of distal biceps tendon avulsion, *Orthop Traumatol Surg Res* 105:861, 2019.

Matzon JL, Graham JG, Penna S, et al.: A prospective evaluation of early postoperative complications after distal biceps tendon repairs, *J Hand Surg Am* 44:382, 2019.

Miyamoto RG, Elser F, Millett PJ: Current concepts review: distal biceps tendon injuries, *J Bone Joint Surg* 92A:2128, 2010.

Prud'homme-Foster M, Louati H, Pollock JW, et al.: Proper placement of the distal biceps tendon during repair improves supination strength-a biomechanical analysis, *J Shoulder Elbow Surg* 24:527, 2015.

Otto A, Mehl J, Obopilwe E, et al.: Biomechanical comparison of onlay distal biceps tendon repair: all-suture anchors versus titanium suture anchors, *Am J Sports Med* 47:2478, 2019.

Park JS, Kim SH, Jung HJ, et al.: A prospective randomized study comparing the interference screw and suture anchor techniques for biceps tenodesis, *Am J Sports Med* 45:440, 2017.

Phadnis J, Flannery O, Watts AC: Distal biceps reconstruction using an Achilles tendon allograft, transosseous EndoButton, and Pulvertaft weave with tendon wrap technique for retracted, irreparable distal biceps ruptures, *J Shoulder Elbow Surg* 25:1013, 2016.

Quach T, Jazayeri R, Sherman OH, Rosen JE: Distal biceps tendon injuries: current treatment options, *Bull NYU Hosp Jt Dis* 68:103, 2010.

Reichert P, Królikowska A, Kentel M, et al.: A comparative clinical and functional assessment of cortical button versus suture anchor in distal biceps brachii tendon repair, *J Orthop Sci* 24:103, 2018.

Sarda P, Qaddori A, Nauschutz F, et al.: Distal biceps tendon rupture: current concepts, *Injury* 44:417, 2013.

Savin DD, Watson J, Youderian AR, et al.: Surgical management of acute distal biceps tendon ruptures, *J Bone Joint Surg Am* 99:785, 2017.

Schmidt CC, Brown BT, Sawardeker PJ, et al.: Factors affecting supination strength after a distal biceps rupture, *J Shoulder Elbow Surg* 23:68, 2014.

Sutton KM, Dodds SD, Ahmad CS, Sethi PM: Surgical treatment of distal biceps rupture, *J Am Acad Orthop Surg* 18:139, 2010.

Vestermark GL, Van Doren BA, Connor PM, et al.: The prevalence of rotator cuff pathology in the setting of acute proximal biceps tendon rupture, *J Shoulder Elbow Surg* 27:1258, 2018.

RUPTURE OF THE TRICEPS TENDON

Bava ED, Barber FA, Lund ER: Clinical outcome after suture anchor repair for complete traumatic rupture of the distal triceps tendon, *Arthroscopy* 28:1058, 2012.

Carpenter SR, Stroh DA, Melvani R, et al.: Distal triceps transosseous cruciate versus suture anchor repair using equal constructs: biomechanical comparison, *J Shoulder Elbow Surg* 27:2052, 2018.

Dimrock RAC, Kontoghiorghe C, Consigliere P, et al.: Distal triceps rupture repair: the triceps pulley-pullover technique, *Arthrosc Tech* 8:e85, 2019.

Dunn JC, Kusnezov N, Fares A, et al.: Triceps tendon ruptures: a systematic review, *Hand (N Y)* 12:431, 2017.

Heikenfeld R, Listringhaus R, Godolias G: Endoscopic repair of tears of the superficial layer of the distal triceps tendon, *Arthroscopy* 30:785, 2014.

Horneff 3rd JG, Aleem A, Nicholson T, et al.: Functional outcomes of distal triceps tendon repair comparing transosseous bone tunnels with suture anchor constructs, *J Shoulder Elbow Surg* 26:2213, 2017.

Kokkalis ZT, Mavrogenis AF, Spyridonos S, et al.: Triceps brachii distal tendon reattachment with a double-row technique, *Orthopedics* 36:110, 2013.

Mirzayan R, Acevdeo DC, Sodl JF, et al.: Operative management of acute triceps tendon ruptures: review of 184 cases, *Am J Sports Med* 46:1451, 2018.

Scheiderer B, Imhoff FB, Morikawa D, et al.: The V-shaped distal triceps tendon repair: a comparative biomechanical analysis, *Am J Sports Med* 46:1952, 2018.

Tom JA, Kumar NS, Cernyik DL, et al.: Diagnosis and treatment of triceps tendon injuries: a review of the literature, *Clin J Sport Med* 24:197, 2014.

Yeh PC, Dodds SD, Smart LR, et al.: Distal triceps rupture, *J Am Acad Orthop Surg* 18:31, 2010.

Yeh PC, Stephens KT, Solovyova O, et al.: The distal triceps tendon footprint and a biomechanical analysis of 3 repair techniques, *Am J Sports Med* 38:1025, 2010.

RUPTURE OF PECTORALIS MAJOR MUSCLE

de Castro Pochini A, Andreoli CV, Belangero PS, et al.: Clinical considerations for the surgical treatment of pectoralis major muscle ruptures based on 60 cases: a prospective study and literature review, *Am J Sports Med* 42:95, 2014.

Edgar CM, Singh H, Obopilwe E, et al.: Pectoralis major repair: a biomechanical analysis of modern repair configurations versus traditional repair configuration, *Am J Sports Med* 45:2858, 2017.

ElMaraghy AW, Devereaux MW: A systematic review and comprehensive classification of pectoralis major tears, *J Shoulder Elbow Surg* 21:412, 2012.

Gregory JM, Klosterman EL, Thomas JM, et al.: Suture technique influences the biomechanical integrity of pectoralis major repairs, *Orthopedics* 38:e746, 2015.

Haley CA, Zacchilli MA: Pectoralis major injuries: evaluation and treatment, *Clin Sports Med* 33:739, 2014.

Merolla G, Paladini P, Artiaco S, et al.: Surgical repair of acute and chronic pectoralis major tendon rupture: clinical and ultrasound outcomes at a mean follow-up of 5 years, *Eur J Orthop Surg Traumatol* 25:91, 2015.

Metzger PD, Bailey JR, Filler RD, et al.: Pectoralis major muscle rupture repair: technique using unicortical buttons, *Arthrosc Tech* 1:e119, 2012.

Pochini Ade C, Ejnisman B, Andreoli CV, et al.: Pectoralis major muscle rupture in athletes: a prospective study, *Am J Sports Med* 38:92, 2010.

Provencher MT, Hardfield K, Boniquit NT, et al.: Injuries to the pectoralis major muscle: diagnosis and management, *Am J Sports Med* 38:1693, 2010.

Rabuck SJ, Synch JL, Guo X, et al.: Biomechanical comparison of 3 methods to repair pectoralis major ruptures, *Am J Sports Med* 40:1635, 2012.

Sherman SL, Lin EC, Verma NN, et al.: Biomechanical analysis of the pectoralis major tendon and comparison of techniques for tendo-osseous repair, *Am J Sports Med* 40:1887, 2012.

Tarity TD, Garrigues GE, Ciccotti MG, et al.: Pectoralis major ruptures in professional American football players, *Phys Sportsmed* 42:131, 2014.

Thompson K, Kwon Y, Flatow E, et al.: Everything pectoralis major: from repair to transfer, *Phys Sports Med* Jul 23, 2019, [Epub ahead of print].

Yu J, Zhang C, Horner N, et al.: Outcomes and return to sport after pectoralis major tendon repair: a systematic review, *Sports Health* 11:134, 2019.

Zacchilli MA, Fowler JT, Owens BD: Allograft reconstruction of chronic pectoralis major tendon ruptures, *J Surg Orthop Adv* 22:95, 2013.

DISPLACEMENT OF PERONEAL TENDONS

Cho J, Kim JY, Song DG, Lee WC: Comparison of outcome after retinaculum repair with and without fibular groove deepening for recurrent dislocation of the peroneal tendons, *Foot Ankle Int* 35:683, 2014.

Draghi F, Bortolott C, Draghi AG, et al.: Intrasheath instability of peroneal tendons: dynamic ultrasound imaging, *J Ultrasound Med* 37:2753, 2018.

Espinosa N, Maurer MA: Peroneal tendon dislocation, *Eur J Trauma Emerg Surg* 41:631, 2015.

Fokin Jr A, Huntley SR, Summers SH, et al.: Computed tomography assessment of peroneal tendon displacement and posteromedial structure entrapment in pilon fractures, *J Orthop Trauma* 30:627, 2016.

Guillo S, Calder JD: Treatment of recurring peroneal tendon subluxation in athletes: endoscopic repair of the retinaculum, *Foot Ankle Clin* 18:293, 2013.

Pesquer L, Guillo S, Poussange N, et al.: Dynamic ultrasound of peroneal tendon instability, *Br J Radiol* 89:20150958, 2016.

Roth JA, Taylor WC, Whalen J: Peroneal tendon subluxation: the other lateral ankle injury, *Br J Sports Med* 44:1047, 2010.

Saragas NP, Ferrao PN, Mayet Z, et al.: Peroneal tendon dislocation/subluxation—case series and review of the literature, *Foot Ankle Surg* 22:125, 2016.

Saxena A, Ewen B: Peroneal subluxation: surgical results in 31 athletic patients, *J Foot Ankle Surg* 49:238, 2010.

Scholten PE, Breugem SJ, van Dijk CN: Tendoscopic treatment of recurrent peroneal tendon dislocation, *Knee Surg Sports Traumatol Arthrosc* 21:1304, 2013.

van Dijk PAD, Gianakos AL, Kerkhoffs GMMJ, et al.: Return to sports and clinical outcomes in patients treated for peroneal tendon dislocation: a systematic review, *Knee Surg Sports Traumatol Arthrosc* 24:1155, 2016.

Zhenbo Z, Jin W, Haifeng G, et al.: Sliding fibular graft repair for the treatment of recurrent peroneal subluxation, *Foot Ankle Int* 35:496, 2014.

The complete list of references is available online at ExpertConsult.com.